Neuromuscular Imaging

Mike P. Wattjes • Dirk Fischer
Editors

Neuromuscular Imaging

Springer

Editors
Mike P. Wattjes, MD
Department of Radiology
VU University Medical Center
Amsterdam, The Netherlands

Dirk Fischer, MD
Division of Neuropaediatrics University
Children's Hospital Basel
Basel, Switzerland

Department of Neurology
University Hospital Basel
Basel, Switzerland

ISBN 978-1-4614-6551-5 ISBN 978-1-4614-6552-2 (eBook)
DOI 10.1007/978-1-4614-6552-2
Springer New York Heidelberg Dordrecht London

Library of Congress Control Number: 2013936737

Printed on acid-free paper

Springer is part of Springer Science+Business Media (www.springer.com)

To Anja and Ole (MPW)

*To Elgin, Anna-Lotta, Josephine,
and Lasse (DF)*

Preface

Enormous progress has been made regarding genetic diagnosis of inherited neuromuscular diseases in recent years. A large number of new genetic abnormalities associated with dystrophic or nondystrophic myopathies have been identified, leading to new insights into understanding the pathological aspects of these heterogeneous disorders. The classic three pillars of the diagnostic process for neuromuscular diseases have been the neurological examination to determine the clinical phenotype, the neurophysiological assessment, and diagnostic muscle biopsies. It seems that a fourth pillar, neuromuscular imaging, is becoming increasingly important as a tool for detecting muscular involvement and describing the degree and pattern of involvement. Muscle imaging techniques have thus made their entrance into clinical practice. Neuromuscular imaging has become particularly helpful in supporting the clinical diagnosis, confining the complex range of differential diagnoses, and guiding interventional diagnostic procedures, such as muscle biopsy. This book was inspired by the great success and the recent developments in neuromuscular imaging. There is definitely a need to summarize and categorize the increasing amount of data that have accumulated during the past few years in a precise and comprehensive way. Creating a completely new book that deals with a rather new discipline of imaging—including aspects of neuroimaging as well as musculoskeletal imaging—we aimed to provide a comprehensive overview of the available imaging modalities and the genetic, clinical, and pathological backgrounds of acquired and inherited neuromuscular disorders. To make it as clinically useful as possible, we created a standardized structure for the chapters that includes illustrations, figures, and summarizing key points.

It has been a great pleasure for us to collaborate with so many internationally well-known experts, colleagues, and friends. We trust that this work will guide you through the huge and complex field of neuromuscular disorder (differential) diagnosis and we hope that you will find this book comprehensive and informative enough to use it in your daily practice for clinical and research purposes.

Amsterdam, The Netherlands — Mike P. Wattjes
Basel, Switzerland — Dirk Fischer

How to Use This Book?

The main focus of this book is the use of neuromuscular imaging in the clinical setting of inherited and acquired neuromuscular diseases. We aimed to create a practical guide that is useful in the daily clinical practice rather than an all-embracing reference book that most of the time is in a bookcase. The role of imaging in inherited and acquired neuromuscular disorders has been extensively investigated by many researchers and has become increasingly important in the routine clinical setting, particularly in terms of supporting the clinical (differential) diagnosis before interventional procedures take place. The vast majority of publications in this field of research have described single disease entities. To our mind, it is now time to collect, categorize, and present this knowledge in the context of differential diagnostic considerations. We believe that there is a need for a comprehensive book as a guidance in the diagnosis and differential diagnosis of neuromuscular disorders with special regard to imaging findings.

The organization of this book starts with descriptions of the imaging modalities that are currently used as standard techniques in the field of neuromuscular imaging or experimental applications that might become important in the near future. The second part focuses on the anatomical and histopathological backgrounds, which aids in the understanding of the underlying pathogenesis and anatomical distribution patterns of neuromuscular disorders. The various neuromuscular disease entities are subdivided into three parts: hereditary muscle diseases; acquired muscles diseases; and diseases of the neurons/peripheral nerves. Given the multi-modality approach to diagnosing neuromuscular disorders—in particular inherited muscle diseases—brief but important background information on their clinical presentation, genetics, and histopathology are addressed. The descriptions of the muscle disease entities are structured in a certain way, focusing on genetics, pathophysiology, histopathology, clinical presentation, imaging findings, and differential diagnosis. For readers who are interested in more detailed information suggestions of further reading sections are provided at the end of each chapter. Although the main emphasis of this book is on primary muscle diseases, it also includes important, often underrated aspects of neuromuscular imaging, such as muscle neoplasms and peripheral nerve imaging. Particularly the latter benefits from the advances in magnetic resonance imaging and has gained increasing interest among neuroradiologists.

Once again, this book does not represent an encyclopedia of imaging of neuromuscular diseases. It is the first approach to collect, categorize, and summarize the most clinically relevant aspects of this group of diseases. On behalf of all the contributors, we would very much appreciate comments and suggestions to improve this book and make it even more comprehensive for future editions.

Mike P. Wattjes and Dirk Fischer

Acknowledgements

The editors would like to thank the publisher Springer, in particular Andrew Moyer and Connie Walsh for their support and help. We also gratefully acknowledge Angelique Mathilda for the excellent assistance in compiling the book. We are also very grateful to our colleague, Ulrike Bonati, for critical reading of the book.

This book was only possible because of the support and tremendous contributions of many colleagues and friends in sharing ideas and images. The editors are particularly grateful to all contributing authors and the following collaborators and colleagues:

Frederik Barkhof
Ludwig Kappos
Thomas Klockgether
Anneke J. van der Kooi
Leroy ten Dam
Marjo S. van der Knaap
Jeroen Vermeulen
Peter Weber
Michael Wiederholt
Nicole Wolf
Rolf Schröder
Michael Sinnreich

Abbreviations

AB	Adductor brevis muscle
ABD	Actin-binding domain
ACE	Angiotensin-converting-enzyme
ACTA1	α(Alfa)-1 actin
AD	Autosomal dominant
AFAM	Actin filament aggregate myopathy
AL	Adductor longus muscle
ALS	Amyotrophic lateral sclerosis
ALSFRS	ALS functional rating scale
AM	Adductor magnus muscle
AM	Actin myopathy
AN	Anconeus muscle
ANO5	Anoctamin 5
AON	Antisense oligonucleotides
APC	Adenomatous polyposis coli
APL	Abductor pollicis longus muscle
APP	Amyloid precursor protein
AR	Autosomal recessive
AS	Anterior scalenus muscle
ASL	Arterial spin labelling
ATP	Adenosine triphosphate
BAF	Barrier-to-autointegration factor
BF	Biceps femoris short head
BH	Biceps humeri muscle
BIN1	Amphiphysin 2 encoding gene
BIPAP	Bilevel positive airway pressure
BL	Biceps femoris long head
BM	Bethlem myopathy
BMD	Dystrophinopathy type Becker
BR	Brachioradialis muscle
Bra	Brachialis muscle
CB	Coracobrachialis muscle
CCD	Central core disease
CD	Cluster of differentiation
cDNA	Complementary DNA
CFTD	Congenital fiber type disproportion

CK	Creatine kinase
CM	Congenital myopathy
CMD	Congenital muscular dystrophy
CMD1A	Dilated cardiomyopathy with conduction defects
^{13}C-MRS	13-Carbon magnetic resonance spectroscopy
CMS	Congenital myasthenic syndrome
CMT	Charcot–Marie–Tooth
CNM	Centronuclear myopathy
CNS	Central nervous symptoms
CNTF	Ciliaryneurothrophic factor
CoA	Coenzyme A
COL6	Collagen 6
CONTICANET	European connective tissue cancer network
COX	Cytochrome oxidase
CPAP	Continuous positive airway pressure
CPEO	Chronic progressive external ophthalmoplegia
CPT	Carnitine-palmitoyltransferase
CRIM	Cross-reactive immunological material
CSA	Cross sectional area
CT	Computed tomography
CTD	Connective tissue disease
CTS	Carpal tunnel syndrome
CYP	Cytochrome P450
dB	Decibel
DDLS	Dedifferentiated liposarcoma
DE	Debranching enzyme
DEXA	Dual energy X-ray absorptiometry
DG	Digastric muscle
DGC	Dystrophin associated glycoprotein complex
DM	Dermatomyositis
DM1	Myotonic dystrophy type 1
DM2	Myotonic dystrophy type 2
DMAT	Distal myopathy with anterior tibial onset
DMC	Dominant myotonia congenita
DMD	Duchenne muscular dystrophy
DMRV	Distal myopathy with rimmed vacuoles
DNA	Deoxyribonucleic acid
DNM2	Dynamin 2
DTI	Diffusion tensor imaging
DTPA	Diethylene triamine pentaacetic acid
DWI	Diffusion weighted imaging
ECM	Extracellullar matrix
ECR	Extensor carpi radialis muscle
ECU	Extensor carpi ulnaris muscle
ED	Extensor digitorum muscle
EDB	Extensor digitorum brevis
EDL	Extensor digitorum longus muscle
EDM	Extensor digiti minimi muscle

EDMD	Emery Dreifuss muscular dystrophy
EM	Electron microscopy
EMG	Electromyography
EPL	Extensor pollicis longus muscle
ER	Endoplasmic reticulum
ERT	Enzyme replacement therapy
FA	Fractional anisotropy
FCMD	Fukuyama congenital muscular dystrophy
FCR	Flexor carpi radialis muscle
FCU	Flexor carpi ulnaris muscle
FDA	American Food and Drug Administration
^{18}F-FDG	Fluodeoxyglucose
FDL	Flexor digitorum longus muscle
FDP	Flexor digitorum profundus muscle
FDS	Flexor digitorum superficialis muscle
FHL	Flexor hallucis longus muscle
FHL1	Four and a half LIM domain 1 protein
FISH	Fluorescent in situ hybridization
FKRP	Fukutin related protein
FPLA	Familial partial lipodystrophy of the Dunnigan type
FPLD	Familial partial lipodystrophy
FSE	Fast spin echo
FSHD	Facioscapulohumeral dystrophy
FSHD1	Facioscapulohumeral dystrophy type 1
FSHD2	Facioscapulohumeral dystrophy type 2
FTD	Frontotemporal dementia
GAA	Acid α(alfa)-glucosidase
GCG	Guanin–cytosin–guanin (repeat)
GCN	Guanin–cytosin–any (repeat)
GCTTS	Giant cell tumor of the tendon sheath
Gd	Gadolinium
GH	Growth hormone
GL	Gastrocnemius lateral head
GM	Gastrocnemius medial head
GMa	Gluteus maximus muscle
GMe	Gluteus medius muscle
GMm	Gluteus minimus muscle
GNE	UDP-*N*-acetylglucosamine 2-epimerase/*N*-acetylmannosamine kinase
GOT	Glutamic-oxaloacetic transaminase
GPC	Glycerophosphocholine
GPE	Glycerophosphoethanolimine
GPT	Glutamate pyruvate transaminase
GR	Gracilis muscle
GrH	Gonadotropic releasing hormone
GSDs	Glycogen storage diseases
γGT	Gamma-glutamyltransferase
Gy	Gray

H&E	Hematoxylin and eosin
HIBM	Hereditary inclusion body myopathy
HIV	Human immunodeficiency virus
HLA	Human leukocyte antigen
^{1}H-MRS	Proton magnetic resonance spectroscopy
HM	Hamstring muscles
HMERF	Hereditary myopathy with early respiratory failure
HMG-CoA	3-Hydroxy 3-methyl glutaryl coenzyme A
HU	Hounsfield unit
HyperPP	Hyperkalemic periodic paralysis
HypoPP	Hypokalemic periodic paralysis
IBM	Inclusion body myositis
IBMPFD	Inclusion body myopathy with Paget and frontotemporal dementia
IC/ICL	Iliocostalis lumborum muscle
ICD	Implantable cardioverter defibrillator
IF	Intermediate filament
IFSHD	Infantile facioscapulohumeral dystrophy
IFSHD	Infantile FSHD
IGF-1	Insulin-like growth factor-1
IHC	Immunohistochemistry
IIM	Idiopathic inflammatory myopathies
IL	Iliacus muscle
IL	Iliacus muscle
IL-1β	Interleukin-1 β
IL-6	Interleukin-6
INIs	Intranuclear inclusions
INM	Inner nuclear membrane
Ins	Myoinositol
IR	Inversion recovery
IRM	Intranuclear rod myopathy
IS	Infraspinatus muscle
IS	Interspinosus muscle
IvIg	Intravenous immunoglobulin
kDa	Kilo Dalton
LAMA2	Alpha2 laminin = merosin
LAP	Lamina-associated polypeptide
LARGE	Like-acetylglucosaminyltransferase
LC	Longus colli muscle
L-CMD	Lamin A/C related congenital muscular dystrophy
LD	Latissimus dorsi muscle
LGMD	Limb girdle muscular dystrophy
LH	Luteinizing hormone
LHBF	Long head biceps femoris
LHG	Lateral head of gastrocnemius
LMNA	Lamin A/C
LPt	Lateral pterygoid muscle
LsC	Longissimus colli muscle

LSc	Levator scapulae muscle
LT	Longissimus thoracis muscle
MA	Masticator muscle
MC	Myotonia congenital
MD	Mean diffusivity
MDC	Muscular dystrophy congenital = congenital muscular dystrophy
MEB	Muscle–eye–brain disease
MELAS	Mitochondrial encephalomyopathy, lactic acidosis, and stroke-like episodes
mEq	Milliequivalents
MERFF	Myoclonic epilepsy and ragged red fibers
MF	Multifidus muscle
MFH	Malignant fibrous histocytoma
MFM	Myofibrillar myopathy
MH	Malignant hyperthermia
MHC	Major histocompatibility complex
MHG	Medial head of gastrocnemius
MHz	Megahertz
MIRS	Muscular impairment rating scale
MMD1	Miyoshi myopathy/Miyoshi muscular dystrophy
mm	Millimeter
μm	Micrometer
mM	Millimolar
MMD	Miyoshi muscular dystrophy
MmD	Multi-minicore disease
MND	Motor neuron diseases
MRC	Medical research council
MRI	Magnetic resonance imaging
mRNA	Messenger ribonucleic acid
MRS	Magnetic resonance spectroscopy
ms	Milliseconds
MS	Middle scalenus muscle
MSA	Myositis specific antibodies
mtDNA	Mitochondrial DNA
MTM1	Myotubularin 1 gene
MYH7	Myosin heavy chain 7
NAA	*N*-acetylaspartate
NAAG	*N*-acetylaspartylglutamate
NADH-TR	Nicotinamide adenine dinucleotide–tetrazoliumreductasestain
NB	Nemaline bodies
NCAM	Neural cell adhesion molecule
NCS	Nerve conduction studies
NEB	Nebuline
NM	Nemaline myopathy
nm	Nanometer
NMDA	*N*-methyl-D-aspartate

NMJ	Neuromuscular junctions
NMR	Nuclear magnetic resonance
NPV	Negative predictive value
OAE	Obliquus abdominis externus muscle
OAI	Obliquus abdominis internus muscle
OAM	Obliquus abdominis internus, externus and transversusabdominis muscles
OCI	Obliquus capitis inferior muscle
OI	Obturator internus muscle
OMD/OPMD	Oculo-pharyngeal-muscular dystrophy
OMIM	Online mendelian inheritance in man
ONM	Outer nuclear membrane
OPDM	Oculo-pharyngeodistal-muscular dystrophy
PABPN1	Polyadenylate binding protein nuclear 1
PAM	Potassium-aggravated myotonia
PAS	Periodic acid Schiff
PB	Peroneus muscle short head
PC	Paramyotonia congenita
PCr	Phospocreatine
PDE	Phoshodiester
PE	Pectineus muscle
PET	Positron emission tomography
PFK	Phosphofructokinase
pH	Potential hydrogen
PI	Piriformis muscle
Pi	Inorganic phophates
PIN	Posterior interosseous nerve
PL	Palmaris longus muscle
PL	Peroneus muscle long head
PLA	Plantaris muscle
^{31}P-MRS	31-Phosphorus magnetic resonance spectroscopy
PM	Polymyositis
PMa	Pectoralis major muscle
PME	Phosphomonoester
Pmi	Pectoralis minor muscle
PNS	Peripheral nerve system
POMT1	Protein-O-mannosyltransferase 1
POMT2	Protein-O-mannosyltransferase 2
POMGnT1	Protein O-linked mannose beta1,2-*N*-acetylglucosaminyltransferase
POP	Popliteus muscle
PPAR	Peroxisome proliferator-activated receptor
ppm	Parts-per-million
PROMM	Proximal myotonic myopathy
PS	Posterior scalenus muscle
PS	Psoas muscle
PT	Pronator teres muscle
PVNS	Pigmented villonodularsynovitis

QF	Quadratus femoris muscle
QL	Quadratus lumborum muscle
QSM	Quadriceps sparing myopathy
RA	Rectus abdominis muscle
RCP	Rectus capitis posterior muscle
RF	Rectus femoris muscle
RH	Rhomboid muscle
RMC	Recessive myotonia congenita
RNA	Ribonucleic acid
RNAi	RNA interference
RRF	Ragged red fibers
RSMD1	Rigid spine syndrome type 1
RYR1	Ryanodine receptor type 1
SA	Sartorius muscle
SA	Serratus anterior muscle (Chap. 10)
SCM	Sternocleidomastoid muscle
SEPN1	Selenoprotein 1 gene
SG	Sarcoglycan
SGCA	Alpha-sarcoglycan
SGCB	Beta-sarcoglycan
SGCD	Delta-sarcoglycan
SGCG	Gamma-sarcoglycan
SH	Sternohyoid muscle
SLE	Systemic lupus erythematodus
SM	Semimembranosus muscle
SMA	Spinal muscular atrophy
SMN	Survival motor neuron
SNR	Signal-to-noise ratio
snRNP	Small nuclear ribonucleoproteins
SO	Soleus
SOD	Superoxide dismutase
SP	Splenius capitis muscle
SP	Serratus posterior muscle
SPECT	Single-photon-emission-computed tomography
SPMA	Scapuloperoneal muscular atrophy
SPMD	Scapuloperoneal muscular dystrophy
SR	Sarcoplasmic reticulum
SREBP1	Sterolregulatory element-binding protein-1
SS	Semispinalis capitis and semispinalis cervicis muscles
SSp	Supraspinatus muscle
SSc	Subscapularis muscle
SSFP	Steady-state free precession
ST	Semitendinosus muscle
STIR	Short-tau inversion recovery
STS	Soft tissue sarcomas
SU	Supinator muscle
TA	Tibialis anterior muscle
TARDBP	TAR DNA binding protein

^{99m}Tc-PYP	^{99m}Technetium pyrophosphate
TE	Echo time
TFL	Tensor fasciae latae muscle
TGC	Time gain control amplification
TIRM	Turbo inversion recovery magnitude
TMD	Tibial muscular dystrophy
TMi	Teres minor muscle
TNFα	Tumor necrosis factor-α
TOS	Neurogenic thoracic outlet syndrome
TP	Tibialis posterior muscle
TPM2	Tropomyosin 2
TR	Repetition time
TSE	Turbo spin echo
TrA	Transversus abdominis muscle
TrH	Triceps humeri muscle
T1w	T1-weighted
T2w	T2-weighted
UCMD	Ullrich type congenital muscular dystrophy
ULN	Upper limit of normal
UNEE	Ulnar nerve entrapment at the elbow
US	Ultrasound
VBM	Voxel-based morphometry
VCP	Valosin containing protein
VI	Vastus intermedius muscle
VL	Vastus lateralis muscle
VM	Vastus medialis muscle
VV	Vasti muscles
WDLS	Well-differentiated liposarcoma
WDM	Welander distal myopathy
WHO	World Health Organization
WWS	Walker Warburg (lissencephaly) syndrome
XR	Plain radiography
XLMTM	X-linked myotubular myopathy
ZASP	Z-band alternatively spliced PDZ-motif containing protein
3T	3 Tesla
6AP	6-Aminophenathridine

Contents

Contributors

Daniela Avila-Smirnow Servicio de Pediatría, Unidad de Neurología, Las Condes, Santiago, Chile

Umesh A. Badrising Department of Neurology, Leiden University Medical Center, Leiden, The Netherlands

Jorge A. Bevilacqua Department of Neurology and Neurosurgery, Hospital Clinico Universidad de Chile, Santiago, Chile

Nicola Carboni Neuromuscular Unit, Multiple Sclerosis Center, University of Cagliari, Sardinia, Italy

Robert-Yves Carlier Pole neuro-locomoteur, Service d'imagerie medicale, Hopital Raymond Poincare, Garches, France

Jean-Michel Coindre Department of Pathology, Institut Bergonie, Bordeaux Cedex, France

Fieke M. Cox Department of Neurology, Leiden University Medical Center, Leiden, The Netherlands

Marianne de Visser Department of Neurology, Academic Medical Center, Amsterdam, The Netherlands

Dirk Fischer Division of Neuropaediatrics, Children's Hospital Basel, Basel, Switzerland

Department of Neurology, University Hospital Basel, Basel, Switzerland

Arne Fischmann Department of Radiology, University of Basel Hospital, Basel, Switzerland

Hans H. Goebel Neuropathology Department, Johannes Gutenberg-University Medical Center, Mainz, Germany

Kieren G. Hollingsworth Newcastle Magnetic Resonance Centre, Institute of Cellular Medicine, Newcastle University, Newcastle upon Tyne, UK

Barbara H. Janssen Department of Radiology, Radboud University Nijmegen Medical Center, Nijmegen, The Netherlands

Karin Jurkat-Rott Division Neurophysiology, University of Ulm, Ulm, Germany

Hermien E. Kan C.J. Gorter Center for High Field MRI, Department of Radiology, Leiden University Medical Center, Leiden, The Netherlands

Arnold Kang Division of Neuroradiology, Department of Radiology, University of Washington, Seattle, WA, USA

Michèle Kind Radiology Department, Institut Bergonie, Bordeaux Cedex, France

Rudolf Andre Kley Department of Neurology, Neuromuscular Center Ruhrgebiet, University Hospital Bergmannsheil, Ruhr-University Bochum, Bochum, Germany

Michel Kliot Department of Neurological Surgery, University of California San Francisco, San Francisco, CA, USA

Cornelia Kornblum Universitätsklinikum Bonn, Klinik und Poliklinik für Neurologie, Bonn, Germany

Marco Mura Complex Operative Unit of Radiology, AOU Cagliari, Policlinico di Monserrato, Cagliari, Sardinia, Italy

Montse Olivé Institute of Neuropathology, Department of Neurology and Neuromuscular Unit, Department of Neurology, IDIBELL-Hospital de Bellvitge, Hospitalet de Llobregat, Barcelona, Spain

Sören Peters Berufsgenossenschaftliches Universitätsklinikum Bergmannsheil, Institut für Radiologische Diagnostik, Interventionelle Radiologie und Nuklearmedizin, Bochum, Germany

Anna Pichiecchio Department of Neuroradiology, C. Mondino National Institute of Neurology Foundation, IRCCS, Pavia, Italy

Sigrid Pillen Child Development and Exercise Center, Wilhelmina Children's Hospital, University Medical Center Utrecht, Utrecht, The Netherlands

Susana Quijano-Roy Garches Neuromuscular Center (GNMH), Raymond Poincare Hospital, Paris Ile-de-France Ouest Univesity Hospitals (APHP), Versailles Saint-Quentin-en-Yvelines University (UVSQ), Garches, France

Norma Beatriz Romero Morphology Neuromuscular Unit of the Myology Institute, Pitie-Salpetriere University Hospital, UPMC, Paris, France

Christopher D.J. Sinclair MRC Centre for Neuromuscular Diseases, UCL Institute of Neurology, London, UK

Werner Stenzel Neuropathology Department, Charite-Universitatsmedizin Berlin, Berlin, Germany

Volker Straub Neurology, The Harold Macmillan Chair of Medicine, Institute of Genetic Medicine, University of Newcastle upon Tyne, International Centre for Life, Newcastle upon Tyne, UK

Eleonora Tavazzi Department of Neuroradiology, C. Mondino National Institute of Neurology Foundation, IRCCS, Pavia, Italy

Bjarne Udd Neuromuscular Research Center, Tampere University Hospital, Tampere, Finland

Nens van Alfen Department of Neurology and Clinical Neurophysiology, Radboud University Nijmegen Medical Center, Nijmegen, The Netherlands

Baziel van Engelen Department of Neurology, Radboud University Nijmegen Medical Center, Nijmegen, The Netherlands

Jan Verschuuren Department of Neurology, Leiden University Medical Center, Leiden, The Netherlands

Nicoline Berendina Maria Voet Department of Rehabilitation/Nijmegen Center for Evidence Based Practice, Radboud University Nijmegen Medical Center, Nijmegen, The Netherlands

Maggie C. Walter Friedrich-Baur-Institute, Department of Neurology, Ludwig-Maximilians, University of Munich, Munich, Germany

Marc-André Weber Department of Diagnostic and Interventional Radiology, University Hospital of Heidelberg, Heidelberg, Germany

Tracey A. Willis Neuromuscular Department, The Robert and Agnes Hunt Orthopaedic Hospital, NHS Foundation Trust, Oswestry Shropshire, UK

Mike P. Wattjes Department of Radiology, VU University Medical Center, Amsterdam, The Netherlands

Part I

Imaging Modalities

Introduction

1

Mike P. Wattjes

The choice and use of certain imaging modalities in the diagnostic workup of patients with inherited or acquired myopathies has changed during the past decades. Whereas computed tomography (CT) was introduced and used during the 1980s and early 1990s for this purpose, during the past two decades magnetic resonance imaging (MRI) has become increasingly available and has been used in the diagnostic process and monitoring of neuromuscular disorders. This has led to almost complete replacement of CT by MRI in this field. CT is still valuable, however, for studying certain disease entities such as neoplasms and under specific conditions (e.g., diseases for which MRI is contraindicated, claustrophobic patients).

Despite the fact that MRI is the imaging modality of choice for many neuromuscular disorders, ultrasonography, a rather "old fashioned" imaging technique, is still extremely valuable. Progress in the technical development of ultrasonography enables high-resolution and even dynamic imaging of muscles and peripheral nerves. These improvements make it indispensable for neuromuscular imaging, particularly in children.

Newer advanced imaging techniques dealing with the functional assessment of muscle tissue have recently been introduced, including perfusion MRI, diffusion MRI, and MR spectroscopy. Most of these imaging methods are available but are not yet used routinely in the clinical setting.

Peripheral nerve imaging is increasingly becoming an important part of neuromuscular imaging in various disease entities. It joins a broad selection of imaging modalities including MRI, CT, ultrasonography, and positron emission tomography.

This section of the book focuses on the various imaging techniques that are available and used in clinical and research settings. All of the chapters discuss the strengths, challenges, and limitations of each method. They also provide a perspective of possible future roles for the technique in the field of neuromuscular imaging.

M.P. Wattjes (✉)
Department of Radiology, Nuclear Medicine
& PET Research, VU University Medical Center,
De Boelelaan 1117, 1081 HV Amsterdam,
The Netherlands
e-mail: m.wattjes@vumc.nl

M.P. Wattjes and D. Fischer (eds.), *Neuromuscular Imaging*, DOI 10.1007/978-1-4614-6552-2_1,

2 Ultrasonography

Sigrid Pillen and Nens van Alfen

2.1 Introduction

Ultrasonography (US) was first used in human medical practice during the 1950s and has since developed into a well-established diagnostic imaging method. In 1980, dystrophic muscle tissue was found to show typical US changes. Over the next three decades, muscle US has developed into a reliable screening tool for childhood neuromuscular disorders that can also be used to select an optimal biopsy site. In addition to its application in the field of neurology, muscle US is used in oncology for diagnosing soft tissue tumors and in sports medicine and physical therapy for imaging muscle and tendon injuries.

During the 1990s, with the advent of more advanced US machines and software, imaging of peripheral nerves has become feasible for everyday clinical use. Initially, nerve US was mainly used by anesthesiologists to facilitate and help prevent complications during peripheral nerve blocks, but soon the imaging of nerve entrapments—especially carpal tunnel syndrome—became routine practice in many neurology and radiology departments.

S. Pillen (✉)
Child Development and Exercise Center, Wilhelmina Children's Hospital, University Medical Center Utrecht, P.O. Box 85090, 3508AB, Utrecht, The Netherlands
e-mail: sigridpillen@gmail.com

N. van Alfen
Department of Neurology and Clinical Neurophysiology, Radboud University Nijmegen Medical Center, P.O. Box 9101, 6500 HB Nijmegen, The Netherlands
e-mail: n.vanalfen@neuro.umcn.nl

The main advantage of US over other imaging modalities is the possibility of capturing moving (real time) images. Muscle US can help analyze muscle contractions and corresponding pennation angles, and it can show finer intramuscular movements such as fasciculations and even fibrillations. Fasciculation screening is easy and reliable with muscle US, which makes the technique a valuable noninvasive tool for diagnosing disorders such as motor neuron disease. Further advanced applications, such as power Doppler and contrast-enhanced US, provide opportunities to not only image muscle and nerve tissue itself but also its vascularization, which helps diagnose inflammatory and infectious conditions such as myositis or leprosy.

2.2 Principles of Ultrasonography in Relation to Neuromuscular Imaging

2.2.1 Transducer Types

Transducers, or "probes," are nowadays made of rows of electronically steered ceramic polymer piezoelectric elements that can usually send out and receive a range of US frequencies. These so-called broadband transducers come in different shapes and sizes, such as rectangular or curved forms, each with its own special advantages and purpose. For neuromuscular imaging, a linear probe with a frequency ranging between of 5 to 20 MHz that produces a rectangular image is most practical, except for deep structures such as

M.P. Wattjes and D. Fischer (eds.), *Neuromuscular Imaging*, DOI 10.1007/978-1-4614-6552-2_2,

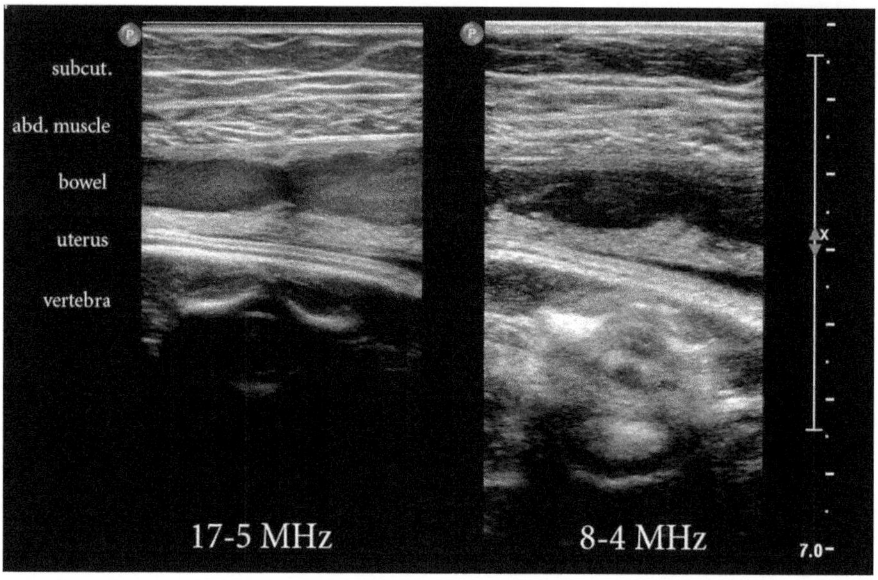

Fig. 2.1 Measurement of the abdominal wall and underlying structures in an 8 months pregnant woman with a high-frequency transducer (17–5 MHz, *left panel*) and a lower-frequency transducer (8–4 MHz, *right panel*). The high-frequency transducer depicts superficial structures such as the abdominal wall muscles with high resolution, whereas deeper structures are more difficult to visualize. Only highly reflective structures such as bone remain visible. The low-frequency probe results in lower resolution, but deeper structures such as the fetal vertebra in utero are visible (*subcut.* subcutaneous tissue, *abd. muscle* abdominal muscle)

the diaphragm or sciatic nerve where a sector-scanning or curvilinear probe may be more convenient.

2.2.2 Attenuation, Resolution, and Transducer Choice

Ultrasonography is less capable of displaying deep tissues than other imaging techniques such as magnetic resonance imaging (MRI). The reason for this is attenuation. That is, there is a progressive reduction in amplitude of the US beam as it travels through a medium such as muscle. Attenuation results from the loss of sound waves from the penetrating US beam by absorption of wave energy and other mechanisms such as reflection and scattering. The amount of absorption depends on the type of tissue (e.g., attenuation is very high in bone). Absorption increases with the use of higher transducer frequencies (Fig. 2.1), just as the higher tones in music are lost before the bass tones when the sound moves farther away from its source. For average soft tissues, the loss of US energy amounts to approximately 1 dB per 10 mm tissue depth for each megahertz. This means that a 50 MHz transducer can image tissue at up to 12 mm depth, whereas a 3 MHz probe can reach approximately 200 mm deep.

It is tempting to use a low-frequency transducer to prevent image loss due to attenuation. To do so, however, would compromise the maximum image resolution when scanning a tissue more superficial than the maximum image depth. The resolution of US images must be considered separately for the axial direction (i.e., depth along the beam) and lateral direction (i.e., transversely across the beam). Axial resolution is linearly related to transducer frequency and at best approaches the wavelength of the sound emitted. Neuromuscular imaging uses frequencies ranging from 5 to 20 MHz, with corresponding wavelengths—and therefore resolution—of 0.3–0.08 mm. The lateral resolution of US is limited by the beam width and is several times larger than the axial resolution. For optimal resolution, the highest possible transducer frequency is preferable. However, this choice contradicts using the lowest possible frequency to prevent beam attenuation. Thus, choosing a transducer is always a

Table 2.1 Transducer frequencies for various tissues

Exam	Transducer frequency (MHz)
Transcranial	2–3
Abdominal organs	3–7
Deep muscles	4–8
Superficial muscles	7–17
Eye	30–100

Table 2.2 Sound velocity in various tissue types

Tissue	Sound velocity (m/s)
Air	330
Fat	1,450
Water	1,540
Connective tissue	1,540
Blood	1,570
Muscle	1,585
Bone	4,080

trade-off depending on the depth and type of tissue under investigation (Table 2.1; Fig. 2.1). Modern broadband US equipment facilitates adjusting the frequency, which is done by imaging software based on the depth, focus, and resolution required for the measurement.

2.2.3 Effects of Tissue Properties: Acoustical Impedance and Anisotropy

The amount of sound reflection depends on the difference in acoustical impedance between tissues. Acoustical impedance is determined by a combination of the tissue density and the sound velocity within that tissue (Table 2.2). It varies according to the tissue type. The larger the impedance difference, the larger is the degree of reflection of the US beam. For example, the difference in acoustical impedance of air and skin is large, which makes it impossible to produce US images without gel or another contact medium placed between the transducer and the skin. Without a suitable contact medium, all sound would be reflected at the air–skin surface before it could penetrate the skin. A muscle-to-bone transition or intramuscular calcifications also cause a strong reflection with a typical "acoustic shadow" underneath because no sound gets through (Fig. 2.2). Conversely, a small difference in acoustical impedance, such as in normal muscle tissue, results in little to no sound reflection and almost no image signal as most of the US beam is transmitted to deeper layers. Therefore, normal muscle tissue usually appears relatively black on US images (Fig. 2.3).

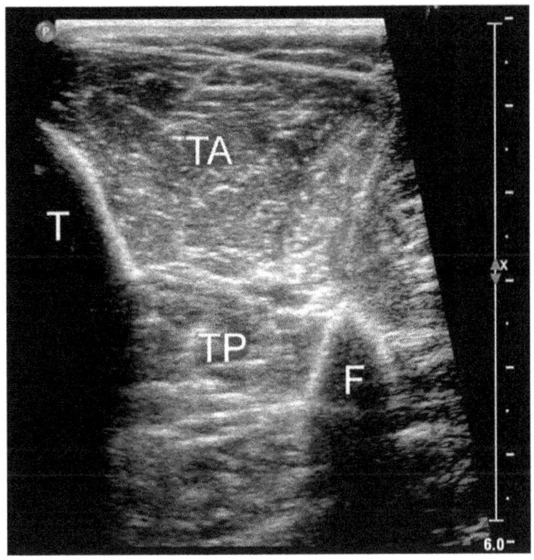

Fig. 2.2 Transverse image of the lower leg shows the tibialis anterior muscle (*TA*) and the tibialis posterior muscle (*TP*) between the tibia (*T*) and fibula (*F*). The bone reflections are very strong, resulting in clear *white lines* with a typical bone shadow underneath

Anisotropy is the property of soft tissues to vary in the amount of US reflection depending on the angle of insonation. It is caused by the amount of parallel, usually collagen-type structures present in a tissue, which reflect only sound that is perpendicular to their fibers. Anisotropy is present particularly in healthy tendon and other connective tissues and to a lesser degree in peripheral nerves and skeletal muscle (Fig. 2.4).

2.2.4 Image Formation

The same transducer that creates sound waves of the desired frequency and sends them to the target tissue also receives their echoes (reflections). US differs from other imaging modalities in that it does not display tissue itself but the transitions between two adjacent tissue

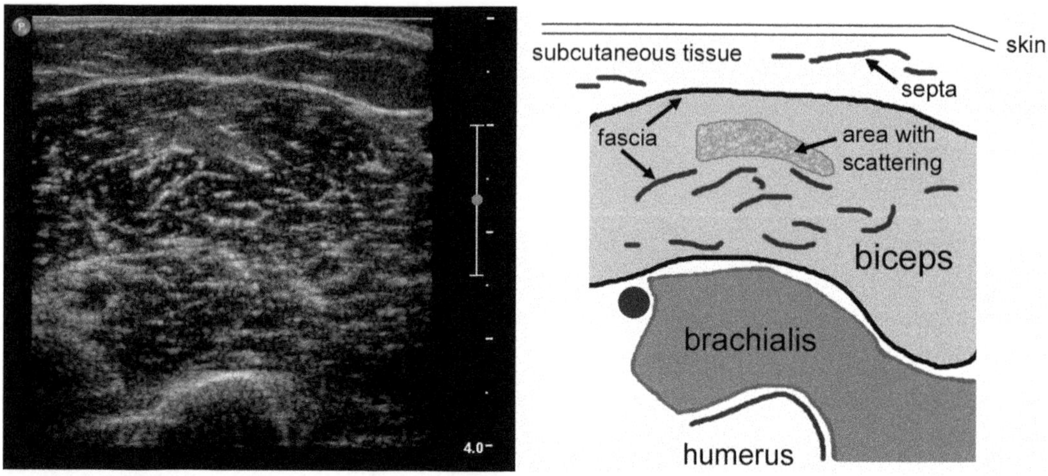

Fig. 2.3 Transverse image of the upper arm at one-third of the way from the elbow to the acromion shows a healthy biceps brachii and brachialis muscle. Healthy muscle appears relatively *black* with a few *white lines* caused by the reflections of fascia. Depending on the angle of insonation, a part of the muscle can have a homogeneous *gray appearance* caused by scattering of sound on some of the muscle fascicles. Some *bright white lines* can also be visible in the subcutaneous tissue. These are connective tissue septa between the fat lobules

types. When high-frequency sound waves sent by the transducer interact with tissue, four things can happen to the US beam: The sound waves are reflected, deflected, scattered, or absorbed (Figs. 2.5 and 2.6). Only sound waves that return to the transducer by direct reflection or as part of the scattering can form an image on the screen. Reflection or deflection of the US beam depends on the angle of impact. A 90° angle results in reflection of all sound back to the transducer, resulting in an image signal (Fig. 2.5). A smaller or larger angle of impact leads to deflection of a part or all of the sound waves. The tissue transition that caused them is not displayed in the image (Fig. 2.5). For example, an intermuscular fascia that is parallel to the direction of the US beam (i.e., at a 180° angle) is displayed as a black area (no signal) or as an interrupted line (Fig. 2.5). Conversely, these anisotropic fascial structures are highly echogenic when they lie perpendicular to the beam. Because of their anisotropy, though, even slightly oblique scanning results in diminished echo intensity (Fig. 2.4). When the US beam encounters structures smaller than the US wavelength, the sound waves are scattered (Fig. 2.6). Thus, only a small portion of this sound returns to the transducer, resulting in only a small increase in signal strength in the image. Typical scattering occurs in the liver and thyroid, which contain many small ducts and veins (Fig. 2.6), giving healthy liver and thyroid tissue a homogeneous aspect. Little scattering occurs in healthy muscle (Fig. 2.3).

2.2.5 Image Quality Optimization and Postprocessing Techniques

The final step is building an image based on the reflections received by the transducer. The equipment software calculates to which parts of the image the shades of white, gray, and black are allocated. These allocations are based on how long it took for the sound wave to return to the transducer (i.e., signal depth), from which direction it came, and how strong the returning signal is in decibels (i.e., signal brightness).

Next, several postprocessing techniques incorporated into the US machine hardware and software are applied to create the optimal image. First, the US echoes have to be amplified for further processing by a mechanism called *gain*. Because of the attenuation that occurs in deeper

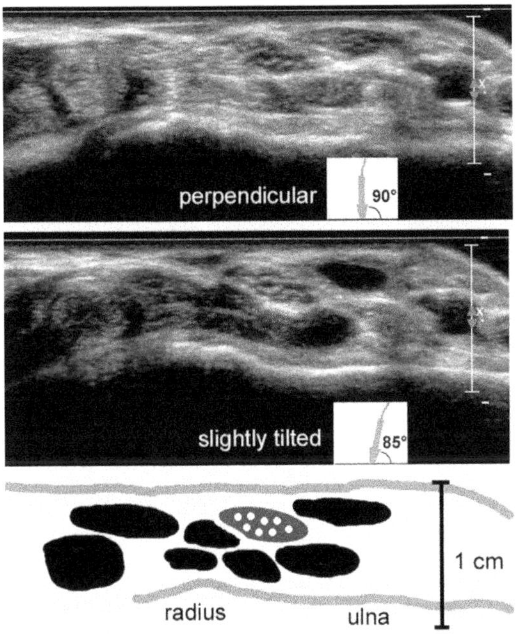

Fig. 2.4 Transverse image of the distal forearm shows the median nerve (*gray oval with white dots* in schematic picture) surrounded by several tendons. The nerve has a coarse granular "honeycomb" appearance, whereas the internal structure of the tendons is finer. Angulation of the transducer can help distinguish nerve and tendon as nerve is less anisotropic than tendon. When measuring tendons perpendicularly, all reflections of their internal structure return to the transducer, causing a finely *speckled pattern*. However, scanning at even slightly oblique angles causes all sound to be deflected, resulting in a *black image* (*middle panel*). Nerves show less anisotropy, so their internal structure remains preserved even when scanning at slightly oblique angles

layers, returning signals from deeper layers have to be amplified more than echoes from superficial layers to achieve an even image. This is achieved by *time gain control amplification* (TGC).

The returning tissue echoes have a large dynamic range (i.e., large variation in signal amplitude). As this would translate to more gray values than can be processed by the human visual system, signals are usually compressed to 256 gray values, which is about the maximum the human eye can discern. As most clinically relevant information lies in the lower- and mid-range signals, compression settings are chosen to show most contrast in these lower ranges. The final compression pattern is often called a *gray map* or *look-up table*. Most US machines have different preset gray maps to suit optimal imaging of the structure of interest.

Compound imaging is frequently applied for nerve US. It combines successive frames using different steering angles to form a single image on the screen. In this way, compounding diminishes the effects of single-angle beam signal deflection, resulting in fewer image artifacts, smoother image texture, and improved delineation of tissue boundaries, especially in a direction parallel to the US beam (Fig. 2.7).

Other US techniques include *panoramic*, or *extended field-of-view*, *imaging*. With this technique, the probe motion and echoes are tracked during real time, and the complete image is gradually built on screen. Panoramic view technology requires special software but allows, for example, tracking of nerve abnormalities over a long distance (Fig. 2.8).

Recent advances in *Doppler flow imaging* technology make it possible to detect signals from low-flow vasculature, such as intramuscular arterioles or epineural blood vessels. Power Doppler indirectly measures the number of red blood cells, creating the Doppler frequency shift, in contrast to normal color Doppler, which measures the mean frequency shift (or velocity) of blood cells (Fig. 2.9). Its main advantage is that any flow is assigned a color, improving sensitivity for low-flow signals. It allows us to measure the degree of tissue vascularization and to detect hyperemia (Fig. 2.9), which in turn can help detect locally increased blood flow in patients with inflammatory conditions (e.g., myositis, leprous neuropathy). Because Power Doppler is independent of the angle of insonation, however, it cannot discern between arterial and venous flow.

Microvascular imaging can be enhanced by the use of intravenous contrast fluids containing US reflectors. Most commonly, small (1–5 μm) lipid or protein capsules (microbubbles) containing an inert gas are used. These microbubbles are then imaged during destruction using high-energy US pulses or by imaging the harmonics of their oscillations using lower-energy pulses. Contrast-enhanced imaging is highly sensitive for measuring capillary perfusion and can even be used to deliver specific drugs to a particular site. The drug is then released upon insonation.

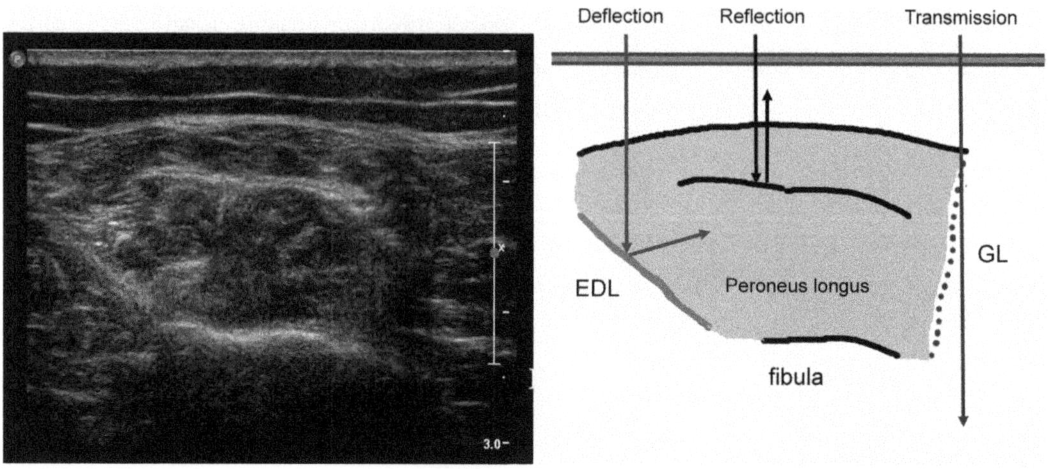

Fig. 2.5 Transverse image of the lower leg shows the peroneus longus muscle over the fibula. Bright fascia is visible within the peroneus longus. This structure is perpendicular to the ultrasonography (US) beam and is therefore highly reflective. Part of the extensor digitorum longus (EDL) is visible on the *left side*. The boundary between the EDL and the peroneus longus is askew with respect to the direction of the US beam. Therefore a large part of the beam is deflected from this boundary, which makes it difficult to see. The fascia between the peroneus longus and the lateral head of the gastrocnemius (GL) is not visible because it is parallel to the US beam and no sound is reflected, which results in a *broad black line*

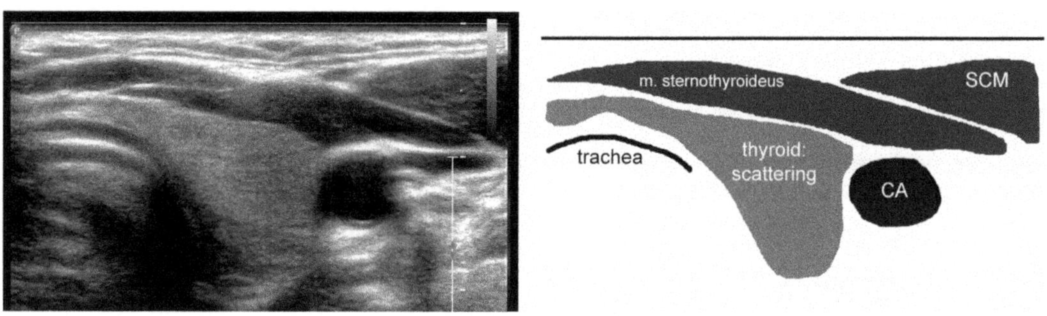

Fig. 2.6 The thyroid is an example of tissue that scatters the US beam, resulting in a homogeneous *gray appearance*. The surrounding muscle structures show little scattering and only some reflections, which leads to a *black image* with a few *white spots* and *lines* (*CA* carotid artery, *SCM* sternocleidomastoid muscle)

2.3 Ultrasonography of Normal Neuromuscular Tissue

2.3.1 Muscle Appearance in Transverse and Longitudinal Planes

Skeletal muscles are composed of bundles of muscle fibers (Fig. 2.10, see also Chap. 9). Each muscle fiber is surrounded by thin connective tissue called the endomysium. Bundles of muscle fibers are surrounded by the epimysium, which also contains small blood vessels and nerve fibers. The muscle as a whole is covered by the epimysium or fascia that also forms the tendons and aponeuroses.

Healthy muscle tissue has low echo intensity; that is, it appears black on a US scan. When measured in a transverse plane, it has a speckled appearance (Fig. 2.3). The intramuscular reflections originate from the perimysium, intramuscular fascia, and veins. The epimysium, or surrounding fascia, is normally thin, consisting

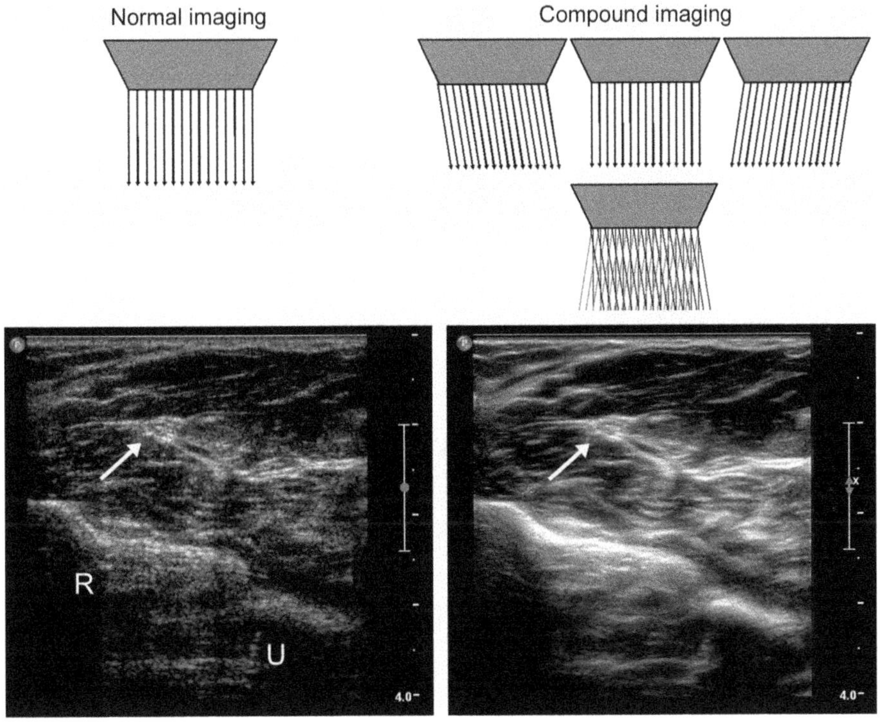

Fig. 2.7 Transverse image of the forearm, halfway between the elbow and the wrist, shows the median nerve (*arrow*) between the superficial and deep finger flexor muscles. With compound imaging the fascia surrounding the muscle a more visible and have a rounder appearance. The nerve is also easier recognizable (*R* radius, *U* ulna)

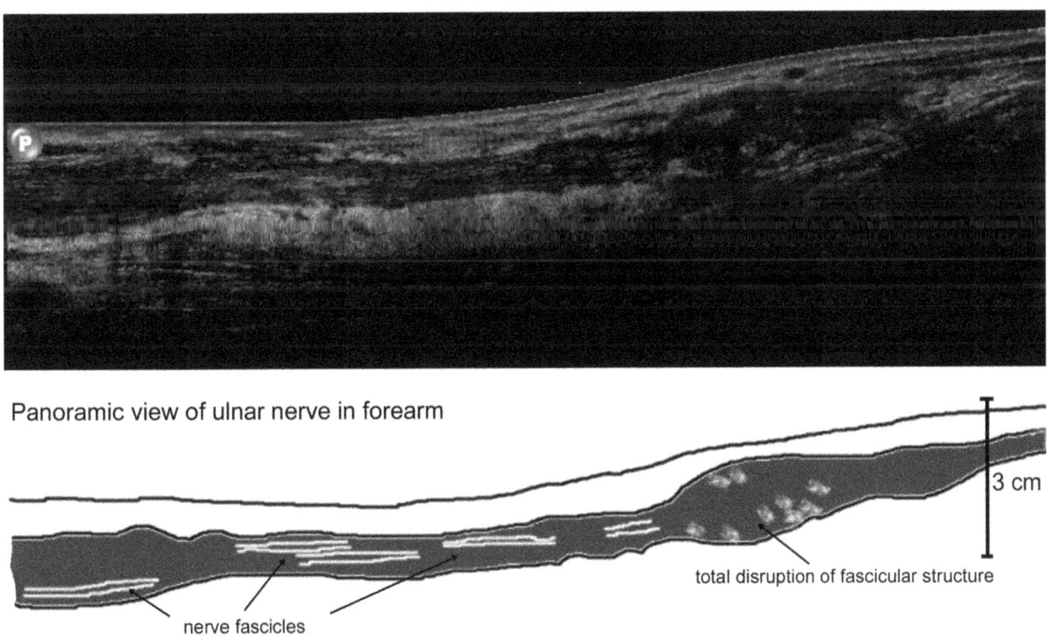

Fig. 2.8 Longitudinal image of the ulnar nerve in the forearm of a patient with an inflammatory nerve disorder, which has led to gross swelling of the nerve. The fascicular structure is still visible in some parts of the nerve, although the nerve fascicles are wider apart than normal. Other nerve parts are even more disrupted, leading to a very thick nerve without any visible internal structure. Panoramic imaging makes it possible to visualize a longer stretch of the nerve in a single image, although it comes at the cost of reduced image resolution

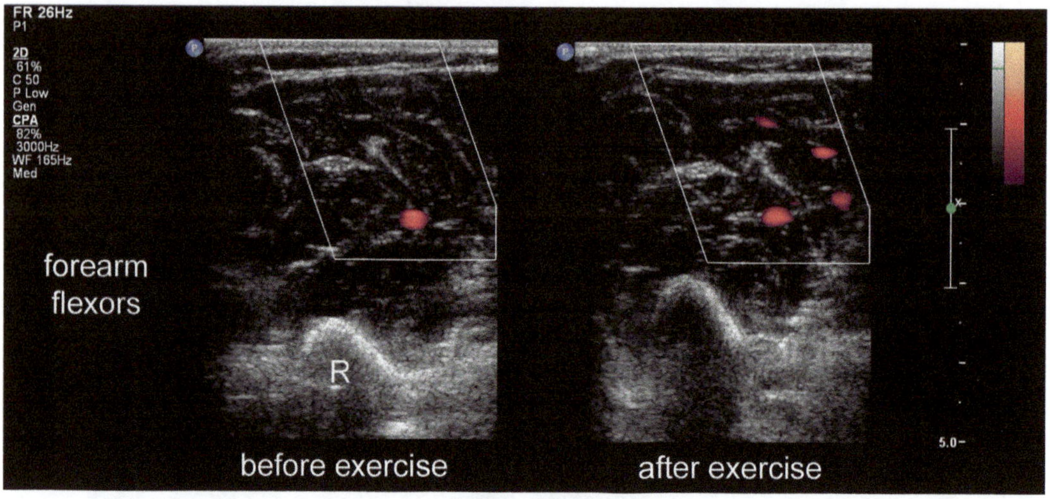

Fig. 2.9 Transverse image of the forearm with power Doppler applied before exercise (*left panel*) and directly after 20 s of maximum voluntary muscle contraction (finger flexion), resulting in hyperemia

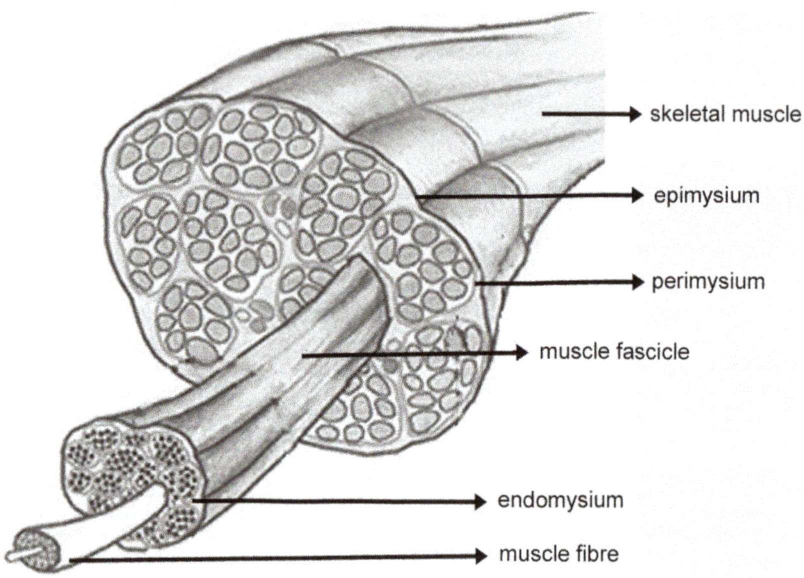

Fig. 2.10 Overview of normal muscle architecture

of one or a few layers that are strongly reflective and sharply demarcated. In a longitudinal plane, the fascicular organization of muscle becomes visible. For example, the tibialis anterior muscle has a pennate, feather-like structure in which the muscle fibers are attached to a central aponeurosis, and the biceps brachii exhibits uniform parallel tissue organization (Fig. 2.11). Scanning muscle in a longitudinal direction makes it possible to visualize the muscle architecture and measure pennation angles. In case of suspected muscle pathology, longitudinal imaging can visualize disruption of muscle structures caused by tears, hematomas, or tumors.

Muscle tissue echo intensity is relatively low In children and young adults, although obese

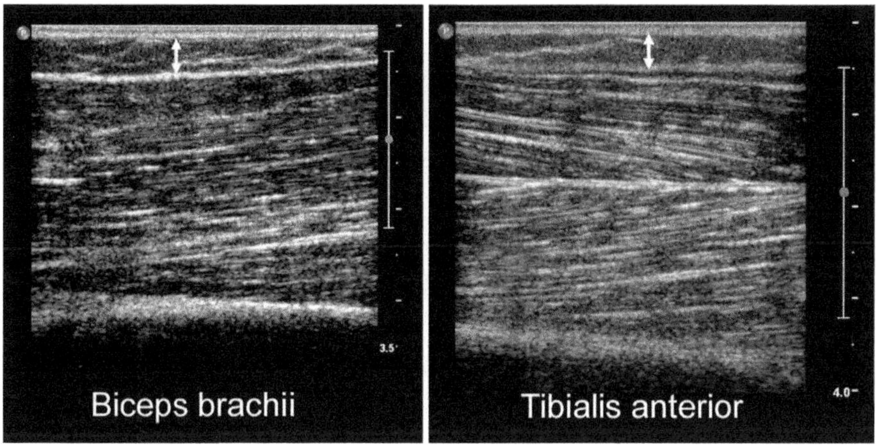

Fig. 2.11 Longitudinal image of the biceps brachii and tibialis anterior muscle. The biceps brachii has a parallel structure, whereas the tibialis anterior is a bipennate muscle, meaning that the muscle fascicles are attached to a central aponeurosis, which gives the muscle a feather-like appearance (*Double arrow* = subcutaneous tissue)

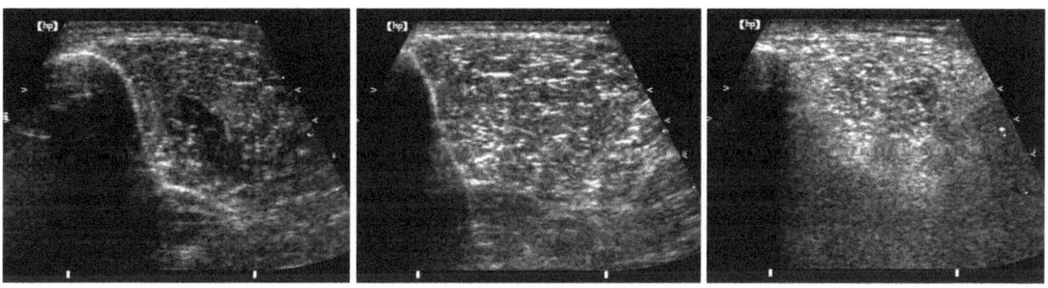

Fig. 2.12 Transverse image of the tibialis anterior muscles of three healthy men from one family, ages 20, 50, and 80 years. All images were made at the same anatomical location and with identical US settings. Note the increasing echo intensity with older age caused by sarcopenia

people may show slightly increased echo intensity, probably caused by the increased intramuscular fat content. With advancing age, especially in people over 60 years, muscle tissue becomes increasingly whiter with higher echo intensity. It is caused by age-related muscle changes called sarcopenia, which lead to a higher connective tissue content (Fig. 2.12) and a steady age-related decrease in muscle thickness. Finally, muscle echo intensity and US morphology also differ between relaxation (muscle resting state) and contraction. Contraction leads to increased cross-sectional muscle thickness, a blacker appearance (i.e., decreased echo intensity), and a change in the pennation angle.

Because each muscle has a different architecture, the specific echo intensity varies per muscle. Thus, each muscle has its own set of age-specific reference values for echo intensity.

2.3.2 Ultrasonography of Nerves

Peripheral nerves are composed of fascicles: bundles of myelinated and unmyelinated axons lying in endoneurial connective tissue and surrounded by a dense layer of perineurium, which also contains the nervi and vasa nervorum. A single nerve contains one to several fascicles, grouped together by an epineurial sheath (Fig. 2.13). Peripheral

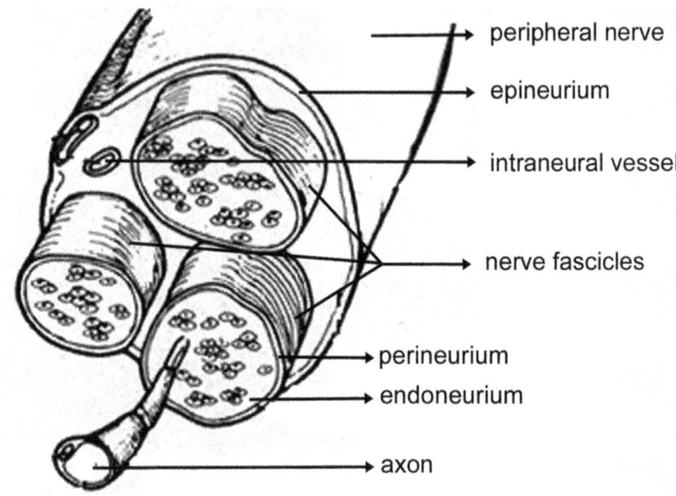

Fig. 2.13 Overview of normal nerve architecture

nerves run between the muscle fascia or next to bone (just as blood vessels do) and have shapes to suit their environment. Current high-resolution US allows imaging of the individual fascicles within a nerve. As the perineurium is strongly reflective, it usually makes the demarcation of the nerve quite clear.

The proximal nerve roots and trunks have few fascicles and little epineurium. They often appear on transverse images as a single round structure with low echo intensity (Fig. 2.14a). In the brachial plexus, the nerve roots form multifascicular strands in the supraclavicular area that resemble a cluster of grapes (Fig. 2.14b). More distally, the limb nerves appear as oval, round, or triangular structures with a honeycomb appearance (Fig. 2.14c). On longitudinal images the nerves are visible as tube-like structures containing several parallel lines that represent the perineural fascicle sheaths (Fig. 2.15).

2.3.2.1 Ultrasonography Appearance of Structures Surrounding Muscle and Nerves

The skin (i.e., epidermis and dermis) is visible as two thin straight lines just below the transducer surface. The deepest line demarcates the transition to the subcutaneous layer. The subcutaneous tissue consists of fat (relatively black). Between the fat lobules are several connective tissue septa also containing the lymphatic vessels. Septa appear as bright, sharp lines (Fig. 2.3). Especially in the case of muscle atrophy one should take care not to mistake these septa for muscle tissue or fascia. To differentiate between fat and muscle, the patient can perform a muscle contraction, or longitudinal scanning can assess the extent of the connective tissue structure.

Differentiation of nerves and tendons can be challenging during nerve US. In a transverse plane, tendons also have a round or oval shape with a granular internal pattern, but this pattern tends to be finer compared to the coarse granular honeycomb appearance of nerves (Fig. 2.4). In longitudinal orientation, tendons appear as finer, more fibrillar parallel structures that are less compact than those of nerves, although the difference can be difficult to see (Fig. 2.15). Tendons are also more anisotropic than nerves owing to the strong longitudinal orientation of their connective tissue fibers. Angulation of the transducer leads to a larger variation in echo intensity (Fig. 2.4).

Blood vessels are visible as black dots or tubes depending on the image angle. Arterial pulsations are usually visible during scanning. If there is any doubt, Doppler imaging can help identify the nature of a round or tube-like structure. Bone has high acoustical impedance, causing a strong reflection and a typical acoustical shadow underneath (Fig. 2.2). The same is seen in the case of tissue calcifications.

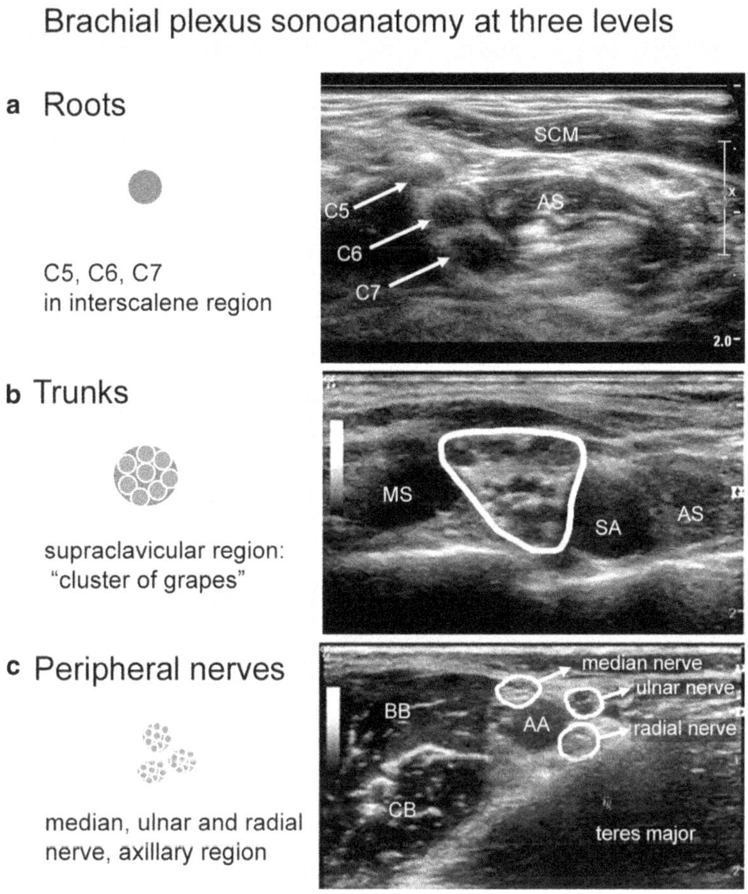

Fig. 2.14 The US appearance of nerves at several levels of the brachial plexus. The roots consist of a single bundle of axons and contain little connective tissue, appearing as *black circles* on US (**a**). A little more distally the nerve fascicles appear in the trunks. They become visible at the supraclavicular level as a compact granular structure that resembles a cluster of grapes (**b**). Even more distally, at the axillary level, the individual nerves emerge with their typical honeycomb-like appearance (**c**). *AA* axillary artery, *AS* anterior scalene muscle, *BB* biceps brachii muscle, *CB* coracobrachialis muscle, *MS* middle scalene muscle, *SA* subclavian artery, *SCM* sternocleidomastoid muscle

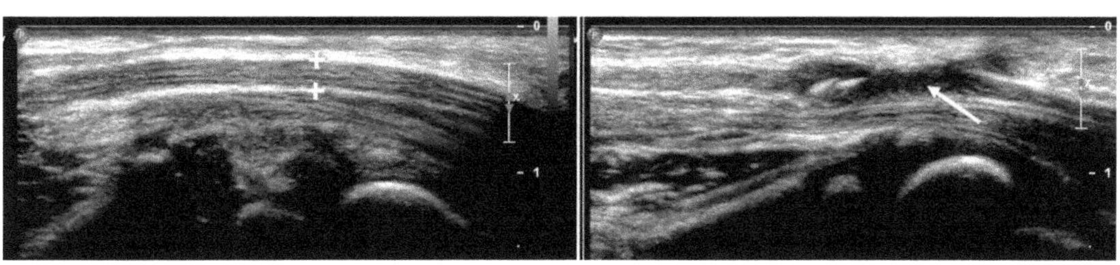

Fig. 2.15 Longitudinal image of the median nerve (between "+.….+") in a healthy subject (*left*) and a patient with a traumatic nerve lesion (*right*). The fascicles are visible with parallel organization. A tendon is visible directly below the median nerve. Although tendons normally have a slightly finer structure, differentiation based on the US appearance alone can be difficult. On the *right*, interruption of the longitudinal structure is seen that corresponds to a partial nerve tear caused by trauma. Courtesy of T. T. M. Claessen-Oude Luttikhuis, Department of Neurology, Canisius Wilhelmina Hospital, Nijmegen, The Netherlands

2.4 General Aspects of Muscle Ultrasonography in Neuromuscular Disorders

Many neuromuscular disorders are characterized by increased muscle echo intensity caused by a gradual replacement of healthy muscle tissue by fibrosis and fatty infiltration. Such change increases the number of tissue transitions and thus the number of reflections (Fig. 2.16). These changes in echo intensity and morphology (e.g., atrophy, hypertrophy) aid in the diagnostic workup of patients with a suspected neuromuscular disorder. Depending on the type of pathology, the muscle may appear diffusely gray as in Duchenne muscular dystrophy (DMD) (Fig. 2.16), or it may develop a moth-eaten appearance as seen in motor neuron disorders. Inflammatory changes blur normal muscle architecture, leading to a fuzzy appearance of the intramuscular fascia (Fig. 2.17). Inflammation probably also increases muscle echo intensity although not as much as fibrosis does.

2.4.1 Quantification of Muscle Echo Intensity

A marked increased of muscle echo intensity can be easily identified. However, as muscle echo intensity increases with age and varies individually per muscle, visual distinction of healthy and diseased muscles can be unreliable. Unreliability also occurs during early stages of a neuromuscular disease, when muscle echo intensity might be only slightly increased. Consequently, the sensitivity of visual muscle US evaluation for detecting neuromuscular disorders in children is relatively low (67–81 %, depending on operator experience).

Standardized techniques for quantifying echo intensity produce more objective results and increase the reliability and sensitivity of muscle US. There are several established ways to quantify muscle US images, such as backscatter, the luminosity ratio, or gray scale analysis. Of these methods, gray scale analysis has been studied most extensively and has proven to be sensitive and reliable in patients with neuromuscular

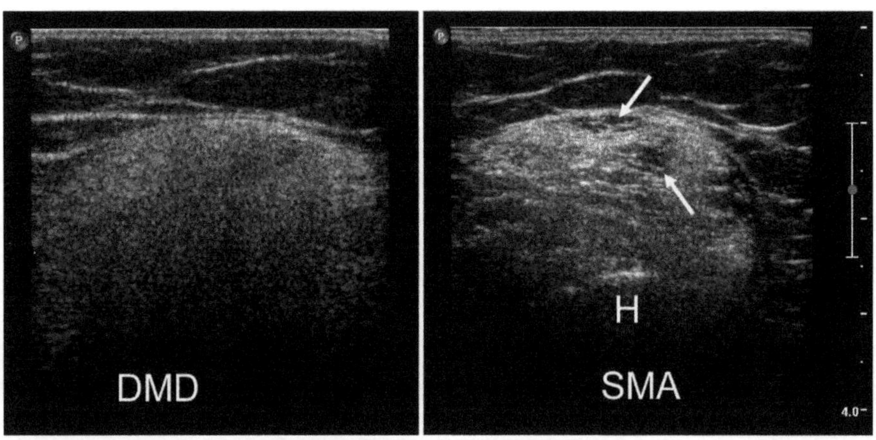

Fig. 2.16 Transverse image of the biceps brachii muscle in a patient with Duchenne muscular dystrophy (DMD) and a patient with spinal muscular atrophy. In both images, muscle echo intensity is severely increased with a loss of internal muscle architecture. In DMD, the muscle echo intensity is homogeneously increased with a strong attenuation of the US beam. Therefore the humerus (*H*) can no longer be visualized. In SMA a moth-eaten pattern is visible with very *white spots* caused by severely atrophic fibers and *black spots* caused by groups of hypertrophic muscle fibers (*arrow*)

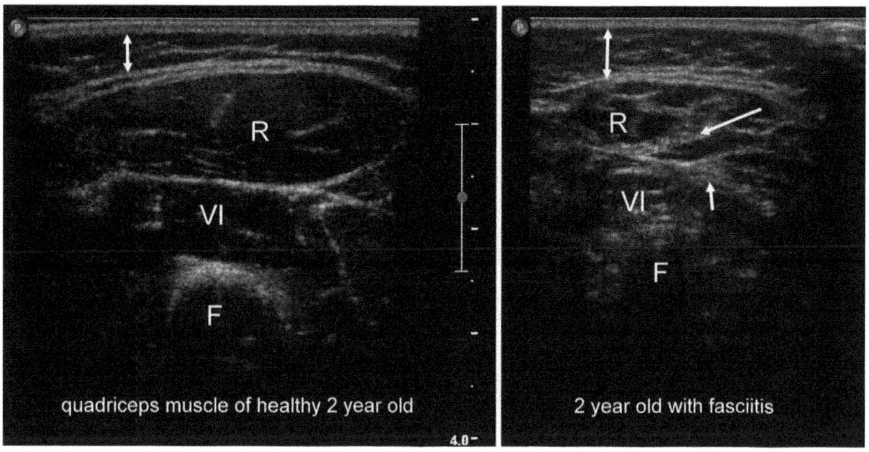

Fig. 2.17 Transverse US scan of the quadriceps muscle of a healthy 2-year-old child (*left*) and a 2-year-old suffering from fasciitis (*right*). Note the atrophy and increased echo intensity in the rectus femoris muscle. The intramuscular fascia are thickened and fuzzy (*long arrow*), as is the fascia between the rectus femoris muscle and the vastus intermedius muscle (*short arrow*) (*Double arrow* = subcutaneous tissue, *F* femur, *R* rectus femoris muscle, *VI* vastus intermedius muscle)

disorders. Quantitative gray scale analysis is conducted as follows: A region of muscle in the image is selected, and subsequently an average gray value that describes the degree to which the muscle is black, gray, or white is calculated. This value can then be compared to the corresponding reference value for that specific muscle and patient. To use reference values reliably, the same measurement protocol should be used each time, including the measurement location and the position of the patient. Care must be taken to measure muscles in a relaxed position as contraction leads to increased muscle thickness and decreased muscle echo intensity. Measurements must be performed in a transverse plane, avoiding too much pressure on the skin as compression increases muscle echo intensity. As system settings strongly influence echo intensity, it is important to keep all settings that influence the gray value (e.g., the gain, compression, focus, TGC) constant throughout the measurements. Gray scale analysis is performed offline by selecting a region of interest in the output image and running a standard histogram function, which is widely available in commercial software programs for image editing. To facilitate clinical use, customized gray scale analysis software has been developed that already incorporates reference values (Fig. 2.18).

The main difficulty with implementing quantitative muscle US in different centers is the need for specific reference values for each US machine because each device has its own characteristics that are incorporated into the machine and cannot be adjusted (e.g., beam frequency, transducer shape, gray map, and several other postprocessing techniques that transform the signal). Copying the user-adjustable system settings to another US device therefore does not lead to a similar range of muscle echo intensities.

Device-specific reference values can be obtained by establishing one's own or by using degradable muscle phantoms (i.e., meat) and calculating a conversion equation between machines. The gray value analysis technique is a sufficiently robust measurement to transpose reference values reliably to other US devices after application of such a conversion factor. Both methods are somewhat cumbersome, so new developments in US and phantom technology that focus on the device-independent interpretation of echo intensities would be most welcome.

Other quantification techniques that are supposedly less US device-dependent have been proposed. One is the luminosity ratio, which compares muscle echo intensity to that of subcutaneous tissue. Another is backscatter analysis, which compares the measured echo intensity to

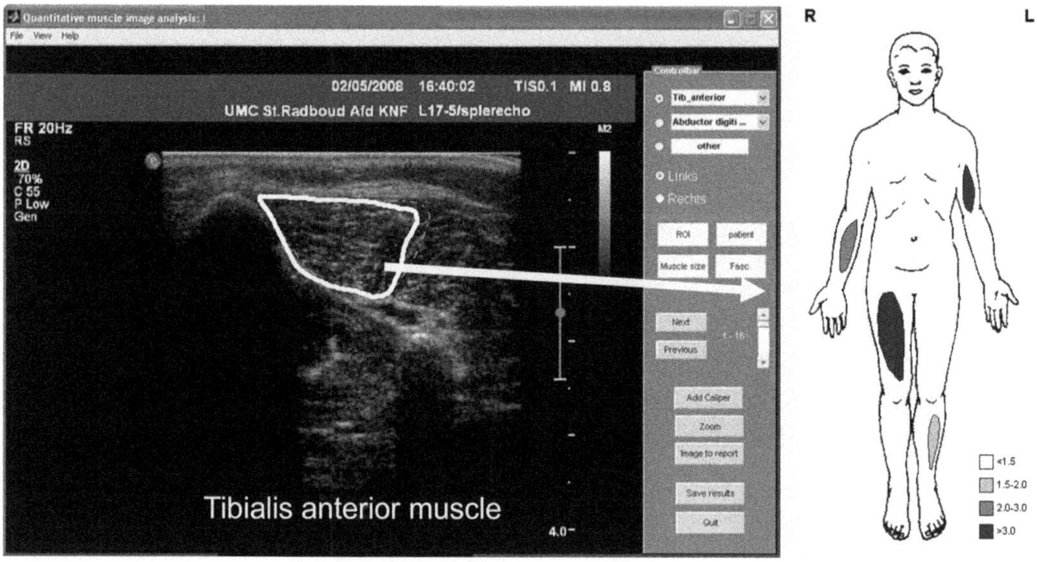

Fig. 2.18 QUMIA software and its output format. The mean echo intensity can easily be calculated and compared to muscle- and age-specific normal values using this customized quantitative muscle image analysis program. The output consists of a diagram showing which muscles were measured and how (ab-)normal their echo intensity is. With this format it is easy to appreciate the pattern of muscle involvement and chose an optimal site for muscle biopsy

that of a calibrated phantom. These techniques, however, also depend on several system settings and transducer characteristics, and they have not yet been proven to be as sensitive or reliable as plain gray scale analysis.

2.4.2 Dynamic Muscle Ultrasonography

The main advantage of US compared to other imaging techniques (e.g., MRI, CT) is that it is dynamic: The image is formed online and can be tracked in real time. US can thus help detect both physiological and pathological muscle movements.

Although individual motor units or muscle fibers cannot be visualized with current US resolutions, simultaneous contraction of several muscle fibers causes enough displacement of surrounding tissue to be visible. Contractions lead to a change in shape, resulting in an increased diameter or cross-sectional area (Fig. 2.19) and a slight decrease in echo intensity. Both voluntary and involuntary movements (e.g., cramps, tremor, clonus) can easily be visualized. Because all contractions look similar, it is not possible to discern voluntary from involuntary contractions by dynamic muscle US alone. Different patterns with certain clinical significance can be observed, however. Tremor, for example, is recognized as a rhythmic contraction of the entire muscle, and dynamic muscle US can be used to estimate tremor frequency.

Smaller, intramuscular movements are also visible with dynamic imaging. Fasciculations—involuntary random contractions of single motor units (an area of ≈2–8 mm)—are easily detected with dynamic US and with higher sensitivity than when using needle electromyography (EMG) or clinical examination. This is because a larger muscle area is screened with dynamic US than with EMG, and deeper muscle parts can be examined that are not visible from the outside. Interobserver agreement is good (0.85—comparable to that for EMG). Fasciculations, caused by spontaneous depolarization somewhere along the motor neuron or axonal membrane, are a hallmark of motor neuron disease. They appear on US as spontaneous focal jerky movements that occur

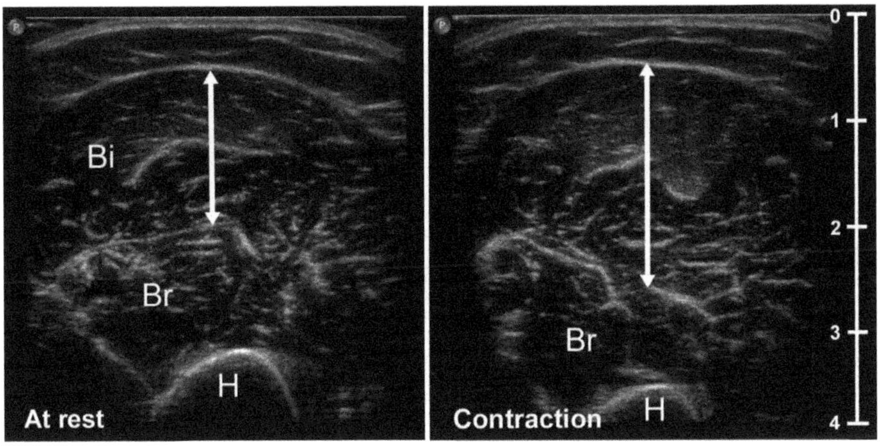

Fig. 2.19 Muscle US image of the upper arm showing the biceps brachii (*Bi*) and brachialis muscle (*Br*) at rest (*left panel*) and during isometric elbow flexion with the forearm supinated (*right panel*). The US image shows that the biceps brachii is more active (i.e., more contracted) during this movement as its diameter clearly increases, whereas the diameter of the brachialis muscle is unchanged. *H* humerus

irregularly and randomly throughout the muscle. Fasciculations are best recognized in a transverse plane, appearing as focal muscle thickening in both horizontal and vertical directions.

With its increasing resolution and frame rate, US is now able to detect fibrillations. Although a fibrillation is spontaneous activity of a single muscle fiber (~40–80 μm), multiple fibrillating muscle fibers cause sufficient displacement of their surroundings to be detectable. Fibrillations appear on US scans as small, irregularly oscillating movements within an overall preserved muscle shape. The skin and subcutaneous tissue are not displaced. Fibrillations are caused by spontaneous depolarization of individual muscle fiber membranes when a fiber loses contact with its innervating axon. This makes fibrillations an important sign of axonal damage in peripheral nerve disorders and of muscle inflammation (with fiber breakage) in inflammatory myopathies. It is important to know that fibrillations are very temperature-dependent and are best detected in limbs warmed to at least 34 °C.

2.4.3 Diagnostic Value of Muscle Ultrasonography

In children, quantitative muscle US using gray scale analysis is capable of detecting a neuromuscular disorder with an overall positive predictive value of 91 % and a negative predictive value (NPV) of 86 %. Muscle US is even more reliable (NPV 95 %) in patients over age 3 years. Below the age of 3 years more false-negative results are found (sensitivity 75 % in patients younger than 3 years), as often during the early stages of a neuromuscular disorder few structural muscle changes are present. False-negative US results are also seen in children with mitochondrial myopathy in which an energy disturbance in muscle metabolism affects function before it affects structure. It thus presents in only 25–46 % with increased echo intensities.

No prospective studies of muscle US as a screening tool for adult neuromuscular disorders are available yet, although recently it was shown that quantitative muscle US can aid in diagnosing amyotrophic lateral sclerosis. Apart from increased echo intensities in affected regions, US can confirm the presence of lower motor nerve involvement by detecting fasciculations. US is more sensitive for detecting fasciculations than EMG or clinical evaluation. It has a specificity of 86 %, which equals that of visual inspection. US criteria similar to the El Escorial criteria for EMG have been established to describe the likelihood of a motor neuron disorder being present.

In other adult manifestations of neuromuscular disorders, muscle US usually shows increasing echo intensity and atrophy as the disease progresses. However, the exact diagnostic value for specific neuromuscular disorders is not yet known.

2.5 General Ultrasonographic Aspects of Nerve Pathology

Many peripheral nerves are accessible to US provided they are not located too deep. The best images are obtained from relatively superficial nerves that can be reached with high-frequency probes. For example, the median nerve at the wrist can be imaged using a 17–5 MHz broadband transducer with better resolution than when using 7-tesla MRI. Conversely, the lumbar and sacral plexus are almost impossible to image with sufficient resolution using US.

Nerve US is most commonly used to detect entrapment neuropathies, such as carpal tunnel syndrome, compression neuropathy of the ulnar nerve at the elbow, or entrapment of the peroneal nerve at the fibular head. Nerves can also be scanned for inflammation, a neoplasm, or traumatic lesions. The most basic US abnormality in patients with nerve pathology is focal thickening leading to a hypoechogenic appearance and loss of the internal fascicular ("honeycomb") structure (Fig. 2.20). These abnormalities, which are

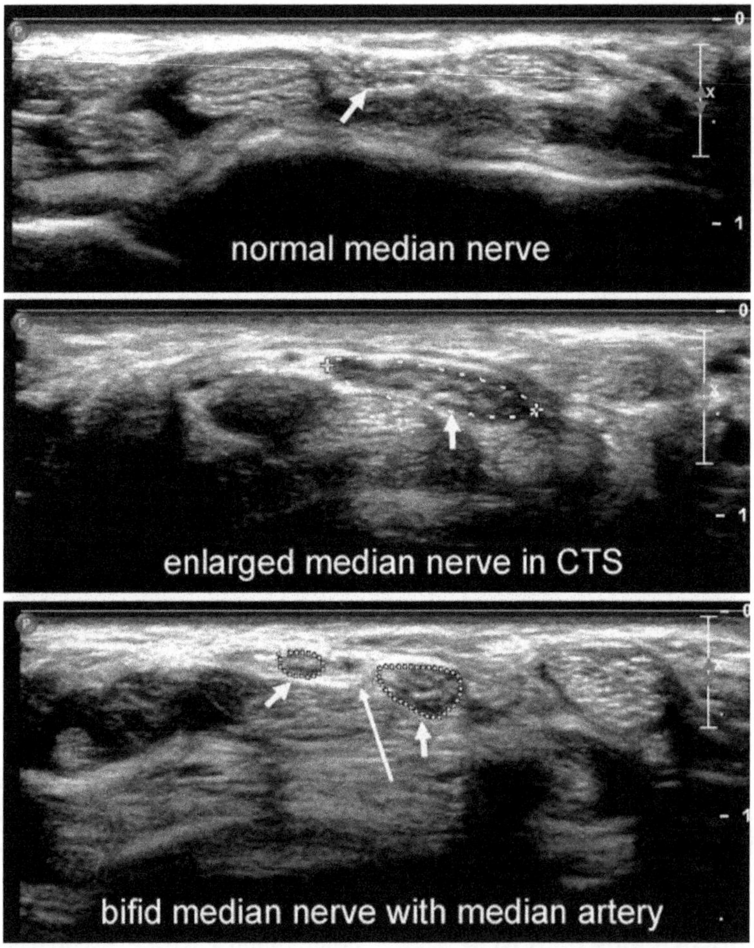

Fig. 2.20 Transverse US image of the distal forearm just proximal to the carpal tunnel. In the *upper panel* a normal median nerve is visible (*short arrow*). *Middle panel* shows an enlarged median nerve (with preservation of the fascicular architecture) caused by carpal tunnel syndrome. *Lower panel* shows a bifid median nerve with a persistent median artery in between (*long arrow*). Courtesy of T. T. M. Claessen-Oude Luttikhuis, Department of Neurology, Canisius Wilhelmina Hospital, Nijmegen, The Netherlands

probably caused by edema and accumulation of axonal flow, can be seen just proximal to the entrapment site (whereas relative thinning occurs at the entrapment site itself) and in inflamed or traumatically injured nerve segments. In trauma patients, interruption of the fascicular lines or gap between adjacent segments can be seen in a longitudinal or panoramic scan (Fig. 2.15).

Ultrasonography can assess both nerves and their surrounding structures, which is useful in case of nerve entrapment by synovial thickening in patients with rheumatoid arthritis, tendon ganglia, or misaligned fracture segments. Additional anatomical information can help when planning a surgical intervention for carpal tunnel syndrome when (in a few percent of the population) a persistent median artery is found to be present between both segments of a bifid median nerve (Fig. 2.20).

Because nerve pathology usually appears as focal nerve thickening, reference values have been established for a number of nerves and sites. As nerves are often not round or symmetrical, using a simple diameter is somewhat problematic. Most commonly, the cross-sectional area (CSA) of the nerve, traced within the hyperechogenic epineural rim, is used as a measure. Other parameters such as proximal to distal segment ratios or semiquantitative texture analysis can also be helpful as adjuncts to the CSA. So far, no single method has been found superior with respect to diagnostic accuracy. Nerve size is dependent on other parameters, such as height, body weight, and whether the nerve is measured proximally or distally. Currently, no reference values are available for children or patients of extreme height or weight. Therefore, good clinical judgment is imperative when using nerve US for diagnostic purposes in these patients.

Dynamic imaging with nerve US can also be useful, such as when looking for ulnar nerve luxation from the cubital tunnel with hyperflexion of the elbow as a cause of cubital tunnel syndrome. Doppler imaging can be used when inflammation is suspected in patients with vasculitis, leprous neuropathy, or chronic inflammatory demyelinating neuropathy. It can also demonstrate increased blood flow surrounding a schwannoma or other peripheral nervous system tumor.

Imaging Modalities: Ultrasonography

Key Points

- Ultrasonography has excellent capabilities for imaging muscle and nerve, especially in superficial tissue layers.
- Ultrasonography techniques such as compound imaging and panoramic imaging help with easy identification of specific muscles and nerves.
- The advantages of ultrasonography over other imaging modalities are its easy access, bedside availability, and noninvasive character. It is also patient-friendly. Ultrasonography can be used for dynamic, real-time imaging to detect normal and pathological muscle and nerve movement.
- Quantitative muscle ultrasonography using gray scale analysis is a reliable technique for confirming the presence of a neuromuscular disorder, with high sensitivity and specificity.
- In patients with myopathies, the ultrasonographic appearance of muscles becomes increasingly more white (i.e., echogenic) as normal muscle tissue is replaced by fat and fibrosis. Because the same process happens during normal aging, quantitative analysis using age-specific reference values is the optimal method for assessing echo intensity and following it over time.
- Nerve ultrasonography is mainly used in neurology to detect nerve entrapment (e.g., carpal tunnel syndrome). It can also be used to screen for hereditary or inflammatory neuropathy and to assess nerve trauma.

Suggestions for Further Reading

Adler RS, Garofalo G. Ultrasound in the evaluation of the inflammatory myopathies. Curr Rheumatol Rep. 2009; 11:302–8.

Bianchi S, Martinoli C. In: Baert AL, Knauth M, Sartor K, editors. Ultrasound of the musculoskeletal system, Springer series diagnostic imaging. Berlin: Springer; 2007.

Cartwright MS, Passmore LV, Yoon JS, Brown ME, Caress JB, Walker FO. Cross-sectional area reference values for nerve ultrasonography. Muscle Nerve. 2008; 37:566–71.

Koenig RW, Pedro MT, Heinen CP, Schmidt T, Richter HP, Antoniadis G, Kretschmer T. High-resolution ultrasonography in evaluating peripheral nerve entrapment and trauma. Neurosurg Focus. 2009; 26:E13.

Peer S, Bodner G, editors. High resolution sonography of the peripheral nervous system. 2nd revised ed. Springer diagnostic imaging series. Berlin: Springer; 2008.

Pillen S, Verrips A, van Alfen N, Arts IM, Sie LT, Zwarts MJ. Quantitative skeletal muscle ultrasound: diagnostic value in childhood neuromuscular disease. Neuromuscul Disord. 2007;17:509–16.

Pillen S, Arts IMP, Zwarts MJ. Muscle ultrasound in neuromuscular disorders. Muscle Nerve. 2008;37:679–93.

Pillen S, Van Dijk JP, Weijers G, Raymann W, De Korte CL, Zwarts MJ. Quantitative grey scale analysis in skeletal muscle ultrasound: a comparison study of two ultrasound devices. Muscle Nerve. 2009;39:781–6.

Van Alfen N, Nienhuis M, Zwarts MJ, Pillen S. Detection of fibrillations using muscle ultrasound: diagnostic accuracy and identification of pitfalls. Muscle Nerve. 2011;43:178–82.

Walker FO, Cartwright MS, editors. Neuromuscular ultrasound. Elsevier expert consult series. Philadelphia: Elsevier Saunders; 2011.

Computed Tomography

3

Mike P. Wattjes

3.1 Introduction

The use of computed tomography (CT) for diagnosing inherited and inflammatory muscle disease using second-generation whole-body CT systems was first described during the late 1970s and early 1980s. These first reports focused on the normal appearance of the skeletal muscle in terms of size, shape, and soft tissue densities. They also described pathological changes such as atrophy, abnormal appearance in general, and focal changes in muscle tissue architecture ("moth-eaten appearance"). Compared to the image quality today, the initial results were disappointing. With the development of newer generations of whole-body (spiral) CT systems using multi-detector rows, the quality and applicability of CT to imaging muscle improved dramatically. However, since the development of whole-body magnetic resonance imaging (MRI) systems during the 1990s, CT imaging in inherited and inflammatory muscle disease became less important. This chapter gives a brief overview of CT applications in the field of neuromuscular imaging in the past and present, including the advantages and disadvantages of this imaging modality compared to ultrasonography (US) and MRI.

3.2 Imaging Protocol

Standardized imaging protocols are not available for evaluating inherited or inflammatory muscle disease. The exact protocol (i.e., tube voltage, tube output, collimation, pitch) has to be adjusted and optimized according to the individual CT scanner. Currently, multi-detector row spiral CT systems are widely available and used in clinical practice, allowing multi-planar reconstructions. However, for the evaluation of patients with inherited or inflammatory muscle diseases, CT imaging should be limited to certain (e.g., clinically affected) muscles or certain important anatomical regions (e.g., pelvis, thigh, calf) to limit the radiation dose. Whole-body imaging protocols are therefore not recommended for CT. As with MRI (see Chap. 4), intravenous contrast administration is not recommended in patients with suspected muscular dystrophy or inflammatory muscle disease. Intravenous contrast administration is helpful only in patients with suspected soft tissue tumors. In addition to visualizing the local expansion and infiltration of the tumor, further tumor staging can be performed via lymph node and/or organ metastasis evaluation.

M.P. Wattjes (✉)
Department of Radiology, Nuclear Medicine & PET Research, VU University Medical Center, De Boelelaan 1117, 1081 HV Amsterdam, The Netherlands
e-mail: m.wattjes@vumc.nl

M.P. Wattjes and D. Fischer (eds.), *Neuromuscular Imaging*, DOI 10.1007/978-1-4614-6552-2_3,

3.3 Image Analysis of Muscle Tissue on CT

The macroscopic tissue architecture of the striated muscle with its subcomponents such as connective and fat tissues can be easily identified on CT. The tissue radiodensity is described using a quantitative Hounsfield unit (HU) scale. The radiodensity of water is per definition 0. The striated muscle tissue has a CT attenuation of approximately 40–50 HU and fat has one of −100± 20 HU depending on tube voltage. For image analysis, early CT studies used a window center of 50 HU and a window width of 250 HU, which is also appropriate for the current generation of CT scanners. Alternatively, a window center of 40 HE and a width of 400 HE can be used.

The appearance of various muscles seen on MRI (see Chap. 10) can also be identified on CT. According to the radiodensity values, lipomatous tissue appears more hypodense than normal muscle tissue. Atrophy and secondary fatty replacement leads to increased fatty tissue between the muscle bundles, whereas dystrophic fatty degeneration leads to destruction of muscle tissue and secondary fatty replacement. Examples of different degrees of fatty degeneration in muscular dystrophy patients are presented in Figure 3.1a–d. First reports on muscle CT used a rather rough four-point rating scale established by Bulcke and colleagues.

- *Normal*: normal appearance and attenuation of the striated muscle
- *Atrophy*: reduced muscle area, abnormally clear delineation and/or areas of decreased attenuation
- *Moth-eaten*: patchy areas of low attenuation
- *Washed-out*: generalized low attenuation without focal abnormalities

The term "moth-eaten" refers to fatty replacement and degeneration. Because the image quality has been substantially improved during the past two decades, the imaging criteria for these phenomena are the same on MRI and CT. Also, the established MRI rating scales for semi-quantitative assessment of these changes (see Chap. 4, Table 4.1) can be applied to CT images. However, based on the lower soft tissue contrast on CT, the visual rating of fatty replacement and degeneration on CT is probably less sensitive than that on MRI (Fig. 3.2).

Regarding inflammatory changes, CT is much less sensitive when compared to MRI. Discrete muscle inflammation, as seen during the early stages of muscle degeneration, is missed on CT. Severe and chronic muscle inflammation leads to low attenuation of the muscle or muscle groups because of the larger amount of water in terms of muscle edema. This has also been described as "washed-out" during the early days of CT imaging for muscle disease. "Washed-out" changes have also been observed in dystrophic muscles.

3.4 Value of CT Compared to MRI and US

In general, CT is an operator-independent imaging technique that allows fast, reproducible image acquisition. In the daily practice of radiology, CT is a highly valuable tool for diagnosing many disease entities. In the field of neuromuscular imaging, CT allows fast, reproducible assessment of the skeletal muscle in terms of shape and degeneration (e.g., fatty degeneration) even of the deeper muscle groups. In addition, when adjacent bones have to be evaluated, CT is superior to MRI. However, when compared to MRI and US, the most relevant drawback of CT is inferior soft tissue contrast and exposing the patient to ionizing radiation. The latter makes application of CT in young patients, particularly children, inappropriate. Also, whole-body protocols are not ethical because of the high radiation dose and the broad availability of whole-body MRI systems. The detection of edematous muscle changes is crucial in many regards. CT shows low sensitivity in the detection of muscle edema and inflammation and is not the imaging modality of choice. US and particularly MRI are more suited to these purposes. Hybrid CT imaging approaches, such as positron emission tomography (PET)-CT, can aid in the diagnosis of inflammatory and neoplastic diseases of striated muscle.

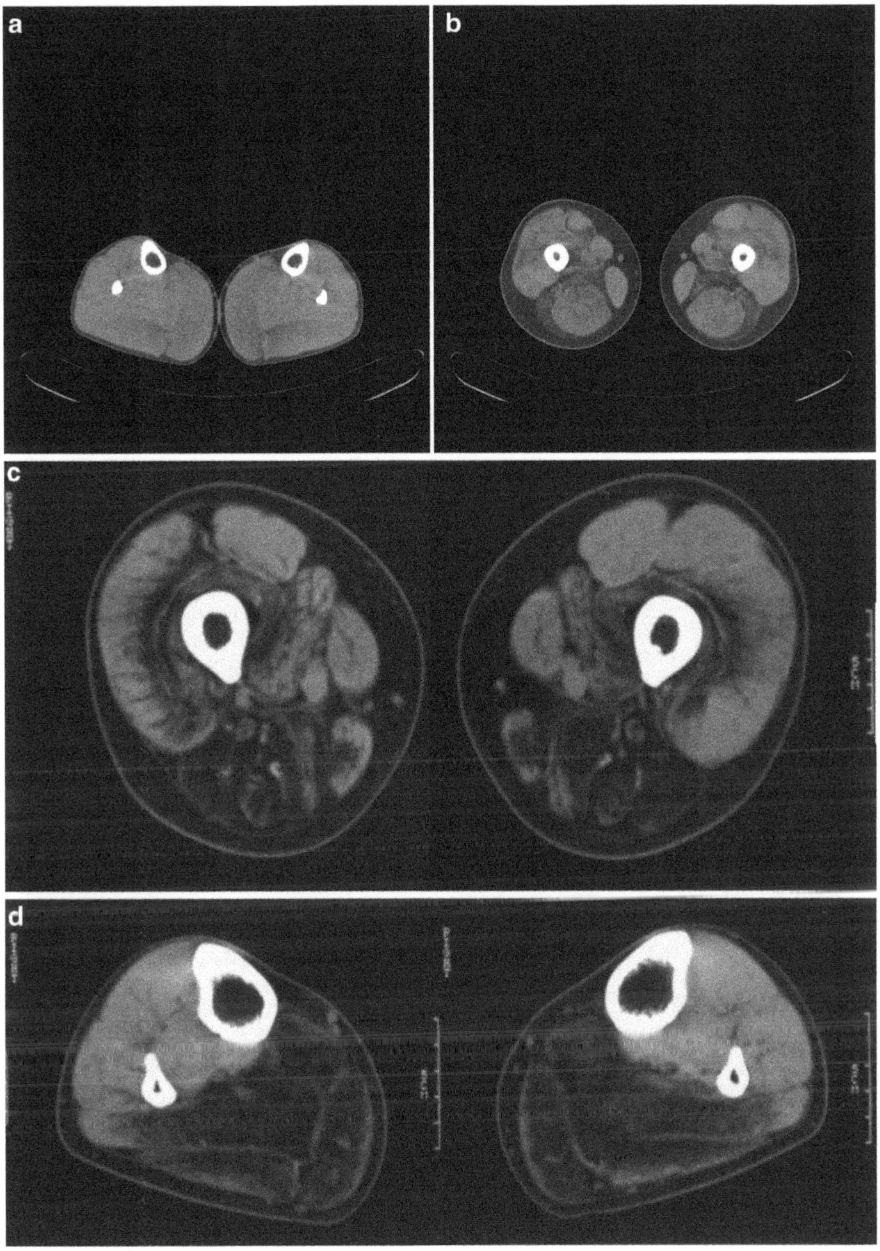

Fig. 3.1 Axial computed tomography (CT) images of the thigh and lower leg in a patient with Becker muscular dystrophy (**a**, **b**) and a patient with limb-girdle muscular dystrophy, autosomal recessive (LGMD2) (**c**, **d**). Note the different degrees of fatty degeneration (with low density) of distinct muscle groups depending on the underlying disease entity. The soft tissue contrast is lower when compared to magnetic resonance imaging (MRI) scans. Muscle edema cannot be assessed. Courtesy of L. ten Dam, M. de Visser and A.J. van der Kooi, Academic Medical Center, Amsterdam, The Netherlands

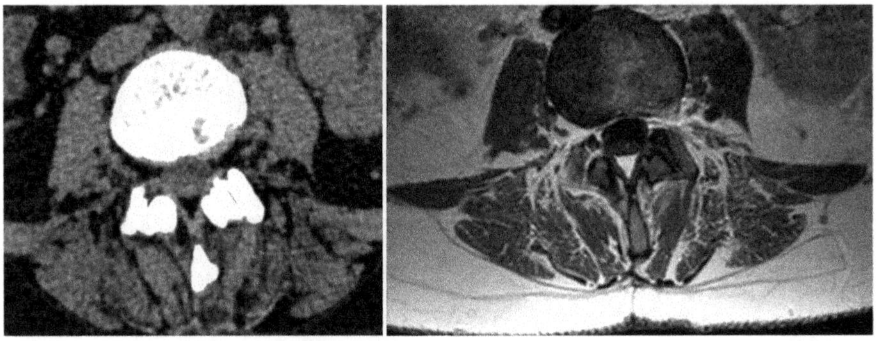

Fig. 3.2 Axial CT (*left*) and T1-weighted MRI (*right*) scans of the paraspinal muscles at the lumbar level in a 50-year-old man. Note the significant increase in soft tissue contrast on MRI. Even small depositions of fat in the muscle can be easily identified on MRI

Imaging Modalities: Computed Tomography

Key Points

- CT has been replaced by MRI and US for many purposes in the field of neuromuscular imaging.
- CT can assess dystrophic muscle changes with an acceptable image quality when MRI cannot be performed (e.g., presence of a pacemaker, patients with claustrophobia).
- Image-reading guidelines and recommended visual rating scales are comparable to those for MRI.
- Discrete inflammatory changes and muscle edema can be easily missed on CT.
- Hybrid CT imaging approaches (e.g., PET-CT) can be helpful for detecting inflammatory and neoplastic diseases of striated muscle.

Suggestions for Further Reading

Bulcke JA, Termote JL, Palmers Y, Crolla D. Computed tomography of the human skeletal system. Neuroradiology. 1979;17:127–36.

Bulcke JA, Crolla D, Termotte JL, et al. Computed tomography of muscle. Muscle Nerve. 1981;4:67–72.

Calò M, Crisi G, Martinelli C, Colombo A, Schoenhuber R, Gibertoni M. CT and the diagnosis of myopathies. Preliminary findings in 42 cases. Neuroradiology. 1986;28:53–7.

Schedel H. Imaging techniques in myotonic dystrophy. A comparative study of ultrasound, computed tomography and magnetic resonance imaging of skeletal muscles. Eur J Radiol. 1992;15:230–8.

Swash M, Brown MM, Thakkar C. CT Muscle imaging and the clinical assessment of neuromuscular disease. Muscle Nerve. 1995;18:708–14.

Termote JL, Baert A, Crolla D, Palmers Y, Bulcke JA. Computed tomography of the normal and pathologic muscular system. Radiology. 1980;137:439–44.

Wallgren-Peterson C, Kivisaari L, Jääskeläinen J, Lamminen A, Holmberg C. Ultrasonography, CT and MRI of muscles in congenital nemaline myopathy. Pediatr Neurol. 1990;6:20–8.

4 Conventional Magnetic Resonance Imaging

Mike P. Wattjes

4.1 Introduction

During the past decades, magnetic resonance imaging (MRI) has become crucial for diagnosing soft tissue diseases. Particularly in the field of neuromuscular imaging, MRI has dramatically influenced and improved the diagnostic workup. The diagnostic value of MRI has been conclusively and convincingly demonstrated in regard to inherited and inflammatory neuromuscular diseases. In fact, it has almost completely replaced computed tomography (CT) in this field. In addition to the clinical neurological examination and neurophysiological studies, neuromuscular MRI has developed into a valuable complementary diagnostic tool that allows assessment of the degree and, more importantly, the pattern of involvement. This imaging method can therefore be helpful for supporting a clinical diagnosis, limiting the complex range of differential diagnoses, and guiding interventional diagnostic procedures, such as muscle biopsy.

This chapter focuses on the possibilities and challenges of conventional neuromuscular MRI in the diagnosis and monitoring of patients with inherited (dystrophic and nondystrophic) and inflammatory muscle diseases. MRI applications for imaging muscle/soft tissue tumors are presented in Chap. 28. MRI techniques for evaluating peripheral nerves and diseases affecting peripheral nerves are discussed in Chaps. 7 and 30.

M.P. Wattjes (✉)
Department of Radiology, Nuclear Medicine & PET Research, VU University Medical Center, De Boelelaan 1117, 1081 HV, Amsterdam, The Netherlands
e-mail: m.wattjes@vumc.nl

4.2 Imaging Protocol

There are no MRI guidelines available for the diagnostic workup of patients with suspected inherited or acquired muscle diseases. The most relevant standard sequences used for these patients are

- Axial T1-weighted (turbo/fast) spin echo and
- Axial T2-weighted (turbo/fast) spin echo with fat suppression.

There are various techniques of fat suppression available including spectral fat suppression and relaxation time-dependent fat suppression [e.g., short tau inversion recovery (STIR)]. Many groups prefer STIR sequences because of the rather homogeneous fat suppression.

There are no general recommendations whether conventional spin echo or turbo/fast spin echo sequences should be used. However, turbo/fast spin echo sequences can considerably reduce the scan time without impairing the image quality in terms of the signal-to-noise ratio, particularly when higher magnetic field strengths are used.

The exact sequence parameters have to be adjusted and optimized according to the magnetic field strength and other characteristics of the MRI system used. MRI acquisition in the axial plane is

M.P. Wattjes and D. Fischer (eds.), *Neuromuscular Imaging*, DOI 10.1007/978-1-4614-6552-2_4,

sufficient in most patients. If necessary, the image acquisition can be performed in other anatomic orientations (e.g., coronal, sagittal). The spatial resolution is strongly dependent on the clinical situation. For detecting dystrophic and edematous muscle changes in patients with myopathies/muscular dystrophies, a slice thickness of 5–8 mm, interslice gap of 1–2 mm, and in-plane resolution of 1–2 mm are sufficient. The signal-to-noise ratio (SNR) is not a crucial issue for these diagnostic purposes when using magnetic field strengths of ≥1.5 T. Therefore, the standard body coil can be used to obtain adequate image quality. If possible, surface coils are recommended to improve the SNR.

4.2.1 Contrast-Enhanced MRI

The diagnostic benefit of contrast (gadolinium)-enhanced MRI for inherited muscle diseases (e.g., muscular dystrophies) has not yet been investigated. The late contrast enhancement phenomenon might have some value for assessing connective tissue that replaces normal muscle tissue in degenerative myopathies. In animal studies, tissue-specific contrast agents that enter affected muscle tissue can be helpful for distinguishing normal, unaffected muscle from damaged muscle. Furthermore, it can help to describe the extension and mechanism of muscular damage in dystrophic disorders. These applications are still in the experimental phase (see Chap. 5). However, based on the limited data, lack of evidence with regard to possible diagnostic benefits, longer scan time, and potential adverse effects of gadolinium-based contrast agents (e.g., systemic nephrogenic sclerosis, allergic reaction), contrast-enhanced MRI is not recommended on a regular basis in clinical practice.

Contrast-enhanced MRI can be helpful for evaluating acute inflammatory processes (e.g., connective tissue diseases, inflammatory myopathies; see Chap. 26). It can detect inflammatory changes, which appear as focal and/or diffuse enhancement in muscle tissue, perifascial septa, and in subcutaneous connective tissue septa. However, these inflammatory changes result also in edematous changes that can be detected with great sensitivity on fat-suppressed T2-weighted sequences. The benefit of contrast medium administration is thus limited for evaluating aseptic inflammatory diseases. In patients presenting with clinical findings suggestive of septic inflammation (e.g., abscess) or muscle neoplasm (see Chap. 28), however, contrast-enhanced MRI should be considered mandatory.

4.2.2 Whole-Body MRI

The first reports describing degenerative findings in skeletal muscles—particularly those in patients with inherited dystrophic muscle diseases—used MRI protocols focusing on certain anatomical regions (e.g., pelvis, thigh). More recently, whole-body MRI protocols have been introduced allowing evaluation of almost all relevant muscle groups beyond the pelvis and proximal lower extremities, including the trunk, shoulder girdle, neck, and distal parts of the upper and lower extremities (Fig. 4.1). It allows an almost complete description of the involvement pattern, which can support the clinical (differential) diagnosis. In addition, pathological changes of tissues and organs beyond the striated muscle, such as the parenchymatous organs in the abdomen, esophagus, and heart, all of which may be affected in patients with inherited neuromuscular diseases such as myotonic dystrophies can be detected by whole body MRI (see Chap. 22, Fig. 22.4).

4.3 Image Analysis

For image analysis, the most relevant tissue types are muscle and fat. The signal intensity of skeletal muscle tissue on T1-weighted images is slightly higher than that of water and substantially lower than that of fat. On T2-weighted images, the signal intensity of muscle tissue is much lower than that of water or fat tissue. Because of its short T1 relaxation time, the signal intensity of fat tissue is bright on T1-weighted MRI images (Figs. 4.2 and 4.3). Fat also shows high signal intensity on T2-weighted images.

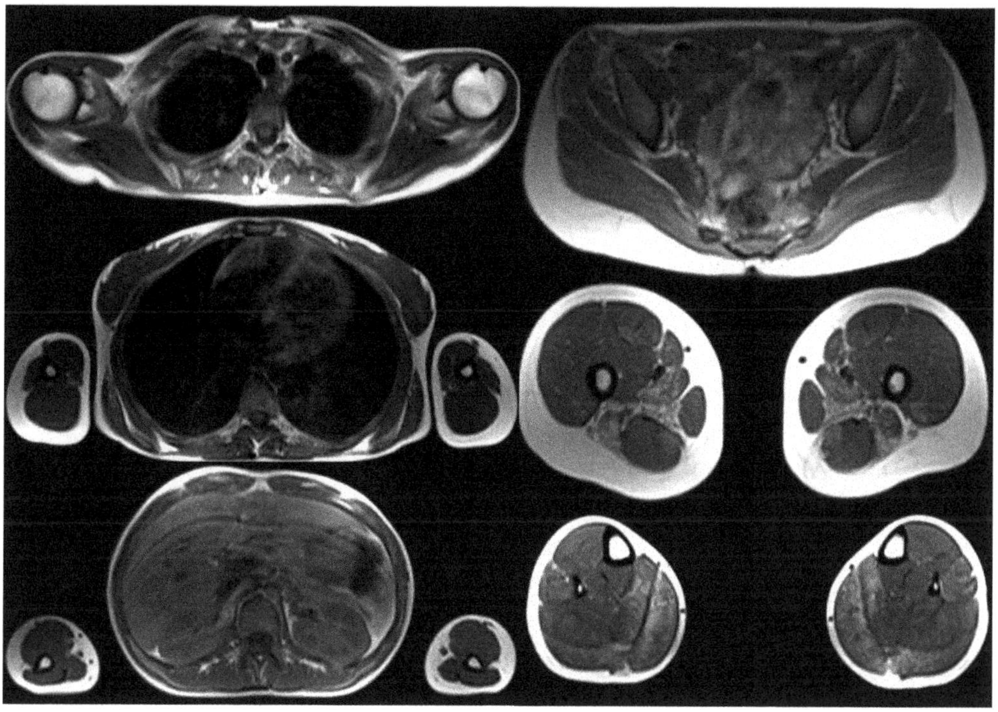

Fig. 4.1 Axial T1-weighted magnetic resonance imaging (MRI) scans using a whole-body MRI protocol in a patient with suspected limb girdle dystrophy. Note that the shoulder girdle,upper extremities, and the paraspinal muscles can be evaluated, as well as the parenchymatous organs (e.g., liver)

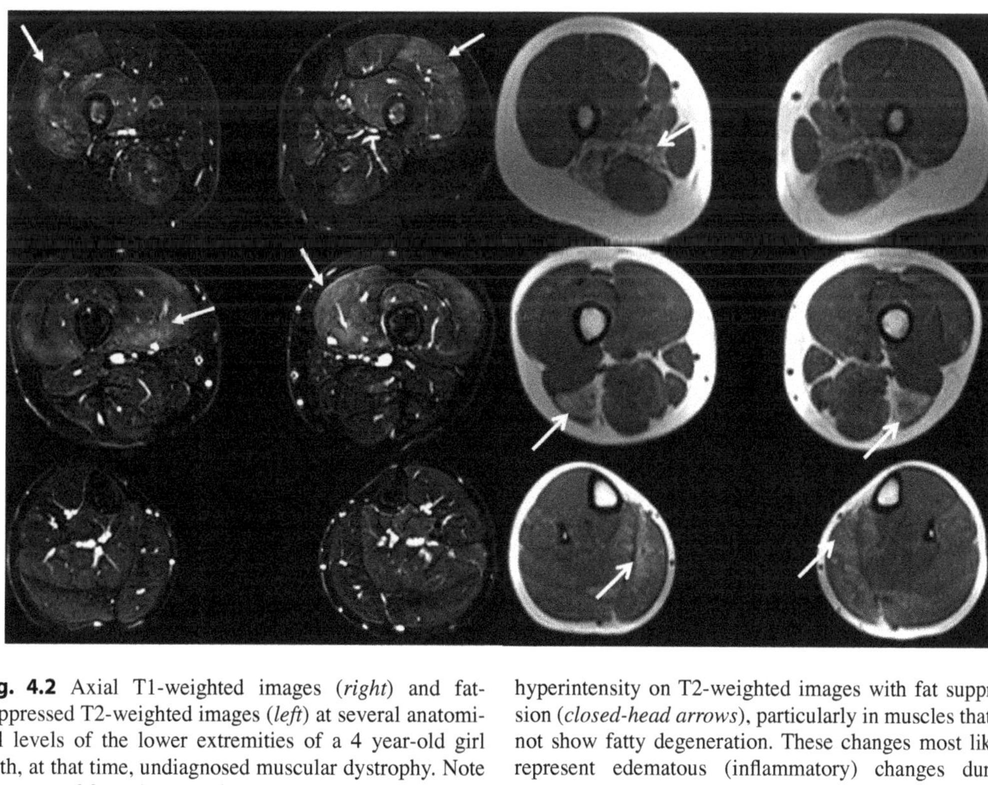

Fig. 4.2 Axial T1-weighted images (*right*) and fat-suppressed T2-weighted images (*left*) at several anatomical levels of the lower extremities of a 4 year-old girl with, at that time, undiagnosed muscular dystrophy. Note the areas of fatty degeneration involving several muscles (*open-head arrows*) and the areas of high signal hyperintensity on T2-weighted images with fat suppression (*closed-head arrows*), particularly in muscles that do not show fatty degeneration. These changes most likely represent edematous (inflammatory) changes during active muscle degeneration

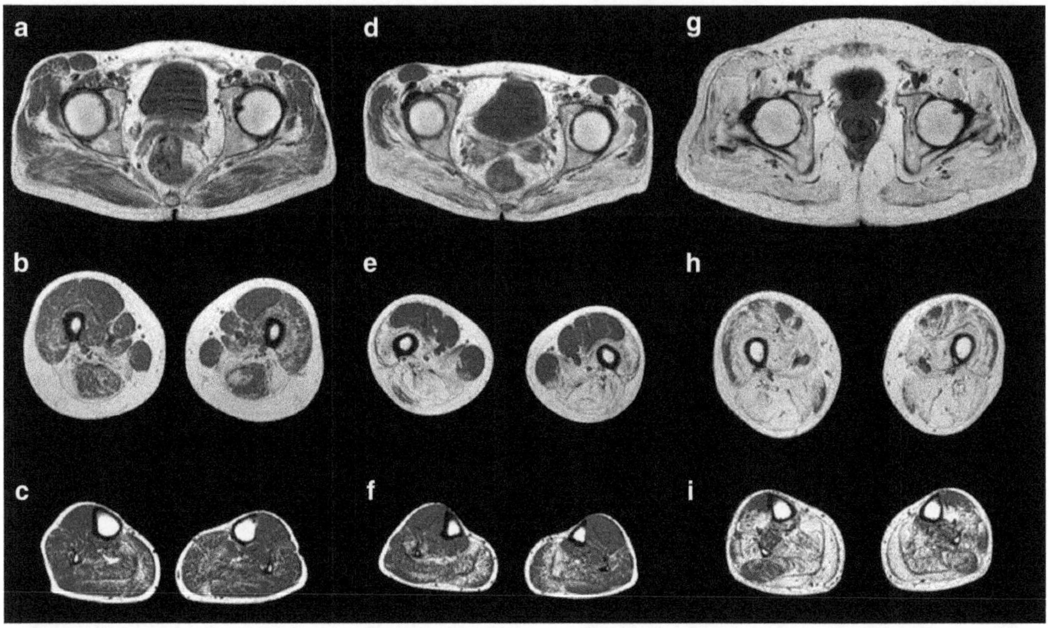

Fig. 4.3 Axial T1-weighted MRI scans obtained from three limb-girdle muscular dystrophy (LGMD-2I) patients. The scans were obtained on the pelvic (**a**, **d**, **g**), thigh (**b**, **e**, **h**), and lower leg (**c**, **f**, **i**), levels and demonstrated different degrees of fatty muscle degeneration. The MRI findings correspond well with the clinical phenotype. In the mild clinical phenotype (**a, b, c**), fatty degeneration is most obvious in the adductor and biceps femoris muscles. In the patient with a rather moderate clinical phenotype (**d, e, f**), additionally changes are present in the semimembranosus and semitendinosus, vastus intermediolateralis, and gluteus maximus muscles. In the patient with a severe clinical phenotype (**g, h, i**), an almost diffuse involvement can be observed. From Fischer et al. (2005). Diagnostic value of muscle MRI in differentiating LGMD2I from other LGMDs. J Neurol 252: 538–547. Reprinted with permission from Springer-Verlag

A simple way to distinguish between fat and water on T2-weighted images is to apply fat suppression. On fat-suppressed T2-weighted images, muscle signal intensity is lower than that of water and slightly lower than that of fat tissue. Simply speaking, both, fat and muscle tissue show rather low signal intensities when compared to that of water, leading to high tissue contrast between fat/muscle and water which improves the sensitivity of detecting intracellular and extracellular free water (muscle edema) (Fig. 4.2).

In general, image analysis of neuromuscular MRI images does not substantially differ from the analysis of CT or ultrasonography (US) images and include

- Shape—e.g., normal configuration, deformation
- Size—normal, atrophic, hypertrophic
- Tissue architecture—homogeneous, signs of (fatty) degeneration, adjacent connective tissue
- Focal lesions—calcifications, soft/mixed tissue lesions
- Signal abnormalities—edema

The first three aspects of image analysis described above should be performed on T1-weighted imaging. Shape and size of muscles differ among individuals, depending on several factors (e.g., nutrition, exercise, age, sex). The normal tissue architecture of skeletal muscle differ among muscle groups and anatomical locations. Chap. 9 gives an overview of macroscopic anatomy and the variations in different muscle groups according to the anatomical location.

4.3.1 Fatty Degeneration

The term "fatty degeneration" (synonym: fatty replacement) describes the replacement of muscle tissue by fat, which can be observed in

Table 4.1 Overview of well-established rating scales on MRI concerning the visual rating of dystrophic changes (fatty degeneration) of striated muscle tissue

Grade	Mercuri et al. 2002	Kornblum et al. 2006	Fischer et al. 2008
0		Normal appearance	Normal appearance
1	Normal appearance	Discrete moth-eaten appearance with sporadic T1 hyperintense areas	Mild: traces of increased signal intensity on the T1-weighted MRI sequences
2	Mild involvement: Early moth-eaten appearance with scattered small areas of increased signal or with numerous discrete areas of increased signal with beginning confluence, comprising < 30 % of the volume of the individual muscle	(a) Moderate moth-eaten appearance with numerous scattered T1 hyperintense areas (b) Late moth-eaten appearance with numerous confluent T1 hyperintense areas	Moderate: increased T1-weighted signal intensity with beginning confluence in < 50 % of the muscle
3	Moderate involvement: Late moth-eaten appearance with numerous discrete areas of increased signal with beginning confluence, comprising 30–60 % of the volume of the individual muscle	Complete fatty degeneration, replacement of muscle by connective tissue and fat	Severe: increased T1-weighted signal intensity with beginning confluence in > 50 % of the muscle
4	Severe involvement: Washed-out appearance, fuzzy appearance due to confluent areas of increased signal, or an end-stage appearance, with muscle replaced by increased-density connective tissue and fat, and only a rim of fascia and neurovascular structures distinguishable		End-stage appearance, entire muscle replaced by increased-density connective tissue and fat

Reprinted from Wattjes MP, et al. (2010) Neuromuscular imaging in inherited muscle diseases. Eur Radiol 20: 2447–2460 with permission from Springer

various conditions—e.g., muscle aging, inactivity, disuse, denervation (chronic stage), drug use (steroids), degenerative/dystrophic muscle diseases. The term "fatty degeneration" should be used to describe a primary degenerative process such as in chronic denervation and (inherited) dystrophic muscle diseases. The term "fatty replacement" is more suited for aging and other possibly reversible underlying processes.

Fatty degeneration and fatty replacement can occur focally or diffusely. They are often associated with muscle atrophy. The assessment and grading of fatty degeneration in skeletal muscles is important particularly in patients who present with clinical symptoms that suggest an inherited muscle disease. In these patients, identifying a certain pattern of involvement can be helpful in supporting the clinical diagnosis by narrowing the differential diagnosis (Fig. 4.3). For these purposes, several semi-quantitative visual rating scales have been developed and used in a considerable number of studies. Table 4.1 gives an overview of the most established and frequently used scales for visual rating of fatty degeneration in inherited muscle diseases.

4.3.2 Muscle Edema

Skeletal muscle edema (myoedema) is defined as increased extracellular and/or intracellular water that leads to prolonged T2 tissue relaxation time and high signal intensity on T2-weighted images. These signals are most sensitively detected on fat-suppressed T2-weighted MRI (Fig. 4.2). The spectrum of imaging findings of muscle edema ranges from focal edema involving certain parts of a single muscle to diffuse edema involving several muscle groups, as in rhabdomyolysis. Similar to the evaluation of fatty degeneration,

Table 4.2 Rating scale on skeletal muscle edema according to Poliachik and colleagues

Rating scale on skeletal muscle edema (myoedema)
• Myoedema absent
• Slight, interfascicular myoedema
• Slight, intrafascicular, segmental myoedema of individual muscle
• Slight, intrafascicular, global myoedema of individual muscle
• Moderate, intrafascicular, segmental myoedema of individual muscle
• Moderate, intrafascicular, global myoedema of individual muscle

From Poliachik SL, Friedman SD, Carter GT, Parnell SE, Shaw DW. (2012) Skeletal muscle edema in muscular dystrophy: clinical and diagnostic implications. Phys Med Rehabil Clin Am 23: 107–122. Reprinted with permission from Elsevier Limited

several ratings scales have been introduced to classify and quantify skeletal muscle edema. The one developed by Poliachik and colleagues is shown in Table 4.2.

It is important to realize that muscle edema is a rather unspecific finding and can be observed in an abundance of (heterogenic) clinical circumstances including muscle denervation, autoimmune (aseptic) inflammatory myopathies (polymyositis, dermatomyositis) (see Chap. 26), infectious muscle disease or infections of the adjacent structures, muscle trauma, treatment-related conditions (e.g., irradiation), rhabdomyolysis (e.g., toxic, drug-induced) (see Chap. 27), and inherited myopathies/muscular dystrophies. Muscle edema is also a physiological phenomenon that can be observed in healthy persons during or after exercise, probably due to extracellular (intercellular) water accumulation.

The role of muscle edema in patients with inherited muscle disease has been increasingly investigated during the past few years. In addition to degenerative changes in terms of fatty degeneration, some muscles/muscle groups show signs of edema on MRI. Histopathological studies have suggested that muscle edema reflects loss of muscle fiber integrity, leading to primarily intracellular water accumulation as a first sign of degeneration followed by degeneration of muscle fibers, which are subsequently replaced by fat and connective tissue during later disease stages. Interestingly, the skeletal muscle edema in dystrophic muscle tissue is frequently combined with inflammatory changes as shown by immunohistochemistry in biopsy samples. The severity of edematous changes in a dystrophic muscle can be provoked and further aggravated by muscle exercise. These findings suggest that muscle cell edema in dystrophic muscle disease might be the first manifestation of muscle tissue degeneration on MRI. Therefore, muscle MRI has increasingly been used to guide muscle biopsy to obtain muscle tissue with active disease.

4.4 Pitfalls in Image Analysis

When assessing and interpreting fatty replacement and degeneration of skeletal muscle, it is important to differentiate between true fatty degeneration and other imaging findings associated with increased fat deposition. Possible confounders are soft tissues including lipomas, hemangiomas, and other soft tissue tumors containing lipomatous tissue (see Chap. 29). Also, particularly in elderly and/or immobilized patients, it is crucial to differentiate between muscle changes due to aging, non-use, and immobilization (e.g., atrophy with fatty replacement), and abnormalities due to a primary degenerative disease of the skeletal muscle such as late-onset inherited muscle dystrophies or sporadic inclusion body myositis. In clinical practice, this can be challenging. Atrophy with fatty replacement is observed in "normally aging" skeletal muscle. It appears homogeneously and symmetrically in almost all skeletal muscle in these patients (see Chap. 11). In immobilized patients with non-used muscles, determining the underlying cause (e.g., degenerative changes in the spine, postoperative changes) can lead to the correct diagnosis. Degenerative muscle changes in patients with muscle dystrophies may be symmetrical. Although, particularly during the early stages, fatty infiltration manifests in a rather "moth-eaten" appearance that does not involve all muscle homogeneously. In most cases, more than one muscle group is involved.

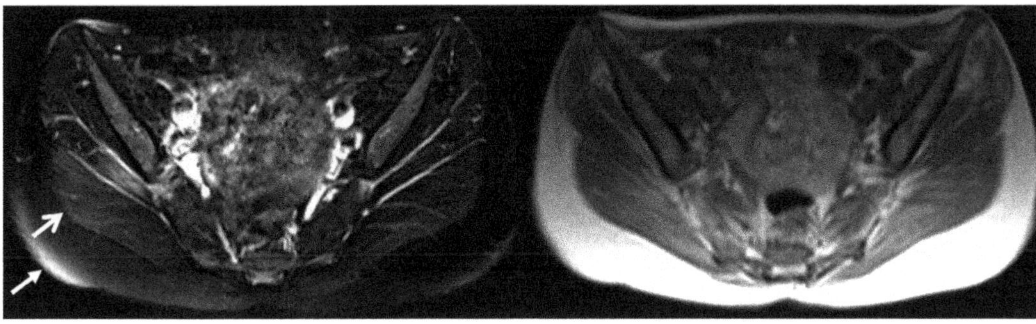

Fig. 4.4 Axial T1-weighted images (*right*) and fat-suppressed T2-weighted images (*left*) from the pelvis region. Note the high signal intensity in the subcutaneous fat (*closed head arrow*) and adjacent gluteus maximus muscle (*open head arrow*), which is due to inhomogeneous fat suppression

When assessing muscle edema, the most relevant pitfall is based on inhomogeneous and/or insufficient fat suppression on T2-weighted images. Inhomogeneous fat suppression is most often due to insufficient magnetic field homogeneity, particularly in the peripheral region of the field of view (Fig. 4.4). When high signal changes on fat-suppressed T2-weighted images are seen in skeletal muscle, it is important to evaluate the adjacent tissue (e.g., subcutaneous fat). If the adjacent structures show inhomogeneous signal intensity and insufficient suppression of subcutaneous fat, these muscle changes should not be considered "real" muscle edema. Other important reasons for insufficient fat suppression include susceptibility artifacts particularly close to material containing metal (e.g., a joint prosthesis).

4.5 Strengths and Challenges of Structural MRI for Neuromuscular Imaging

The strengths of MRI as a diagnostic tool to evaluate neuromuscular diseases are obvious: high soft tissue contrast; high-resolution imaging; tissue signal manipulation due to multi-sequence imaging (e.g., application of T1- and T2-weighted images with and without fat suppression); lack of radiation exposure. These advantages has led to almost complete replacement of CT by MRI. The latter aspect—no radiation exposure—is particularly important for young adults and children. Because of the rather long acquisition time required for MRI, however, it is sometimes necessary to sedate children to avoid movement artifacts. Ultrasonography is a good alternative imaging modality in these patients, allowing high-resolution dynamic imaging of muscle tissue (see Chap. 2). Ultrasonography can have difficulty assessing pathology in deep muscles, however, this can be easily evaluated with MRI.

Using whole-body imaging protocols, MRI provides the possibility of an almost "one-stop shop" strategy for evaluating patients with suspected inherited muscle diseases, inclusive tissues and organ systems other than skeletal muscle. Using advanced quantitative MRI methods, e.g. functional imaging, MRI can even more improve our understanding of the underlying pathophysiological mechanisms. Chap. 5 focuses on these advanced MRI methods.

Imaging Modalities: Conventional MRI

Key Points

- Structural MRI is one of the most important imaging modalities in the diagnosis of muscle pathology.
- Axial T1-weighted and fat-suppressed T2-weighted sequences are the workhorses of structural MRI in the routine clinical setting.
- Contrast enhanced MRI is only recommended in inflammatory and infectious muscle disease, and to detect soft tissue tumors.
- A standardized image analysis in terms of muscle shape, size, tissue architecture, focal lesions and diffuse signal abnormalities is crucial.
- Visual rating scales for rating fatty degeneration/replacement and muscle edema can aid in quantifying and describing the disease manifestation in terms of patterns of involvement.
- Assessment of the pattern of involvement based on MRI-attained information from patients with suspected inherited muscle diseases can support the clinical diagnosis.
- Whole-body MRI is useful to show distinctive generalised involvement patterns and for assessing co-morbidities in nonmuscle tissue and parenchymatous organs.
- Muscle edema assessed by MRI can represent the first stage of muscle degeneration in patients with (inherited) muscle diseases. This can be also helpful in directing the muscle biopsy.

Suggestions for Further Reading

Fischer D, Kley RA, Strach K, et al. Distinct muscle imaging patterns in myofibrillar myopathies. Neurology. 2008;71:758–65.

Fleckenstein JL, Crues III JV, Reimers CD. Muscle imaging in health and disease. New York: Springer; 1996.

Goodwin DW. Imaging of skeletal muscle. Rheum Dis Clin North Am. 2011;37:245–51.

Kamath S, Venkatanarasimha N, Walsh MA, Hughes PM. MRI appearance of muscle denervation. Skeletal Radiol. 2008;37:397–404.

Kornblum C, Lutterbey G, Bogdanow M, Kesper K, Schild H, Schröder R, Wattjes MP. Distinct neuromuscular phenotypes in myotonic dystrophy types 1 and 2: a whole body highfield MRI study. J Neurol. 2006;253:753–61.

May DA, Disler DG, Jones EA, Balkinson AA, Manaster BJ. Abnormal signal intensity in skeletal muscle at MR imaging: patterns, pearls and pitfalls. Radiographics 2000;20 Spec No:S295–315.

Mercuri E, Jungbluth H, Muntoni F. Muscle imaging in clinical practice: diagnostic value of muscle magnetic resonance imaging in inherited neuromuscular disorders. Curr Opin Neurol. 2005;18:526–37.

Mercuri E, Pichiecchio A, Allsop J, Messina S, Pane M, Muntoni F. Muscle MRI in inherited neuromuscular disorders: past, present and future. J Magn Reson Imaging. 2007;25:433–40.

Peters SA, Köhler C, Schara U, et al. Muscular magnetic resonance imaging for evaluation of myopathies in children. Klin Padiatr. 2008;220:37–46.

Poliachik SL, Friedman SD, Carter GT, Parnell SE, Shaw DW. Skeletal muscle edema in muscular dystrophy: clinical and diagnostic implications. Phys Med Rehabil Clin N Am. 2012;23:107–22.

Schmidt GP, Reiser MF, Baur-Melnyk A. Whole-body MRI of the musculoskeletal system: the value of MR imaging. Skeletal Radiol. 2007;36:1109–19.

Schulze M, Kötter I, Ernemann U, et al. MRI findings in inflammatory muscle diseases and their noninflammatory mimics. AJR Am J Roentgenol. 2009;192:1708–16.

Wattjes MP, Kley RA, Fischer D. Neuromuscular imaging in inherited muscle diseases. Eur Radiol. 2010;20: 2447–60.

Advanced and Quantitative Magnetic Resonance Imaging Techniques

5

Kieren G. Hollingsworth and Marc-André Weber

5.1 Introduction and Classification

In addition to the conventional magnetic resonance imaging (MRI) methods presented in Chap. 4, there are a number of advanced and quantitative MRI methods that can be used to further characterize skeletal muscle changes in neuromuscular diseases. This chapter considers the use of spectroscopy, sodium MRI, diffusion and perfusion measurements, measurement of T1 and T2 relaxation times, the three-point Dixon method for quantifying fat infiltration, and the use of novel contrast agents.

5.2 Magnetic Resonance Spectroscopy

Magnetic resonance spectroscopy (MRS) permits assessment and quantification of metabolite concentrations in striated muscle tissue, which can be useful biomarkers in neuromuscular disease. For a given nucleus and magnetic field strength, there is a defined resonance frequency. For MRI, we encode the spins, regardless of chemical species, so water or fat from a specific location is accurately represented in the image. However, the magnetic field strength experienced by the individual nuclei is modified very slightly by the electron cloud that surrounds it. Hence, the precise resonance frequency depends on the chemical bonding of that nucleus. This means that different chemical species resonate at slightly different frequencies and can be distinguished from each other using MRS. The differences in the frequency between compounds are expressed as a fraction of the main resonance frequency in parts per million (ppm).

Spectroscopy can be performed on compounds of several nuclei, most commonly protons (hydrogen) with standard MRI systems (designed for routine imaging). With additional hardware—broadband radiofrequency amplifiers and specialized coils tuned to other frequencies (neither are routinely supplied with scanners)—studies of energy metabolism by phosphorus-31 and of glycogen storage by carbon-13 are also possible.

5.2.1 Proton Magnetic Resonance Spectroscopy

Figure 5.1 shows proton spectra acquired from a voxel in the soleus muscle of a healthy subject and that of a patient with limb-girdle muscular dystrophy 2I (LGMD-2I) with fat having replaced part of the soleus muscle. The water peak at 4.7 ppm is dominant, followed by the resonance at 1.3 ppm, which represents the CH_2 groups in fatty acid

K.G. Hollingsworth (✉)
Newcastle Magnetic Resonance Centre,
Institute of Cellular Medicine, Newcastle University,
Newcastle upon Tyne NE4 5PL, UK
e-mail: k.g.hollingsworth@ncl.ac.uk

M.-A. Weber
Department of Diagnostic and Interventional Radiology,
University Hospital of Heidelberg, Im Neuenheimer
Feld 110, D-69120 Heidelberg, Germany
e-mail: marcandre.weber@med.uni-heidelberg.de

M.P. Wattjes and D. Fischer (eds.), *Neuromuscular Imaging*, DOI 10.1007/978-1-4614-6552-2_5,

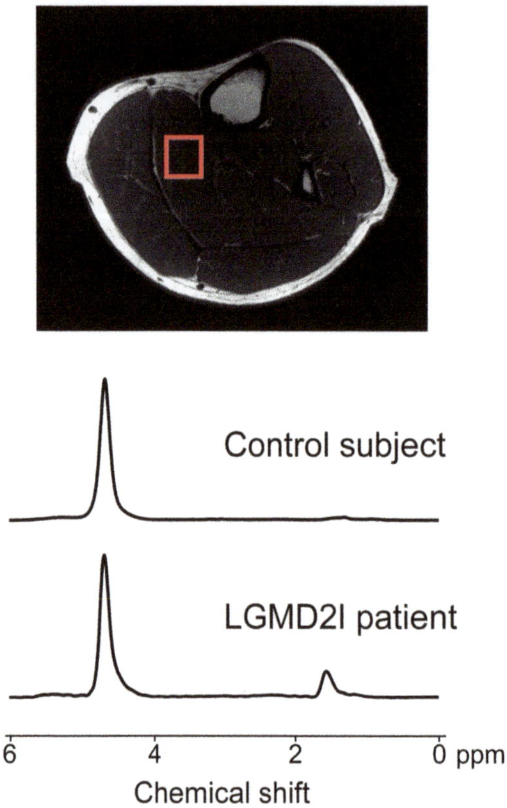

Fig. 5.1 Proton spectra from the soleus of a healthy control subject *(top)* and a patient with limb-girdle muscular dystrophy 2I (LGMD2I) *(bottom)* at 3.0 T

chains. Fat replacement in the LGMD2I soleus is reflected in the higher amplitude of this CH_2 peak relative to the water peak, whereas it is barely visible in healthy muscle. The proton spectrum can also yield the concentrations of total choline (choline + phosphocholine) and total creatine (creatine + phosphocreatine) in muscle. The total choline resonance is affected by changes in the metabolism of membrane phospholipids. It is often found to be present in high concentraions in tumor cells, where there is rapid cell turnover. An in vivo study of Duchenne muscular dystrophy (DMD) soleus muscle tissue, however, demonstrated a lower concentration than in controls. A reduction in the total creatine pool is associated with abnormal membrane permeability, which was also observed in the same study. Seeing these finer details in vivo requires good water suppression, and distinguishing these signals in significantly fat-infiltrated muscle may be difficult.

Proton (^{1}H)-MRS can be used to quantify the fat concentration in muscle and measure the T2

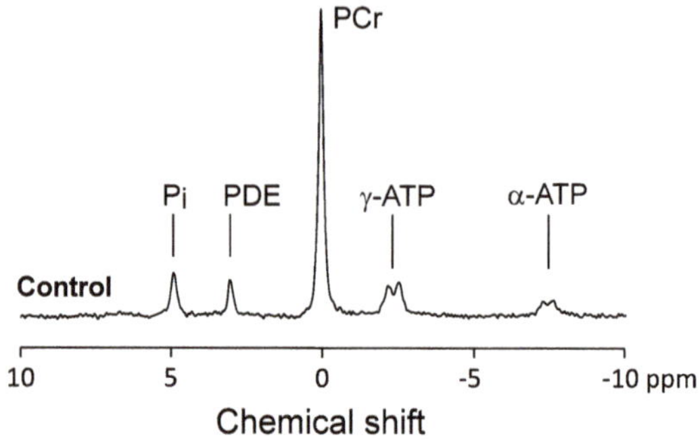

$$\text{ATP} \longrightarrow \text{ADP} + \text{P}_i + \text{Energy}$$

$$\text{PCr} + \text{ADP} \longleftrightarrow \text{ATP} + \text{Cr}$$

Fig. 5.2 A phosphorus spectrum from the gastrocnemius and soleus of a healthy control at 3.0 T. It shows the relative concentrations of inorganic phosphate (*Pi*), phosphodiesters (*PDE*), phosphocreatine (*PCr*) and adenosine triphosphate (*ATP*). The equations underneath show the relations between these metabolites when energy is released from ATP to form ADP and P_i. The concentration of ADP is too low to be perceived in the spectrum. ATP concentrations are buffered by transfer of a phosphate group from PCr to ADP, as indicated

relaxation times of water and fat in the selected voxel (see Sect. 5.6). Generally, researchers have preferred to use cross-sectional imaging for these purposes, where region of interest (ROI) analysis can be used to derive fat concentrations and T2 values from image-defined, whole-muscle regions of interest, although the drawing of the regions is rather labor-intensive.

5.2.2 Phosphorus-31 Magnetic Resonance Spectroscopy

Figure 5.2 shows a phosphorus spectrum acquired from the gastrocnemius and soleus muscles of a healthy subject. The dominant resonance is that of phosphocreatine (PCr) at 0 ppm and adenosine triphosphate (ATP) represented by the three high-energy phosphate groups (γ, α, β) at −2.4, −7.6, and −16.0 ppm respectively. At 4.8 ppm, the inorganic phosphates (labeled Pi) are represented, with the phosphodiester (PDE) group at 2.9 ppm. This group includes catabolic products such as glycerophosphocholine (GPC) and glycerophosphoethanolamine (GPE). Because these latter resonances would be expected to increase with active muscle degradation, they are of particular interest in neuromuscular disease. At 6.9 ppm are the phosphomonoesters (PME), which are usually present at low concentration in healthy muscle. They include phosphocholine, phosphoethanolamine, and the glycolysis intermediate glucose-6-phosphate, which is difficult to detect under normal metabolic conditions because of its relatively low concentration. Because the chemical shift of the Pi peak is dependent on pH but that of PCr is not, the difference in chemical shift between these resonances can be used to estimate tissue pH. Although absolute quantification of spectra is possible by reference to external calibrated standards, most research studies either quote metabolite ratios or assume the concentration of ATP to be 8.2 mM. Phosphorus spectra can be collected at rest. Alternatively, by designing exercise devices that fit in the scanner and keep the muscle of interest in the center of the MRI system, we can study phosphorus metabolites during exercise and recovery with a time resolution of seconds (Fig. 5.3). This allows us to probe pH handling and maximal mitochondrial function.

^{31}P-MRS of skeletal muscle at rest has been performed for a number of neuromuscular diseases, including Duchenne (DMD), Becker (BMD), limb girdle (LGMD), and fascioscapulohumeral (FSHD) muscular dystrophies. The patterns of findings have been similar, although the pattern is the most markedly abnormal in DMD, with increased concentrations of PDE and Pi and reduced PCr. The abnormalities increase with increasing age of DMD boys. Abnormalities have been found to be less marked in conditions other than DMD. In a mixed group of LGMD patients, impaired PCr concentration and elevated pH were associated with the degree of fat replacement in muscles. In FSHD, the same metabolic alterations have been found to be associated with fat replacement.

The data concerning exercising conditions are limited. There is evidence, however, that the rate of recovery of phosphocreatine after exercise (a surrogate for maximal mitochondrial ATP generation) is normal in the muscular dystrophies but that pH handling may be affected, with reduced acidosis during exercise suggesting defective glycolytic activity, as shown in BMD patients. Such measurements can be used to determine whether

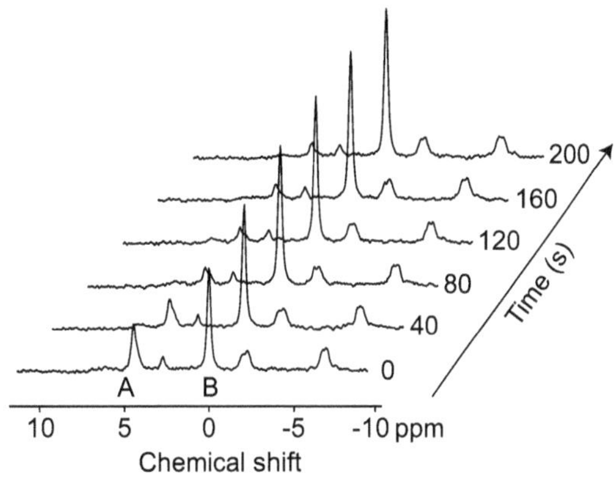

Fig. 5.3 Selection of phosphorus spectra acquired from the gastrocnemius and soleus of an LGMD-2I patient at 3.0 T during recovery from a plantar flexion exercise. The decreasing concentration of inorganic phosphate (*A*) and replenishment of phosphocreatine (*B*) can be measured. The rate of recovery of the phosphocreatine acts as a surrogate measure for maximal mitochondrial function

such a deficit is consistent with reduced glucose availability rather than a defect of glycogenolysis. This aspect of analysis can also be used to quantify the absence of glycolytic ATP formation in phosphofructokinase deficiency, where PME levels rise sharply on commencing exercise but pH does not decline and where there is no independent evidence of mitochondrial dysfunction. By contrast the reduced oxidative function found in polymyositis and dermatomyositis, combined with reduced proton efflux rates, might be evidence of an impaired blood supply.

In summary, phosphorus spectroscopy allows scientific questions about muscle energetics to be answered. Because of the specialized hardware involved, ^{31}P-MRS is not as widely used as ^{1}H-MRS. To date, no longitudinal studies have proved its value as a longitudinal outcome measure in clinical trials. Other than DMD, studies of the muscular dystrophies do not yet suggest that ^{31}P-MRS provides early evidence for muscle degradation before the appearance of increases in T2 relaxation times.

5.2.3 Carbon-13 Magnetic Resonance Spectroscopy

When abnormal glycogen storage is suspected, it is possible to quantify it with carbon-13

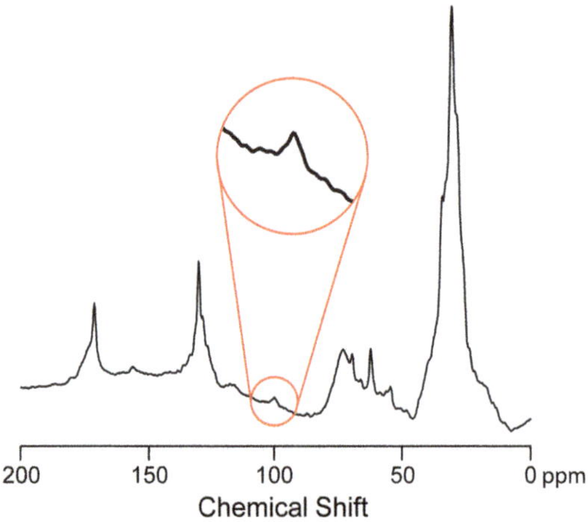

Fig. 5.4 Carbon-13 spectrum from a posterior lower leg muscle of a control subject at 3.0 T. The inset highlights the principal glycogen resonance. Courtesy of Dr. P.E. Thelwall, Newcastle University

(^{13}C)-MRS. However, the signal-to-noise ratio (SNR) for endogenous glycogen is low, even at magnetic field strengths of 3 or 4 T (Fig. 5.4). The hardware required is specialized, and patient safety considerations regarding radiofrequency heating must be taken into account. As no vendor has met these requirements in a standard package, such measurements remain firmly in specialized research centers. The technique has been applied to measure excess glycogen in glycogenosis type III disorder alongside phosphorus measurements of reduced mitochondrial function. The researchers were able to gain further insight into this dysfunction by simultaneous measurements of impaired muscle perfusion by magnetic resonance, a technique we consider in Sect. 5.4.

Imaging Modalities: MR Spectroscopy

Key Points

- ^{1}H-MRS can measure the concentration of water and fat in skeletal muscle within a defined region of tissue.
- ^{31}P-MRS can measure the concentrations of key energy metabolites in skeletal muscle including ATP, PCr, and Pi, as well as tissue pH.
- Several metabolites can be quantified at rest or during an exercise intervention.
- The rate of PCr regeneration after recovery from an exercise period is a surrogate marker for maximal mitochondrial function.
- ^{13}C-MRS can be used to quantify muscle glycogen content, but it remains technically challenging.

5.3 Sodium (^{23}Na) Magnetic Resonance Imaging

The principle of conventional MRI is based on proton (^{1}H) signals from water and lipid compounds. ^{23}Na-MRI is an innovative technique that offers the possibility of detecting sodium ions (Na^+) in vivo. In a healthy muscle cell, Na/K-ATPase moves Na^+ out of the cytoplasm and K^+ into the cytoplasm with a stoichiometry of 3:2—thus helping to maintain a constant membrane potential and a Na^+ concentration gradient. In healthy tissue, the extracellular Na^+ concentration ($[Na^+]_{ex}$) of 145 mM is about 10-fold higher than the intracellular concentration ($[Na^+]_{in}$) of 10–15 mM. ^{23}Na-MRI allows noninvasive volume- and relaxation-weighted measurements of these Na^+ compartments.

The membrane potential is necessary to allow contraction of muscle cells. Muscular Na^+ channels within the cell membrane auxiliary control Na^+ homeostasis. In muscle channelopathies (see Chap. 13), patients are affected by incomplete inactivation of these muscular Na^+ channels. The resulting Na^+ leak leads to an inward Na^+ current that causes ongoing depolarization of muscle fibers and an increased intracellular Na^+ concentration. This leads to an elevated total Na^+ concentration compared to that in healthy muscle tissue. ^{23}Na-MRI is able to measure noninvasively this pathological increase in the Na^+ concentration.

^{23}Na-MRI unfortunately poses several challenges. First, the physical nuclear magnetic resonance (NMR) sensitivity of ^{23}Na is only about 9 % of the sensitivity of ^{1}H for an equivalent number of nuclei. The 1,000- to 5,000-fold lower in vivo concentration compared to that of ^{1}H leads to an 11,000- 55,000-fold lower muscular ^{23}Na signal. Second, the ^{23}Na signal in vivo decays biexponentially, with a fast (0.5–3.0 ms) and a slow (15–30 ms) component. To measure the total ^{23}Na signal, sequences with ultra-short echo times are necessary. Specialized acquisition techniques, which combine both short echo times and high SNR efficiency are essential for quantitative ^{23}Na-MRI. As for phosphorus and carbon spectroscopy, specific nonstandard scanner hardware is needed (e.g., radiofrequency coils that are able to work with the resonance frequencies of sodium nuclei and protons). Third, the amount of intracellular Na^+ (responsible for the muscle membrane potential) is about 10 times lower than the extracellular amount of Na^+. This complicates the noninvasive quantification of intracellular Na^+. It is a further challenge to discriminate between intra- and extracellular sodium amount via noninvasive techniques such as MRI. Paramagnetic shift reagents allow a clear separation between intra- and extracellular sodium in preclinical models. Unfortunately, they cannot be applied in humans because of their toxicity.

Current research in ^{23}Na-MRI has demonstrated the possibility of reducing the signal from extracellular sodium compartments such as vasogenic edema. A ^{23}Na inversion recovery (IR) sequence (TE/TR 0.3/124 ms, inversion time 34 ms, voxel size $6\times6\times6$ mm^3, acquisition time 10 min) based on a three-dimensional radial sequence was developed to reduce the ^{23}Na signal emitted by free Na^+ (e.g., from cerebrospinal fluid or vasogenic edema as well as the ^{23}Na signal received from the extracellular space) to achieve a weighting toward the intracellular ^{23}Na amount. The 3-Tesla ^{23}Na-MRI protocol used at the German Cancer Research Center Heidelberg currently includes two special ^{23}Na pulse sequences with an ultra-short echo time of < 0.5 ms to minimize T2*-weighting because the ^{23}Na T2* signal decays biexponentially with a fast component ($T2^*_{fast}$) of 0.5–3.0 ms. With spin density image contrast (TE/TR 0.3/100 ms, flip angle 90°, voxel size $5\times5\times5$ mm^3, acquisition time 8 min 20 s), a volume-weighted average of the intracellular and extracellular Na^+ concentrations is measured. As the extracellular Na^+ concentration at 140 mM is 10-fold higher than that of the intracellular Na^+ concentration at 10–15 mM, the analysis of intracellular ^{23}Na is limited when using the aforementioned sequence. Thus, the ^{23}Na inversion recovery (IR) sequence in each patient is used to suppress the ^{23}Na signal emitted by extracellular edema and vessels. Although the IR-prepared Na^+ measurement enables weighting of the measurement toward intracellular ^{23}Na, it would still have a significant contribution from the extracellular pool, and it does not provide a clear separation between intracellular and extracellular ^{23}Na.

^{23}Na MRI is effectively of value in the radiological management of muscular Na^+ channel diseases (see Chap. 13). Recently, the development of ^{23}Na-MRI at higher magnetic field strengths of 3–7 T permits greater SNR efficiency and maybe more precise quantification of intracellular ^{23}Na homeostasis in healthy volunteers and in patients (see Fig. 5.5a–d). The potential of ^{23}Na MRI at 7 T can be expected to generate a high level of acceptance for this new technique in the near future.

Imaging Modalities: Sodium ^{23}Na-MRI

Key Points

- Sodium ^{23}Na-MRI is an innovative technique that offers the possibility of detecting sodium ions (Na^+) in vivo.
- To measure the total ^{23}Na signal in muscle tissue, sequences with ultra-short echo times (< 0.5 ms) are necessary.
- The ^{23}Na inversion recovery sequence achieves a weighting toward the intracellular ^{23}Na amount in muscle tissue.
- ^{23}Na-MRI has effectively achieved value in the radiological management of muscular Na^+ channel diseases (paramyotonia congenita, hyperkalemic periodic paralysis, hypokalemic periodic paralysis) and most recently in DMD.

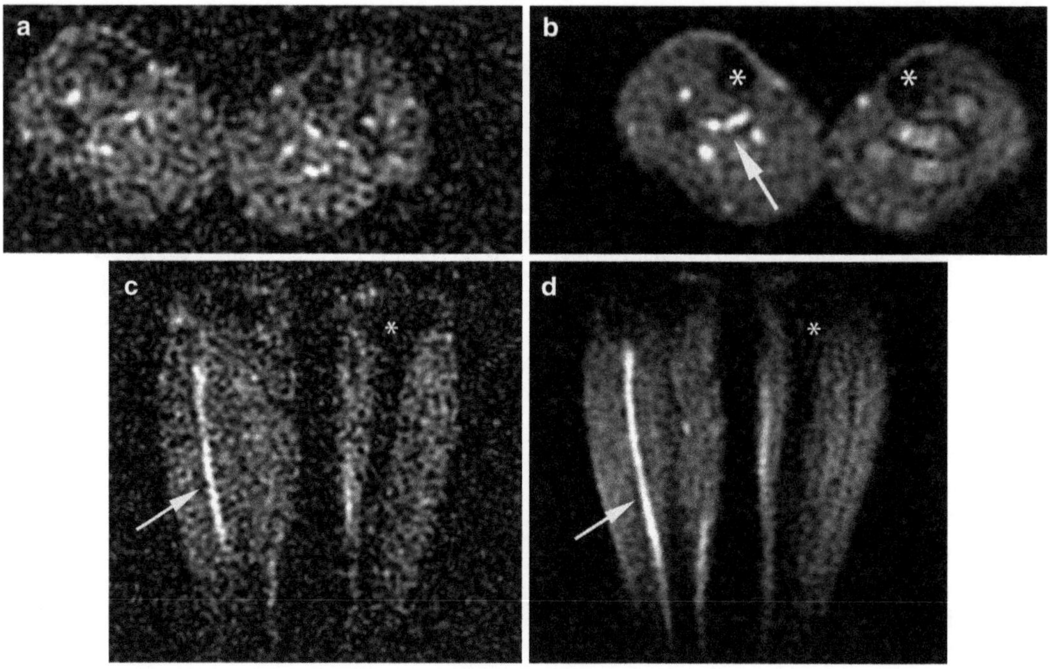

Fig. 5.5 Comparison of axial ^{23}Na-MRI scans of the lower legs of a healthy volunteer acquired with a 3-Tesla (T) (**a**) and a 7-T MRI system (**b**). Also shown are the corresponding coronal ^{23}Na-MRI scans acquired with 3-T (**c**) and 7-Tesla (**d**) MRI. *Asterisks* mark the tibial bones as structures with low signal intensity. *Arrows* point to vessels with high signal intensity. Clearly visible is the higher signal-to-noise ratio (SNR) at 7-T and the reduced background noise outside the lower legs. Courtesy of Armin Nagel, PhD, Department of Medical Physics in Radiology, German Cancer Research Center, Heidelberg

5.4 Diffusion- and Perfusion-Weighted Magnetic Resonance Imaging

MRI offers the possibility of making noninvasive measurements of (1) muscle perfusion and tissue level blood flow and (2) diffusion, the measurement of Brownian motion of water molecules within muscle cells to probe muscle structure and permeability. The use of these techniques in the brain is well established, but there are relatively few data using these techniques in skeletal muscle.

5.4.1 Magnetic Resonance Perfusion

Being able to measure blood flow at the tissue level can be valuable for distinguishing inflammatory processes (where we expect microvascular perfusion to increase) and degenerative processes. Blood flow in vessels can be measured by standard phase-contrast methods, but measuring perfusion at the tissue level requires a different approach. We need to be able to label a bolus of blood arriving at the volume of interest and determine how much of that blood reaches a given piece of tissue in a specified time, analogous to radioactive tracer methods. We can do it in two ways: (1) using a gadolinium contrast agent to label the blood and perform rapid T1-weighted imaging of the muscle concerned to measure the arrival of the blood, or (2) we can use magnetic labeling of the protons themselves as our tracer—arterial spin labeling (ASL)—thus avoiding the need for injection.

For method (1), a rapid series (at least every 3 s) of T1-weighted images are acquired at the muscle of interest before, during, and after administration of gadolinium contrast. As gadolinium circulates through the arteries, the signal intensity of the arteries increase (as the T1 relaxation time

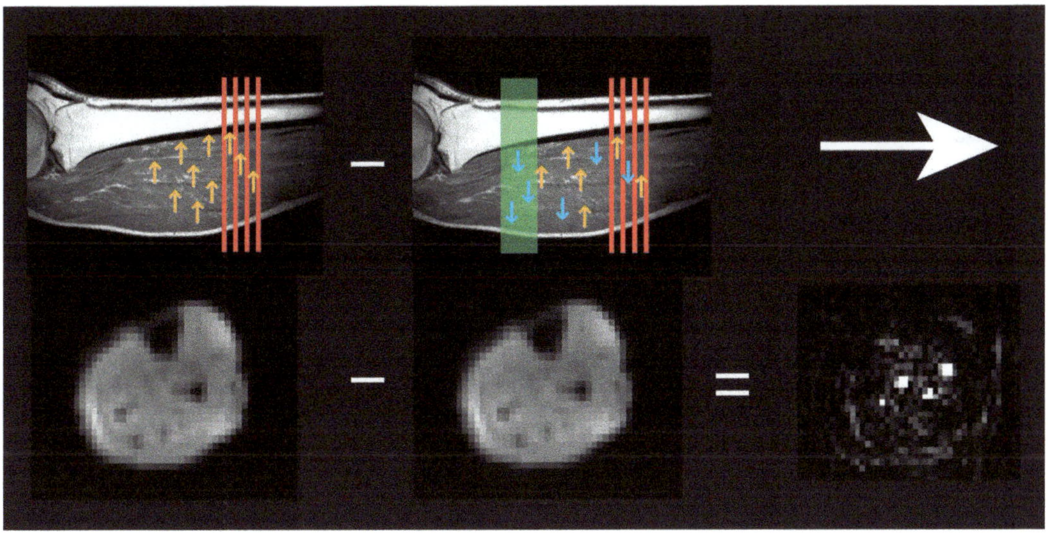

Fig. 5.6 Perfusion measurement sequence using endogenous contrast. In a control image (*left*) we measured the signal intensity with blood and tissue spins starting from equilibrium. Spins are inverted upstream of the desired imaging plane and we allow sufficient time for blood to travel to the imaging plane. Subtraction of the two images removes signal corresponding to stationary material, leaving a map with signal intensity representing blood flow. The example shown along the bottom is for a single acquisition of resting-state blood flow. The difference image (*bottom right*) has a low SNR, and many repetitions were needed. Courtesy of Dr J. He, Newcastle University

of the blood is reduced), followed by an increase in the signal intensity of the muscle as the gadolinium is distributed to the extracellular space. The initial rate of uptake (known as the "first pass") and hence of tissue perfusion can be estimated using a mathematical model that is well known from nuclear tracer studies. The accuracy of such measurements may be reduced when cell membranes are not impervious to gadolinium (e.g., muscular dystrophies) as gadolinium not only enters and leaves the extracellular space by perfusion but may also diffuse into the cell. The method has found the most use in peripheral arterial disease, where not only can perfusion be quantified from the first pass but the contrast material can be used to acquire an angiogram of the region.

For method (2), ASL, special pulse sequences are required. While there are many different types of perfusion pulse sequences, the basic principle is the same (Fig. 5.6). When attempting to measure blood flow at the tissue level, incoming blood is magnetically inverted, such that when it reaches the tissue level and an image is obtained the MR signal of the blood that has flowed into the tissue, but not the stationary tissue, is altered. Subtraction from an equivalent image where this preparation has not been performed yields the amount of blood from the inverted region that has passed into the imaging slice. We can then estimate the perfusion rate from these data.

The difference in signals so generated is small, typically about 0.5 2.0 %. Therefore, patient immobilization must be meticulous. It has proved possible, however, to make viable measurements of muscle perfusion in healthy subjects and in some subjects with impaired perfusion, including older healthy people and glycogenosis type III patients, where impaired perfusion responses suggested the limiting factor for impaired mitochondrial function. The perfusion technique is one of the more exciting that has not been widely exploited for neuromuscular disease. It can be combined with phosphorus spectroscopy to examine metabolic and blood flow responses to aerobic and ischemic exercise. Perfusion sequences have traditionally not been supplied with commercial scanners, although this situation is beginning to change and sequences suitable for brain perfusion are now being included.

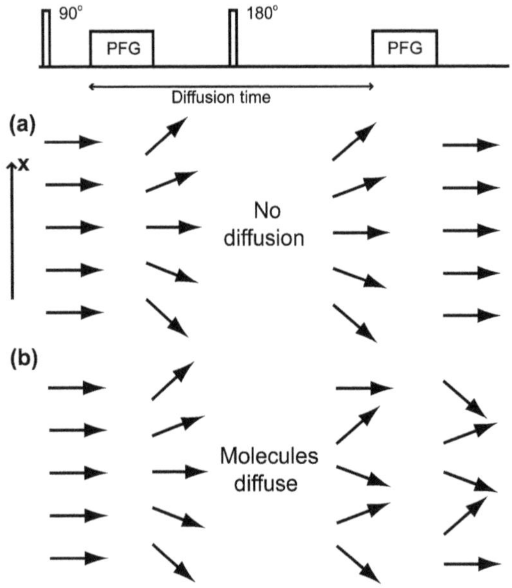

Fig. 5.7 A diffusion measurement experiment showing the pulse sequence at the top and the behavior of five water molecules (or spins) at different spatial positions. After excitation, all the spins are aligned with the same phase (*1st column*). After the pulsed field gradient (PFG) is applied, the spins have a phase angle proportional to their distance from the center (*2nd column*). (**a**) If no molecules move, the second PFG reverses the phase angles exactly. The spins added together produce a maximum signal (*4th column*). (**b**) In real life, the molecules undergo diffusion, taking their relative phase with them. The second PFG does not restore the original phase alignment, and when the spins are summed the signal is reduced in proportion to how far they have moved. *Note*: The effect of relaxation and the spin rotation induced by the 180° pulse is ignored in this figure

5.4.2 Magnetic Resonance Diffusion

Diffusion imaging of the muscle by magnetic resonance is the measurement of Brownian motion of water molecules in muscle tissue. Such measurements can be used to probe muscle cell structure indirectly below the resolution of a conventional MR image (~0.3 mm). Imagine a large glass of water placed in the MRI scanner. If we excite the magnetization, all the spins are initially aligned (Fig. 5.7). A field gradient applied causes spins to precess faster in proportion to their position along the direction of the gradient. When the gradient ceases, there is a phase difference proportional to the location. If no spins move and we apply the opposite gradient, all spins realign and we recover the full signal. However, during the time between the gradients—the diffusion time—individual spins move by Brownian motion. When the second gradient is applied, there is over- or under-compensation for the original phase offset, and the amplitude of the measured signal is reduced.

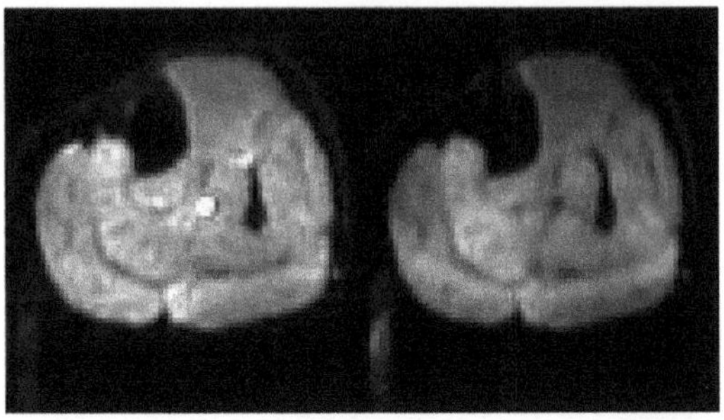

Fig. 5.8 Non diffusion-weighted (*left*) and diffusion-weighted (*right*) images of lower leg muscles in a control at 3.0 T showing fat suppression artifact below the muscle

With a large volume of fluid, few molecules are restrained by the sides of the container in which they reside. However, for a water molecule in the muscle cell, there are many obstructions to Brownian motion, including cell membranes and organelles. As the individual muscle cell has much greater length then breadth, the difference in intracellular diffusion properties caused by the constraints of the cell membranes can be detected. Muscle cells are also not impermeable to water; and with appropriate modeling, cell permeability may also be measured. The signal from extracellular water diffusing between the muscle structures is measured as well.

Diffusion measurements are potentially difficult to carry out in muscle. The diffusion sequence is based on fast echo-planar imaging, which limits the overall image quality and makes good fat saturation essential but difficult to achieve in skeletal muscle (Fig. 5.8). Standard vendor-supplied sequences use a spin echo sequence with a long echo time. Therefore, because the T2 relaxation time of muscle tissue is short (compared with that of brain), the SNR can be limiting.

Taken to its logical conclusion, this technique should be capable of quantifying muscle cell size, arrangement, and permeability. With gross muscle injury (i.e., a tear), we can determine any increases in the distance water is diffusing. In the inflammatory myopathies, inflammation is detectable as an increase in water diffusion. There have been sophisticated attempts to model both intracellular and extracellular water diffusion in a structure of packed muscle cells to try to explain the diffusion patterns found. One attempt fitted intracellular and extracellular contributions to the diffusion and quantified their relative contribution, showing that the intracellular component was dominant under the conditions used. However, such models rely on a number of assumptions and have not yet been successfully applied to models of pathological processes in neuromuscular disease. This area remains challenging. Another approach is to estimate muscle fiber directions by tracking the direction in which diffusion is least restricted from pixel to pixel. The utility of this measure in neuromuscular disease remains to be elucidated. There are few demonstrations of this technique in other neuromuscular diseases (e.g., muscular dystrophies). The twin difficulties of complex mathematical interpretation and fat infiltration mean that this technique is unlikely to find widespread clinical application in the foreseeable future.

Imaging Modalities: Diffusion- and Perfusion-Weighted MRI

Key Points

- Perfusion measurements in skeletal muscle at rest and during exercise are feasible.
- Using MR perfusion, valuable information about pathological change can be gained, particularly when combined with the assessment of muscle energetics using phosphorus spectroscopy.
- Diffusion measurements make the intensity of the MR signal sensitive to the Brownian motion of water in tissue.
- Although diffusion measurements can provide information about muscle cell integrity and altered muscle structure and permeability, the detailed interpretation of these measures remains complex and challenging.

5.5 Three-Point Dixon Technique for Intramuscular Fat Quantification

Although T1-weighted images provide rapid visualization of fat infiltration and replacement in skeletal muscle, it is extremely difficult to quantify the fat content in a robust way. In clinical treatment trials, where we may be looking for small changes during the course of muscle degradation, the use of broad qualitative grades and semi-quantitative rating scales are unlikely to be sensitive enough. The problem of quantification arises because, unlike CT, the signal intensity in an MRI scan is not absolute, being affected by imperfections. Notably, the amount of radiofrequency power (B_1) delivered to all parts of the tissue is not equal, effectively delivering different flip angles to different areas and causing different signal intensities. Figure 5.9 shows the changes in intensity in fat and muscle tissues of a healthy subject. Such inhomogeneities are dependent not only on the original anatomy of the patient but the individual magnet used and the positioning of the patient within it. In a multi-center trial, it would clearly be difficult to control all of these parameters at all centers.

The three-point Dixon technique provides an alternative method for quantitative assessment of fatty degeneration. As observed in Sect. 5.2, dealing with magnetic resonance spectroscopy, there is a frequency difference between the water resonance and the CH_2 resonance of fat. In a spoiled gradient echo scan this means that, like two cars going round

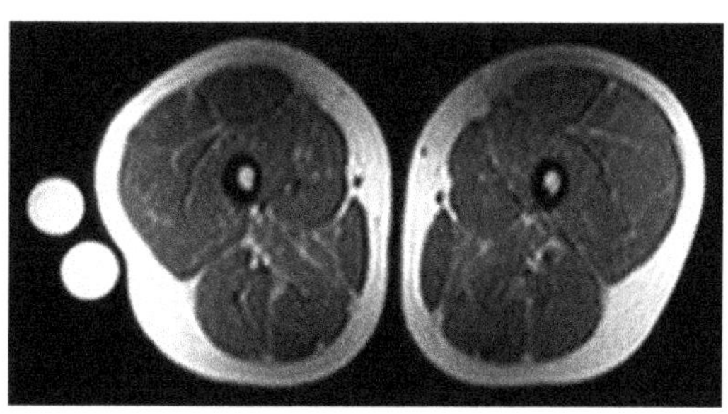

Fig. 5.9 B_1 inhomogeneity of T1-weighted imaging of thigh muscles. This is a typically inhomogeneous area at 3.0 T. Note that the signal intensity at the anterior (near the rectus femoris) for both muscle and fat is lower than at the outer edge of the image, making quantification challenging

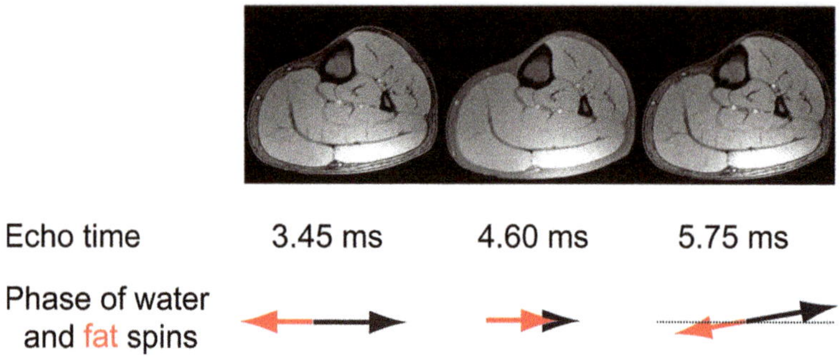

Fig. 5.10 Three-point Dixon acquisition, showing how the echo time influences the relative phase of the water and fat protons (spins). These are lower-leg images acquired at 3.0 T. At the time of the first echo, water and fat are out of phase, and voxels containing water and fat suffer subtraction of signal (see muscle–fat boundaries). At twice the first echo time, they are in phase (*middle image*), and at the third they are out of phase. If there are no B_0 inhomogeneities, the phases of the first and third scans are identical; otherwise, the phase offset allows a phase map to be constructed and allowed for when calculating the fat percentage

a racetrack at slightly different speeds, there is an echo time during which the signals from fat and water are 180° out of phase (analogous to the time when the cars are on the opposite sides of the track. By doubling that time, we can bring the two signals back in phase (Fig. 5.10). In principle, therefore, we can calculate the fat and water content of an image by subtracting the pair of images and adding them to produce images of the fat components and water components, respectively. Such a calculation would be "two-point" Dixon calculation ("in-phase and out-of-phase imaging") as two echo times are used.

How does this help accurate quantification? The water and fat images that have been produced still contain B_1 inhomogeneity. Provided that we have used a sufficiently long TR and low flip angle to make sure there is no T1 weighting, however, the inhomogeneity profile is the same in both images. Therefore, we can cancel it by calculating the percentage of separated fat signal over the total signal. The image produced is then independent of the B_1 profile experienced.

Why use three points instead of two? The frequency separation of water and fat depends on the local main magnetic field (B_0), which is not homogeneous within a patient, between patients, or indeed for the same patient repositioned within the scanner for a follow-up scan. By acquiring a third echo, we can correct for the variation in B_0 across the subject, making our final fat percentage map truly independent of specific placement, the magnet, and B_1 inhomogeneity. By drawing an ROI on the muscle of choice, we can evaluate the percentage of the signal due to fat in that muscle. We can compare this measurement robustly among patients, longitudinally, and among centers. The separation of water and fat highlights early fat infiltration more strikingly than conventional T1-weighted imaging, where healthy muscle is mid-intensity. It also permits detailed discrimination of fat infiltration patterns (Fig. 5.11).

Is this truly a fat percentage? It is the percentage of fat in the MRI visible signal, certainly. Certain components of tissue (e.g., macromolecules) are not visible by MRI due to short T2 relaxation times and are thus not counted. The three-point Dixon technique provides a fast, robust method for tracking longitudinal change. With careful repositioning of anatomy between scans, reproducibility coefficients of < 0.5 % can be achieved. This method was first applied to a cross-sectional study of DMD and has recently been used in studies of oculopharyngeal muscular dystrophy. Notably, the first longitudinal study of LGMD-2I to examine the progression of individual muscle groups using the three-point Dixon technique found that increases in fat fraction could be sensitively detected in nine muscle groups (Fig. 5.12). With the increasing activity in therapy trials moving to clinical practice for DMD or the inherited neuromuscular dieases in general, it seems likely that this modality will be adopted.

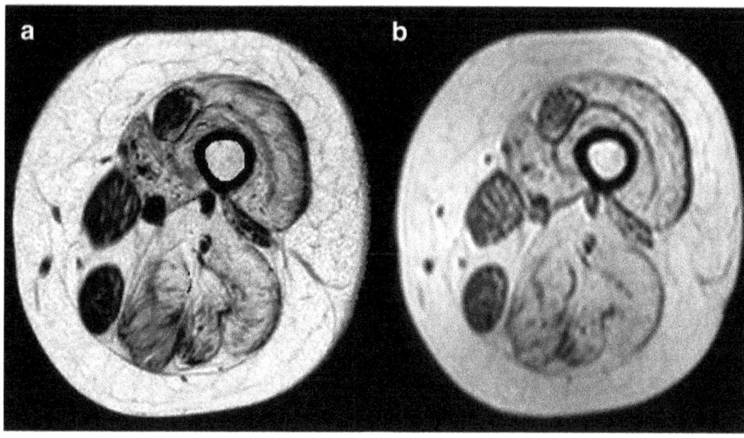

Fig. 5.11 Comparison of (**a**) three-point Dixon technique and (**b**) T1-weighted images of the mid-thigh of an LGMD-2I patient at 3.0 T. Not only does the three-point Dixon method offer a quantitative image free from inhomogeneities, the complete separation of water and fat makes more obvious the pattern of fat infiltration and the early involvement of the gracilis and sartorius muscles

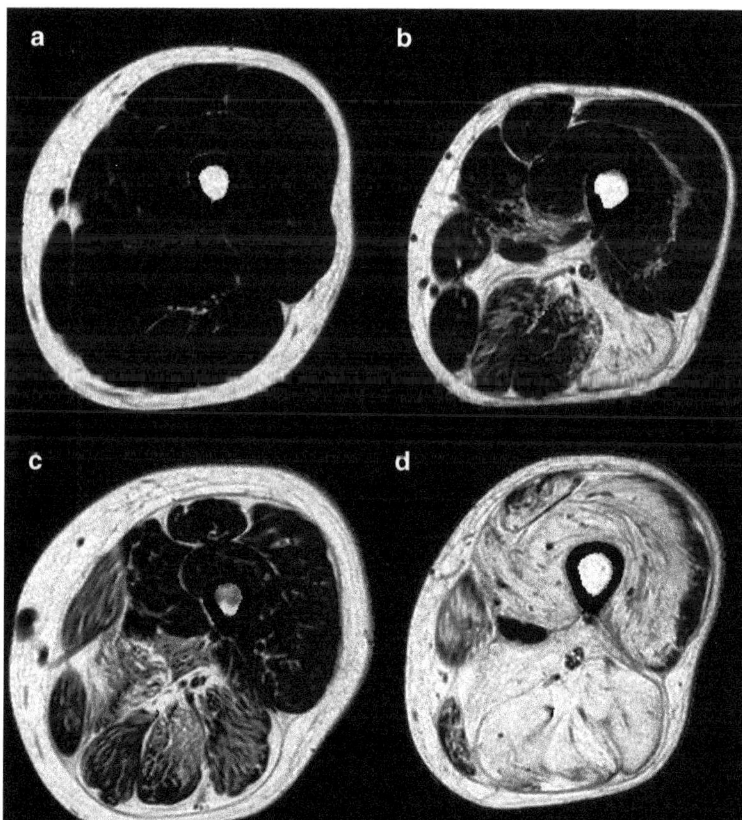

Fig. 5.12 Quantitative fat percentage images from a three-point Dixon acquisition from the mid-thigh at 3.0 T for (**a**) a healthy control and (**b–d**) LGMD-2I patients with differing degrees of fat infiltration

The three-point Dixon and related sequences are becoming more widely available on commercial MRI scanners, with two of the three major vendors (Philips Medical Systems and General Electric) supporting full implementation at the time of this writing. A two-point Dixon method is available on Siemens MR systems. Various refinements are available, such as recognition that the fat resonance is not a single peak but, rather, consists of multiple peaks. This refinement adds accuracy to the measurement but is not yet widely available commercially. It is also not necessary to adopt purely in-phase and out-of-phase echo times, and the related iterative decomposition of water and fat with echo asymmetry and least-squares estimation (IDEAL) sequence uses echo times that put the fat and water signals at three different angles to each other: There are advantages in the distribution of noise for tissues with 50 % fat infiltration (where one of the Dixon images would be completely nulled), but the principle remains the same.

The increasing availability of these sequences and their utility in performing longitudinal comparison studies in multi-center settings mean that the use of three-point Dixon sequences to evaluate neuromuscular diseases is likely to increase markedly.

Imaging Modalities: 3-Point Dixon for Intramuscular Fat Quantification

Key Points

- Standard T1-weighted imaging is good for qualitative analysis, but it is difficult to use for quantitative analyses.
- Three-point Dixon methods can eliminate the effects of inhomogeneity in both the main magnetic field (B_0) and the applied radiofrequency pulses (B_1). This means that we can produce images showing the percentage of fat in the muscle, which can be compared in longitudinal studies and among centers.
- Several implementations of the three-point Dixon method exist—including such variations as IDEAL—that are increasingly available on commercial MRI scanners.
- Because fat has a shorter T1 relaxation time than water, it is essential that the images be acquired without T1 weighting (long TR, low flip angle) to obtain accurate data.
- The fat percentage produced is a percentage of fat in the visible MRI signal (i.e., macromolecules that are MRI-invisible are not accounted for).
- Fat percentages calculated from the three-point Dixon method are highly reproducible within and among centers with careful patient positioning.

5.6 T1 and T2 Relaxation Time Measurements

Measurement of the T2 relaxation time of water is an attractive endpoint in muscular dystrophy studies because it is affected by early changes in muscle integrity, before fat infiltration begins. The T2 relaxation time of water is physically a measure of how fast coherence of phase between spins is lost. Physiologically, the T2 relaxation time of a muscle increases if there is a greater proportion of free fluid present. This situation occurs with damage due to exercise and edema. It is also a well-known characteristic of many neuromuscular diseases, often preceding structural degenerative neuromuscular changes, such as fatty degeneration.

The simplest way to measure T2 relaxation times is by ^{1}H-MRS (Fig. 5.13, see also Sect. 5.2). By acquiring spectra at multiple echo times from a defined volume of muscle and fitting the area under the curve, the T2 component of water can be speedily calculated. Such an approach has been taken in preclinical models of LGMD and DMD. In these diseases, MR spectroscopy was used to determine that the reintroduction of the γsg gene

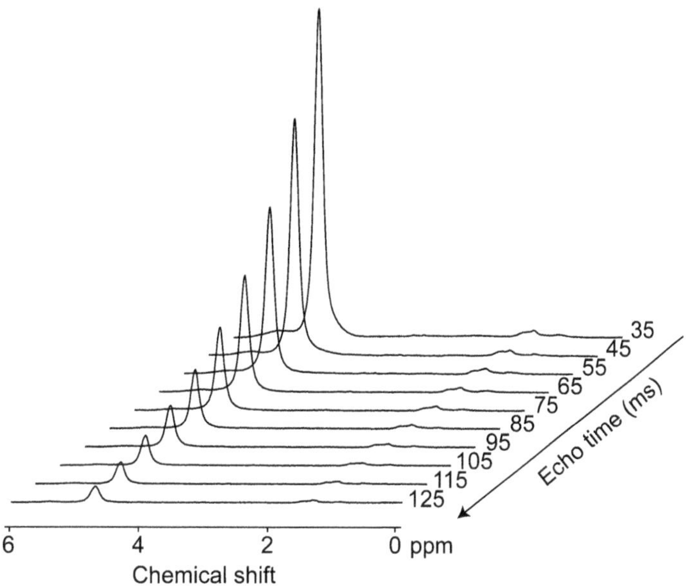

Fig. 5.13 T2 relaxation time in healthy tibialis anterior muscle as measured by proton spectroscopy at 3.0 T. The spectra were acquired at 10 echo times from 35 to 125 ms. The water resonance is dominant on the left, with a small fat resonance clearly separated on the right. The T2 relaxation time of the water is 29 ms in this instance

into γsg–/– mice could reduce the number of voxels with enhanced T2 relaxation time.

However, most clinicians and investigators prefer to measure T2 relaxation times from a defined ROI on an image of skeletal muscle. Although every commercial MR system has an imaging sequence that can produce data to plot a curve of T2 decay, few are truly quantitative, and still fewer could be accurately compared in a multi-center trial. Why is this true, and can it be overcome?

First, most commercial sequences are designed to indicate only T2-weighted contrast (mid-intensity muscle, bright fat, bright edema). A gold standard measurement of T2 relaxation time requires accurate delivery of a 90° excitation pulse followed by 180° refocusing pulses to produce the echoes. Not only must we contend with radiofrequency inhomogeneity affecting the size of the flip angles but the slice selective refocusing pulses tend not to deliver a full 180° pulse across the slice.

Second, the presence of fat infiltration presents issues for T2 relaxation time measurements—unlike spectroscopic methods—as the signals measured become composite measures of water T2 and fat T2. Therefore, if the concentration of fat increases in a muscle between two measurements, the apparent T2 relaxation time increases even if the T2 relaxation time of water in the muscle does not increase. Although this is not important for some diseases and disease models (such as the *mdx* mouse, where fat accumulation occurs late in the disease course), it is of great practical concern in human studies (Fig. 5.14). Fat saturation studies do not provide the answer because the efficiency of the saturation is not uniform across the image (Fig. 5.15).

Is spectroscopy our only robust way of measuring muscle T2 relaxation time, free from the confounding influence of fat? The answer is "no." Recently, water/fat separation using IDEAL (see Sect. 5.5) has been incorporated within the multi-echo turbo spin echo sequence required to produce T2 measurements. This delivers separate images from which the T2 of water and fat can be separately deduced. The sequence provides coverage of eight sections during a 10 min scan time. Simultaneous measurement of fat and T2 relaxation time was demonstrated in a patient with inclusion body myositis (Fig. 5.16). The implementation of such a sequence by commercial vendors (not presently available) would be of immense value to longitudinal research on determining the interplay between changes in T2 and changes in fat infiltration in neuromuscular disorders.

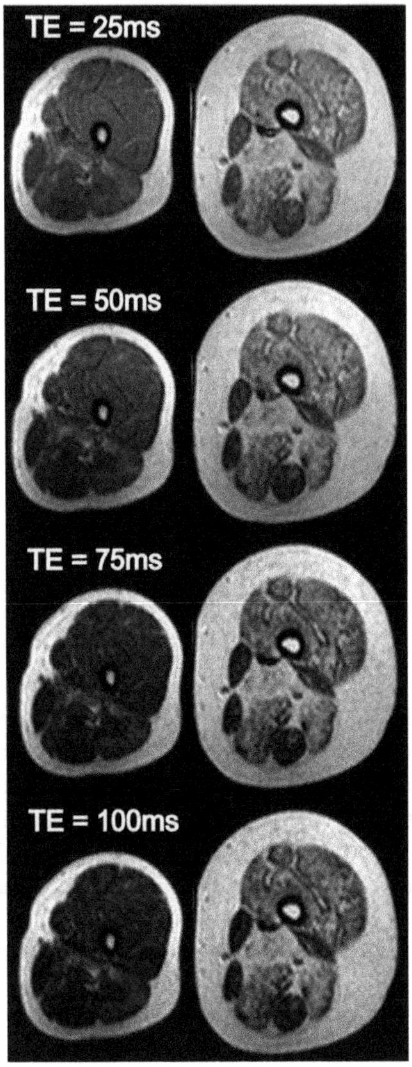

Fig. 5.14 T2 measurement performed by imaging mid-thigh muscles at 3.0 T without fat saturation in two individuals with Duchenne muscular dystrophy (DMD). One had moderate fat infiltration (*left*), and the other had substantial fat infiltration (*right*). Images at four echo times are shown. Note the relatively slow T2 decay of the fat-infiltrated muscles (vastus lateralis) on the right compared to noninfiltrated muscles (gracilis, sartorius). Measured T2 values are as follows: gracilis 47 ms (*left*) and 68 ms (*right*); vastus lateralis 47 ms (*left*) and 86 ms (*right*); rectus femoris 60 ms (*left*) and 73 ms (*right*)

T1 relaxation time measurements in neuromuscular diseases are used less frequently. During the early course of DMD, muscle T1 rises because of degeneration and increased water in muscle. However, with increasing fat infiltration, the overall T1 relaxation time falls, the T1 of fat being much shorter than that of muscle water. The fat infiltration can be measured more simply and accurately by three-point Dixon imaging (see Sect. 5.5). In addition, although muscle T1 can increase with membrane damage similarly to T2, the relative degree of change is less. Also, T1 measurement sequences are typically longer than those for T2. The difference in the T1 relaxation times of fat and water is exploited qualitatively with STIR imaging to eliminate the fat signal from T2-weighted images. However, it is difficult to fully quantify such measurements, and they are less useful for longitudinal studies.

Imaging Modalities: T1 and T2 Relaxation Time Measurements

Key Points

- T2 relaxation time measurements are useful endpoints for neuromuscular disease as increased T2 is indicative of edema and structural muscle damage, which alters the local free water distribution.
- T2 relaxation times in a specific muscle region can be measured by ^{1}H-MRS, resolving the water and fat components.
- Most vendors provide T2-weighted sequences to produce T2 relaxation curves, but they may not be fully quantitative without modification.
- Fat infiltration can confound T2 measurements, and robust fat suppression is difficult to achieve.
- T2 relaxation time measurements can also be indicative of muscle damage but are rarely performed because there are easier methods for determining fat infiltration.

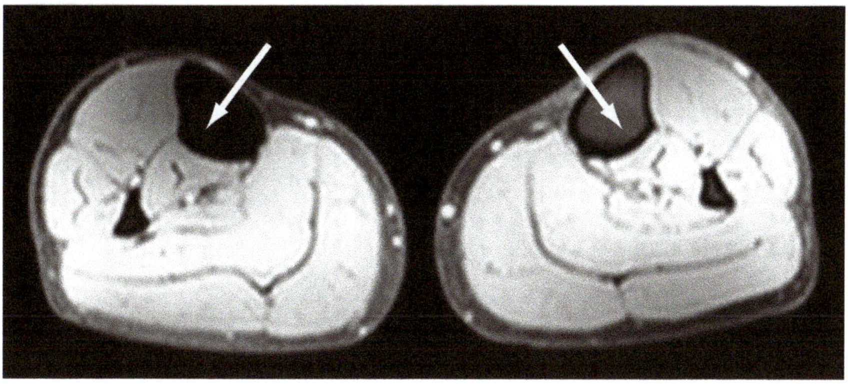

Fig. 5.15 Image from a T2 measurement performed in a healthy subject with fat saturation at 3.0 T. Note the gross inhomogeneity of fat saturation in the lower leg. There is clear asymmetrical intensity of the bone marrow (*arrows*) and tibialis anterior. This is an extreme case, but the inability to predict the uniformity of fat saturation makes quantification of T2 relaxation times difficult

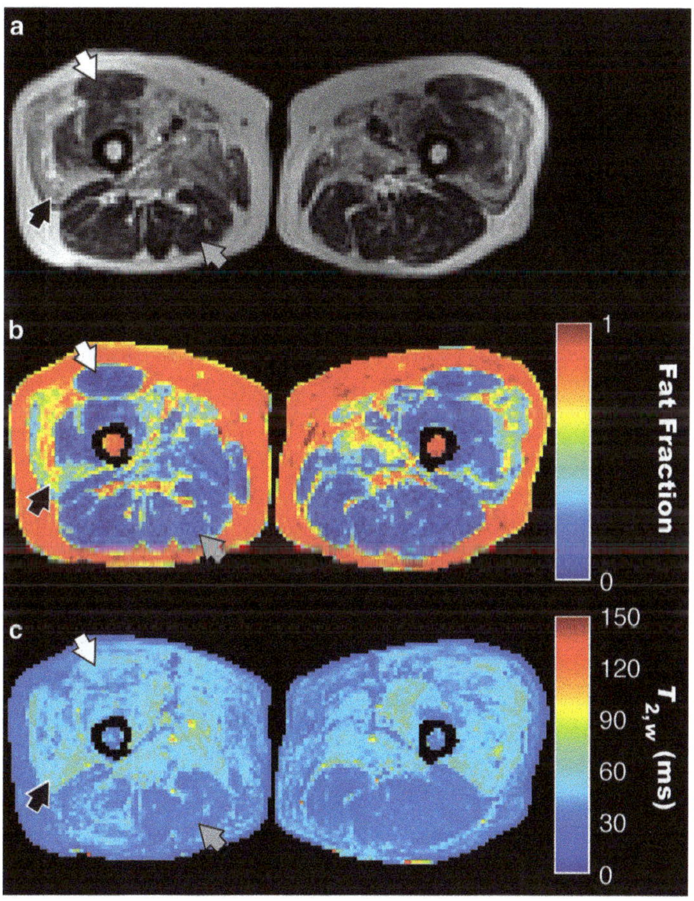

Fig. 5.16 IDEAL-CPMG imaging results from a 61-year-old patient with inclusion body myositis. T2-weighted image at TE = 80 ms (**a**) corresponds to the T2-corrected fat fraction map (**b**) and the T2 map of the water component $T2_w$ (**c**). *White*, *black*, and *gray arrows* indicate the rectus femoris, vastus lateralis, and semimembranosus, respectively. A large variation in inflammation and fat infiltration can be seen between the different muscle groups, and the presence of one does not imply the presence of the other. A fat/water swap artifact can be seen at the base of the legs near the air interface caused by a large field-inhomogeneity gradient. Courtesy of Dr. R.L. Janiczek, UCL. From Janiczek RL, et al (2011) Simultaneous T2 and lipid quantitation using IDEAL CPMG. Magn Reson Med 66:1293–1302. Reprinted with permission from John Wiley and Sons

5.7 Experimental Contrast-Enhanced Magnetic Resonance Imaging

This section discusses the off-label use of clinical contrast agents and the use of experimental preclinical contrast agents in research. The availability of such agents for clinical or research use varies by jurisdiction and over time. The reader must establish their local legal framework for the use of contrast agents in clinical practice and for research.

There are various properties of the MR signal that can be used to quantify fat infiltration noninvasively, such as detecting edema by recording the changes in T2 relaxation times. These properties are indirect indicators, however, and we would ideally use an MR biomarker that reflects microstructural changes, such as those at the sarcolemmal level. We need an agent that alters the MR signal intensity according to our chosen measure of muscle degradation—hence, contrast agents. Most MR contrast agents are based on the paramagnetic ion gadolinium (Gd), which decreases the T1 relaxation time of surrounding water protons. Within a defined concentration range, the change in the reciprocal of this relaxation time (1/T1) is linearly proportional to the concentration of contrast agent present, allowing some degree of quantification of the contrast agent concentration in the tissue by imaging with appropriate T1-weighted sequences.

Common low-molecular-weight contrast agents (e.g., Gd-DTPA) show greater uptake in dystrophic muscle than in controls (Fig. 5.17), as shown in DMD. A study using the golden retriever muscular dystrophy model—a good model system for DMD—revealed increased uptake in dystrophic muscle (double that of control subjects), suggesting that this low-molecular-weight contrast agent may extravasate rapidly into dystrophic tissue. Determining whether the contrast agent

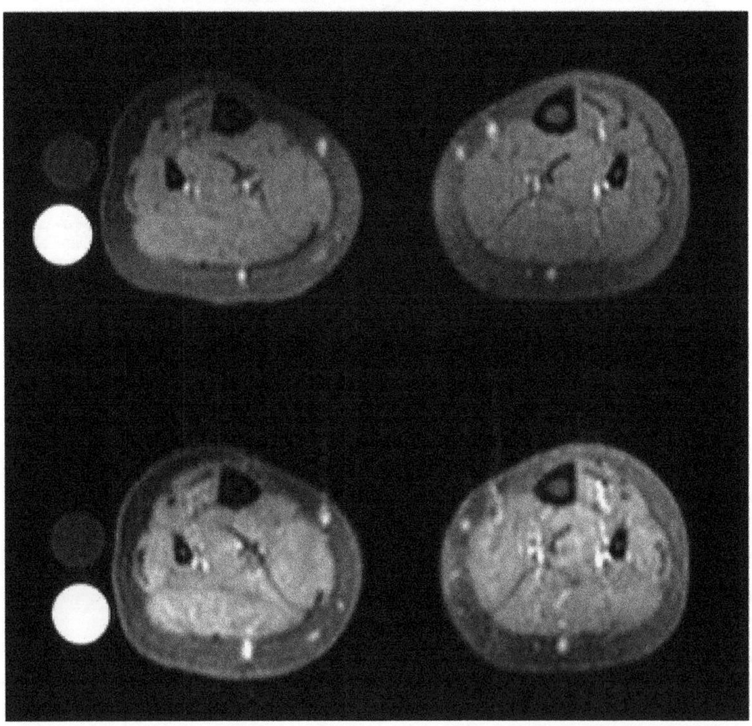

Fig. 5.17 T1-weighted images of the lower leg of a male child with DMD. They were acquired before (*top*) and 5 min after (*bottom*) administration of Gd-DTPA. Muscles show an average signal enhancement of 40 % (compared to 20 % in healthy adults)

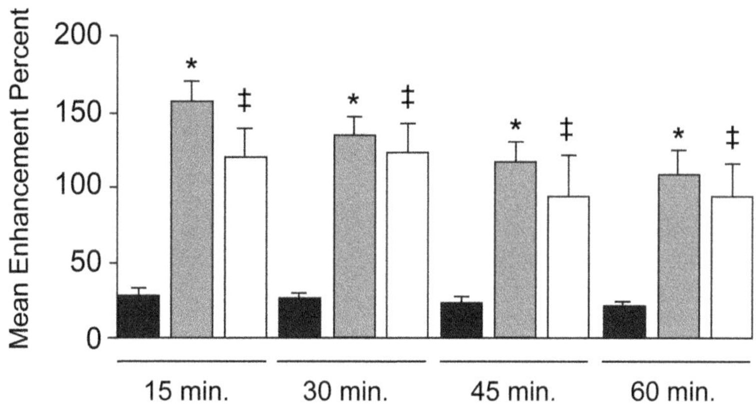

Fig. 5.18 The increase in signal enhancement in skeletal muscle lesions as a mean enhancement percent was calculated from the mean signals in a region of interest before and after intravenous injection of MS-325. The mean enhancement in *mdx* (*gray columns*) and *Sgca*-null (*white columns*) mice was significantly higher during all four analyzed time points compared to that of the control mice (*black columns*) (*$P<0.001$; ‡$P<0.017$). The signal enhancement in control mice was due to MS-325 in the vessels and reflected the long blood half-life of the contrast agent. Courtesy of Prof. V. Straub, Newcastle University. From Straub V, et al (2000) Contrast agent enhanced magnetic resonance imaging of skeletal muscle damage in animal models of muscular dystrophy. Magn Reson Med. 44:655–659. Reprinted with permission from John Wiley and Sons

enters the muscle cells and accumulates at areas of advanced fibrosis, inflammation, or clusters of damaged muscle fibers or merely accumulates in the extracellular space is not straightforward because of its fast clearance and the lack of an established assay for Gd-DTPA.

To circumvent these problems, we need more specific high molecular-weight contrast agents. The accumulation of serum albumin in damaged muscle fibers in dystrophic muscle has been well described. Recent work has concentrated on Gd-based contrast agents that (1) are directly bound to exogenous albumin or (2) interact strongly with endogenous albumin. In the first class, human albumin was bound to Gd-DTPA and was injected into wild-type and dystrophic *mdx* mice. Enhancement after 4 and 15 h was found only in skeletal muscle. Also, postmortem anti-human albumin antibody analysis showed intracellular accumulation of the contrast agent in clusters of damaged *mdx* muscle fibers. Thus, MR signal enhancement can illuminate the pattern of muscle damage. Such a long duration of residence in the body, however, is a problem for clinical use, where rapid clearance is preferred to avoid possible metabolism of the contrast agent and release of free Gd.

A second approach—the use of amphiphilic contrast agents that interact strongly with endogenous albumin—has been explored. Contrast agents such as gadofosveset trisodium (MS-325), also known as Vasovist™, have been developed for use as blood pool agents for the diagnosing vascular disease by magnetic resonance angiography. Transient binding to albumin lengthens the transit time of the agent, but greater relaxivity is also achieved by slowing the rotation of the gadolinium chelate, giving greater image contrast per unit agent. Signal enhancement in the *mdx* and *sgca*-null mouse models (for Duchenne and sarcoglycan-deficient LGMD, respectively) has been demonstrated to be greater than 100 % compared with 25 % for control mice, believed to result from contrast agent in small vessels (Fig. 5.18). This contrast agent was then used to demonstrate the effect of adenovirus-mediated gene transfer to restore expression of α-sarcoglycan in 3- or 4-day-old *sgca*-null mice (which could be sustained for 7 months). Significantly reduced enhancement (50 %) could be demonstrated with treatment and corresponded with the results obtained using Evans blue dye, a gold standard for probing sarcolemmal permeability.

In a preclinical study of dysferlin-deficient muscle, the contrast agent Gadofluorine M, an amphilic gadolinium complex that interacts with albumin and extracellular matrix proteins, was shown to cause differential enhancement of dysferlin-deficient muscle compared to wild-type muscle. The mechanism of contrast specificity again was thought to be albumin binding. Although it was shown that the contrast agent had entered the cell, the mode of entry could not be confirmed. There has been no further characterization of this agent in other dystrophy or neuromuscular disease models.

Other contrast agents may target necrotic tissue specifically. Porphyrin Gd agents have been identified, among others, as having value in identifying necrosis in acute myocardial infarction and liver tissues. However, there appear to be no studies of the value of this type of contrast agent in neuromuscular diseases.

Imaging Modalities: Experimental Contrast-Enhanced MRI

Key Points

- Contrast agents allow modification of tissue T1 relaxation times in regions the agents penetrate.
- Routine low-molecular-weight agents cause general signal enhancement in dystrophic muscle. The precise distribution of such agents within the dystrophic muscle is unclear.
- Contrast agents that are bound to albumin or interact with endogenous albumin have been shown in preclinical models to be specific for probing sarcolemmal permeability.

Suggestions for Further Reading

Allamand V, Donahue KM, Straub V, Davisson RL, Davidson BL, Campbell KP. Prevention of muscular dystrophy in alpha-sarcoglycan-deficient mice by early adenoviral-mediated gene transfer. Neuromuscul Disord. 2001;11:674.

Amthor H, Egelhof T, McKinnell I, et al. Albumin targeting of damaged muscle fibers in the mdx mouse can be monitored by MRI. Neuromuscul Disord. 2004;14:791–6.

Cea G, Bendahan D, Manners D, et al. Reduced oxidative phosphorylation and proton efflux suggest reduced capillary blood supply in skeletal muscle of patients with dermatomyositis and polymyositis: a quantitative P-31-magnetic resonance spectroscopy and MRI study. Brain. 2002;125:1635–45.

Chang G, Wang L, Schweitzer ME, Regatte RR. 3D ^{23}Na MRI of human skeletal muscle at 7 tesla: initial experience. Eur Radiol. 2010;20:2039–46.

Englund EK, Elder CP, Xu Q, Ding ZH, Damon BM. Combined diffusion and strain tensor MRI reveals a heterogeneous, planar pattern of strain development during isometric muscle contraction. Am J Physiol Regul Integr Comp Physiol. 2011;300:R1079–90.

Garrood P, Hollingsworth KG, Eagle M, et al. MR imaging in Duchenne muscular dystrophy: quantification of T-1-weighted signal, contrast uptake, and the effects of exercise. J Magn Reson Imaging. 2009;30:1130–8.

Gloor M, Fasler S, Fischmann A, et al. Quantification of fat infiltration in oculopharyngeal muscular dystrophy: comparison of three MR imaging methods. J Magn Reson Imaging. 2011;33:203–10.

Glover GH, Schneider E. Three-point Dixon technique for true water/fat decomposition with B_0 inhomogeneity correction. Magn Reson Med. 1991;18:371–83.

Grehl T, Muller K, Vorgerd M, Tegenthoff M, Malin JP, Zange J. Impaired aerobic glycolysis in muscle phosphofructokinase deficiency results in biphasic post-exercise phosphocreatine recovery in P-31 magnetic resonance spectroscopy. Neuromuscul Disord. 1998;8:480–8.

Hollingsworth KG, de Sousa PL, Straub V, Carlier PG. Towards harmonization of protocols for MRI outcome measures in skeletal muscle studies: consensus recommendations from two TREAT-NMD NMR workshops, 2 May 2010, Stockholm, Sweden, 1–2 October 2009, Paris, France. Neuromuscul Disord. 2012 Oct 1;22 Suppl 2:S54–67.

Hsieh TJ, Jaw TS, Chuang HY, Jong YJ, Liu GC, Li CW. Muscle metabolism in Duchenne muscular dystrophy assessed by in vivo proton magnetic resonance spectroscopy. J Comput Assist Tomogr. 2009;33:150–4.

Janiczek RL, Gambarota G, Sinclair CD, et al. Simultaneous T(2) and lipid quantitation using IDEAL-CPMG. Magn Reson Med. 2011;66:1293–302.

Kan HE, Klomp DWJ, Wohlgemuth M, et al. Only fat infiltrated muscles in resting lower leg of FSHD patients show disturbed energy metabolism. NMR Biomed. 2010;23:563–8.

Karampinos DC, King KF, Sutton BP, Georgiadis JG. Myofiber ellipticity as an explanation for transverse asymmetry of skeletal muscle diffusion MRI in vivo signal. Ann Biomed Eng. 2009;37:2532–46.

Lim TH, Choi SI. MRI of myocardial infarction. J Magn Reson Imaging. 1999;10:686–93.

Liu CY, McKenzie CA, Yu H, Brittain JH, Reeder SB. Fat quantification with IDEAL gradient echo imaging: correction of bias from T_1 and noise. Magn Reson Med. 2007;58:354–64.

Lodi R, Muntoni F, Taylor J, et al. Correlative MR imaging and P-31-MR spectroscopy study in sarcoglycan deficient limb girdle muscular dystrophy. Neuromuscul Disord. 1997;7:505–11.

Lodi R, Kemp GJ, Muntoni F, et al. Reduced cytosolic acidification during exercise suggests defective glycolytic activity in skeletal muscle of patients with Becker muscular dystrophy: an in vivo P-31 magnetic resonance spectroscopy study. Brain. 1999;122:121–30.

Nagel AM, Laun FB, Weber MA, Matthies C, Semmler W, Schad LR. Sodium-MRI using a density adapted 3D radial acquisition technique. Magn Reson Med. 2009;62:1565–73.

Nagel AM, Amarteifio E, Lehmann-Horn F, Jurkat-Rott K, Semmler W, Schad LR, Weber MA. 3 Tesla sodium inversion recovery magnetic resonance imaging allows for improved visualization of intracellular sodium content changes in muscular channelopathies. Invest Radiol. 2011;46:759–66.

Nielles-Vallespin S, Weber MA, Bock M, Bongers A, Speier P, Combs SE, Wöhrle J, Lehmann-Horn F, Essig M, Schad LR. 3D radial projection technique with ultrashort echo times for sodium MRI: clinical applications in human brain and skeletal muscle. Magn Reson Med. 2007;57:74–81.

Qi J, Olsen NJ, Price RR, Winston JA, Park JH. Diffusion-weighted imaging of inflammatory myopathies: polymyositis and dermatomyositis. J Magn Reson Imaging. 2008;27:212–7.

Raynaud JS, Duteil S, Vaughan JT, et al. Determination of skeletal muscle perfusion using arterial spin labeling NMRI: validation by comparison with venous occlusion plethysmography. Magn Reson Med. 2001;46:305–11.

Schmidt S, Vieweger A, Obst M, et al. Dysferlin-deficient muscular dystrophy: gadofluorine M suitability at MR imaging in a mouse model. Radiology. 2009;250: 87–94.

Straub V, Donahue KM, Allamand V, Davisson RL, Kim YR, Campbell KP. Contrast agent-enhanced magnetic resonance imaging of skeletal muscle damage in animal models of muscular dystrophy. Magn Reson Med. 2000;44:655–9.

Thibaud JL, Monnet A, Bertoldi D, Barthelemy I, Blot S, Carlier PG. Characterization of dystrophic muscle in Golden Retriever muscular dystrophy dogs by nuclear magnetic resonance imaging. Neuromuscul Disord. 2007;17:575–84.

Walter G, Cordier L, Bloy D, Sweeney HL. Noninvasive monitoring of gene correction in dystrophic muscle. Magn Reson Med. 2005;54:1369–76.

Wary C, Nadaj-Pakleza A, Laforet P, et al. Investigating glycogenosis type III patients with multi-parametric functional NMR imaging and spectroscopy. Neuromuscul Disord. 2010;20:548–58.

Willis TA, Hollingsworth KG, Sveen ML, et al. Assessing muscle pathology by MRI in LGMD2I. Neuromuscul Disord. 2010;20:666.

Wray DW, Nishiyama SK, Monnet A, et al. Antioxidants and aging: NMR-based evidence of improved skeletal muscle perfusion and energetics. Am J Physiol Heart Circ Physiol. 2009;297:H1870–5.

Wren TAL, Bluml S, Tseng-Ong L, Gilsanz V. Three-point technique of fat quantification of muscle tissue as a marker of disease progression in Duchenne muscular dystrophy: preliminary study. Am J Roentgenol. 2008;190:W8–12.

Younkin DP, Berman P, Sladky J, Chee C, Bank W, Chance B. P-31 NMR-studies in Duchenne muscular-dystrophy: age-related metabolic changes. Neurology. 1987;37:165–9.

Nuclear Medicine Methods

6

Mike P. Wattjes

6.1 Introduction

In nuclear medicine radioactive substances (radiopharmaceuticals, tracers) are used for the diagnosis and treatment of several disease entities. These well-established imaging methods include scintigraphy, single photon emission computed tomography (SPECT), and positron emission tomography (PET). Newer developments include hybrid scanning techniques such as PET-computed tomography (CT), SPECT-CT, and PET-magnetic resonance imaging (MRI). In contrast to the other presented imaging modalities such as ultrasonography (US), (see Chap. 2), CT (see Chap. 3), and MRI (see Chap. 4), the data and experience concerning nuclear medicine methods in the diagnosis of inherited muscle diseases are limited. There are few other clinical conditions in which particularly PET, in addition to other imaging modalities, might be useful in supporting the clinical diagnosis (e.g., inflammatory muscle diseases) or as a screening and staging tool (e.g., malignancies). This chapter gives a brief overview of the clinical applications of nuclear medicine methods used in (neuro)muscular diseases mainly focusing on PET and scintigraphic methods.

M.P. Wattjes (✉)
Department of Radiology, Nuclear Medicine & PET Research, VU University Medical Center, De Boelelaan 1117, 1081 HV Amsterdam, The Netherlands
e-mail: m.wattjes@vumc.nl

6.2 Modalities

The most relevant PET tracer used for muscle PET imaging is ^{18}F-fluorodeoxyglucose (^{18}F-FDG). It is an imaging marker for glucose metabolism because it measures glucose uptake. During the past decade PET imaging has been performed using a hybrid imaging approach (PET-CT), combining a full-ring PET scanner and a multidetector spiral CT system in a single gantry. PET and CT imaging data sets can be fused when performing the PET examination directly after CT scanning. This combination provides substantially improved anatomical localization of the PET findings, thereby increasing the diagnostic accuracy for several purposes.

6.3 PET of Normal Muscle Tissue

Normal muscle tissue at rest shows homogeneous uptake of ^{18}F-FDG-PET (PET-CT), suggesting homogeneous glucose metabolism. In a small number of patients, however, ^{18}F-FDG-PET reveals an enhanced curvilinear area in the neck and supraclavicular region, although there is no clinical or radiological evidence of pathological metabolism (e.g., inflammation, malignancy). The underlying pathophysiological mechanism is still not completely understood. As these changes have disappeared on a repeat PET scan and after administration of muscle relaxants, increased muscle activity has been suggested as the underlying

M.P. Wattjes and D. Fischer (eds.), *Neuromuscular Imaging*, DOI 10.1007/978-1-4614-6552-2_6,

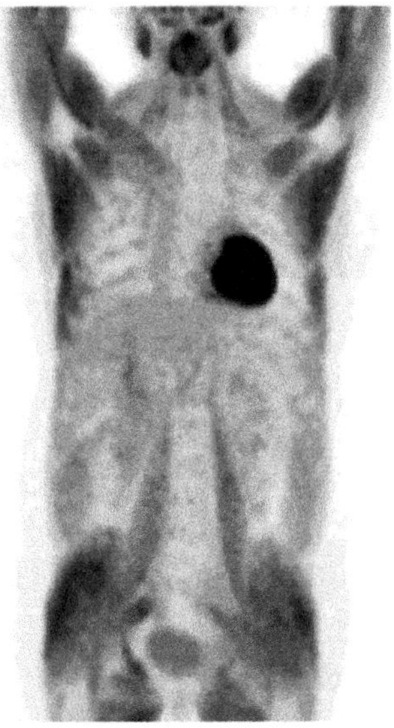

Fig. 6.1 Coronal image obtained from whole-body ^{18}F-fluorodeoxyglucose positron emission tomography (^{18}F-FDG-PET) examination (maximum intensity image) in a male patient after a heavy physical workout directly prior to the ^{18}F-FDG injection. Note the diffusely increased metabolic activity in the muscle. From Al-Nahhas and Jawad (2011) PET/CT imaging in inflammatory myopathies. Ann NY Acad Sci 1228:39–45. Reprinted with permission from John Wiley and Sons

cause. More recent data, however, suggest that the increased glucose uptake might be located in the brown fat tissue and not exclusively in the adjacent muscle tissue. Physical exercise leads to higher metabolic activity of the skeletal muscle, which is reflected in increased ^{18}F-FDG uptake. The pattern of ^{18}F-FDG uptake is strongly associated with the mode of exercise and the involved muscle groups (Fig. 6.1).

Compared to striated skeletal muscle, the myocardium shows rather high ^{18}F-FDG uptake owing to its higher metabolic activity.

6.4 Imaging of Inflammation

6.4.1 PET of Muscle Inflammation

Detection of inflammation in muscle tissue is the most relevant nononcological clinical condition for which PET is a well-established method in the clinical setting. Muscle inflammation (infectious and noninfectious) is associated with the presence of metabolically highly active inflammatory cells including macrophages (activated), lymphocytes, and granular tissue, all of which show increased uptake of ^{18}F-FDG. PET has detected muscle inflammation in several disease entities including sarcoidosis, infections, vasculitis, granulomas, graft versus host disease, chronic idiopathic inflammatory myopathies (e.g., dermatomyositis) (see Chap. 26), as well as in drug-induced myopathies (see Chap. 27) (Figs. 6.2, 6.3, 6.4). The clinical use of PET in these diseases goes beyond the detection of inflammatory disease activity. PET can also be used for monitoring disease, in particular for demonstrating response to treatment.

The sensitivity of PET for detecting high-grade inflammation, especially infectious muscle inflammation, is high. In contrast, low-grade inflammation, as seen in idiopathic inflammatory myopathies, can be missed. In those cases, multi-modality imaging approaches, including MRI with fat-suppressed T2-weighted images, might be helpful. The detection of muscle edema can lead to the correct diagnosis (see also Chap. 4).

6.4.2 Scintigraphy in Muscle Inflammation

In addition to ^{18}F-FDG PET, scintigraphy techniques can be helpful for diagnosing skeletal muscle pathology, particularly inflammatory changes. These methods include gallium-67 (^{67}Ga) citrate scintigraphy, anti-myosin scintigraphy, and technetium-99m (^{99m}Tc) pyrophosphate scintigraphy.

6.4.2.1 ^{67}Ga Citrate Scintigraphy

Gallium-67 citrate is a tracer that binds to transferrin receptors on activated macrophages and lymphocytes. It can be used to detect inflammation/infection, neoplastic diseases of the lymphoid tissue (lymphomas), and granulomatous disease entities. Particularly regarding muscle inflammation, ^{67}Ga citrate scintigraphy has been used in focal myositis, myofasciitis, and sarcoid-associated inflammation to show their different involvement

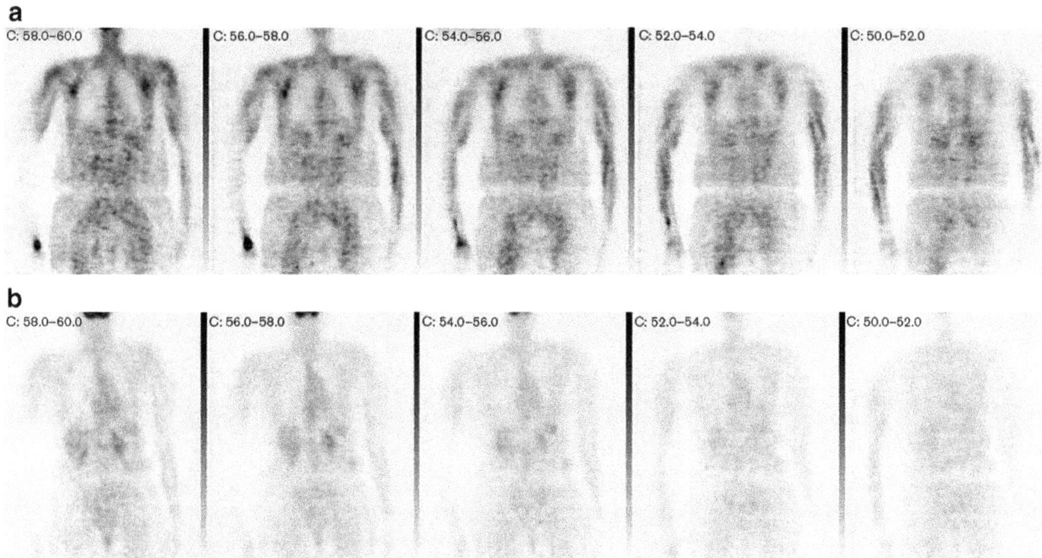

Fig. 6.2 (**a**) Coronal ^{18}F-FDG PET images in a patient with statin-induced necrotizing myopathy demonstrate increased metabolic activity in the muscles of the upper extremities and limb girdle (e.g., gluteus muscles). (**b**) Coronal ^{18}F-FDG-PET images of the same patient after therapy show complete resolution of the increased metabolic activity. From Harari OA, et al (2008) ^{18}F-fluorodeoxyglucose-positron emission tomography imaging in idiopathic inflammatory myositis. Nucl Med Commun 29:838–840. Reprinted with permission from Wolters Kluwer Health

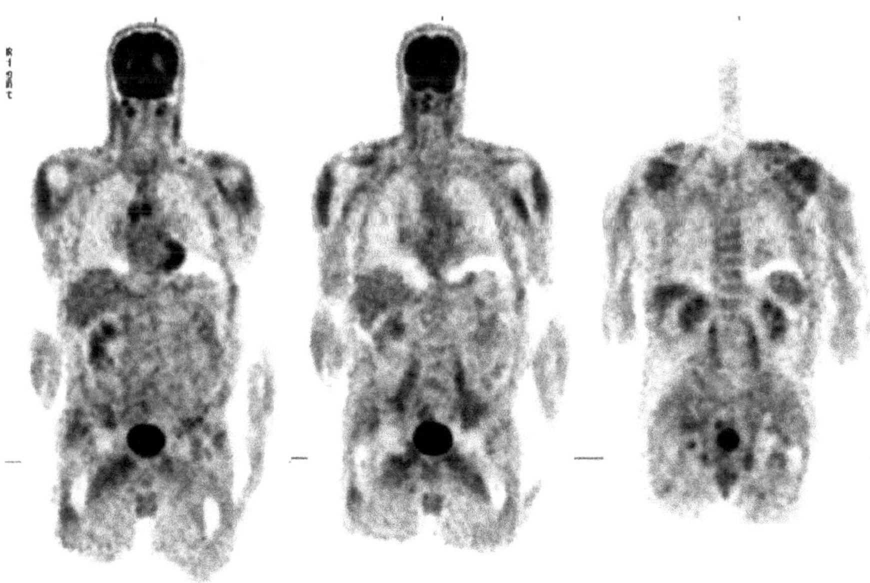

Fig. 6.3 Coronal ^{18}F-FDG-PET images of a 76-year-old patient presenting with dermatomyositis. The PET images 1 h after intravenous injection of ^{18}F-FDG-PET show symmetrical, low-grade metabolic activity in the proximal muscles of the upper extremities, iliopsoas, and hip addcutors. Two foci show high ^{18}F-FDG accumulation in the mediastinum, representing malignant tissue (lymph nodes) from an adenocarcinoma of the lung. From Liau N, et al (2007) F-18 FDG PET/CT detection of mediastinal malignancy in a patient with dermatomyositis. Clin Nucl Med 32:304–305. Reprinted with permission from Wolters Kluwer Health

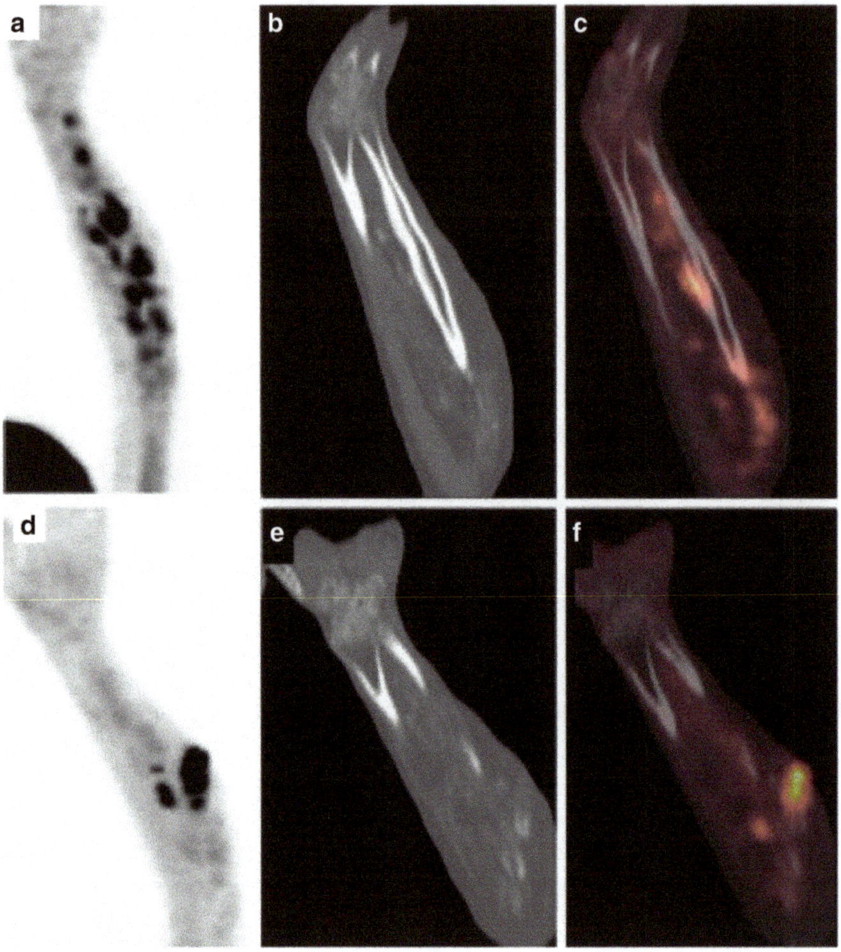

Fig. 6.4 ^{18}F-FDG-PET/CT images of the forearm performed on two different days in a patient with myositis ossificans. The increased tracer uptake indicates osteoblastic activity and inflammatory activity. From Agrawal K, et al (2011) [^{18}F]fluoride and [^{18}F]flourodeoxyglucose PET/CT in myositis ossificans of the forearm. Eur J Nucl Med Mol Imaging 38:1956. Reprinted with permission from Springer

patterns, which can contribute to the correct diagnosis. ^{67}Ga citrate scintigraphy can be helpful in conditions in which MRI findings are normal.

6.4.2.2 Anti-myosin Scintigraphy

Indium-111 (^{111}In)-labeled anti-myosin antibodies or antigen-binding fragments bind to damaged muscle tissue. This isotope has been used to detect muscle inflammation such as in polymyositis and dermatomyositis as well as in myocardial inflammation. However, it is rather unspecific as it also binds to damaged muscle in general. Therefore, it is not suited to differentiate specifically between muscle inflammation and muscle necrosis and (fatty) degeneration.

6.4.2.3 ^{99m}Technetium Pyrophosphate Scintigraphy

Technetium-99m pyrophosphate (^{99m}Tc-PYP) is also a rather unspecific tracer, accumulating in mitochondria and sarcoplasmic reticulum of damaged muscle cells as well as in inflammatory cells. ^{99m}Tc-PYP has been used in idiopathic inflammatory myopathies (e.g., polymyositis) to detect inflammatory activity, which to a certain degree correlates with clinical and laboratory markers of disease activity. However, ^{99m}Tc-PYP also accumulates in tissues from patients with noninflammatory muscle diseases. In neither inflammatory nor noninflammatory disease is ^{99m}Tc-PYP accumulation a sensitive marker: It is positive in about 50 % of patients with inflammatory disease and 39 % of patients with noninflammatory disease.

6.5 Imaging of Neuromuscular Neoplasm

The most established nuclear medicine imaging method for musculoskeletal oncology is PET, preferably PET/CT. ^{18}F-FDG is the most widely used PET tracer for these purposes, demonstrating the increased glucose metabolism (cellular glycolysis) in tumor cells. In general, ^{18}F-FDG PET is helpful for detecting soft tissue metastasis, soft tissue primary tumors, and nerve tumors (Figs. 6.5 and 6.6a, b). Clinical experience is rather limited in regard to soft tissue tumors as they comprise a heterogeneous group of diseases with mixed cell types and different grades of malignancy (see Chap. 28). There is increasing evidence that ^{18}F-FDG-PET/CT can contribute substantially to the diagnosis of muscle and nerve neoplasms as an adjunct to conventional MRI and CT.

It has been shown that the degree of ^{18}F-FDG activity (standardized uptake value, or SUV) correlates to some degree with the grade of malignancy. It can be useful for differentiating high-grade tumors from low-grade and benign tumors. Certain soft tissues have a heterogeneous appearance in terms of cell types and grading, and ^{18}F-FDG-PET/CT might therefore display heterogeneous activity. The latter is helpful for

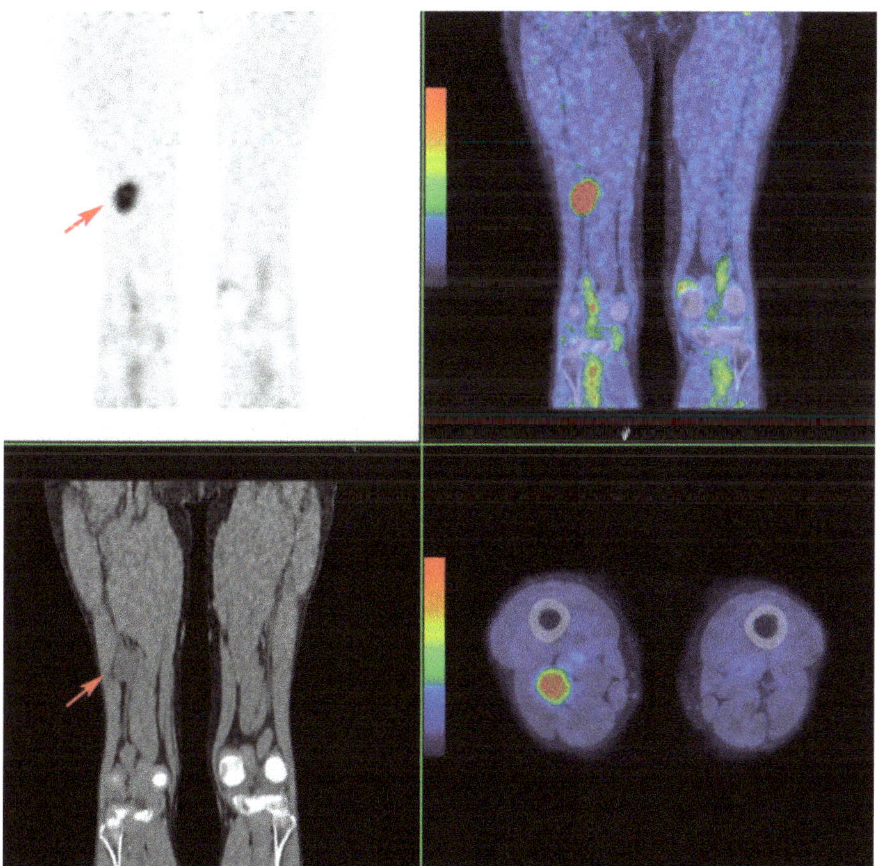

Fig. 6.5 Coronal ^{18}F-FDG-PET/CT of a patient presenting with neurofibromatosis. Note the sciatic nerve neurofibroma. The increased tracer uptake was suggestive of malignant transformation, which was histopathologically confirmed. From Lakkaruji A, et al (2010) PET/CT in primary musculoskeletal tumours: a step forward. Eur Radiol 20:2959–2972. Reprinted with permission from Springer

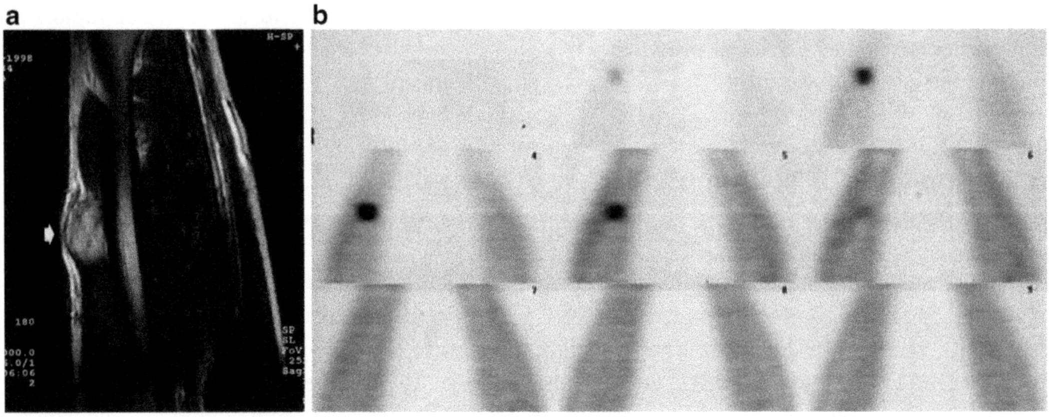

Fig. 6.6 (**a**) Coronal T2-weighted MRI scan of the right forearm of a 38-year-old man shows a focal lesion resembling a desmoid tumor. (**b**) The lesion shows high uptake on ^{18}F-FDG-PET images. From Aoki J, et al (2003) FDG-PET for preoperative differential diagnosis between benign and malignant soft tissue masses. Skeletal Radiol 32:133–138. Reprinted with permission from Springer

the surgeon to choose a biopsy site in the most metabolically active areas. Beyond the detection of neuromuscular neoplasms, ^{18}F-FDG can be used to monitor disease, particularly the response to treatment.

The degree of FDG uptake can provide some prognostic information and is correlated with overall and recurrence-free survival in patients with resectable soft tissue sarcomas. ^{18}F-FDG-PET can be crucial for detecting tumor recurrence and is more sensitive than MRI alone.

6.6 Future Directions

Nuclear medicine is one of the most innovative imaging disciplines today. The diagnostic value is continuously increasing based on novel developments including that of novel tracers and modern hybrid imaging techniques.

^{18}F-FDG is a rather unspecific tracer, measuring the metabolic activity in terms of glucose metabolism. Novel, more-specific tracers are needed. Such tracers currently being evaluated in preclinical and clinical trials are ^{18}F-fluorothymidine (FLT), ^{18}F-α-methyl tyrosine (FMT), ^{18}F-misonidazole (MISO), and ^{11}C-methionine. ^{18}F-FLT, a tracer for DNA synthesis and therefore mitotic activity and cellular proliferation, is promising for detection of sarcomas. It shows a better association between tracer uptake and histopathological tumor grade than does ^{18}F-FDG. It has promising potential particularly for monitoring the response to treatment. ^{11}C-methionine has been used in musculoskeletal neoplasms and provided results in line with those produced by ^{18}F-FDG. It is therefore debatable whether this tracer has any additional value in the future.

The most well-established hybrid imaging technique used in nuclear imaging is PET/CT. The next generation of hybrid imaging, PET/MRI, has recently been introduced and promises interesting developments and (functional) imaging possibilities. Compared to PET/CT, PET/MRI has the crucial advantage that radiation exposure is substantially reduced, which is important in young adults and pediatric patients. For detecting muscle neoplasms, the better soft tissue contrast on MRI scans may lead to a more sensitive and specific diagnosis. However, the drawbacks of MRI (e.g., longer acquisition times, exclusion of patients with a pacemaker or who are claustrophobic) must be considered. Nevertheless, PET/MRI is the hybrid imaging technique of the future and will likely improve the diagnostic and prognostic classifications of muscle diseases, particularly in patients with inflammatory and neoplastic muscle diseases.

Imaging Modalities: Nuclear Medicine Methods

Key Points

- Data on nuclear medicine methods for investigating muscle tissue in neuromuscular diseases is rather limited.
- Positron emission tomography (particularly PET/CT) and scintigraphy have been used in inflammatory and, more frequently, neoplastic muscle diseases.
- ^{18}F-FDG PET is helpful in the diagnosis, prognostic classification, and disease monitoring of musculoskeletal tumors.
- New promising developments including new tracers and hybrid imaging techniques (PET/MRI) become increasingly important.

Suggestions for Further Reading

Ahmad N, Welch I, Grange R, et al. Use of imaging biomarkers to assess perfusion and glucose metabolism in the skeletal muscle of dystrophic mice. BMC Musculoskelet Disord. 2011;12:127.

Al-Nahhas A, Jawad ASM. PET/CT imaging in inflammatory myopathies. Ann N Y Acad Sci. 2011; 1228:39–45.

Aoki J, Watanabe H, Shinozaki T, et al. FDG-PET for preoperative differential diagnosis between benign and malignant soft tissue masses. Skeletal Radiol. 2003;32:133–8.

Cook GJ, Fogelman I. The role of positron emission tomography in skeletal disease. Semin Nucl Med. 2001;31:50–61.

Emmering J, Vogel WV, Stokkel PM. Intramuscular metastases on FDG PET-CT, a review of the literature. Nucl Med Commun. 2012;33:117–20.

Feldman F, van Heertum R, Manos C. ^{18}FDG PET scanning of benign and malignant musculoskeletal lesions. Skeletal Radiol. 2003;32:201–8.

Harari OA, Al-Nahhas A, Jawad A. ^{18}F-fluorodeoxyglucose-positron emission tomography imaging in idiopathic inflammatory myositis. Nucl Med Commun. 2008;29: 838–9.

Jadvar H, Gamie S, Ramanna L, et al. PET in the musculoskeletal system. Semin Nucl Med. 2004;34:254–61.

Lakkaraju A, Patel CN, Bradley KM, et al. PET/CT in primary musculoskeletal tumours: a step forward. Eur Radiol. 2010;20:2959–72.

Liau N, Ooi C, Reid C, et al. F-18 FDG PET/CT detection of mediastinal malignancy in a patient with dermatomyositis. Clin Nucl Med. 2007;32:304–5.

Walker UA. Imaging tools for the clinical assessment of idiopathic inflammatory myositis. Curr Opin Rheumatol. 2008;20:656–61.

Yeung HW, Grewal RK, Gonen M, Schröder H, Larson SM. Patterns of (18)F-FDG uptake in adipose tissue and muscle: a potential source of false-positives for PET. J Nucl Med. 2003;44:1789–96.

Peripheral Nerve Imaging

7

Arnold Kang and Michel Kliot

7.1 Introduction

Imaging modalities that might be considered when imaging peripheral nerve pathology include plain radiography (XR), computed tomography (CT), positron emission tomography (PET), high-resolution ultrasonography (US) and magnetic resonance imaging (MRI). This chapter focuses on methods that have shown the greatest utility because of recent technological advances.

7.2 Diagnostic Imaging Modalities

7.2.1 Plain Radiography

Although conventional radiography is unable to demonstrate peripheral nerves directly, it is nevertheless an important baseline test in the overall imaging work-up. It can be of significant value as an initial screen to rule out potentially relevant considerations such as traumatic lesions (e.g. recent or old radiopaque foreign bodies, post-traumatic calcifications involving adjacent structures), predispositions to neural impingement or traction (e.g. bone spurs, old fracture malunions, joint malalignments instabilities) and tumoral processes (e.g. bone destruction, pressure erosion of bone, tumoral calcification, intramuscular lipoma). See Fig. 7.1.

7.2.2 Computed Tomography

Computed Tomography (with or without the use of iodinated intravenous contrast material) is most helpful in circumstances of tumor assessment (especially with regard to metastatic tumor spread and cortical bone changes) and joint pathology in the spine that may be contributing to nerve root impingement. In some cases, CT may be used as an alternative to MRI for those who are not MR tolerant. CT is also much more sensitive than XR or MRI for detecting calcifications (and other crystal depositions such as gout). CT in combination with myelography can be useful for detecting proximal pathology at the spinal level (e.g. root nerve avulsions at the interface with the spinal cord). Helical CT can be performed using 0.625 mm acquisition and 2.5 mm reconstructions in the axial, coronal and sagittal planes. Standard non-ionic contrast, used for CT abdominal and pelvic studies, should be administered to identify any enhancing components in either the late arterial or portal venous phases. Non-contrast CT can be performed prior to the post contrast study to

A. Kang, MD, FRANZCR (✉)
Division of Neuroradiology, Department of Radiology, University of Washington, 1959 NE Pacific St, Seattle, WA 98195-7115, USA
e-mail: akang79@uw.edu

M. Kliot, M.D.
Department of Neurological Surgery, University of California San Francisco, 500 Parnassus Avenue, M780, San Francisco, CA 94143-0112, USA
e-mail: kliotm@neurosurg.ucsf.edu

M.P. Wattjes and D. Fischer (eds.), *Neuromuscular Imaging*, DOI 10.1007/978-1-4614-6552-2_7,

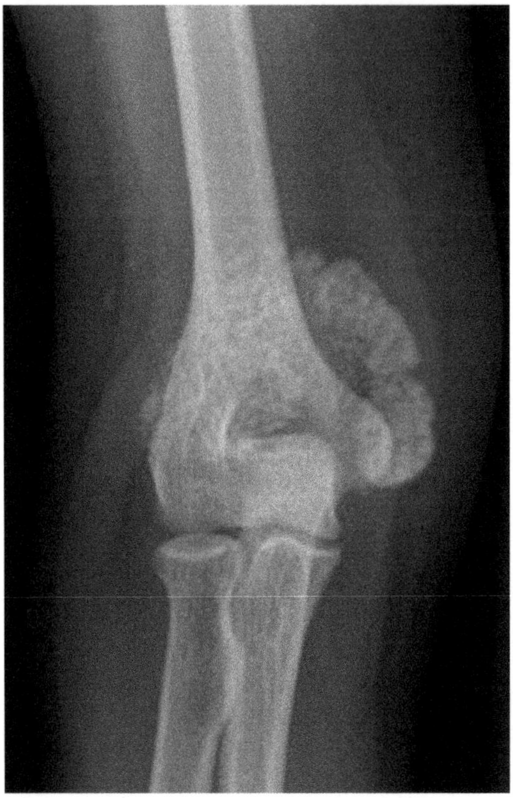

Fig. 7.1 Anteroposterior radiograph demonstrates heterotopic ossification (Source: University of Washington, PACS)

allow better visualization of calcifications and confirm the true presence of enhancement (i.e. ≥20 HU increase in attenuation). The interpreting physician must be cognizant of the pitfalls of streak artifact (near metallic devices), partial voluming (near bone). and pseudo-enhancement (if near vascular structures or organs that enhance).

7.2.3 Positron Emission Tomography

Increased uptake of ^{18}F-fluorodeoxyglucose (^{18}F-FDG) in peripheral nerve tumors suggests malignancy. This test assists in surgical management and can help direct biopsies and distinguish a tumor from radiation- induced changes. If malignancy is proven, adjuvant chemotherapy and/or irradiation can be used. See Fig. 7.2.

7.2.4 Magnetic Resonance Imaging

For peripheral nerve imaging, MRI is the imaging modality of choice in many circumstances. The general advantages of MRI include exceptional soft tissue contrast, high spatial resolution, multiplanar capability and relative safety. The term MR neurography, introduced during the early 1990s, and refers to an MRI application dedicated specifically to visualizing a particular nerve or plexus. It is usually performed on a 1.5-T or 3.0-T magnet using special pulse sequences, multiple phase array coils, and suppressing the signal from fat and vessels. Multi-transmittance is used, and the field of view should be as small as possible to include the area of interest. The inplane resolution can be as low as 0.4 mm.

Images are usually obtained in at least two planes (longitudinal if it is in the coronal or sagittal plane and cross sectional). The planes acquired depend on the area being imaged (e.g. median and sciatic nerves are imaged in the axial and coronal planes whereas the brachial plexus is imaged in the coronal and oblique sagittal planes). The coronal plane allows a global longitudinal assessment of the nerve whereas a cross- sectional plane allows assessment of the size and relation of a lesion to the fascicles of the affected nerve. See Fig. 7.3.

Using multiple phase array coils (which are often custom built) allows integration of signal data from multiple small receiver coils covering the anatomy of interest to produce a single image and increase the field of view. Thus, images with a larger field of view can be obtained without sacrificing signal to noise ratio. Thus, superior resolution and contrast can be obtained simultaneously. The main disadvantage is that surface coils may result in uneven signal distribution across the field of view.

The technique of MR neurography is tissue-selective imaging directed at identifying and evaluating nerve morphology including internal fascicular pattern, longitudinal variations in signal intensity and caliber, and connections/relations to other nerves and plexi. The administration of contrast agent is useful for identifying nerve sheath tumors. Some pulse sequences, including

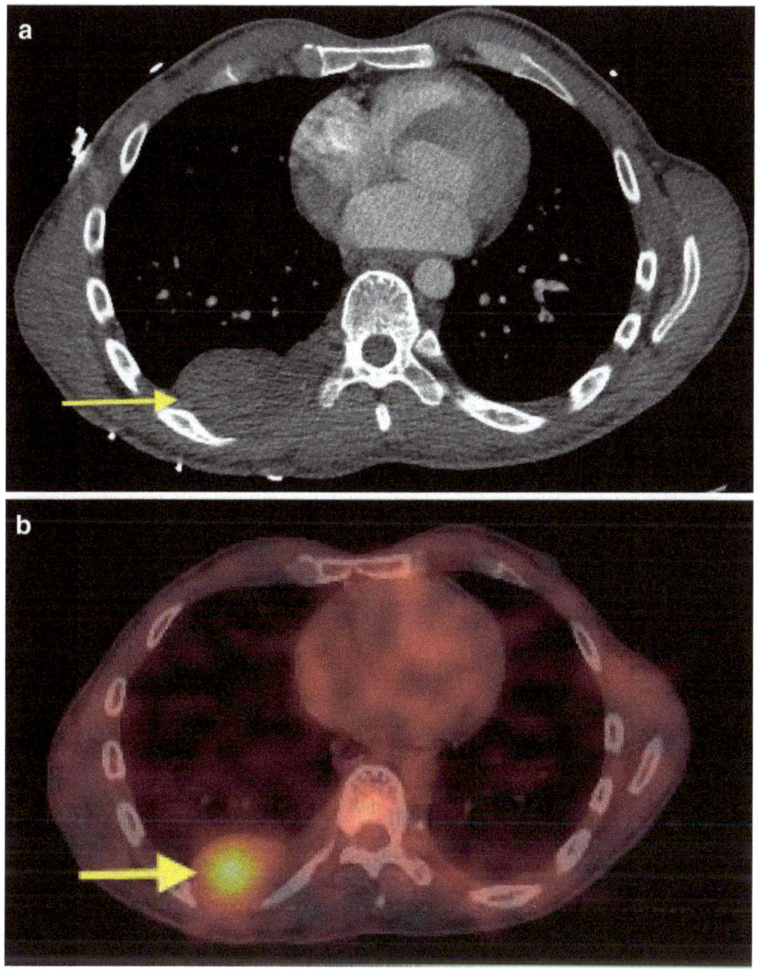

Fig. 7.2 (**a**) Contrast enhanced computed tomography (CT) demonstrates a soft tissue density mass in the location of an intercostal nerve with scalloping of the rib. The patient had a known history of neurofibromatosis type 1. The features are consistent with a neurofibroma. (**b**) Positron emission tomography(PET)/ CT of the same patient demonstrates increased fluorodeoxyglucose uptake at the site of the neurofibroma, consistent with malignant transformation. The diagnosis was confirmed on pathology (Source: University of Washington, PACS)

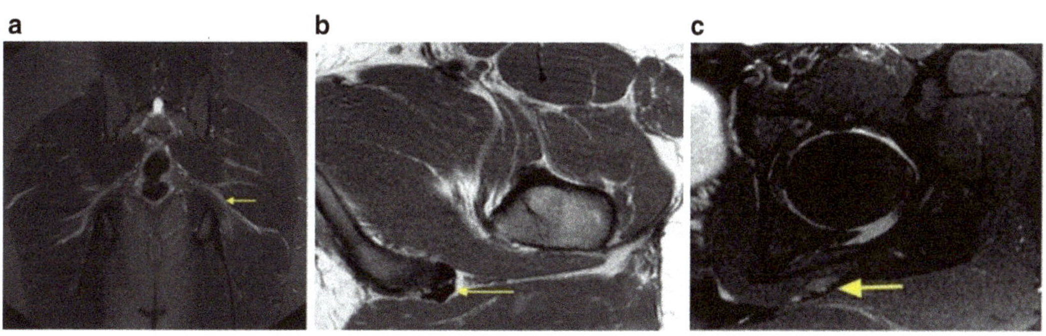

Fig. 7.3 Normal magnetic resonance(MR) neurogram of the left sciatic nerve. (**a**) Coronal short-tau inversion recovery (STIR) demonstrates normal sciatic nerves bilaterally. They are of normal size, normal configuration, and mildly hyperintense to muscle. (**b**) Axial T1-weighted MRI of the left sciatic nerve demonstrates low signal intensity which is normal. Again, the size and configuration are normal. (**c**) Axial T2 with fat saturation also demonstrates normal mild hyperintensity in the left sciatic nerve in comparison to that of the muscle. (Source: University of Washington, PACS)

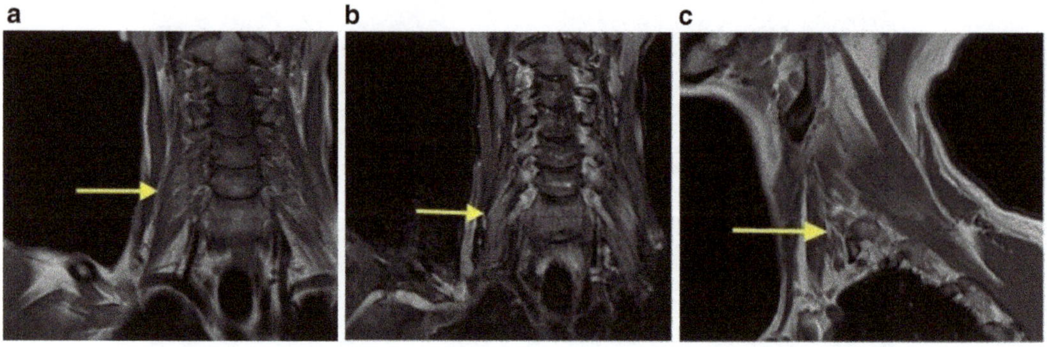

Fig. 7.4 Normal MR neurogram of the right brachial plexus. (**a**) Coronal T1-weighted MRI plexus shows a normal right brachial plexus that displays low to intermediate signal intensity. It is also of normal size and course. (**b**) Coronal STIR of the right brachial plexus. Part of the brachial plexus is imaged because of the oblique nature of the structure. It is mildly hyperintense to muscle and of normal size and course. It has a normal appearance. (**c**) Sagittal oblique T1-weighted image again demonstrates a normal brachial plexus (Source: University of Washington, PACS)

diffusion tensor imaging (DTI), take advantage of the anisotropic properties of nerves.

It cannot be overly stressed that good knowledge of both the histological architecture and the anatomical location of the peripheral nerves is essential to interpreting MRI scans accurately.

T1-weighted imaging shows fine anatomical detail including the internal fascicular structure of nerves. This is the smallest resolvable structure seen on MRI. Normal nerve fascicles demonstrate uniform shape and size and follow the expected course of the nerve. Normal peripheral nerves are isointense to normal muscle on T1-weighted imaging and slightly hyperintense on T2-weighted imaging and short-tau inversion recovery (STIR). This hyperintensity is likely due to endoneurial fluid within the individual fascicles. Normal peripheral nerves including the fascicles and epineurium show no enhancement after gadolinium administration because of the integrity of the blood-nerve barrier. See Fig. 7.4.

7.2.5 Ultrasonography

High-resolution ultrasonography (US) is becoming increasingly important due to improvements in broadband transducer and signal processing technology (see Chap. 2, Sects. 2.3.2 and 2.5). Peripheral nerves are generally well-resolved using 5 to 12 MHz transducers (relatively superficial nerves may be imaged at frequencies of up to 18 MHz). Although spatial compounding suppresses image noise and improves contrast resolution, MRI currently still provides superior contrast resolution. US nevertheless offers better detail resolution and has other distinct advantages that include a real-time interactive aspect. Interactivity allows precise correlation of clinical features, such as tenderness and trigger points with their imaging location and appearance, a dynamic capability that allows assessment of instabilities and impingements in differeny limb positions. Interactivity also provides the ability to assess the entire length of a peripheral nerve in a limb rapidly while comparing it to the contralateral side. US can also be used intra-operatively for localizing a tumor and other pathology. It has the advantages of complete safety, minimal patient discomfort, wide availability, and low cost when compared with MR neurography. The major limitation of US is that it is highly operator-dependent, making this test unreliable in the hands of an inexperienced operator.

Normal peripheral nerve is hypoechoic but has a fascicular appearance because of its the reflective interfaces caused by supporting connective tissues such as endoneurium and perineurium. The number and size of fascicles vary with overall nerve size, location, and type. There is also considerable individual variability and a normal slight difference in nerve caliber between dominant and non-dominant limbs (larger caliber on the non-dominant side). On color flow Doppler imaging, there is generally no detectable intraneuralvascularity. The nerve is thus assessed in its relation to adjacent muscles, tendons, and vessels.

The short-axis plane is the most suitable scanning method when following a nerve throughout the limb. The nerves tend to be much less anisotropic than tendons. Long-axis images can also be obtained with extended field-of-view techniques to produce panoramic images. US is also able to detect muscle denervation changes such as muscle atrophy and fatty infiltration.

Although experience is somewhat limited, intraoperative US has been used to localize lesions and allow a surgical approach that is more limited and "tailored". US does have some disadvantages including a dependence on appropriate equipment and personnel and the increased operative times which may lead to an increase in perioperative complications.

7.2.6 Future Directions of MRI and Ultrasonograhy

Although MR neurography is a well-established technique in large institutions throughout the world, it is difficult to implement optimal imaging techniques in other imaging centers. MR neurography is preferably performed with custom-built coils, which can be time-intensive. Although US has its limitations, in a small institution and with highly trained sonographers and radiologists, US may represent a more viable option for peripheral nerve imaging. A number of novel applications using established techniques have been studied briefly and which may have application in the future after more rigorous study. All of these techniques can be performed on a 1.5-T magnet. In 2008, one study showed that denervated muscles may have increased apparent diffusion coefficient values because of early expansion of the extracellular fluid space in muscles. Thus, by inference, denervation could be identified in an area of interest without direct observation.

Diffusion-weighted MR neurography of the brachial plexus has been performed with the images displayed using a maximum intensity projection technique. Diffusion-weighted imaging (DWI) can give an overview of the brachial plexus and the location of the disease. It also demonstrates excellent conspicuity of the surrounding structures. Three-dimensional diffusion-weighted steady-state free precession imaging (3D DW-SSFP) with isotropic resolution has also been performed to delineate structures of the human lumbosacral plexus. A new type of diffusion weighted MR neurography technique uses the subtraction of unidirectionally encoded images for suppression of heavily isotropic objects (SUSHI). The SUSHI technique can be used to visualize the brachial plexus and single nerves including the sciatic, common peroneal and tibial nerves. Preliminary studies suggest that malignant nerve sheath tumors demonstrate relatively less diffusion than benign nerve sheath tumors, thereby purporting DWI as a promising tool for prospectively differentiating the two.

Diffusion tensor imaging and tractography are established techniques for assessing the orientation of nerve fibers. They require a spin echo single shot diffusion weighted echo planar imaging sequence with fat suppression. They can be used concurrently with motion probing gradients. They have been studied in the brain to assess white matter tracts in the setting of pre-operative planning for tumor resection. Regarding peripheral nerve imaging, there is potential clinical application in entrapment neuropathies (e.g., carpal tunnel syndrome), peripheral nerve injuries —to look for the presence of axons and regeneration of axons as well as intraneural scar tissue (to help distinguish axonotmetic from neurotmetic injury)—and in the preoperative assessment of peripheral nerve tumors especially when planning surgery.

Microstructural parameters including fractional anisotropy values, may be able to be modified earlier than at the time at which the onset of changes is detectable by conventional MRI. MR spectroscopy has not yet been utilized to evaluate of peripheral nerve tumors (as it has in the brain) usually because of the relatively small size of the nerves.

With regard to US, there is the potential for improvement using US contrast agents and new techniques including sonoelastography, particularly in the setting of nerve injury and nerve masses.

Imaging Modalities: Peripheral Nerve Imaging

Key Points

- Plain radiographs, CT, US, MRI and PET can be used to diagnose nerve pathology under varying clinical circumstances.
- US and MRI are the imaging modalities of choice for assessing nerve injury and tumors.
- MR neurography is an established technique that uses phased array coils to image nerves.
- Standard MRI sequences include T1, T2 fast spin echo, STIR, and T1 fat saturation after gadolinium administration.
- US is useful for imaging nerve pathology but requires operator and radiologist expertise and experience.
- Intraoperative US, DWI, and DTI are better able to localize nerve tumors and assess nerve injury. This ability may lead to better patient outcomes.

Suggestions for Further Reading

Aagaard BD, Maravilla KR, Kliot M. MR neurography. MR imaging of peripheral nerves. Magn Reson Imaging Clin N Am. 1998;6:179–94.

Aagaard BD, Maravilla KR, Kliot M. Magnetic resonance neurography: magnetic resonance imaging of peripheral nerves. Neuroimaging Clin N Am. 2001;11:viii, 131–46.

Aagaard BD, Lazar DA, Lankerovich L, et al. High-resolution magnetic resonance imaging is a noninvasive method of observing injury and recovery in the peripheral nervous system. Neurosurgery. 2003;53:199–203; discussion 203–4.

Hyodo T, Sugawara Y, Sakayama K, Kito K. Early stage malignant peripheral nerve sheath tumor arising from a solitary neurofibroma. Br J Radiol. 2012;85(1010): e26–30.

Kästel T, Heiland S, Bäumer P, Bartsch AJ, Bendszus M, Pham M. Magic angle effect: a relevant artifact in MR neurography at 3T? AJNR Am J Neuroradiol. 2011;32:821–7.

Kermarrec E, Demondion X, Khalil C, Le Thuc V, Boutry N, Cotten A. Ultrasound and magnetic resonance imaging of the peripheral nerves: current techniques, promising directions, and open issues. Semin Musculoskelet Radiol. 2010;14:463–72.

Stoll G, Bendszus M, Perez J, Pham M. Magnetic resonance imaging of the peripheral nervous system. J Neurol. 2009;256:1043–51.

Tagliafico A, Altafini L, Garello I, Marchetti A, Gennaro S, Martinoli C. Traumatic neuropathies: spectrum of imaging findings and postoperative assessment. Semin Musculoskelet Radiol. 2010;14:512–22.

Takahara T, Kwee TC, Hendrikse J, et al. Subtraction of unidirectionally encoded images for suppression of heavily isotropic objects (SUSHI) for selective visualization of peripheral nerves. Neuroradiology. 2011;53(2):109–16.

Thawait SK, Chaudhry V, Thawait GK, et al. High-resolution MR neurography of diffuse peripheral nerve lesions. AJNR Am J Neuroradiol. 2011;32:1365–72.

Van de Luijtgaarden A, Flucke U, van der Graaf W, de Rooy J, Bonenkamp H, de Geus-Oei LF. Malignant transformation in an area with elevated F-18 FDG uptake within a low metabolic benign neurofibroma. Clin Nucl Med. 2010;35:271–2.

Part II

Muscle Anatomy and Physiology

Introduction

8

Dirk Fischer and Mike P. Wattjes

The second part of this book focuses on the fundamental anatomy of skeletal muscle tissue. It is important to understand the normal microscopic and macroscopic structure of skeletal muscle and the underlying physiological and pathological processes before focusing on distinct neuromuscular disorders.

The first chapter (Chap. 9) provides a detailed description of the normal microscopic anatomy and ultrastructure of skeletal muscle tissue. In addition, the basic reactions of muscle tissue and histopathological findings to pathological processes are described.

Not all of the readers may be familiar with muscle imaging and macroscopic muscle imaging anatomy. Therefore, Chap. 10 provides a thorough topographical guideline for identifying muscles involved in neuromuscular disorders. Detailed muscle images of the neck, shoulder, upper extremity, trunk, and lower extremity muscles are presented. The "normal" macroscopic muscle anatomy on magnetic resonance imaging (MRI) is not homogeneous and depends on the topographical distribution of several muscle groups. The aim of this chapter is to provide assistance for differentiating between "normal" and pathological muscle appearances on MRI. This chapter should help the reader easily identify certain muscles and muscle groups, which leads to recognizing an anatomical involvement pattern in neuromuscular disorders during one's daily clinical practice.

The histopathological and clinical effects of aging on skeletal muscle tissue, commonly called "sarcopenia," can result in similar changes in the regional muscle mass, muscle function, and muscle imaging. These changes must be distinguished from changes due to pathological conditions. To address this clinically and radiologically important phenomenon, the "normal aging" process of the striated muscle tissue is described in Chap. 11. The complex (patho)physiological mechanism—including many interacting factors such as hormones, nutrition, and physical activity—are discussed. In addition, the effects of "normal aging" on regional muscle mass, muscle fiber size and number, and the clinical consequences with respect to muscle power, strength, and endurance are comprehensively summarized.

D. Fischer
Department of Neuropaediatrics, University Childrens Hospital Basel, 4056 Basel, Switzerland

Department of Neurology, University Hospital Basel, 4031 Basel, Switzerland
e-mail: Dirk.fischer@ukbb.ch

M.P. Wattjes (✉)
Department of Radiology, Nuclear Medicine & PET Research, VU University Medical Center, De Boelelaan 1117, 1081 HV Amsterdam, The Netherlands
e-mail: m.wattjes@vumc.nl

M.P. Wattjes and D. Fischer (eds.), *Neuromuscular Imaging*, DOI 10.1007/978-1-4614-6552-2_8,

Morphology of Skeletal Muscle

9

Hans H. Goebel and Werner Stenzel

9.1 Introduction

Skeletal muscle makes up the largest organ of the body, by both volume and weight, comprising more than 40 %. More than 500 diseases concern muscle tissue, the majority of which originate in muscle, others secondarily affect the muscle, foremost by denervation. The functional and structural dependence of skeletal muscle on innervation—that is, the peripheral and central nervous systems—renders muscle tissue unique and adds a dimension to the nosology, more obviously than in other organs. Therefore, diseases affecting muscle are also termed neuromuscular diseases. Within the nosological spectrum of the muscle parenchyma, which encompasses hereditary and acquired conditions, muscular dystrophies, channelopathies, congenital myopathies, and inflammatory and metabolic disorders, malformations and neoplasms are strikingly absent. Vascular pathology rarely affects skeletal muscle whereas endocrine pathology may do so.

H.H. Goebel (✉)
Neuropathology Department,
Johannes Gutenberg-University Medical Center,
Langenbeckstr. 1, 55131 Mainz, Germany
e-mail: hans-hilmer.goebel@charite.de

W. Stenzel
Neuropathology Department,
Charite-Universitatsmedizin Berlin,
Charite Campus Mitte, Berlin D, Germany
e-mail: werner.stenzel@charite.de

9.2 Normal Histology

The core element of muscle parenchyma is the muscle fiber, a multi-nucleated long stretch of sarcomeres with innumerable nuclei underneath the cell membrane. Within a given muscle, the muscle fibers are usually situated in a parallel fashion. Among the muscle fibers are capillaries and, under normal conditions, very little (endomysial) connective tissue (i.e., fibroblasts and collagen fibrils). Clusters of muscle fibers form fascicles (Fig. 9.1a), which are separated by perimysium, and vessels larger than capillaries (i.e., arterioles, arteries, venules, veins). Muscle fascicles make up the muscle surrounded by the epimysium. Muscle fibers insert at the myotendinous junction and the surrounding fascia. Muscle spindles are occasionally encountered within fascicles.

The neuromuscular contact, or innervation, is characterized by neuromuscular junctions (NMJs), which in each muscle cluster at the motor point and can be recognized by histochemical features and by small nerve twigs spreading within muscle fascicles among the muscle fibers. NMJ areas are characterized by a physiological increase in connective tissue.

Not all muscle fibers are identical. Histochemical—and electrophysiological—techniques have identified types I, IIa, and IIb fibers, corresponding to slow-twitch and fast-twitch fibers. Types I and II muscle fibers are defined by their histochemical—and biochemical—ATPase activities, which require preincubation

M.P. Wattjes and D. Fischer (eds.), *Neuromuscular Imaging*, DOI 10.1007/978-1-4614-6552-2_9,

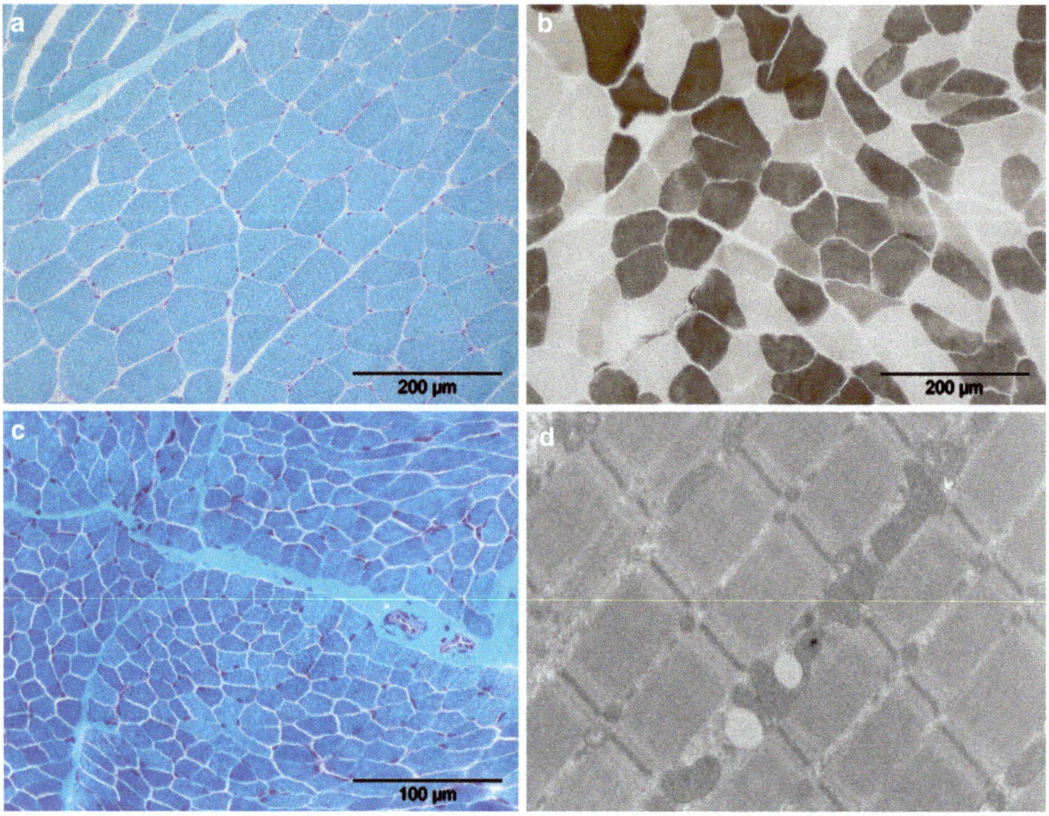

Fig. 9.1 Normal muscle. (**a**) Cross-sectioned polygonal muscle fibers of an adult. (**b**) ATPase preparation at pH 4.6 shows three fiber types: (I) dark; (IIA) nonreacting; (IIB) intermediate. (**c**) Normal muscle of a 1-year-old child. Note the similarity in the shape and packing but the difference in fiber size (compare magnification bars of **a** and **c**) (modified Gomori trichrome). (**d**) Electron micrograph of a longitudinally sectioned muscle fiber shows sarcomeres with Z-discs, I-bands, and A-bands

for subdivision of types I, IIa, and IIb muscle fibers (Fig. 9.1b). The basis of this differentiation of muscle fibers—various isoforms of myosin—can also be recognized by immunohistochemically applying antibodies against fast or slow myosin as well as against further subtypes of type II (fast) muscle fibers. Enzyme histochemical preparations for the oxidative enzymes, phosphorylase and phosphofructokinase also show two types of muscle fiber. Usually in limb muscles types I and II fibers appear in a chess-board pattern with varying ratios of the two types in different muscles. The soleus muscle is largely composed of type I fibers, whereas the extensor digitorum longus muscle contains more type II than type I fibers. These fiber types are not recognizable by muscular imaging.

9.2.1 Normal Skeletal Muscle During Lifespan

At birth, skeletal muscle fibers, though small (Fig. 9.1c), have already reached maturity. Markers of immaturity, including vimentin, developmental and neonatal myosin, and neural cell adhesion molecule (NCAM), among others, are not expressed in mature skeletal muscle fibers. Typing muscle fibers is as easy in neonates as in adult muscle. Muscle fibers grow until about the middle of the second decade, when they reach their adult diameters. The ratio of type I:II fibers in individual muscles is not known to change between birth and adulthood. The only exception is that some rounding of muscle fiber contours is characteristic of infantile muscle.

9.2.2 Age-Related Features in Skeletal Muscle

From early adulthood (i.e., mid-twenties), limb muscles tend to become smaller. Counting the entire population of muscle fibers in the limb muscle shows that the number continuously decreases between early adulthood and senescence. Such loss of muscle fibers may follow the loss of motor neurons by denervation or simply by disappearance of the fibers. The pathogenesis of this loss is not clear, but it affects both fiber types, which can only be ascertained by studying cross sections of entire muscles. However, this loss of fibers is not apparent in biopsied muscle from elderly people. In addition, when muscle fiber diameters decrease in size, type II fibers are preferentially affected. Hence, mild type II fiber atrophy in an aged patient may be the norm rather than evidence of myopathology. The extent to which muscle fibers are lost is not well established, although it varies among the limb, trunk, extraocular, and facial muscles. Apparently, the loss of muscle fibers in skeletal muscle does not leave any trace. Replacement of muscle parenchyma by fatty or connective tissue (i.e., fibrosis) is not a feature of normal aged muscle.

An additional feature of aging muscle is an increase in ragged red fibers and, even more extensive, in cytochrome-c oxidase (COX)-negative muscle fibers. These changes are caused by increasing mutations in the mitochondrial genome. Firm numerical threshold data of such COX-negative and ragged red fibers in different muscles or at different ages have not yet been ascertained.

The topic of normal aging muscle tissue is presented in more detail in Chap. 11.

9.2.3 Muscle Fibers in Various Muscles

Diameters of muscle fibers in limb, axial, and other muscles (i.e., proximal or very distal muscles), including intercostal muscles—irrespective of the length of the muscle—vary between 40 and 70 μm. Type II fibers are often somewhat smaller in females. The differences in fiber size between those at the surface of individual muscles (the usual site of open biopsy) and deeply located muscle fibers (usually the target of needle biopsies) are within < 10 μm. The diameters of muscle fibers in facial muscles are usually 50 % less than those of nonfacial muscles.

The distribution of fiber types (i.e., I and II) may vary considerably among muscles. For instance, the soleus muscle is composed of nearly 90 % type I fibers and the rectus femoris of 70 % type II fibers. Often, however, the I:II fiber ratio approaches 1:1. Considerable differences may also exist among the facial muscles. In the frontalis muscle, for example, type I fibers may make up two-thirds of the muscle fiber population, whereas in the orbicularis oris muscle type I fibers may account for only one-sixth of the fiber population. Other facial muscles show a numerical predominance of type II fibers.

The physiological content of connective tissue and fat cells among muscle fibers seems to be similar in normal limb, axial, and facial muscles. Hence, when aggregates of fat cells and bands of connective tissue are encountered, endomysially and/or perimysially, it indicates the presence of myopathology.

Extraocular muscles comprise six intraorbital muscles, four rectus muscles, and two oblique muscles as well as the extraorbital levator palpebrae muscle. The intraorbital eye muscles have highly complex structures. There are two layers (outer-orbital layer, inner-global layer) and five or six types of muscle fiber (according to the respective classification criteria). The complexity is increased by single or multiple innervation of extraocular muscle fibers with their respective plaque-like or grape cluster-like neuromuscular junctions. The eye muscles are made even more complex with the acetylcholine receptor composition of eye muscle endplates different from those of limb muscle. Ultrastructurally, eye muscles contain many more and even larger mitochondria, have a rich sarcotubular sytem, and may contain more numerous lysosomes as judged by acid phosphatase activity.

9.2.4 Electron Microscopy

Electron microscopy remains an essential component of the diagnostic armamentarium in myopathology. Hence, at biopsy, a separate set of muscles should be sampled, probably fixed in glutaraldehyde, embedded in resin, and either sectioned for electron microscopic investigation or archived for later study. Longitudinally sectioned muscle fibers displaying normal and abnormal details of muscle fibers, especially of the sarcomeres, should be studied, in contrast to light microscopic examination, where cross-sectioned muscle fibers in the tissue section should make up the majority of muscle fibers.

Muscle fibers contain two major groups of components.

1. Those that occur in other cell types (i.e., nucleus, plasma membrane, mitochondria, lysosomes, Golgi complex)
2. Muscle fiber-specific components (i.e., sarcomeres, sarcotubular system)

Each of these cytological components may give rise to pathological features. Sarcomeres are the backbone of the muscle fiber. They extend between two Z-discs and comprise the I-bands of actin filaments and A-bands of myosin filaments. These structures are both nicely visible when extended and—though blurred—when shortened by contraction. The classic sample is a somewhat stretched muscle that is immediately fixed in situ by a clamp extending the length of the muscle fiber. In this configuration, sarcomeres become apparent with conspicuously recognizable I-bands and A-bands (Fig. 9.1d).

9.3 Basic Pathology of the Skeletal Muscle

9.3.1 Macropathology

The spectrum of gross or macroscopic pathology is limited. It largely concerns two features: hypertrophy and atrophy. General hypertrophy is rare, encountered in congenital myotonia or myostatin deficiency. Local or focal hypertrophy is more frequent (e.g., hypertrophy of the calf). Most often, hypertrophy and atrophy are bilateral and symmetrical, only rarely being asymmetrical or unifocal. Focal hypertrophy is a characteristic feature of focal myositis, not infrequently misinterpreted as sarcoma. Atrophy of muscle bulk or parenchyma is more frequent, seen in the muscular dystrophies and especially after denervation.

Disregarding focal trauma to nerves, even generalized diseases causing secondary neurogenic or primary muscle involvement (as in muscular dystrophies) affect different muscles with unequal severity. This is brought out by subtle investigative techniques apart from clinical examination, an important one being myoimaging. Another type of gross pathology, seen at autopsy but locally also at biopsy, is change in color of muscle tissue owing to replacement of muscle parenchyma by fat and connective tissue. Muscle biopsy, not autopsy, is the most thorough investigative technique for learning about and recognizing the myopathology of a neuromuscular disease. A peculiar feature in gross but not microscopic myopathology is the developmental absence of an entire muscle, such as the pectoralis muscle (e.g. Poland's syndrome).

9.3.2 Histopathology

As already mentioned, both diagnostic and scientific data in myopathology have been obtained almost exclusively by muscle biopsy evaluation rather than at autopsy. Over the years, numerous methods have been applied, encompassing not only those addressing general histology but also enzyme histochemistry and immunohistochemistry. Electron microscopy has been a useful tool. This diversity of techniques requires special early prestaining preparations. It is mandatory that for light microscopy muscles remain unfixed and frozen. It further requires orientation of the muscle specimen to obtain cross-sectioned muscle fibers (Figs. 9.1 and 9.2) so the size of muscle fibers and their deviation toward hypertrophic or atrophic fibers can be assessed. Diversity and the panoply of employed investigative techniques, usually available only at specialized laboratories, have prompted the term "muscle biopsy program."

The muscle biopsy site has previously been selected according to the clinical examinations. However, muscles that are too lightly or too

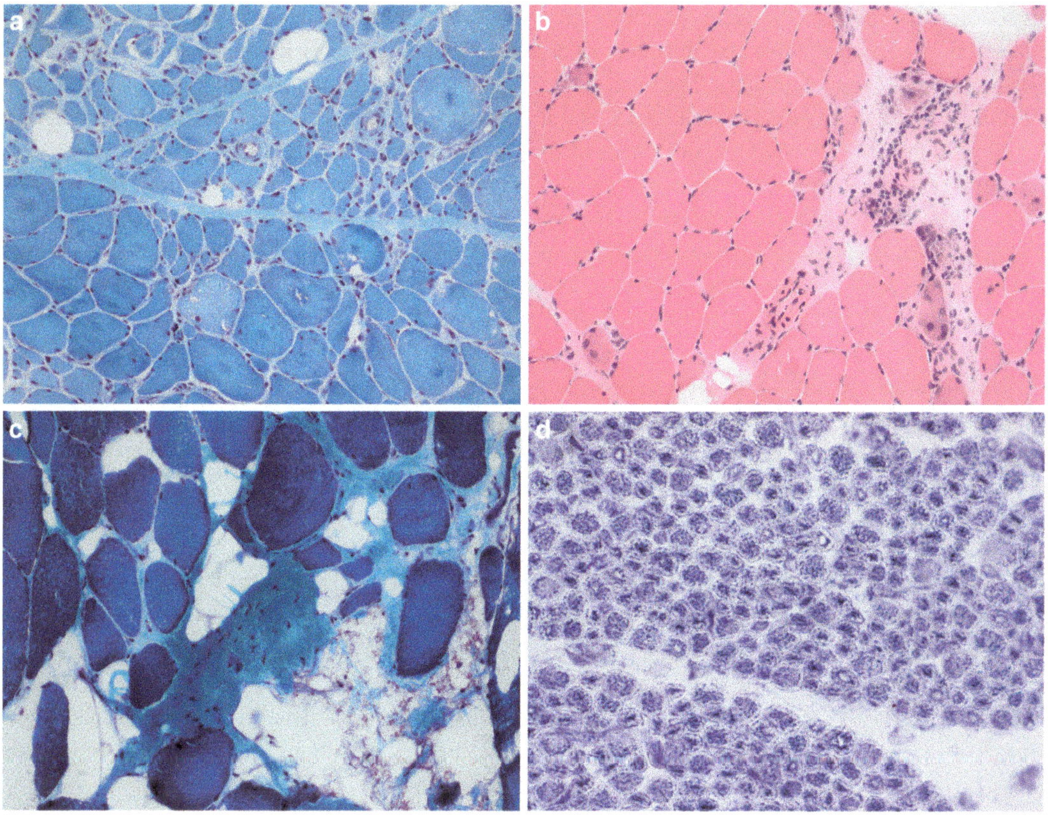

Fig. 9.2 Pathological patterns in skeletal muscle. (**a**) Neurogenic atrophy. Note the groups of polygonal atrophic muscle fibers (modified Gomori trichrome). (**b**) Dermatomyositis with inflammatory infiltrates, especially at the perimysium, and perifascicular atrophy of muscle fibers (H&E). (**c**) Muscular dystrophy with variation in fiber diameters, endomysial fibrosis, and fat cells replacing muscle cells (modified Gomori trichrome). (**d**) Myotubular myopathy in a newborn with small, round fibers displaying central enzyme activity in perinuclear halos or central areas devoid of enzyme activities where nuclei are situated (NADH preparation)

severely affected but in an intermediate range of dysfunction and pathology are more likely today to undergo muscular imaging. Whereas in the past only a limited number of biopsy sites were used—biceps, quadriceps, gastrocnemius, deltoid muscles, and recently axial muscles— imaging now identifies muscles suitable for biopsy based on the degree of involvement. Some of them are rather unusual muscles. Diagnostic needle biopsies are now performed that target a wide range of organs including muscle, especially in children. Stereotactically guided needle biopsy of unusually situated but affected muscles may be prompted by modern muscle imaging.

When properly processed, the myopathological diagnostic armamentarium can detect a wide range of changes in muscle parenchyma, although disease-specific changes are rare. Denervation and reinnervation produce a myopathological pattern of grouped atrophic muscle fibers (Fig. 9.2a), patterns of fibers consisting of one type only, and even patterns of fibers of normal (regrown) size.

Necrosis, followed by regeneration of muscle fibers, is a prominent feature in various groups of muscle diseases and individual diseases. Necrotic muscle fibers are scattered in metabolic diseases. They may form small groups in certain muscular dystrophies, and a perivascular arrangement may be a sign of dermatomyositis. Degeneration is often associated with formation of autophagic/rimmed vacuoles, and mitochondrial abnormalities are obvious from ragged red- and COX-negative muscle fibers. Hypertrophied muscle fibers may be evident because of their large diameters and hypotrophic or atrophic fibers because of their small diameters. The overall loss of muscle fibers in biopsied muscle tissue is not recognized because cross sections of entire muscles and counting of muscle fibers are not performed routinely during a diagnostic biopsy. Pyknotic nuclear clumps are residual evidence of nuclei in severely atrophic muscle fibers. They are the only evidence of profound muscle fiber atrophy.

Inflammatory myopathies (see Chap. 26) (Fig. 9.2b) and to a lesser extent many muscular dystrophies may show inflammatory cell infiltrates among the muscle fibers, often associated with intraparenchymal interstitial fluid accumulation. Necrosis of muscle fibers may add to this deviation from normal histology. With advanced muscle pathology, endomysial fibrosis and appearance of fat cells within fascicles may replace lost muscle fibers or may just indicate continuous damage and transformation of the muscle (Fig. 9.2c), finally resulting in an end-stage myopathy. With certain congenital myopathies (Fig. 9.2d), aggregates of fat cells among intrafascicular muscle fibers with little pathology may be characteristic, lacking a commensurate amount of endomysial fibrosis. Perifascicular or omnifascicular damage and atrophy may be evidence of dermatomyositis. With periodic paralysis abundant vacuoles may be present in muscle fibers, and with lipid myopathies there may be excessive amounts of lipid droplets in the muscle fibers as well. Hemorrhage with subsequent deposition of iron in muscle fascicles and/or calcification are rare myopathological events.

Because of the anatomical complexity and the inaccessibility to biopsy, little is known about the myopathology of extraocular muscles in comparison to that of limb muscles. Clinically, extraocular muscles are frequently affected because of their fine content and the vulnerability of mitochondria in extraocular muscle fibers. Another group of conditions largely affect the levator palpebrae in myasthenic conditions, the foremost being myasthenia gravis. During corrective surgery, occasionally a small sample of the levator palpebrae muscle is biopsied. These specimens usually reveal end-stage myopathy or only fibrosis. Hence, the involvement of extraocular muscles in neuromuscular disorders, other than mitochondrial and myasthenic conditions, has largely been detected at autopsy. Because of the structural (i.e., enzyme and immunohistochemical) complexity, normal controls are needed for comparison to assess true myopathology in an extraocular muscle properly. This is because enzyme and immunohistochemical activity and expression may alter along the length of an individual extraocular muscle fiber. Ignorance about the myopathology of neuromuscular diseases is also on display in regard to the diaphragm. Again, the diaphragmatic muscle is sampled only at autopsies.

9.3.3 Ultrastructural Pathology

Z-disc pathology, a feature of nemaline myopathies (see Chap. 15.6 and 15.7), encompasses the formation of rods, which often cluster underneath the plasma membrane. Occasionally, they occur within nuclei. "Smearing/streaming" of the Z-band and its electron-dense material extends from the Z-band into the adjacent I-band. Such streaming may be confined to one or several scattered sarcomeres or may spread continuously among successive sarcomeres. When it involves several vicinal sarcomeres and mitochondria are absent, cores may form. Small, disseminated cores are called multi-minicores. Larger ones are often located in the center of the muscle fiber along a considerable length of the long axis of the fiber. They are called central cores or, as a morphological variant, eccentric cores. These are the "nonstructured" cores. In contrast, "structured" cores show an absence of mitochondria, their sarcomeric details are preserved, and they are different from the surrounding sarcomeres in both length and in width. They are distinguishable from peripherally located sarcomeres, the morphological lighthouse of core myopathies. Further destruction of the integrity of sarcomeres may result in myofibrillar lesions, another hallmark of myofibrillar myopathies.

Depletion of myofilaments results in attenuation of sarcomeres, such as after denervation. Selective depletion of thick myosin filaments is a hallmark of acute quadriplegic myopathy or critical illness myopathy, an acquired and reversible lesion caused by treatment with steroids or respiration-depressing drugs such as succinylcholine. Destroying the structural integrity of sarcomeres in myofibrils may also result in extralysosomal aggregation of cellular proteins. The existence of some proteins within abnormal aggregates in muscle fibers may become apparent only with such aggregation, for instance β-amyloid, amyloid-precursor protein, or prion protein.

The sarcotubular system may also give rise to variegated ultrastructural pathology. It consists of transverse tubules, an extracellular labyrinthous network of the extracellular space in the multinucleated muscle fiber, and a separate intracellular tubular network that meets transverse tubules at the triads of the terminal sacs. Swelling and enlargement of terminal sacs is a conspicuous feature of certain channelopathies and periodic paralysis. Aggregation of transverse tubules leads to the formation of honeycomb structures with aggregation of the terminal sacs into tubular aggregates of various ultrastructual forms.

The shape of nuclei, normally ovoid or spheroid, may be crenated and lobulated to the point of sarcoplasmic invagination. Intranuclear filaments may accrue (e.g., in oculopharyngeal muscular dystrophy or in a tubulofilamentous pattern) and, when aggregated, as inclusions in inclusion body myositis/myopathy or as intranuclear rods. The latter have been observed in nemaline myopathy (NEM3) owing to mutations in the *ACTA1* gene (see Sect. 15.6) in adult-type nemaline myopathy and in myotilinopathy (see Sect. 20.4) and ZASPopathy (see Sect. 20.6). When situated away from the usual subsarcolemmal position, nuclei may be surrounded by a sarcomere-free halo of mitochondria and sarcoplasm, especially when located at the center of muscle fibers, as in centronuclear myopathies. Nuclei may be large in regenerating muscle fibers and in early-onset myotubular myopathy.

Defects in the plasma membrane are basic features in certain muscular dystrophies (e.g., dysferlinopathy or Duchenne muscular dystrophy (see Chap. 17). In caveolinopathy (see Sect. 19.5), another limb-girdle muscular dystrophy, subsarcolemmal caveolae or vacuoles are the pathological target. Reduplication of the overlying basal lamina may indicate regeneration when forming large loops, and focal segments are seen in autophagic vacuoles with sarolemmal features. In the latter, vacuoles situated deeper inside the muscle fiber may be delimited by the plasma membrane and the basal lamina, indicating some association with the external sarcolemma. The vacuoles may be seen in glycogenoses when sarcoplasmic glycogen accumulates because of degradative failure or within lysosomes in acid maltase deficiency. Autophagic vacuoles may be associated with type II glycogenosis and many other conditions, among them myofibrillar myopathies, inclusion body myositis/myopathy, distal myopathies, and occasionally neurogenic atrophy. Mitochondria are normally scattered across the muscle fiber and form small clusters underneath the plasma membrane. They may proliferate and then form conspicuous subsarcolemmal aggregates or even ragged red fibers. Then, mitochondria may increase in size, vary in shape, and contain abnormally arranged cristae with crystalline inclusions.

Finally, other than the inclusions derived from preexisting organelles or structural components (e.g., rods, tubular aggregates), inclusions such as cylindrical spirals, fingerprint bodies, Zebra bodies, and concentric laminated bodies are still of unknown origin. Some give rise to forms of myopathy. In other instances, inclusion-like patches or plaques form in muscle fibers, such as hyaline bodies consisting of nonfibrillar myosin in hyaline body myopathy due to mutations in the *MYH7* gene. Furthermore, small aggregates of actin filaments in filamentous bodies or larger aggregates of actin filaments in actin filament aggregate myopathy arise because of mutations in the *ACTA1* gene. Caps—subsarcolemmal plaques consisting of fragmentary sarcomeres composed only of Z-discs and biliateral I-bands—are the nosologic basis of cap myopathy/disease.

Neuromuscular junctions are recognized by coincidence or by a targeting motor biopsy. Their pathology is characterized by an absence of terminal axons, the presence of denervation and thus neurogenic atrophy, or flattening of the subneural apparatus (in myasthenia gravis and certain congenital myasthenic syndromes).

Beyond muscle fibers, capillaries may give rise to ultrastructural pathology, such as the destruction and regeneration of endothelial cells, endothelial inclusions (e.g., undulating tubules in dermatomyositis or pathological lysosomal residual bodies in lysosomal diseases), and thickening of the capillary basement membrane up to the appearance of pipestems. Connective tissue may be increased by deposition of collagen fibrils and increased presence of fibroblasts among muscle fibers. Like capillaries, muscle fibers are sometimes surrounded by inflammatory interstitial cells in the presence of an inflammatory myopathy.

Morphology of Skeletal Muscle

Key Points

- Skeletal muscle makes up the largest organ of the body (> 40 %).
- Fibers of types I, IIa, and IIb correspond to slow-twitch and fast-twitch fibers. Distribution of fiber types may vary considerably among muscles.
- Muscle fibers contain two major groups of components: those that occur with other cell types and muscle fiber-specific components, such as sarcomeres and the sarcotubular system.
- The spectrum of gross or macroscopic pathology largely concerns two features: hypertrophy and atrophy.
- A wide range of histopathological changes occur in muscle parenchyma, although disease-specific changes are rare.
- Pathological ultrastructural changes can arise from all cellular components (e.g., defects in the plasma membrane, nuclei, mitochondria, sarcomeres, and sarcotubular system).

Suggestions for Further Reading

Banker BQ, Engel AG. Basic reactions of muscle (chapter 30). In: Engel AG, Franzini-Armstrong C, editors. Myology: basic and clinical, 3rd edn. New York: McGraw-Hill; 2004. p. 691–747.

Dubowitz V, Sewry, CA. Muscle biopsy: a practical approach, 3rd edn. Philadelphia: Saunders Elsevier; 2007.

Engel AG. The muscle biopsy (chapter 29). In: Engel AG, Franzini-Armstrong C, editors. Myology: basic and clinical. 3rd ed. New York: McGraw-Hill; 2004. p. 681–90.

Engel AG, Banker BQ. Ultrastructural changes in diseased muscle (chapter 31). In: Engel AG, Franzini-Armstrong C, editors. Myology: basic and clinical, 3rd edn. New York: McGraw-Hill; 2004. p. 749–887.

Karpati G, Hilton-Jones D, Bushby K, et al. editors. Disorders of voluntary muscle. 7th edn. Cambridge: Cambridge University Press; 2010.

Websites of Use

Online gene table database: http://www.musclegenetable.org

MITOMAP: a human mitochondrial genome database: http://www.mitomap.org/MITOMAP

Neuromuscular Disease Center, Washington University School of Medicine, St. Louis, MO: http://www.neuro.wustl.edu/neuromuscular

Atlas of Topographical Muscle Anatomy

10

Arne Fischmann and Christopher D.J. Sinclair

10.1 Introduction

The aim of this chapter is to provide a topographical guideline for identifying muscles involved in neuromuscular disorders. The scope of the volume cannot include a complete anatomical description of all structures visible on the images. We have therefore decided not to label bones, vessels, nerves and internal organs if they appear on the imaging slices.

All imaging was performed on a clinical 3T scanner with variable spine array and body array coils, depending on the region scanned, as well as peripheral angiography coils for the legs. The subject for this atlas was a healthy 40-year-old male with a moderately obese constitution and a mainly sedentary lifestyle. Axial T1-weighted images were acquired for all body regions as these are currently the standard for neuromuscular imaging.

When evaluating neuromuscular images and especially when assessing fatty replacement/degeneration in muscles, the reader should always be aware of the great variability between muscles in healthy adults. In addition, imaging parameters such as the slice thickness and resolution can influence the appearance of fatty streaks in the slice (Fig. 10.1).

10.2 Neck and Cervical Spine

Imaging of the neck is challenging due to the high variability of the anatomy. Exact reproduction of slice positioning is essential, especially for follow-up studies, otherwise even large muscles like the trapezius can change from the muscle bulk to a small linear configuration in the image.

In most clinical routine MRI examinations, it is difficult to separate the different components of the spinal muscles from each other. As these form a functional unit, it is common to refer to them collectively as the erector spinae muscles. It is also important to realise that degenerative diseases of the spine e.g. herniated discs and immobility can cause localized atrophy of the paraspinal muscles without clinical symptoms (Figs. 10.2, 10.3, and 10.4).

10.3 Shoulder, Upper Arm and Thoracic Wall

Muscle volume in the shoulder girdle and upper arm is especially variable depending on training state and lifestyle. In addition, degenerative disease, especially in elderly patients, can lead to atrophy and fatty replacement which might

A. Fischmann, M.D. (✉)
Department of Radiology, University of Basel Hospital, 4031 Basel, Switzerland
e-mail: arne.fischmann@unibas.ch

C.D.J. Sinclair
MRC Centre for Neuromuscular Diseases, UCL Institute of Neurology, London, UK

M.P. Wattjes and D. Fischer (eds.), *Neuromuscular Imaging*, DOI 10.1007/978-1-4614-6552-2_10,

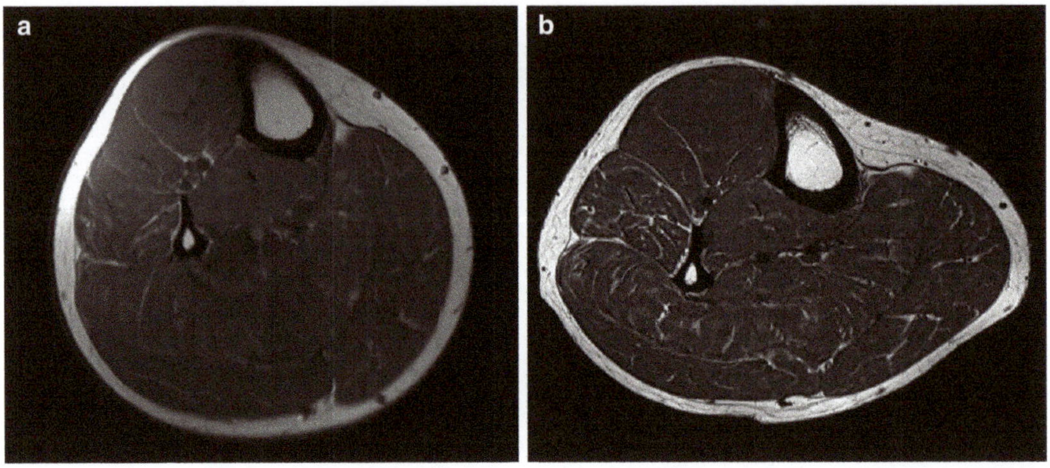

Fig. 10.1 Images of the calf with a slice thickness of 3 mm (**a**) and with a reduced slice thickness of 1 mm (**b**). The extent of fatty replacement in **b** appears to be higher. There is also deformation and compression of the calf in (**b**) due to the use of a knee coil

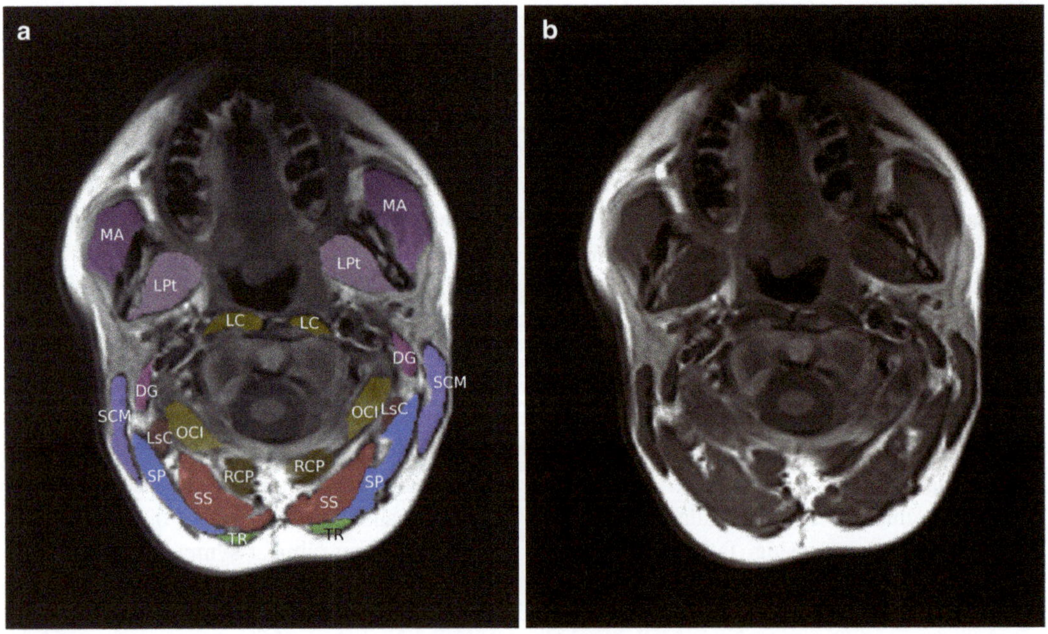

Fig. 10.2 Neck muscles at the level of C1/C2. *DG* digastric muscle, *LC* longus colli muscle, *LsC* longissimus colli, *LPt* lateral pterygoid muscle, *MA* masticator muscle, *OCI* obliquus capitis inferior muscle, *RCP* rectus capitis posterior muscle, *SCM* sternocleidomastoid muscle, *SP* splenius capitis, *SS* semispinalis capitis and cervicis, *TR* trapezius muscle

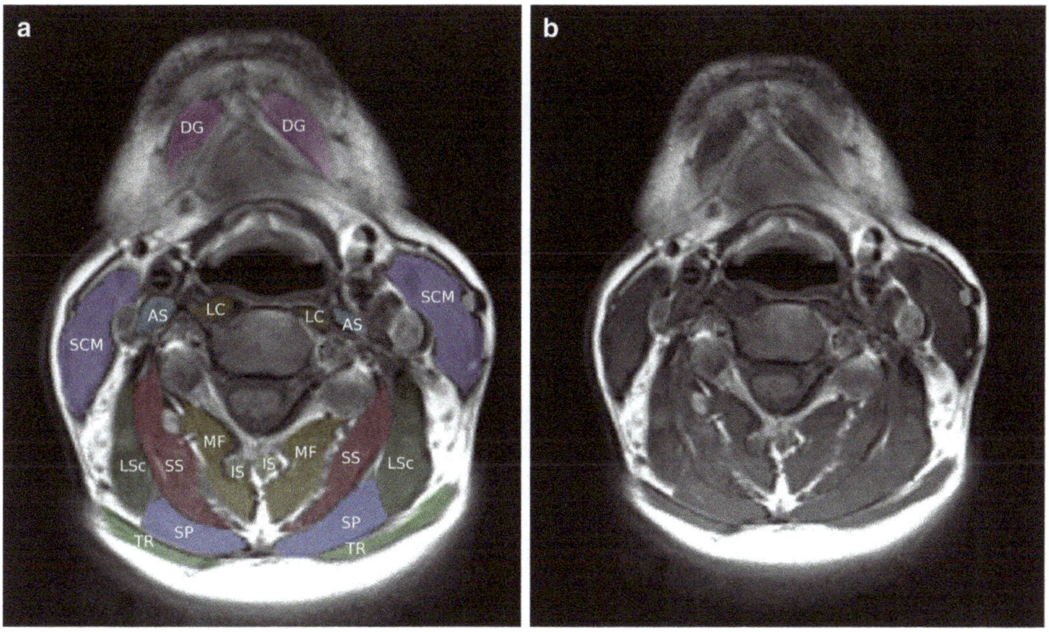

Fig. 10.3 Neck muscles at the level of the hyoid (C3). *AS* anterior scalenus muscle, *DG* digastric muscle; *IS* interspinosus muscle, *LC* longus colli muscle, *LSc* levator scapulae muscle, *MF* multifidus muscle, *SCM* sternocleidomastoid muscle, *SP* splenius capitis, *SS* semispinalis cervicis, *TR* trapezius muscle

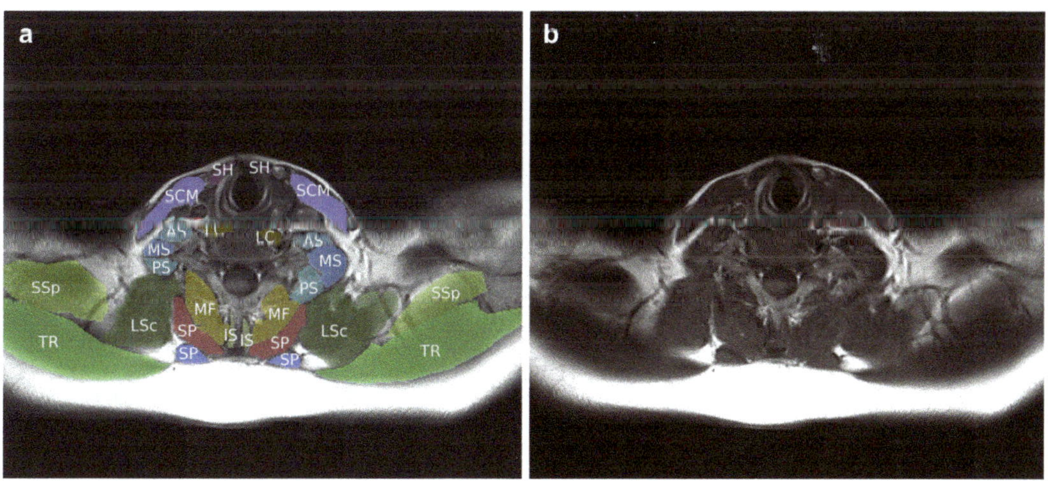

Fig. 10.4 Neck muscles at the level of C6/C7. *AS* anterior scalenus muscle, *IS* interspinosus muscle, *LC* longus colli muscle, *LSc* levator scapulae muscle, *MF* multifidus muscle, *MS* middle scalenus muscle, *PS* posterior scalenus muscle, *SCM* sternocleidomastoid muscle, *SH* sternohyoid muscle, *SP* splenius capitis/cervicis muscle, *SSp* supraspinatus muscle, *TR* trapezius muscle

be misinterpreted as neuromuscular disease involvement. Muscles especially prone to degenerative atrophy are the supraspinatus and the subscapularis.

The deltoid muscle will usually present with multiple small T1-hyperintensities which should not be misinterpreted as fatty replacement/degeneration (Figs. 10.5, 10.6, 10.7, 10.8, 10.9, 10.10, and 10.11).

10.4 Forearm

When imaging and evaluating the muscles of the forearm, special attention should be given to the amount of pronation or supination as these will not only influence anatomy but also muscle tension and therefore cross sectional area. In most scanners, optimal positioning of the arm in the

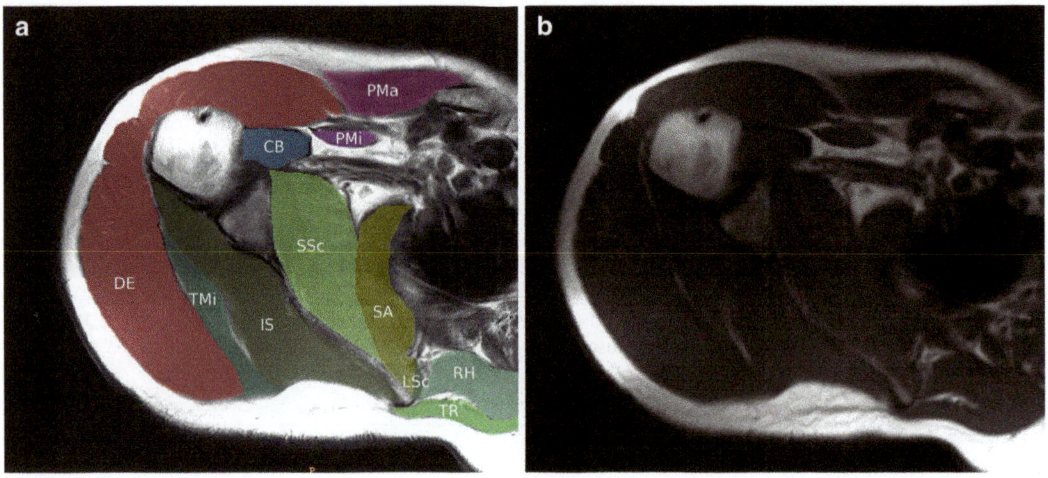

Fig. 10.5 Shoulder muscles at the level Th2. *CB* coracobrachialis muscle, *DE* deltoid muscle, *IS* infraspinatus muscle, *LSc* levator scapulae muscle, *PMa* pectoralis major muscle, *PMi* pectoralis minor muscle, *RH* rhomboideus muscle, *SA* serratus anterior muscle, *SSc* subscapularis muscle, *TMi* teres minor muscle, *TR* trapezius muscle

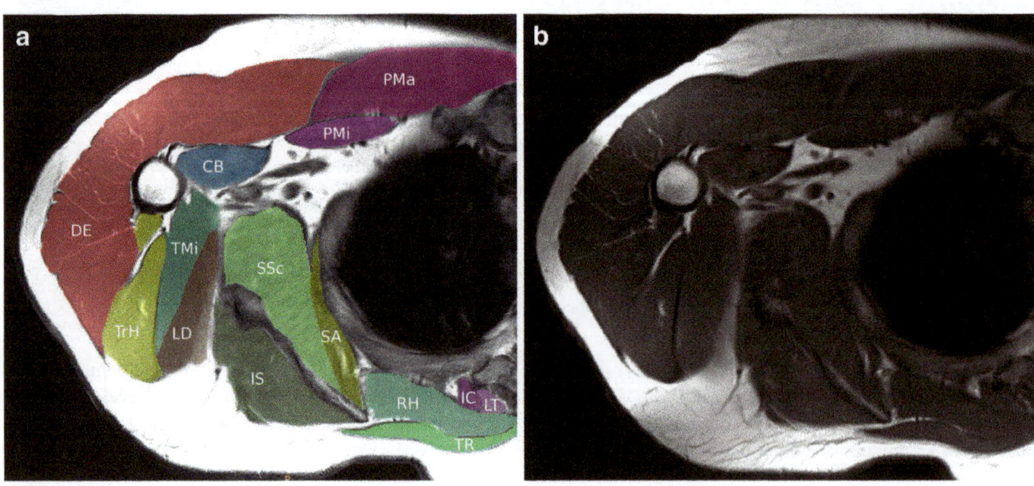

Fig. 10.6 Shoulder muscles at the level Th4. *CB* coracobrachialis muscle, *DE* deltoid muscle, *IC* iliocostalis lumborum muscle, *IS* infraspinatus muscle, *LD* latissimus dorsi muscle, *LSc* levator scapulae muscle, *LT* longissimus thoracis muscle, *MF* multifidus muscle, *PMa* pectoralis major muscle, *PMi* pectoralis minor muscle, *RH* rhomboideus muscle, *SA* serratus anterior muscle, *SSc* subscapularis muscle, *TMi* teres minor muscle, *TR* trapezius muscle, *TrH* triceps humeri muscle

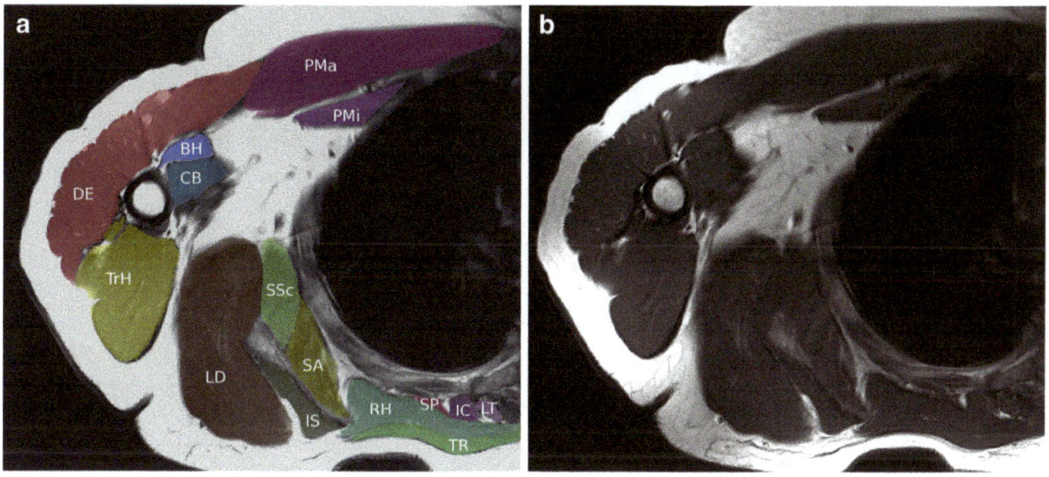

Fig. 10.7 Shoulder muscles at the level Th6. *BH* biceps humeri muscle, *CB* coracobrachialis muscle, *DE* deltoid muscle, *IC* iliocostalis lumborum muscle, *IS* infraspinatus muscle, *LD* latissimus dorsi muscle, *LT* longissimus thoracis muscle, *PMa* pectoralis major muscle, *PMi* pectoralis minor muscle, *RH* rhomboideus muscle, *SA* serratus anterior muscle, *SP* serratus posterior muscle, *SSc* subscapularis muscle, *TR* trapezius muscle, *TrH* triceps humeri muscle

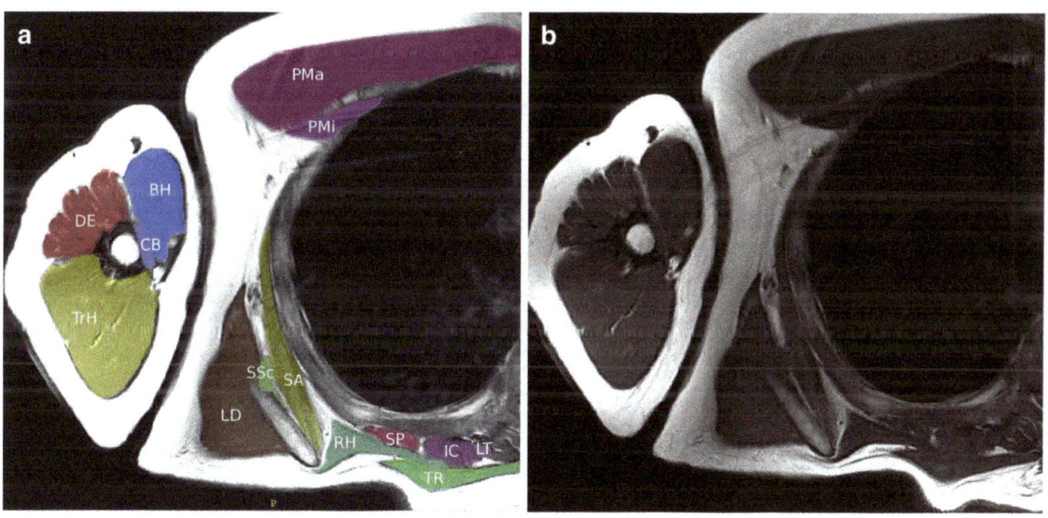

Fig. 10.8 Muscles of the upper arm and thoracic wall. *BH* biceps humeri muscle, *CB* coracobrachialis muscle, *DE* deltoid muscle, *IC* iliocostalis lumborum muscle, *IS* infraspinatus muscle, *LD* latissimus dorsi muscle, *LT* longissimus thoracis muscle, *PMa* pectoralis major muscle, *PMi* pectoralis minor muscle, *RH* rhomboideus muscle, *SA* serratus anterior muscle, *SP* serratus posterior muscle, *SSc* subscapularis muscle, *TR* trapezius muscle, *TrH* triceps humeri muscle

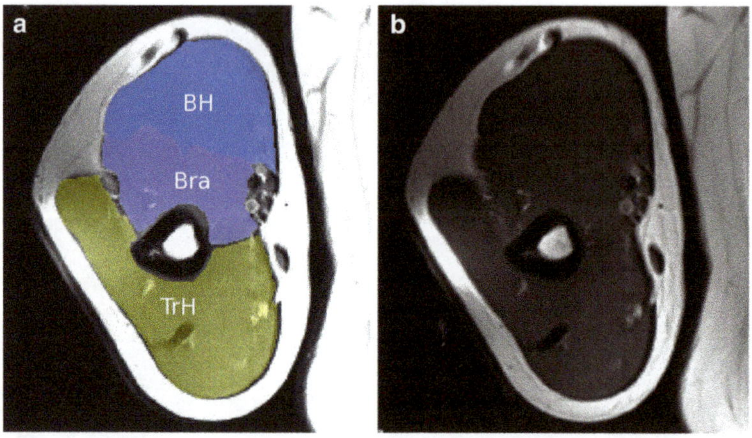

Fig. 10.9 Muscles of the upper arm. *BH* biceps humeri muscle, *Bra* brachialis muscle, *TrH* triceps humeri muscle

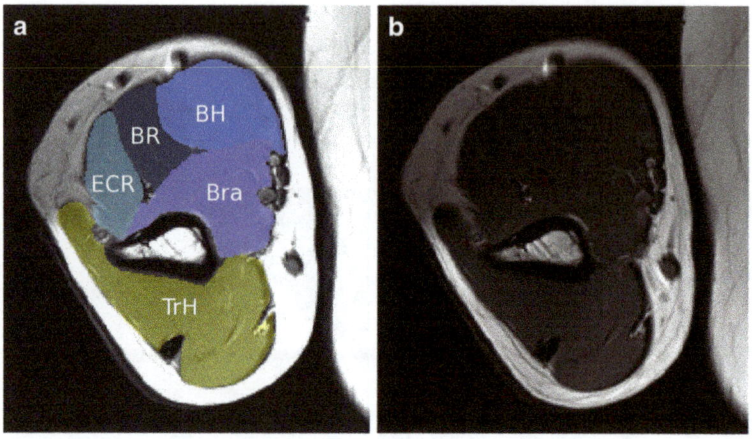

Fig. 10.10 Muscles of the distal upper arm. *BH* biceps humeri muscle, *BR* brachioradial muscle, *Bra* brachialis muscle, *ECR* extensor carpi radialis muscle, *TrH* triceps humeri muscle

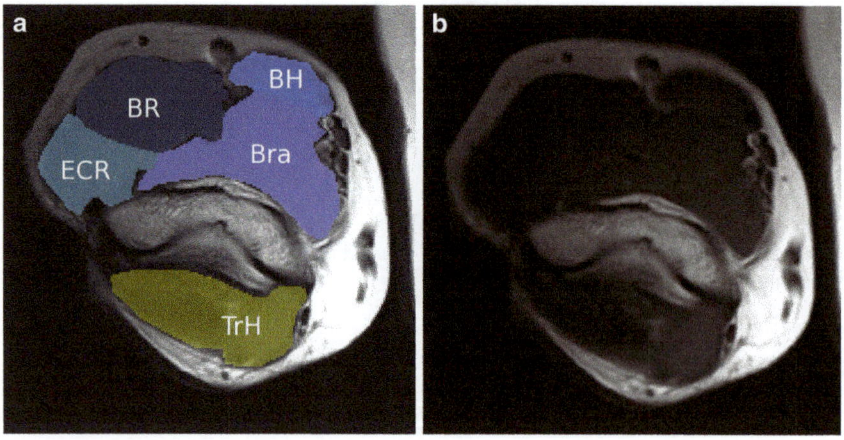

Fig. 10.11 Muscles of the distal upper arm above the elbow. *BH* biceps humeri muscle, *BR* brachioradial muscle, *Bra* brachialis muscle, *ECR* extensor carpi radialis muscle, *TrH* triceps humeri muscle

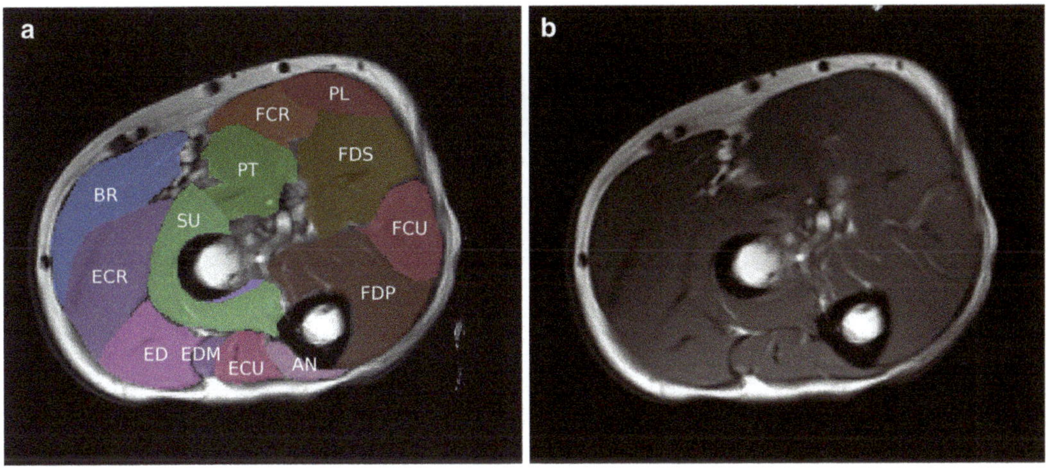

Fig. 10.12 Muscles of the proximal forearm. *AN* anconeus muscle, *BR* brachioradial uscle, *ECR* extensor carpi radialis muscle, *ECU* extensor carpi ulnaris muscle, *ED* extensor digitorum muscle, *EDM* extensor digiti minimi muscle, *FCR* flexor carpi radialis muscle, *FCU* flexor carpi ulnaris muscle, *FDP* flexor digitorum profundus muscle, *FDS* flexor digitorum superficialis muscle, *PL* palmaris longus muscle, *PT* pronator teres muscle, *SU* supinator muscle

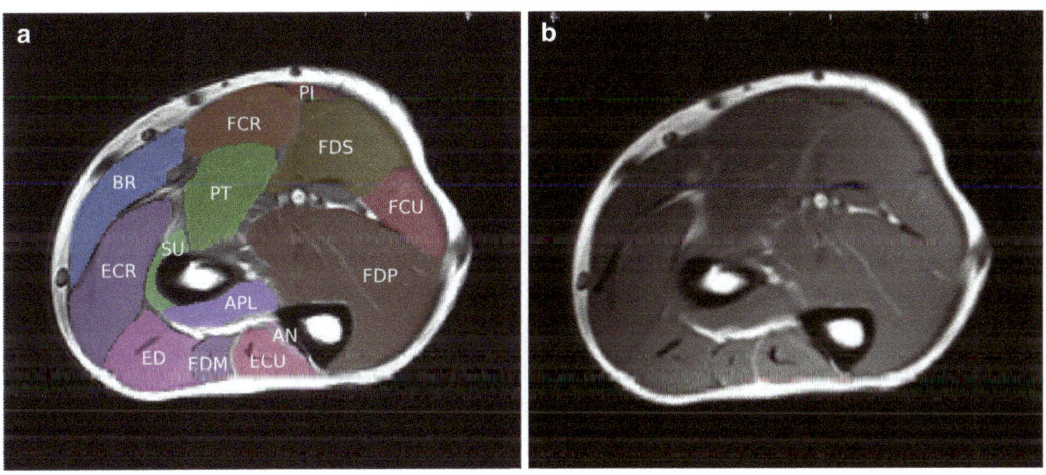

Fig. 10.13 Muscles of the proximal forearm. *AN anconeus muscle*, *APL* abductor pollicis longus muscle, *BR* brachioradial muscle, *ECR* extensor carpi radialis muscle, *ECU* extensor carpi ulnaris muscle, *ED* extensor digitorum muscle, *EDM* extensor digiti minimi muscle, *FCR* flexor carpi radialis muscle, *FCU* flexor carpi ulnaris muscle, *FDP* flexor digitorum profundus muscle, *FDS* flexor digitorum superficialis muscle, *PL* palmaris longus muscle, *PT* pronator teres muscle

centre of the bore requires either a supine position with the arm elevated over the head, or a position with the arm along the body and the patient moved outside the centre of the magnet. As both positioning methods are uncomfortable for the patient, imaging of the forearm is usually restricted to those cases with predominant forearm involvement.

Apart from some smaller muscles like the pronator quadratus, most muscles of the forearm run parallel to the bones and small variations in positioning will have less influence than in the neck or the pelvis. However, the distal third of the forearm mainly contains tendons. Imaging can therefore be limited to the proximal parts (Figs. 10.12, 10.13, 10.14, and 10.15).

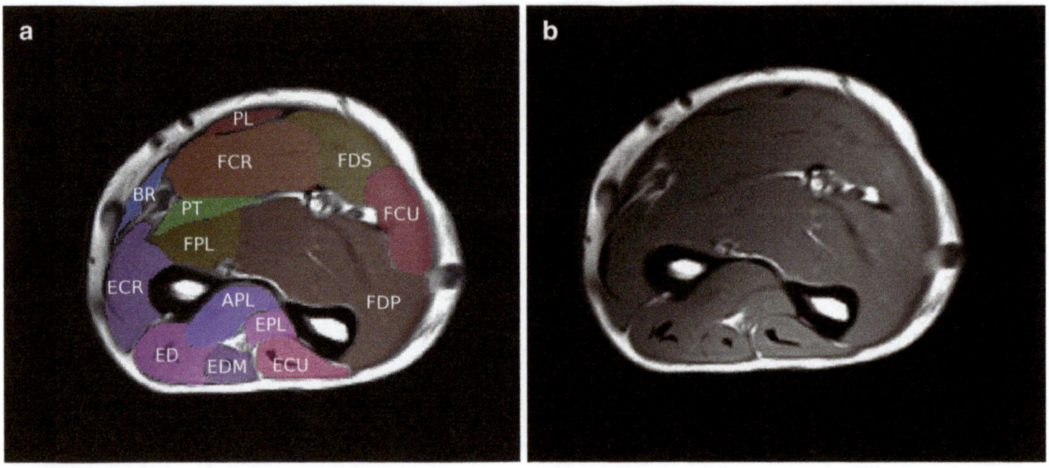

Fig. 10.14 Muscles of the forearm. *APL* abductor pollicis longus muscle, *BR* brachioradial muscle, *ECR* extensor carpi radialis muscle, *ECU* extensor carpi ulnaris muscle, *ED* extensor digitorum muscle, *EDM* extensor digiti minimi muscle, *EPL* extensor pollicis longus muscle, *FCR* flexor carpi radialis muscle, *FCU* flexor carpi ulnaris muscle, *FDP* flexor digitorum profundus muscle, *FDS* flexor digitorum superficialis muscle, *FPL* flexor pollicis longus muscle, *PL* palmaris longus muscle, *PT* pronator teres muscle

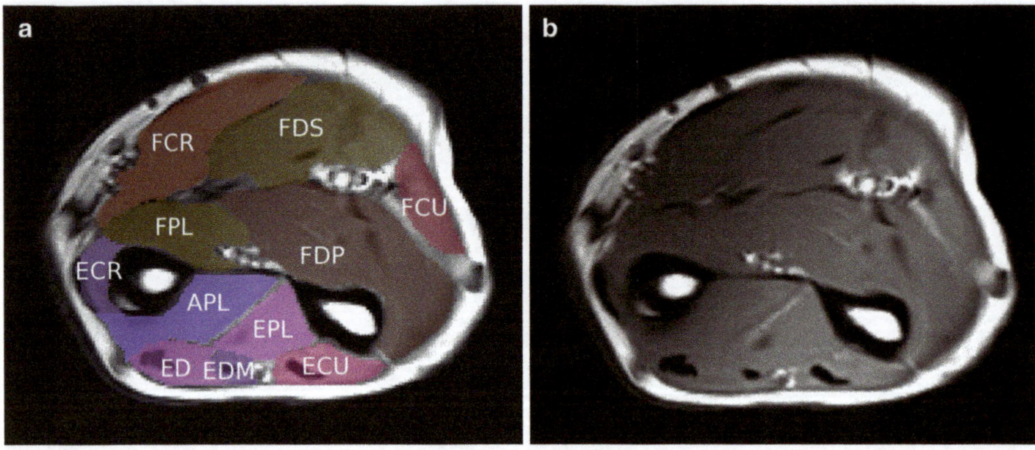

Fig. 10.15 Muscles of the distal forearm. *APL* abductor pollicis longus muscle, *ECR* extensor carpi radialis muscle, *ECU* extensor carpi ulnaris muscle, *ED* extensor digitorum muscle, *EDM*, extensor digiti minimi muscle, *EPL*, extensor pollicis longus muscle, *FCR* flexor carpi radialis muscle, *FCU* flexor carpi ulnaris muscle, *FDP* flexor digitorum profundus muscle, *FDS* flexor digitorum superficialis muscle, *FPL* flexor pollicis longus muscle, *PT* pronator teres muscle

10.5 Lower Abdomen and Pelvis

Muscles of the pelvis and the hip often take a horizontal course and therefore appear highly variable depending on slice positioning in the axial plane. It might therefore be useful to acquire coronal images in selected patients depending on the clinical purpose.

As with the thigh, several muscles of the pelvis will display greater amounts of intramuscular fat even in slim healthy adults. These include the gluteus maximus and the tensor fascia lata muscles especially. The gluteus

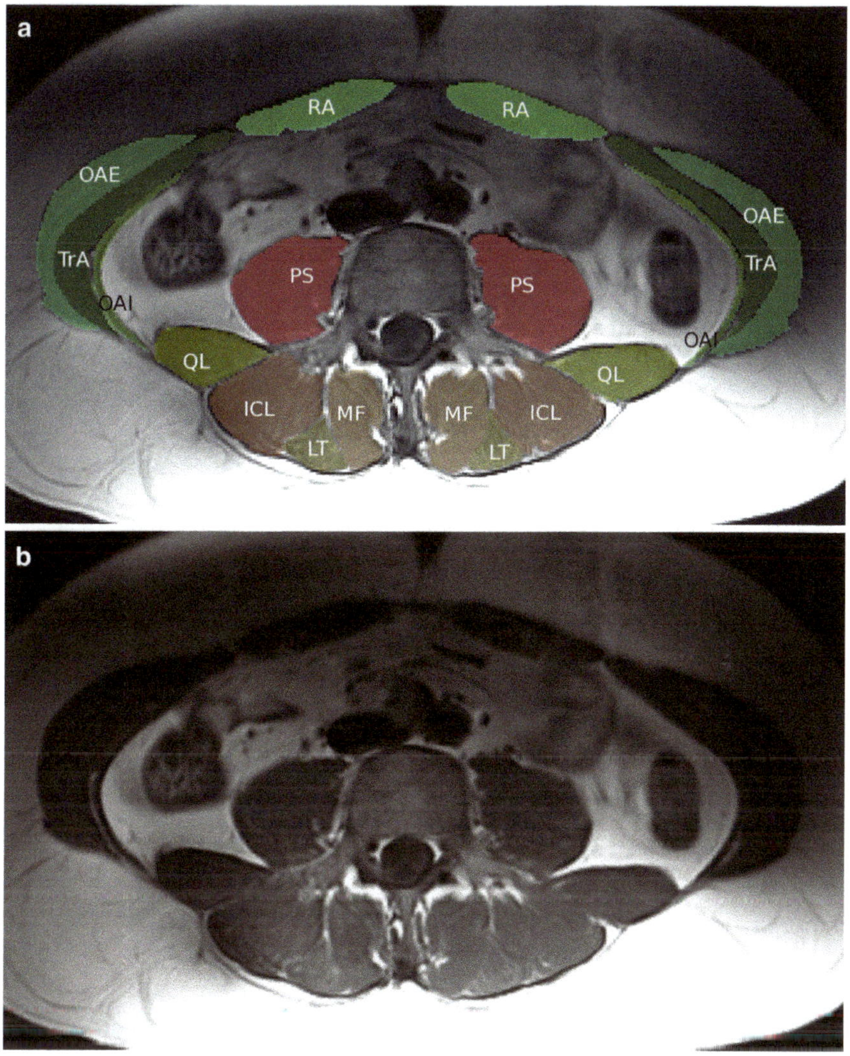

Fig. 10.16 Muscles of the abdominal wall and lumbar spine. *ICL* iliocostalis lumborum muscle, *LT* longissimus thoracis muscle, *MF* multifidus muscle, *OAE* obliquus abdominis externus muscle, *OAI* obliquus abdominis internus muscle, *PS* psoas muscle, *QL* quadratus lumborum muscle, *RA* rectus abdominis muscle, *TrA* transversus abdominis muscle

minimus and medius might also display regional fatty atrophy due to degenerative changes of the hip joint.

Currently there are only few reports of muscular involvement of the pelvis in neuromuscular disease. However, with increasing use of whole body MRI scans, we can expect further patterns to be described in the near future (Figs. 10.16, 10.17, 10.18, 10.19, 10.20, and 10.21).

10.6 Thigh

When evaluating muscles of the thigh, it is especially important to compare any fatty replacement with observations in healthy volunteers as there can be a great variation in the appearance of fatty streaks in specific thigh muscles: e.g. the amount of fat that can be seen in a healthy glutaeus maximus would be abnormal in the quadriceps.

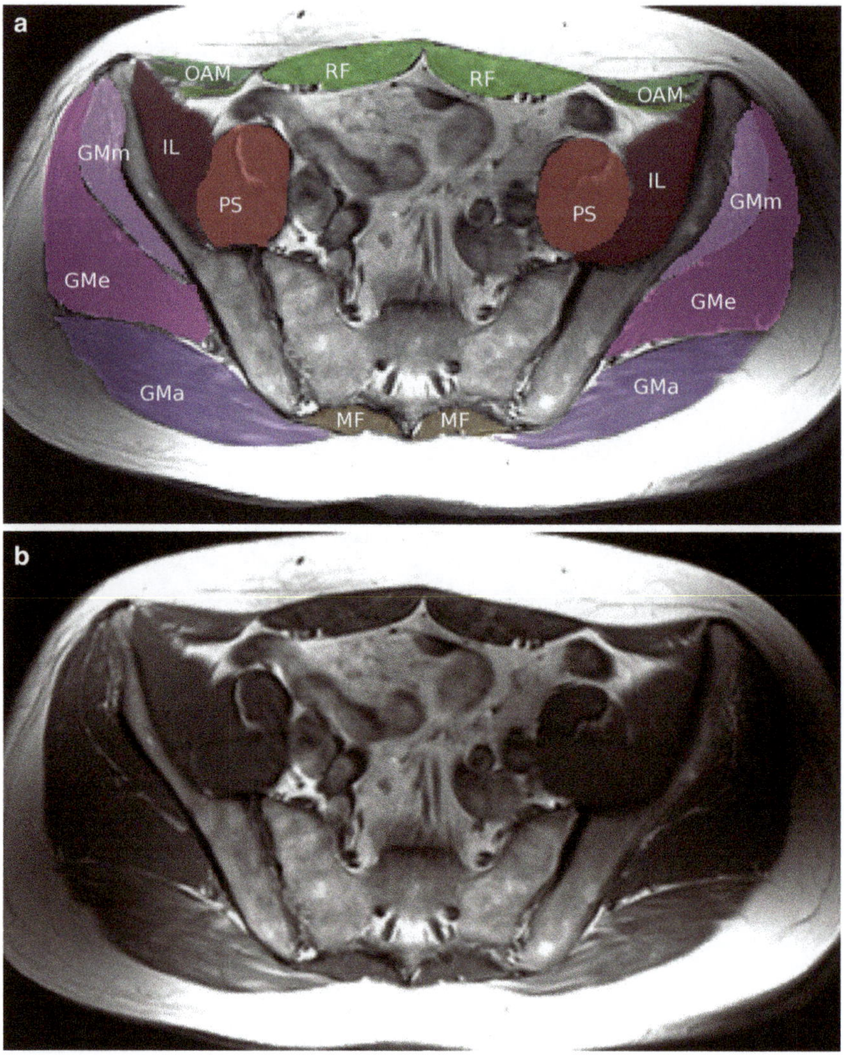

Fig. 10.17 Muscles of the abdominal wall and pelvis. *GMa* glutaeus maximus muscle; *GMe* glutaeus medius muscle; *GMm* glutaeus minimus muscle; *IL* iliacus muscle; *LT* longissimus thoracis muscle; *MF* multifidus muscle; *OAM* obliquus abdominis externus, internus and transversus abdominis muscles; *PS* psoas muscle; *RA* rectus abdominis muscle

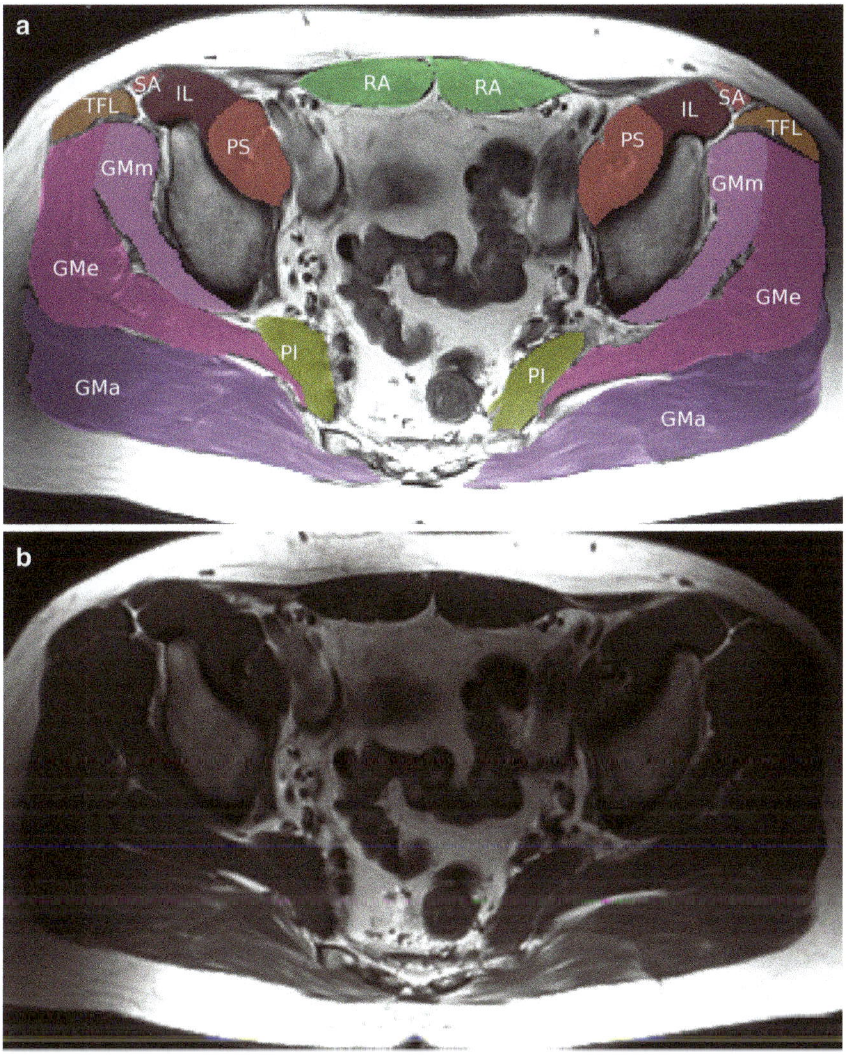

Fig. 10.18 Muscles of the pelvis. *GMa* glutaeus maximus muscle; *GMe* glutaeus medius muscle; *GMm* glutaeus minimus muscle; *IL* iliacus muscle; *LT* longissimus thoracis muscle; *OAM* obliquus abdominis externus, internus and transversus abdominis muscles; *PI* piriformis muscle; *PS* psoas muscle; *RA* rectus abdominis muscle; *SA* sartorius muscle; *TFL* tensor fasciae latae

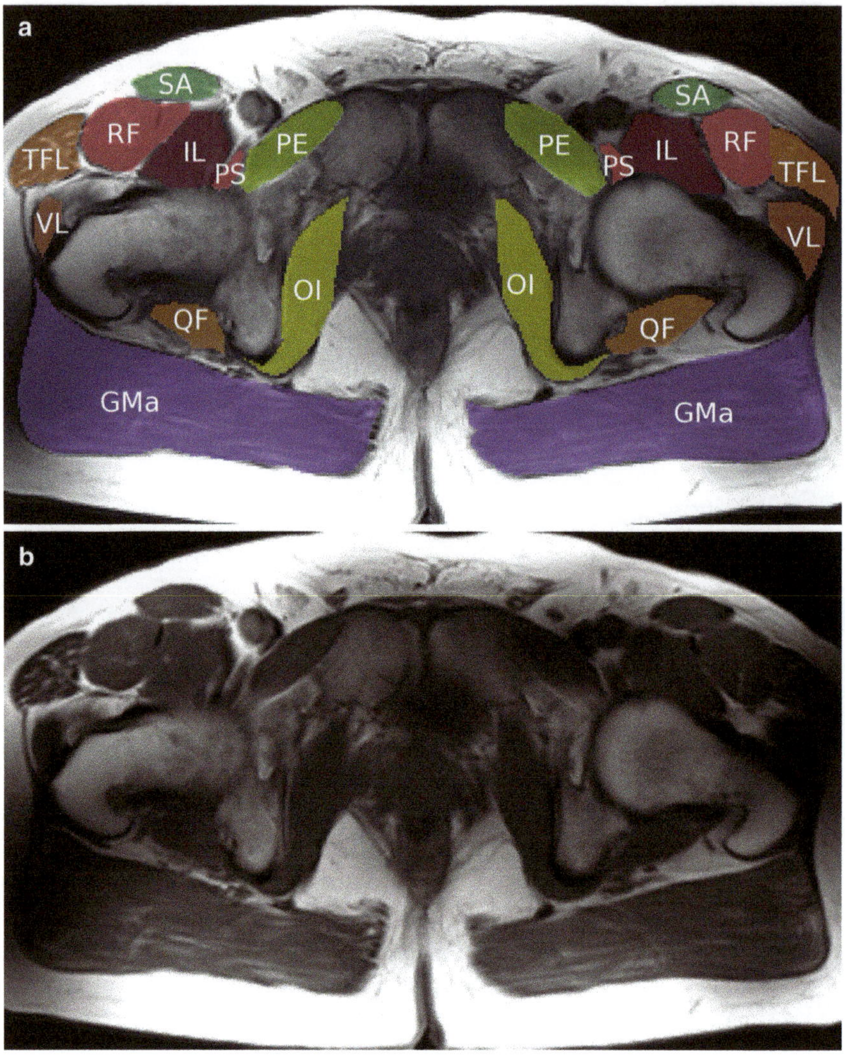

Fig. 10.19 Muscles of the pelvis. *GMa* glutaeus maximus muscle, *IL* iliacus muscle, *OI* obturator internus muscle, *PE* pectineus muscle, *PS* psoas muscle, *QF* quadratus femoris, *RF* rectus femoris muscle, *SA* sartorius muscle, *TFL* tensor fasciae latae, *VL* vastus lateralis muscle

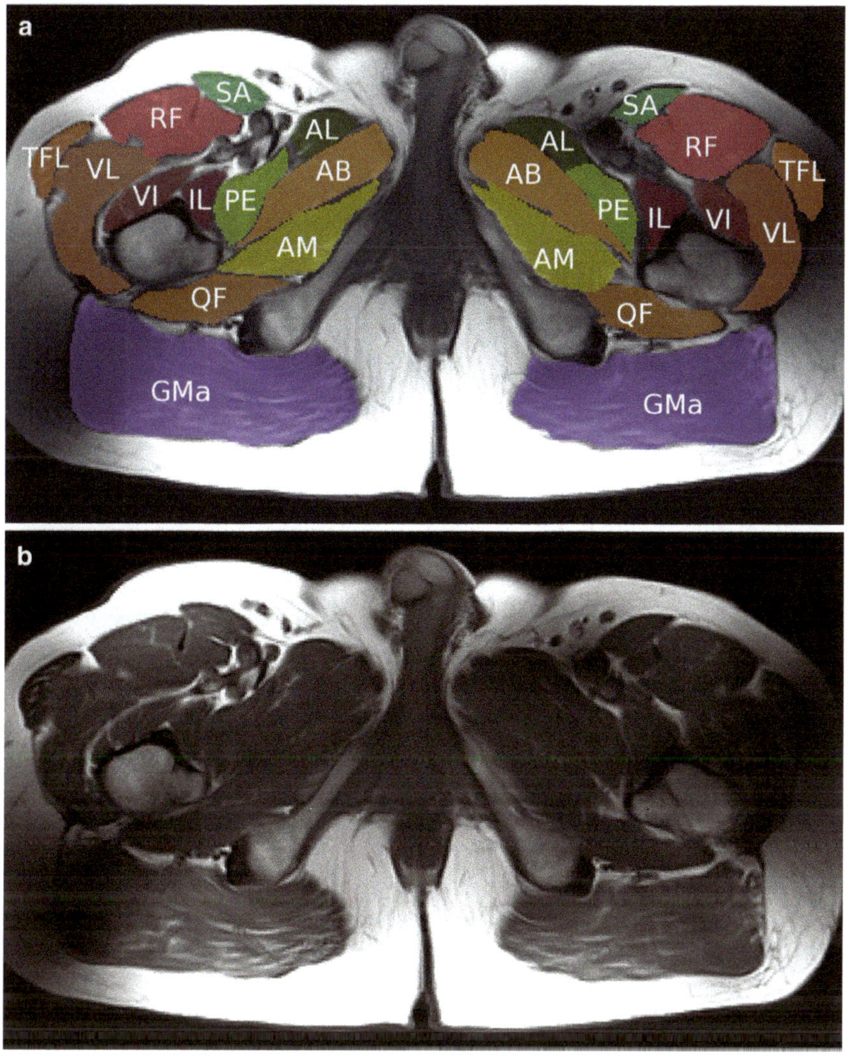

Fig. 10.20 Muscles of the pelvis. *AB* adductor brevis muscle, *AL* adductor longus muscle, *AM* adductor magnus muscle, *GMa* glutaeus maximus muscle, *IL* iliacus muscle, *PE* pectineus muscle, *QF* quadratus femoris, *RF* rectus femoris muscle, *SA* sartorius muscle, *TFL* tensor fasciae latae, *VI* vastus intermedius muscle, *VL* vastus lateralis muscle

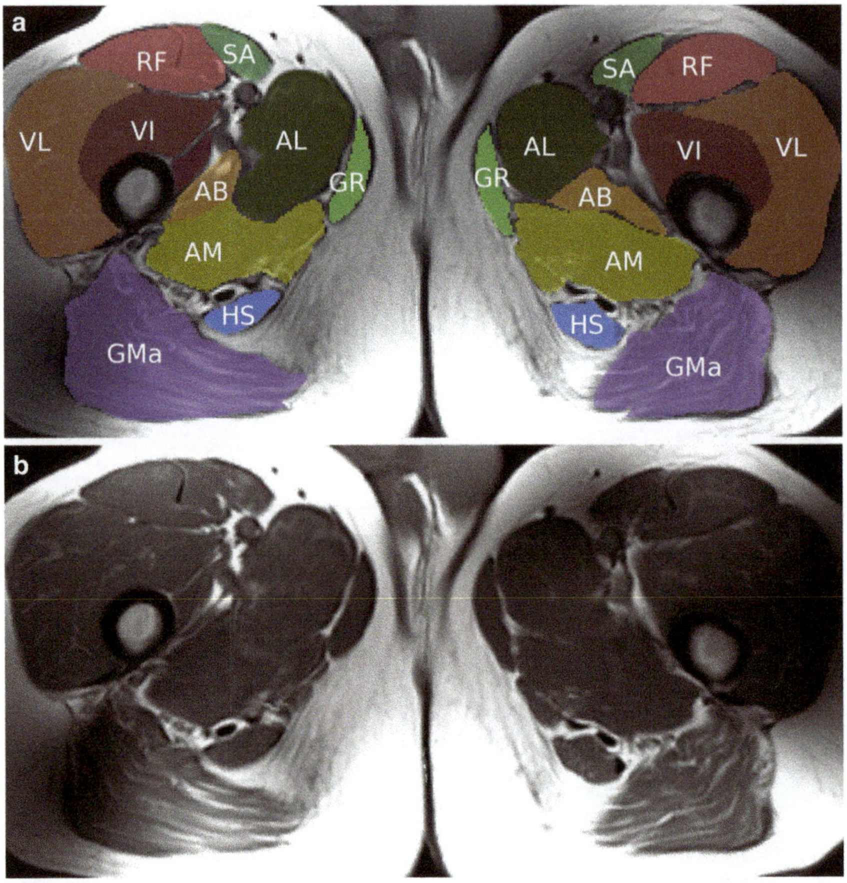

Fig. 10.21 Muscles of the pelvis. *AB* adductor brevis muscle, *AL* adductor longus muscle, *AM* adductor magnus muscle, *GMa* glutaeus maximus muscle, *GR* gracilis muscle, *HS* hamstring muscles, *IL* iliacus muscle, *RF* rectus femoris muscle, *SA* sartorius muscle, *VI* vastus intermedius muscle, *VL* vastus lateralis muscle

The separation of the adductor muscles, especially the adductor magnus from the adductor longus often proves difficult to visualise, as does the separation of the adductor muscles from the proximal semimembranosus.

It is also often difficult to exactly separate the three vasti muscles from each other, although separation might be facilitated by prominent fascia. As many diseases have different involvement of the short and long head of the biceps femoris muscle, these two muscles should usually be evaluated separately (Figs. 10.22, 10.23, 10.24, 10.25, 10.26, and 10.27).

10.7 Lower Leg, Calf

Most muscles of the calf display a relatively homogeneous amount of fat and comparison between muscles in one leg might therefore be helpful in order to assess disease involvement. Usually there are three to five larger fatty streaks in the medial gastrocnemius muscle and several small fatty streaks in the soleus.

The extensor digitorum and hallucis muscles are often difficult to separate from the anterior tibial muscle, especially in patients

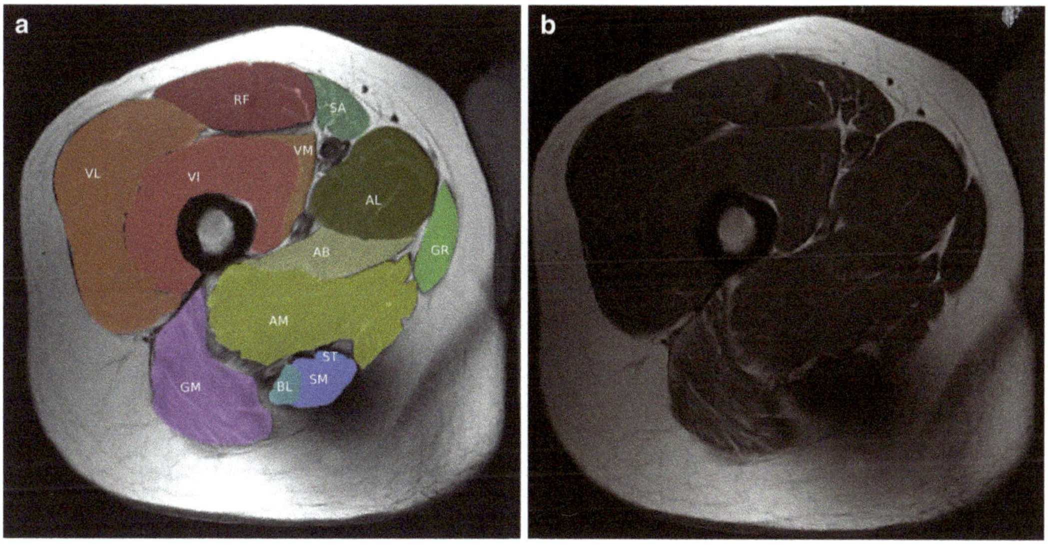

Fig. 10.22 Muscles of the proximal thigh. *AB* adductor brevis muscle, *AL* adductor longus muscle, *AM* adductor magnus muscle, *BL* biceps femoris muscle long head, *GMa* glutaeus maximus muscle, *GR* gracilis muscle, *RF* rectus femoris muscle, *SA* sartorius muscle, *SM* semimembranosus muscle, *ST* semitendinosus muscle, *VI* vastus intermedius muscle, *VL* vastus lateralis muscle, *VM* vastus medialis muscle. Quadriceps muscle in shades of *red*, Hamstrings in *blue*, Adductors in *yellow*, Glutaeus muscles are in shades of *purple*

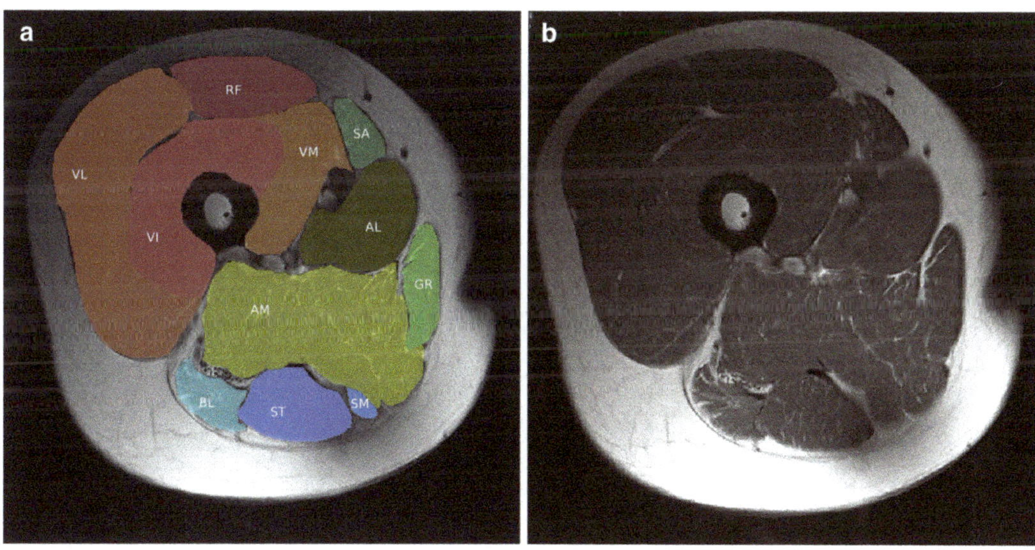

Fig. 10.23 Muscles of the thigh. *AL* adductor longus muscle, *AM* adductor magnus muscle, *BL* biceps femoris muscle long head, *GR* gracilis muscle, *RF* rectus femoris muscle, *SA* sartorius muscle, *SM* semimembranosus muscle, *ST* semitendinosus muscle, *VI* vastus intermedius muscle, *VL* vastus lateralis muscle, *VM* vastus medialis muscle. Quadriceps muscle in shades of *red*, hamstrings in *blue*, adductors in *yellow*

with little subcutaneous fat. In those cases, these muscles might be treated as one unit. In addition, several smaller muscles (e.g. flexor hallucis longus or peroneus brevis) will only be discernible in distal slices even when they are present in more proximal regions of the calf as tendinous structures (Figs. 10.28, 10.29, 10.30, and 10.31).

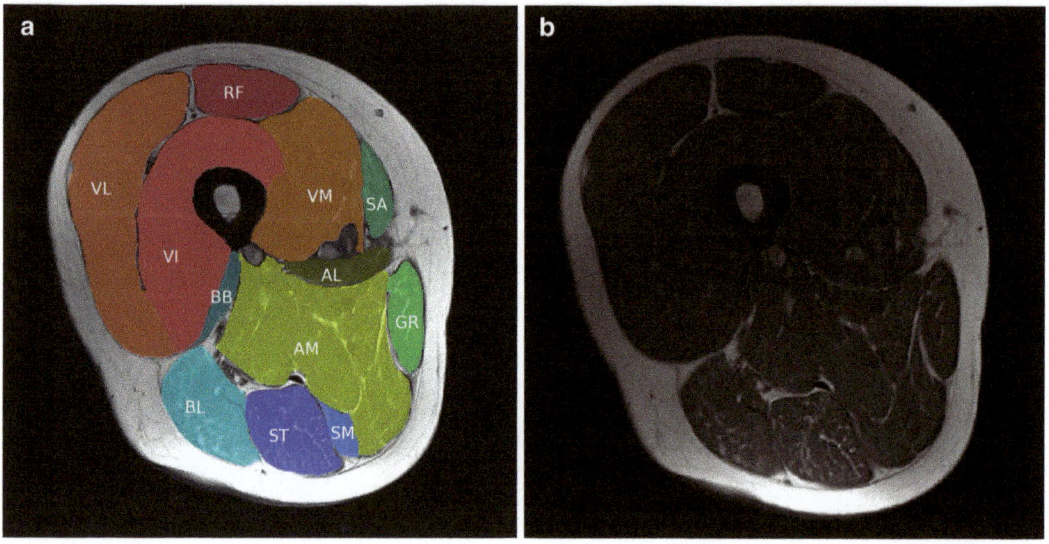

Fig. 10.24 Muscles of the thigh. *AL* adductor longus muscle, *AM* adductor magnus muscle, *BB* biceps femoris muscle short head, *BL* biceps femoris muscle long head, *GR* gracilis muscle, *RF* rectus femoris muscle, *SA* sartorius muscle, *SM* semimembranosus muscle, *ST* semitendinosus muscle, *VI* vastus intermedius muscle, *VL* vastus lateralis muscle, *VM* vastus medialis muscle. Quadriceps muscle in shades of *red*, hamstrings in *blue*, adductors in *yellow*

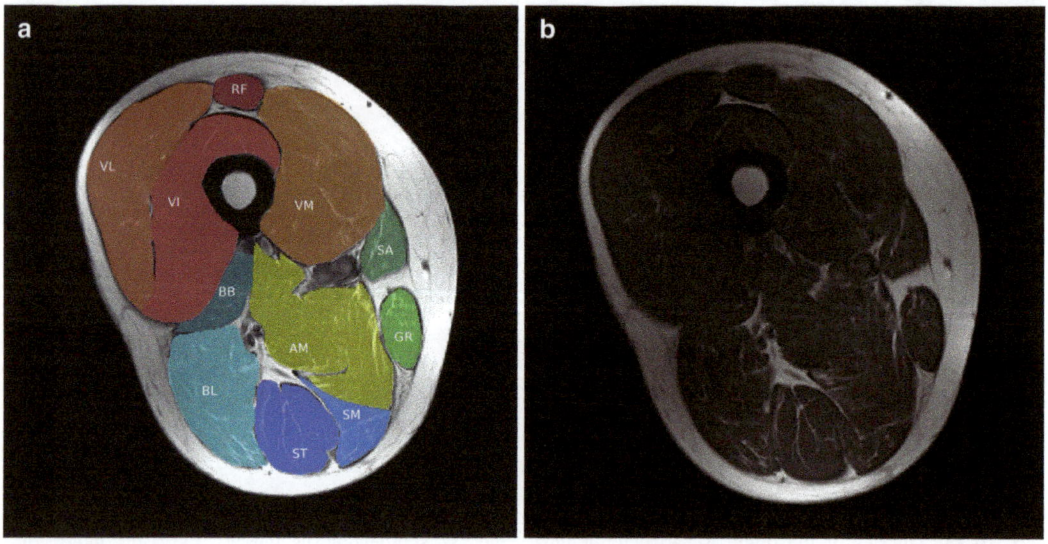

Fig. 10.25 Muscles of the thigh. *AM* adductor magnus muscle, *BB* biceps femoris muscle short head, *BL* biceps femoris muscle long head, *GR* gracilis muscle, *RF* rectus femoris muscle, *SA* sartorius muscle, *SM* semimembranosus muscle, *ST* semitendinosus muscle, *VI* vastus intermedius muscle, *VL* vastus lateralis muscle, *VM* vastus medialis muscle. Quadriceps muscle in shades of *red*, hamstrings in *blue*, adductors in *yellow*

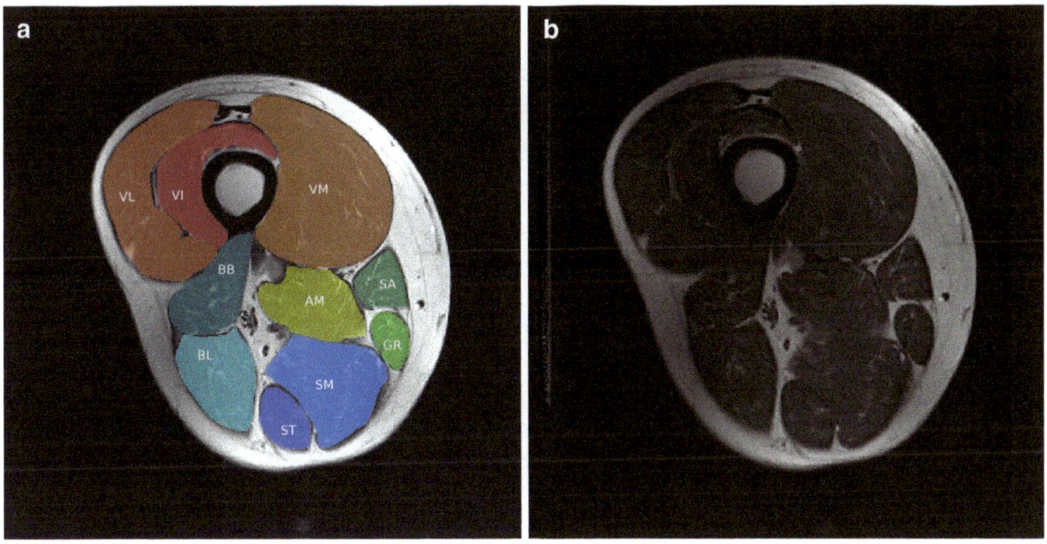

Fig. 10.26 Muscles of the distal thigh. *AM* adductor magnus muscle, *BB* biceps femoris muscle short head, *BL* biceps femoris muscle long head, *GR* gracilis muscle, *SA* sartorius muscle, *SM* semimembranosus muscle, *ST* semitendinosus muscle, *VI* vastus intermedius muscle, *VL* vastus lateralis muscle, *VM* vastus medialis muscle. Quadriceps muscle in shades of *red*, hamstrings in *blue*, adductors in *yellow*

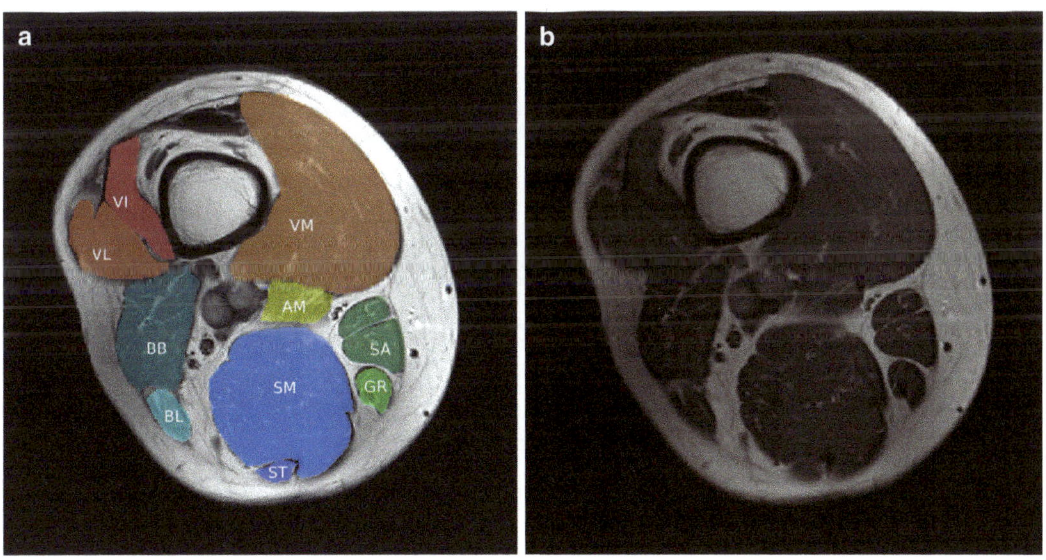

Fig. 10.27 Muscles of the distal thigh. *AM* adductor magnus muscle, *BB* biceps femoris muscle short head, *BL* biceps femoris muscle long head, *GR* gracilis muscle, *SA* sartorius muscle, *SM* semimembranosus muscle, *ST* semitendinosus muscle, *VI* vastus intermedius muscle, *VL* vastus lateralis muscle, *VM* vastus medialis muscle. Quadriceps muscle in shades of *red*, hamstrings in *blue*, adductors in *yellow*

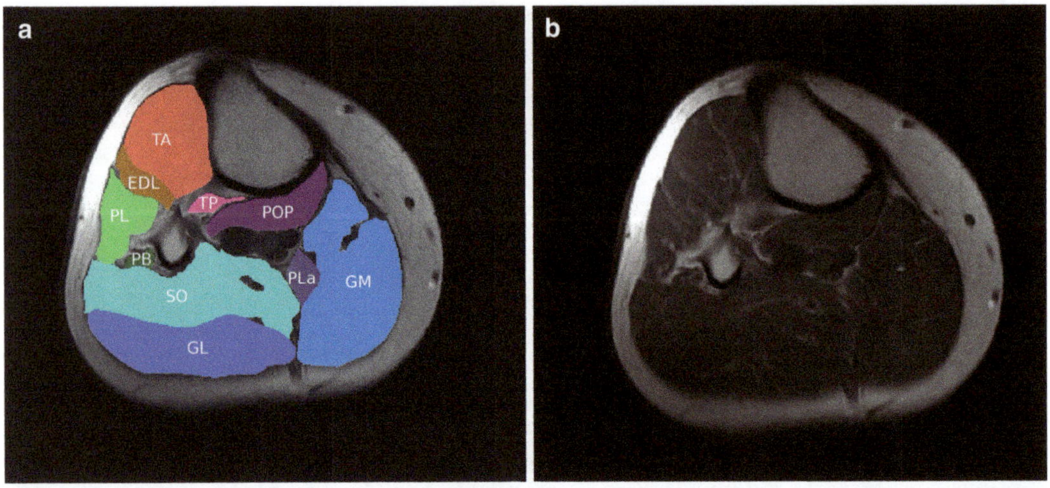

Fig. 10.28 Muscles of the proximal calf. *EDL* extensor digitorum longus, *GM* medial gastrocnemius muscle, *GL* lateral gastrocnemius muscle, *PB* peroneus brevis muscle, *PL* peroneus longus muscle, *PLa* plantaris muscle, *POP* popliteus muscle, *TA* tibialis anterior muscle, *TP* tibialis posterior muscle. Triceps surae in shades of *blue*

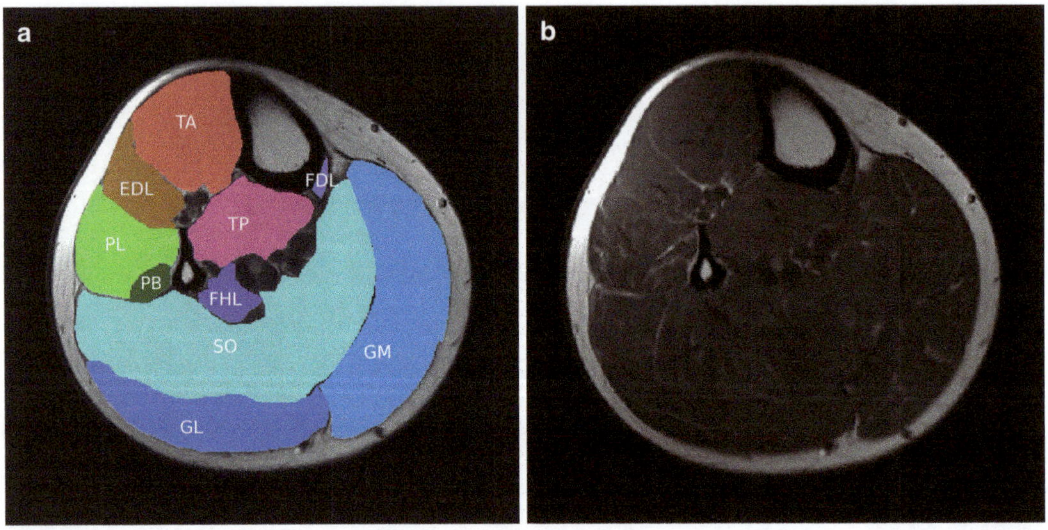

Fig. 10.29 Muscles of the calf. *EDL* extensor digitorum longus, *FDL* flexor digitorum longus muscle, *FHL* flexor hallucis longus muscle, *GM* medial gastrocnemius muscle, *GL* lateral gastrocnemius muscle, *PB* peroneus brevis muscle, *PL* peroneus longus muscle, *TA* tibialis anterior muscle, *TP* tibialis posterior muscle. Triceps surae in shades of *blue*

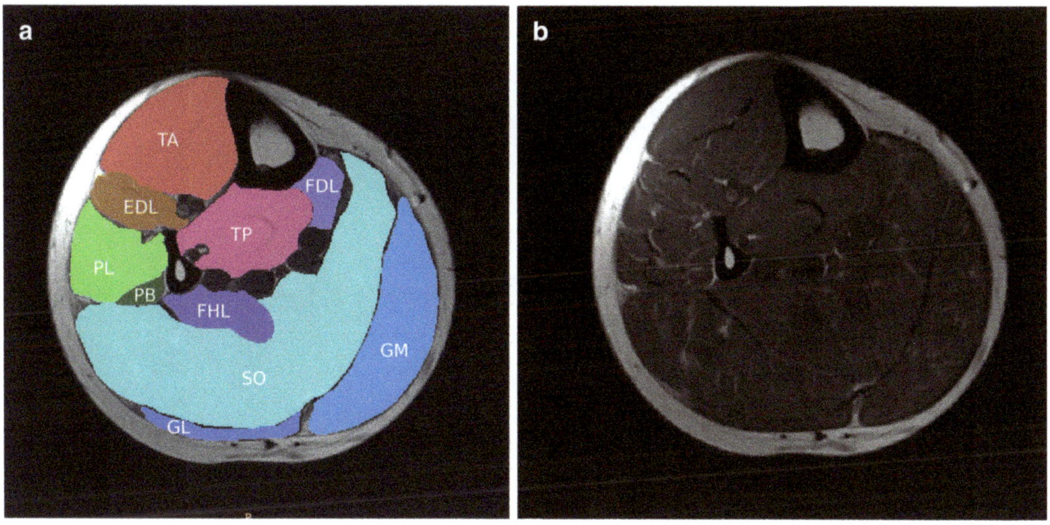

Fig. 10.30 Muscles of the calf. *EDL* extensor digitorum longus, *FDL* flexor digitorum longus muscle, *FHL* flexor hallucis longus muscle, *GM* medial gastrocnemius muscle, *GL* lateral gastrocnemius muscle, *PB* peroneus brevis muscle, *PL* peroneus longus muscle, *TA* tibialis anterior muscle, *TP* tibialis posterior muscle. Triceps surae in shades of *blue*

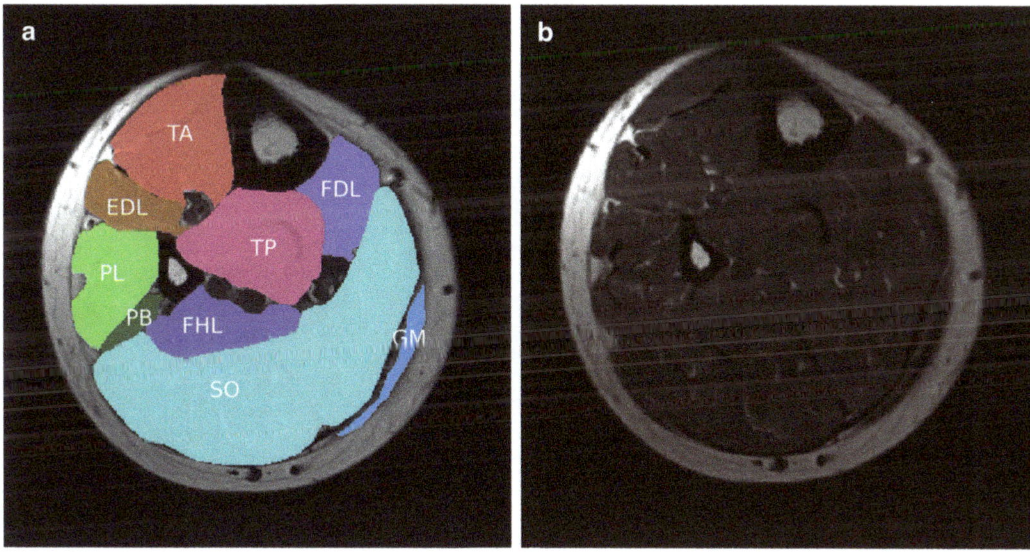

Fig. 10.31 Muscles of the calf. *EDL* extensor digitorum longus, *FDL* flexor digitorum longus muscle, *FHL* flexor hallucis longus muscle, *GM* medial gastrocnemius muscle, *PB* peroneus brevis muscle, *PL* peroneus longus muscle, *TA* tibialis anterior muscle, *TP* tibialis posterior muscle. Triceps surae in shades of *blue*

Normal Aging Muscle Tissue

11

Mike P. Wattjes and Dirk Fischer

11.1 Introduction

The effects of aging on muscle tissue—in terms of total and regional muscle mass, muscle fiber size and number—and its clinical consequences with respect to muscle power, strength, and endurance have been investigated extensively during the past few decades. The aging process of striated muscle tissue is based on a complex (patho)physiological mechanism that includes numerous interacting factors, such as hormones, sex, nutrition, and physical activity. The histopathological, imaging, and functional (clinical) features of the "normal aging muscle" are referred to as "sarcopenia." Although sarcopenia is a normal aging phenomenon, it has a substantial clinical and financial impact on health systems because the human life-span is increasing, particularly in the developed Western countries. Sarcopenia is strongly related to accidental falls and injuries as well as to a higher incidence of other systemic diseases including osteoporosis, obesity, and insulin resistance. Therefore, sarcopenia is substantially influencing the quality of life of the elderly as well as their life-span.

M.P. Wattjes (✉)
Department of Radiology, Nuclear Medicine & PET Research, VU University Medical Center, De Boelelaan 1117, 1081 HV Amsterdam, The Netherlands
e-mail: m.wattjes@vumc.nl

D. Fischer
Division of Neuropaediatrics, University Childrens Hospital Basel, 4056 Basel, Switzerland

Department of Neurology, Petersgraben 4, University Hospital Basel, 4031 Basel, Switzerland
e-mail: Dirk.fischer@ukbb.ch

11.2 Sarcopenia

The literal interpretation of the Greek word sarcopenia is "poverty of flesh." In general, this term describes the age-related changes of striated tissue. Using muscle mass assessment with dual-energy X-ray absorptiometry (DEXA), sarcopenia was defined in research studies as the loss of muscle tissue more than two standard deviations below the mean for young adults. In general, sarcopenia shows a high variability among patients of different ages.

11.3 Loss of Skeletal Muscle Mass

The total muscle mass is strongly age-dependent. It continuously increases until the age of 24 years. During the span from 24 to 50 years of age, the muscle mass decreases only slightly (~10 %). In people older than 50 years, the reduction of muscle mass accelerates, and 30 % of muscle is lost between 50 and 80 years of age. Using imaging techniques—computed tomography (CT), magnetic resonance imaging (MRI), ultrasonography (US)—an annual reduction rate in the whole muscle size ranges from 0.5 % to 0.8 % beyond the age of 50 years based on cross-sectional data and 1.4 % based on longitudinal data (Figs. 11.1, 11.2,

M.P. Wattjes and D. Fischer (eds.), *Neuromuscular Imaging*, DOI 10.1007/978-1-4614-6552-2_11,

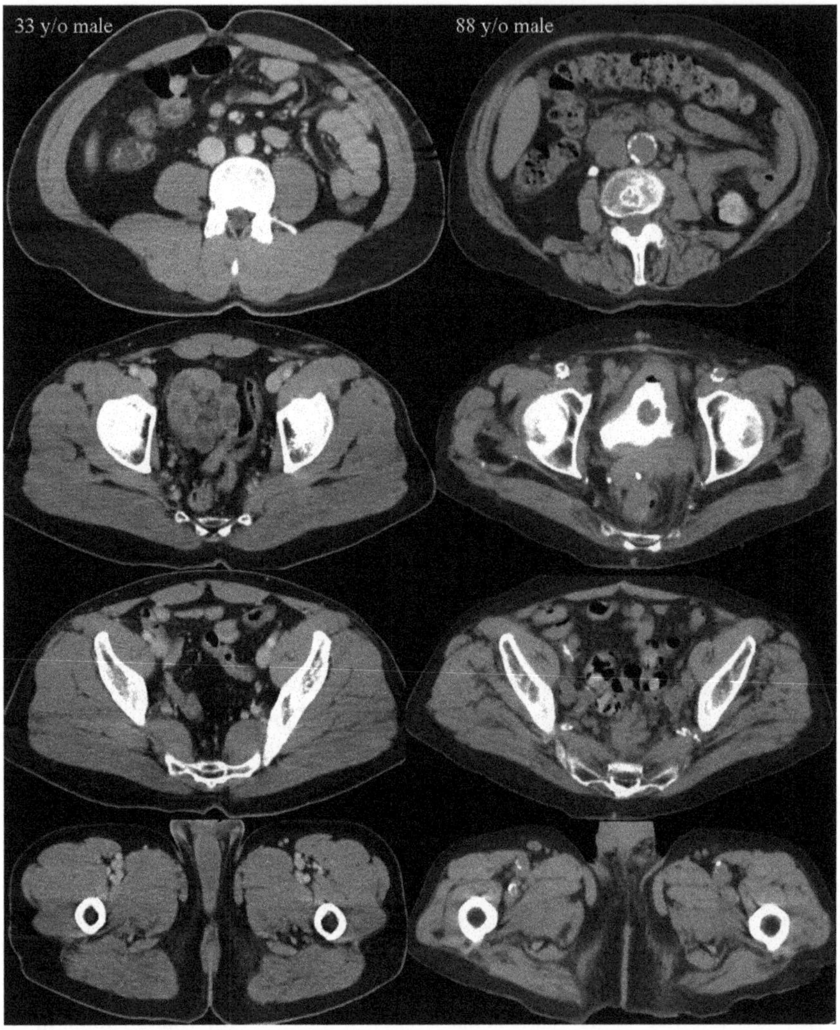

Fig. 11.1 Axial computed tomography (CT) images obtained from a 33-year-old man (*left*) and an 88-year-old man in various anatomical regions. Note the generalized loss of muscle tissue, particularly the decreased muscle thickness in the older subject. Note also the increased amount of intermuscular and intramuscular fat tissue

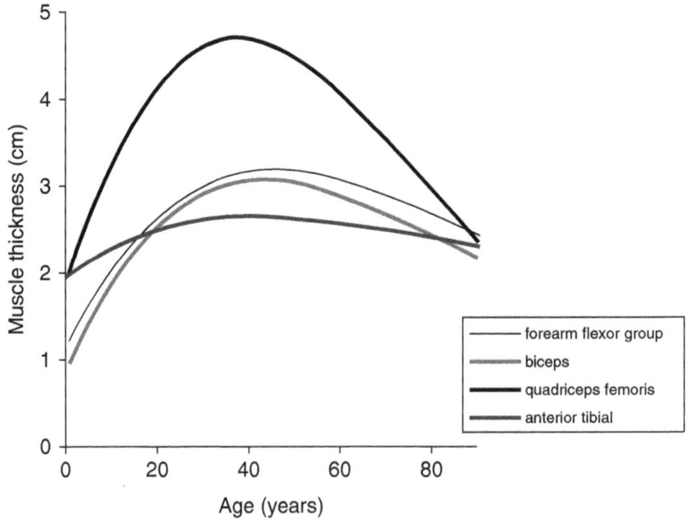

Fig. 11.2 Examples of age-related muscle changes in terms of muscle thickness in men for the biceps brachii, forearm flexor, quadriceps, and anterior tibial muscles. From Pillen S, Arts IMP, Zwarts MJ (2008) Muscle ultrasound in neuromuscular disorders. Muscle Nerve. 37: 679–693. Reprinted with permission from John Wiley and Sons

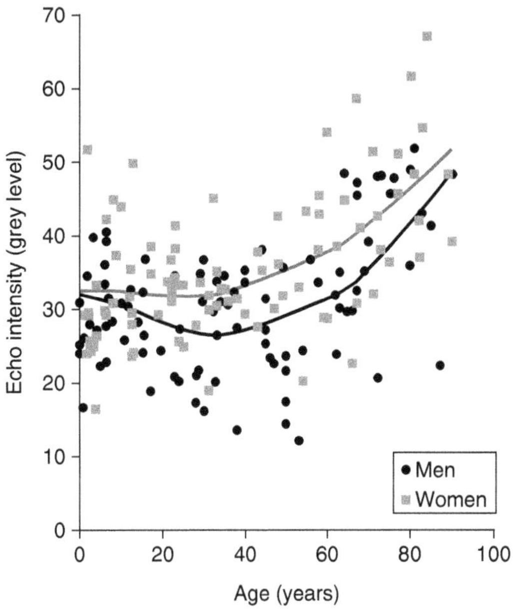

Fig. 11.3 Muscle echo intensity is dependent on age, data on 194 healthy volunteers. The muscle intensity is expressed as a value between 0 (black) and 255 (white). Note that the presented values are specific for the particular ultrasonography system used. During childhood, there are no substantial differences between boys and girls. From early adulthood on, men show lower muscle echo intensity than women. After the age of 40 years, the muscle echo intensity increases continuously. From Pillen S, Arts IMP, Zwarts MJ (2008) Muscle ultrasound in neuromuscular disorders. Muscle Nerve. 37:679–693. Reprinted with permission from John Wiley and Sons

11.3; see Chap. 2, Fig. 2.12). Adjusted for age, height, and body weight, men have more muscle tissue than women. However, men experience a higher degree of loss of muscle tissue during aging than do women. This phenomenon is not fully understood. It is probably due to a complex interaction of multiple factors including hormones (growth hormone, insulin-like growth factor, estrogen, testosterone), exercise, and lifestyle.

The underlying pathophysiological mechanisms include a decrease in fiber size and number. The aging process in terms of fiber size reduction is more prominent in type II fibers. The reduction of the type II fiber area during aging is 20–50 % compared to 1–25 % of the fiber type I area (Fig. 11.4). Even among the type II fibers there seems to be differences in the degree of fiber size reduction. Several studies have conclusively demonstrated that type IIB fibers were more severely affected than type IIA fibers in elderly women and men.

In contrast to the fiber size area, the reduction in fiber number does equally affect type I and type II muscle fibers. Data from postmortem studies have demonstrated that the number of type I and type II fibers has decreased by 50 % at the ninth decade compared to individuals at the age of 20 years. The rate of decrement in fiber number accelerates during the aging process. Between the third and fifth decade a 5 % reduction can be observed compared to a reduction of 35 % between the fifth and the eighth decades of life.

Although normal aging of the muscle tissue does not affect the overall ratio of fiber types in terms of fiber numbers, there is a certain fiber grouping that can be observed in aging muscle tissue. In young muscle tissue, the various fiber types are scattered, resulting in a normal "checkerboard" mosaic appearance, whereas in older muscle tissue several fibers types are arranged in groups. More recent studies focusing on the myosin heavy-chain composition of different muscle fibers showed that the number of so called hybrid fibers, expressing more than a single myosin heavy chain isoform, is increased in aging muscle tissue.

11.4 Pathophysiology of Sarcopenia

Age-related denervation of striated muscle tissue is one of the most important factors leading to loss of muscle fibers/total muscle tissue and associated clinical manifestations in the elderly. It has been conclusively demonstrated that the number of α-motoneurons in the ventral horn of the spinal cord remains almost constant during life until the seventh decade. During the following years of life, the number of α-motoneurons decrease continuously. This leads to progressive denervation of muscle tissue, in turn leading to losses of functional motor units of the proximal and distal muscle in the upper and lower extremities and a subsequent increase in size of the remaining motor units. The chronic denervation process has been linked to possible underlying pathophysiological mechanisms regarding the phenomenon of fiber grouping in aging muscle tissue (described earlier). In addition, the progressive denervation

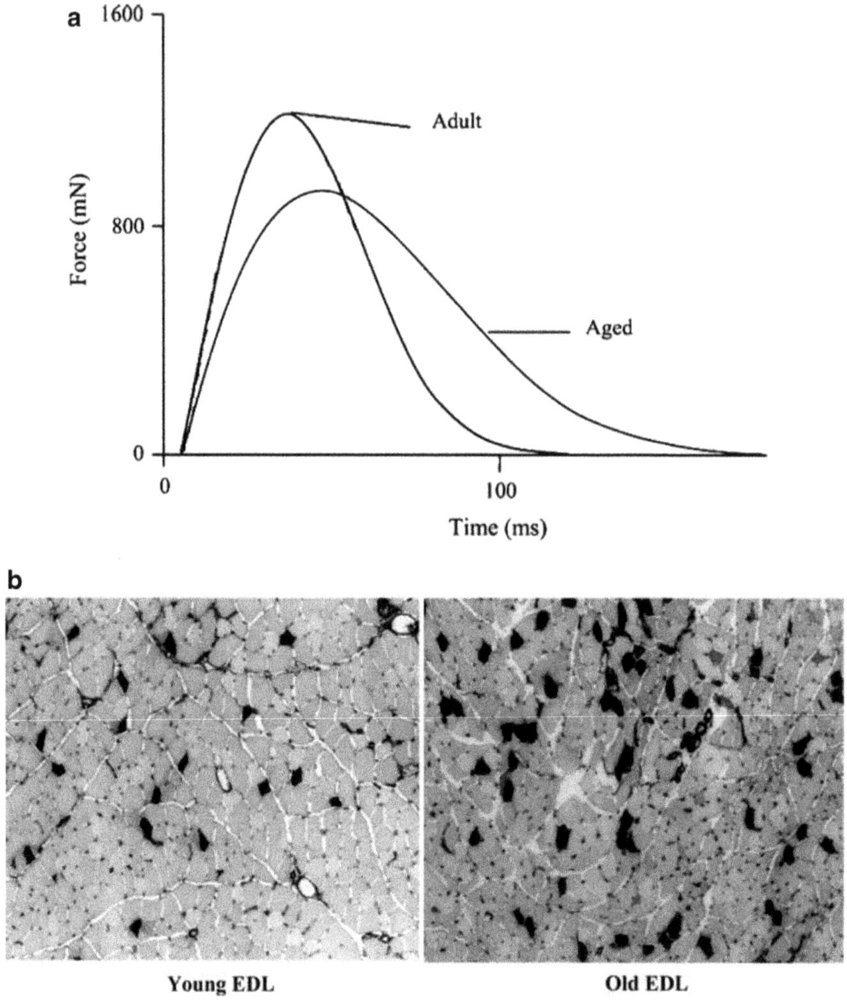

Fig. 11.4 (**a**) Age-related changes in (maximum) muscle force in terms of representative isometric twitch contractile responses. (**b**) Extensor digitorum longus muscle obtained from 16- to 28-month-old rats stained with myosin ATPase. Note the relative increase of the dark-stained type I fibers in the older muscles. From Ryall JG (2008) Cellular and molecular mechanisms underlying age-related skeletal muscle wasting and weakness. Biogerontology 9:213–228. Reprinted with permission from Springer

process explains the acceleration of muscle tissue loss in the elderly and the rather constant muscle tissue volume in middle-aged persons. The underlying reason for the loss of motoneurons is still not understood. Molecules influencing function and survival of motoneurons such as the ciliary neurothrophic factor (CNTF) are currently being investigated.

In addition to chronic denervation, there are other multifactorial pathophysiological pathways that contribute to muscle fiber loss and atrophy in sarcopenia. They include hormonal, metabolic, nutritional, and immunological factors.

11.4.1 Protein Metabolism

Alterations in protein metabolism affect normal aging striated muscle tissue. They can be addressed from various (patho)physiological aspects. First, reduced protein synthesis is observed during the early stages of sarcopenia even in middle-aged persons (50–60 years) before age-related denervation occurs. To a certain extent, this can explain the observation that mild sarcopenia is present before denervation appears. The decline in protein synthesis particularly affects myofibrillar (actin, myosin) and mitochondrial proteins. The assumption that mitochondrial proteins (e.g., aerobic enzymes) are involved is supported by the fact that mitochondria and mitochondrial DNA levels are substantial reduced (approximately 40 %) in normal aging muscle tissue. This decline in oxidative phosphorylation, and therefore adenosine triphosphate (ATP) production, leads to overall impaired protein metabolism with consequences on muscle function.

11.4.2 Hormone Status

The decreasing blood-borne concentrations of anabolic hormones during aging represent an important factor contributing to sarcopenia. In elderly men, the concentrations of total testosterone and, more importantly, unbound testosterone are reduced by 35 % and 50 %, respectively, between the age of 20 to 80 years. The functioning of the hypothalamic-pituitary-gonadal axis influences the status of testosterone, particularly the circadian variation of testosterone concentrations, in elderly men. The multifactorial aspects of anabolic hormone dysfunction affecting the anabolic hormones include impaired secretion of gonadotropin-releasing hormone (GrH) by the hypothalamus, relative insensitivity of Leydig cells to luteinizing hormone (LH) (which normally stimulates testosterone secretion), and reduced responses of several tissue types (e.g., muscle tissue) to anabolic hormones. It has been conclusively demonstrated that adequate replacement of testosterone in elderly men is an effective treatment strategy regarding muscle mass recovery and has clinical benefits in terms of improved muscle strength.

Another important anabolic hormone that influences muscle metabolism, particularly in women, is the growth hormone (GH). Men and women show a 50 % reduction of GH levels between the age of 20 to 70 years, with a substantial effect on muscle mass reduction. GH also regulates the synthesis of insulin-like growth factor-1 (IGF-1). A reduced IGF-1 level is another contributing factor of sarcopenia. IGF-1 plays an important role in the recruitment of satellite cells in muscle tissue. Satellite cells in the muscle represent the proliferative reserve. Stimulation of satellite cells leads to muscle fiber proliferation. Thus, fewer satellite cells during aging limit the proliferative capacity. IGF-1 not only leads to a proliferation of satellite cells but also stimulates satellite cell mitosis. However, in contrast to testosterone replacement, a therapeutic benefit of GH supplementation has not been conclusively shown. GH replacement can lead to increased muscle mass but not to increased muscle strength. It is therefore not recommended as an effective treatment option in sarcopenia.

11.4.3 Nutrition

Nutritional status is an important contributing factor to sarcopenia in the elderly. Aging leads to an impaired nutritional state, for which the term “anorexia of aging” has been coined. The underlying pathophysiological mechanism of anorexia and sarcopenia is not fully understood. The impaired intake of proteins under a certain level is crucial for the maintenance of muscle tissue and the impaired intake of certain aliment that play an important role in muscle homeostasis (e.g., creatine) have been suggested as possible factors. The benefit of anorexia treatment in terms of clinical outcome measures (e.g., muscle strength) is still under debate and has not yet been conclusively demonstrated.

11.4.4 Inflammation

There is increasing evidence that inflammatory reactions in the muscle tissue contribute to sarcopenia. Particularly, increased levels of inflammatory cytokines such as interleukin-6 (IL-6), interleukin-1β (IL-1β), and tumor necrosis factor-α (TNFα) have been observed in aging muscle tissue. These cytokines have some catabolic effects. To what extent these inflammatory changes contribute to sarcopenia is currently under investigation.

11.4.5 Exercise

Reduced physical activity is a well-known phenomenon in the elderly and contributes significantly to sarcopenia. Resistance exercise can reverse age-related changes in muscle tissue in terms of an increase in muscle mass and benefits regarding functional outcome measures such as muscle strength. Exercise-induced increases in muscle mass (cross-sectional area) of up to 40 % have been reported. It is likely that resistance exercise acts in various ways, directly affecting the muscle tissue. Neuronal mechanisms are also being considered.

11.5 Loss of Muscle Function

Age-related loss of muscle strength is the most important clinical manifestation of sarcopenia. In general, the loss involves all domains including concentric, eccentric, and isometric strength, although eccentric strength is relatively preserved. The course of the muscle strength decline corresponds well with the age-related loss of muscle mass (Fig. 11.4). There are no substantial differences in the loss of muscle strength between proximal and distal limb muscles. After reaching 30 years of age, muscle strength shows almost constant values until age 50 years. A rather mild decrease in muscle strength is observed between the ages of 50 and 60 years, followed by a more accelerated loss of muscle strength in people older than 60 years. Men show higher values of muscle mass and strength at baseline, and their absolute loss of muscle strength is greater. However, both men and women show the same rate of age-related muscle strength decline. Several cross-sectional and longitudinal studies have been performed to estimate the rate of muscle strength reduction. The data are difficult to interpret because we are dealing with different baseline ages and different follow-up periods. In general, longitudinal studies show greater declines than do cross-sectional studies. Roughly, a decrease of approximately 15 % per decade is observed in persons beyond the fifth decade of life. Please consider the suggestions for further reading (below) for more detailed information on this topic. Physical activity, particularly resistance training, can influence and recover muscle strength to a certain extent even in very old persons.

In contrast to muscle strength, muscle endurance or, in other words, muscular fatigue is not strongly related to sarcopenia. Studies investigating the effect of aging on muscle endurance are inconclusive, probably due at least partly to methodological differences and difficulties. It has been shown that fatigue in the elderly is not linked to differences of the contractile components in muscle tissue. It has therefore been postulated that fatigue in aged muscle is more likely caused by altered central nervous system factors.

Normal Aging Muscle Tissue

Key Points

- The term sarcopenia describes age-related changes in muscle tissue in terms of muscle mass and muscle strength.
- The age-related changes in muscle tissue accelerate in patients beyond the seventh decade of life.
- The pathophysiology of sarcopenia is complex and multi-factorial, including features of denervation, inflammation, metabolic and hormonal changes, nutritional status, and physical activity.
- Imaging modalities (US, CT, MRI) are useful for assessing and quantifying the degree of sarcopenia in the elderly.
- Physical activity (resistance training) is helpful for slowing down the process of sarcopenia and recovering muscle strength.

Suggestions for Further Reading

Arts IM, Pillen S, Overeem S, et al. Rise and fall of the skeletal muscle over the entire life span. J Am Geriatr Soc. 2007;55:1150–2.

Brown M. Skeletal muscle and bone: effect of steroids and ageing. Adv Physiol Educ. 2008;32:120–6.

Doherty TJ. Invited review: ageing and sacropenia. J Appl Physiol. 2003;95:717–27.

Kanehisa H, Ikegawa S, Tsunoda N, et al. Cross sectional areas of fat and muscle in limbs during growth and middle age. In J Sports Med. 1994;15:420–5.
Roubenhoff R, Hughes VA. Sarcopenia: current concepts. J Gerontol A Biol Sci Med Sci. 2000;55:M716–24.
Ryall JG, Schertzer JD, Lynch GS. Cellular and molecular mechnanism underlying age related skeletal muscle wasting and weakness. Biogerontology. 2008;9:213–28.
Sakuma K, Yamaguchi A. Novel intriguing strategies attenuating to sarcopenia. J Aging Res. 2012;2012: 251217
Wang C, Bai L. Sarcopenia in the elderly: basic and clinical issues. Geriatr Gerontol Int. 2012;12:388–96.
Welle S. Cellular and molecular basis of age-related sarcopenia. Can J Appl Physiol. 2002;27:19–41.

Part III

Clinical Applications in Hereditary Myopathies

Introduction

12

Dirk Fischer

The preceding chapters in this book focused on the basic principles of imaging modalities (Part I) and muscle anatomy and physiology (Part II). Part III deals with the clinical applications of neuromuscular imaging. Neuromuscular disorders comprise a large, heterogeneous group of diseases of the peripheral nervous system. They include hereditary and acquired disorders of the muscles, neuromuscular junction, peripheral nerves, and motor neurons in the spinal cord. They share the presence of positive (cramps, muscle pain) and/or negative (atrophy, weakness) motor symptoms and signs. Periodic or permanent weakness is the most common. Except for peripheral nerve disorders, sensory disturbances are absent in all other neuromuscular disorders.

As neuromuscular imaging has been shown to be most useful for evaluation of various myopathies, these primary disorders of skeletal muscle are described in detail. Part III focuses on hereditary myopathies, which include a large number of disease entities. Genetic, pathological, clinical, and imaging classifications of these disorders are often heterogeneous and overlapping, complicating the clinical and diagnostic approaches to them. As a simple clinical rule of thumb, muscle channelopathies (Chap. 13) and (apart from glycogen storage disorders and some mitochondrial disorders) metabolic myopathies (Chap. 14) most commonly present with episodic and intermittent muscle symptoms. The clinical assessment therefore is often based only on the history presented by the patient. In contrast, other hereditary myopathies present with permanent weakness that can be assessed at the clinical examination. The weakness can be due to structural and morphological disturbances of the muscle fibers such as rods, an increased number of central nuclei, or (central or multiple) cores as seen in congenital myopathies (Chap. 15). In these disorders weakness is often present at birth (congenital), with no or only slow progression. In contrast, muscular dystrophies become clinically evident at various ages of onset, show dystrophic changes in affected muscles with necrotic fibers, often are associated with markedly elevated serum creatine kinase levels, and have a progressive course. Free ambulation is often lost at some stage of the patient's life. Most muscular dystrophies present with predominantly proximal muscle weakness (Fig. 12.1a). Broadly, symptom onset can be at birth in congenital muscular dystrophies (Chap. 16), within the first decade of life as in Duchenne muscular dystrophy (Chap. 17), within the first two decades of life as often observed in the recessive limb girdle muscular dystrophies (Chap. 19). Other forms of muscular dystrophy present with predominantly distal weakness (Fig. 12.1b) including many of the myofibrillar myopathies (Chap. 20) and the distal myopathies (Chap. 21).

D. Fischer (✉)
Division of Neuropaediatrics, University Childrens Hospital Basel, 4056 Basel, Switzerland

Department of Neurology, University Hospital Basel, 4031 Basel, Switzerland
e-mail: Dirk.fischer@ukbb.ch

M.P. Wattjes and D. Fischer (eds.), *Neuromuscular Imaging*, DOI 10.1007/978-1-4614-6552-2_12,

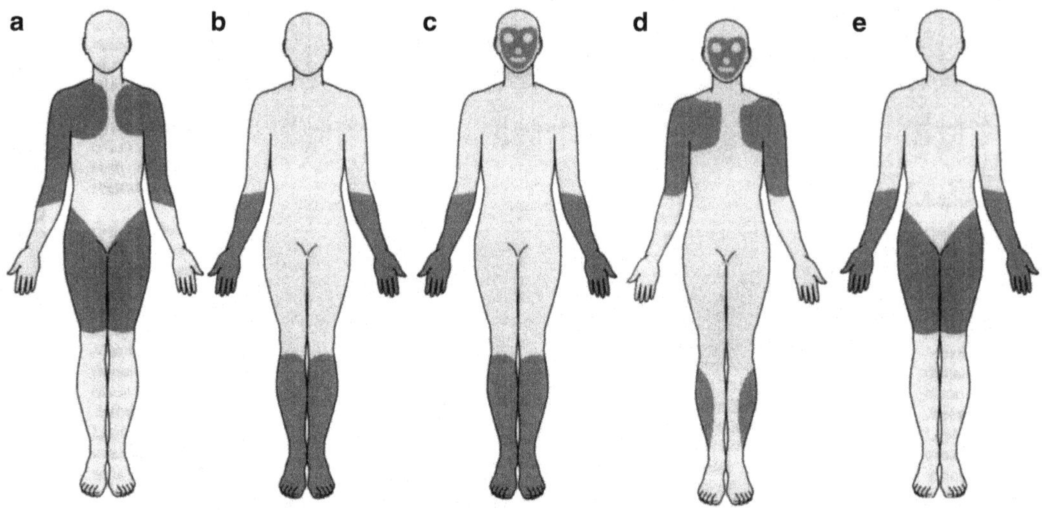

Fig. 12.1 The most common clinical presentations of muscle weakness in myopathies. (**a**) Predominantly proximal weakness, as seen in congenital muscular dystrophies, dystrophinopathies, limb girdle muscular dystrophies, and inflammatory myopathies. (**b**) Predominantly distal weakness in distal myopathies. (**c**) Distal and facial weakness in myotonic dystrophy type Steinert. Facio-scapulo-humero-peroneal weakness in facio-scapulo-humero-peroneal dystrophy (FSHD). (**d**) Often there is asymmetrical weakness of the distal forearm and proximal leg (quadriceps) in sporadic inclusion myositis. From Fischer D. Klinische Neurophysiologie 2006;37:1–9. Reprinted with permission from Georg Thieme Verlag KG

Other, more uncommon presentations of muscular dystrophy include distal and facial weakness (Fig. 12.1c) in myotonic dystrophy type I (Chap. 22), (facio-)scapulo-peroneal weakness (Fig. 12.1d) in facioscapulohumeral dystrophy (Chap. 23) and X-linked Emery–Dreifuss muscular dystrophy (Chap. 18), and oculopharyngeal weakness in oculopharyngeal muscular dystrophy (Chap. 24). Chapter 25 summarizes imaging findings of various hereditary myopathies in flow charts that might be of use in the differential diagnosis of these disorders. Part IV deals with acquired myopathies such as inflammatory myopathies (Chap. 26), toxic and drug-induced myopathies (Chap. 27), and muscle neoplasm (Chap. 28). Part V describes the clinical applications in selected motor neuron disorders (Chap. 29) and peripheral nerve disorders (Chap. 30).

Skeletal Muscle Channelopathies 13

Karin Jurkat-Rott and Marc-André Weber

13.1 Introduction and Classification

Myotonia is an involuntarily slowed relaxation after a forceful voluntary muscle contraction. Patients experience it as muscle stiffness. Electrical hyperexcitability of the muscle fiber membrane is the basis of myotonia, which is apparent in the form of repetitive action potentials on electromyography (EMG). The stiffness recedes with repeated contractions, a phenomenon called warm-up. Patients in whom muscle stiffness worsens with repetition or with cooling suffer from paradoxical myotonia, or paramyotonia. This type of myotonia is associated with episodes of flaccid limb muscle weakness resulting in the adynamia paramyotonia complex.

Patients with periodic paralysis experience episodic spells of weakness with varying intervals of normal muscle function. Electrical inexcitability of the muscle fiber membrane is the basis of periodic paralysis, which is apparent in a lack of activity on EMG. Two dominant episodic types of weakness with or without myotonia are distinguished by the serum K^+ level during the attacks of tetraplegia: hyperkalemic and hypokalemic periodic paralysis. The former is included in the adynamia paramyotonia complex, whereas the latter represents a separate entity. Independent of the severity and frequency of the paralytic episodes, many patients develop a chronic progressive myopathy in their forties, an age at which the attacks of weakness decrease. For an overview of the channelopathies, see Table 13.1.

Routine magnetic resonance imaging (MRI) protocols show normal muscle morphology or may demonstrate edematous or lipomatous changes, atrophy, or hypertrophy. However, these morphological changes are not disease-specific. This chapter describes conventional and modern functional MR imaging methods for evaluating muscular diseases (e.g., ^{23}Na-MRI).

13.2 Nondystrophic Myotonia

13.2.1 Subtypes, Synonyms, Abbreviations

- Thomsen myotonia or dominant myotonia congenita (DMC); Becker myotonia or recessive myotonia congenita (RMC)
- K^+-aggravated myotonia (PAM) with its subtypes: Myotonia fluctuans and Myotonia permanens

K. Jurkat-Rott
Division Neurophysiology, University of Ulm, Albert-Einstein-Allee 11, Ulm, Germany
e-mail: karin.jurkat-rott@uni-ulm.de

M.-A. Weber (✉)
Department of Diagnostic and Interventional Radiology, University Hospital of Heidelberg, Im Neuenheimer Feld 110, 69120 Heidelberg, Germany
e-mail: MarcAndre.Weber@med.uni-heidelberg.de

M.P. Wattjes and D. Fischer (eds.), *Neuromuscular Imaging*, DOI 10.1007/978-1-4614-6552-2_13,

Table 13.1 Overview of the skeletal muscle channelopathies

Entity	Gene chromosome	Protein	Prevalence	Clinical features
Myotonia congenita	*CLCN1* 7q32-qter	Chloride channel ClC1	1:400,000 (recessive) 1:25,000 (dominant)	Autosomal recessive: childhood onset, generalized myotonia, warm-up phenomenon, muscle hypertrophy, transient weakness Autosomal dominant: teenage onset, generalized myotonia, warm-up phenomenon, little muscle hypertrophy
K^+-aggravated myotonia	*SCN4A* 17q23.1-25.3	Sodium channel Nav1.4	1:400,000	Autosomal dominant; onset varies, generalized myotonia of variable severity, warm-up variable, aggravation by K^+ administration, no weakness
Paramyotonia congenita	*SCN4A* 17q23.1-25.3	Sodium channel Nav1.4	1:250,000	Autosomal dominant; childhood onset, paradoxical myotonia, cold-induced muscle stiffness followed by weakness/periodic paralysis, no warm-up
Hyperkalemic periodic paralysis	*SCN4A* 17q23.1-25.3	Sodium channel Nav1.4	1:200,000	Autosomal dominant; childhood onset, episodic attacks of mainly limb weakness, hyperkalemia during episode, triggering by rest after body exertion or K^+ intake, amelioration by glucose intake
Hypokalemic periodic paralysis	*CACNA1S* 1q31-32 *SCN4A* 17q23.1-25.3	Calcium channel Cav1.1 Sodium channel Nav1.4	1:100,000 1:500,000	Autosomal dominant; teenage onset, episodic attacks of mainly limb weakness, hypokalemia during episode, triggering by carbohydrate-rich food or exercise, amelioration by K^+ intake

13.2.2 Genetics and Pathophysiology

Although the two classic forms of Myotonia congenita (MC) are distinguished by their mode of inheritance, they are caused by mutations in the same gene on chromosome 7q, *CLCN1* (i.e., the gene coding for the sarcolemmal voltage-gated Cl^- channel ClC-1). For this reason, they are also referred to as Cl^- channel myotonias. The prevalence of dominant Thomsen disease (DMC) is estimated at ~1:400,000—i.e., much lower than thought in the premolecular era (1:23,000) owing to the fact that many families with dominant myotonia can now be genetically identified as carriers of a Na^+ channel mutation, which results in a clinically overlapping disorder the Potassium-aggravated myotonia (PAM). Other families were found to have recessive Becker myotonia (RMC) with pseudo-dominant inheritance (i.e., affected individuals with two recessive mutations have affected offspring with unaffected spouses carrying one recessive mutation). Conversely, the prevalence of Becker myotonia is now thought to be higher (1:25,000) than Becker's original estimate of 1:50,000.

After-depolarizations of the muscle action potential are normally prevented by Cl^- conducted through homodimeric ClC-1 channels. If this muscle-specific high Cl^- conductance is decreased by ≥ 75 %, after-depolarizations are large and are able to initiate repetitive action potentials. These so-called myotonic runs result in involuntary contractions or slowed relaxation. All DMCs and RMCs are caused by loss-of-function mutations. In DMC, only one allele is mutated, and a typical mutation reduces conductance of mutant/mutant and mutant/wild-type channel complexes in a dominant-negative fashion. In contrast, RMC mutations result in simple loss of function of the mutant/mutant complex only—thus, both alleles

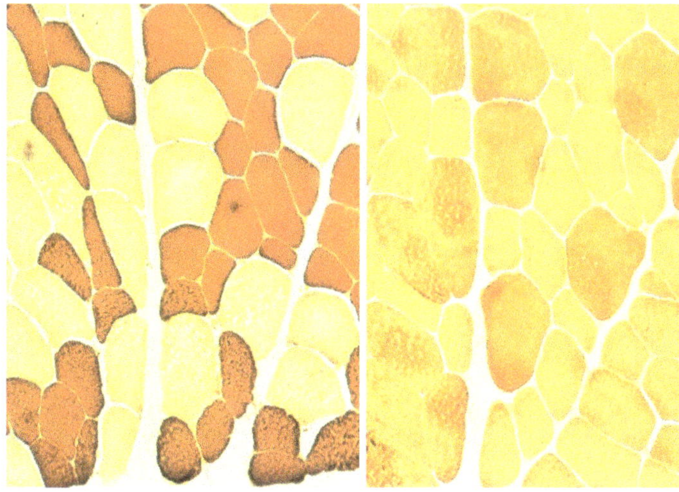

Fig. 13.1 Myofibrillar reactions of muscle fibers from a Myotonia congenita patient. All type 2 fibers are dark in the ATPase preparation at pH 9.4 (*left*). Type 2A fibers in the same biopsy show light staining at pH 4.3, suggesting complete absence of type 2B fibers (*right*). ×100

must be mutated so the Cl^- conductance decrease to < 25 % of its normal value.

PAM is caused by gain-of-function mutations in $Na_v1.4$, the voltage-gated Na^+ channel of skeletal muscle, encoded by *SCN4A* on chromosome 17q. This channel is essential for the generation of the muscle action potential. The mutations cause a pathologically increased inward Na^+ current, which can activate more Na^+ channels, thereby generating action potential bursts. This repetitive activity reflects a dominant-positive effect of the mutations that is enhanced by the preexisting membrane depolarization due to elevated serum K^+ in PAM.

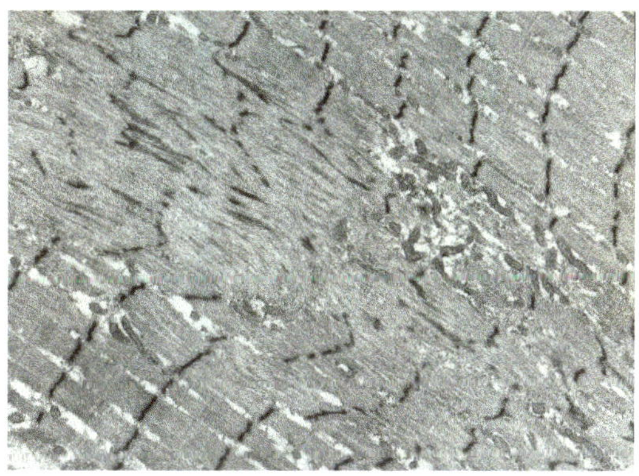

Fig. 13.2 Myofibrillar architecture of a muscle fiber from a Myotonia permanens patient with Potassium-aggravated myotonia. Note the focal disarray of myofibrils and the disappearance of Z discs. Bar = 1 μm

13.2.3 Histopathology

Samples of DMC and RMC muscle tissue sometimes have a normal appearance. Often, however, there are slight myopathic changes with increased occurrence of central nuclei and pathological variation of fiber diameter. Muscle fiber hypertrophy, especially of type 2A fibers, and fiber atrophy may be present. Finally, there may be reduction or complete absence of type 2B fibers (Fig. 13.1).

Despite the widespread range of severity in PAM, the morphological findings are practically the same. In Myotonia fluctuans, the mildest form of PAM, light microscopy may show a normal appearance or increased central nuclei and fiber diameter variation. Subsarcolemmal vacuoles representing a nonspecific enlargement of the T-tubular system may be found by electron microscopy. In Myotonia permanens, the most severe form of PAM, subsarcolemmal myoplasmic space and mitochondria may be increased. There may also be focal disarray or interruption of myofibrils and disappearance of Z-discs, involving one or more sarcomeres (Fig. 13.2). Glycogen particles and elongated or branched mitochondria can be found in these areas. Between the bundles of myofibrils, membrane-bound vacuoles may be visible that are empty or filled with fine granular material or electron-dense whorls.

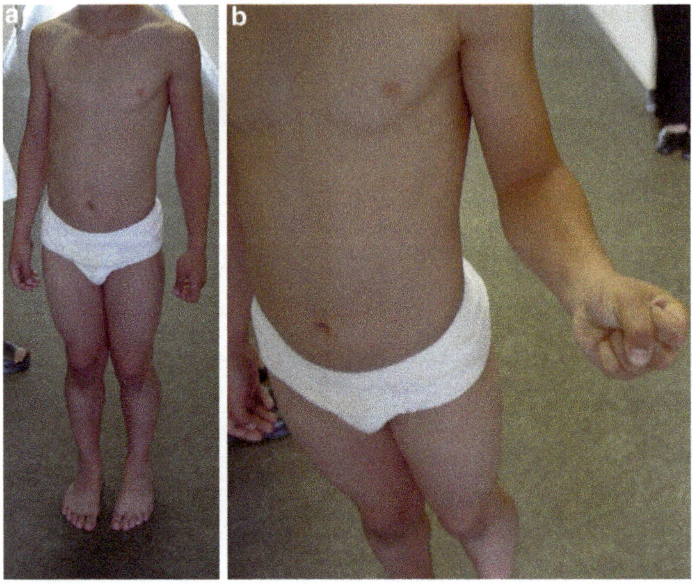

Fig. 13.3 Clinical findings in a RMC patient with generalized muscle hypertrophy (**a**) and grip myotonia (**b**). Courtesy of Dirk Fischer, Basel, Switzerland

13.2.4 Clinical Presentation

Myotonia is characterized by muscle stiffness due to involuntary electrical after-activity following voluntary strong muscle activity. If the myotonia is severe, there may be transient weakness lasting only a few seconds after the first forceful contraction. With MC, the myotonia decreases with continued activity, a phenomenon called warm-up. With PAM, the degree of warm-up is variable, but aggravation by oral potassium loading is indicative. On EMG examination, myotonic muscles exhibit myotonic runs (i.e., action potentials changing frequency and amplitude). In mild cases, myotonia may not be evident on clinical examination, yet EMG may reveal the typical myotonic bursts. This condition is termed latent myotonia. In general, myotonia and corresponding muscle hypertrophy are more prominent in Becker myotonia than in Thomsen's disease or PAM (Fig. 13.3).

13.2.5 Imaging Findings

Myotonia congenita and PAM patients do not generally present with pathological imaging findings. In PAM, T1- and T2-weighted MRI scans of the lower legs were normal in a study of six patients (median age 43 years). In a recent study, three severely affected RMC patients were examined using multisequence (T1-weighted, T2-weighted, fat-suppressed T2-weighted sequences) whole-body 3T MRI. None of the patients showed skeletal muscle signal changes indicative of fatty muscle degeneration or edema, but two patients showed muscle bulk hypertrophy of the thighs and calves in line with their clinical appearance (Fig. 13.4). Therefore, imaging can be used to differentiate DMC and RMC from myotonic dystrophy, in which reduced muscle mass and edema are present. Likewise, the prominent muscle bulk in MC is due to genuine muscle hypertrophy and not to pseudo-hypertrophy—which may be used for differentiating it from other muscular dystrophies.

13.2.6 Therapy

Myotonia congenita can be partially managed by keeping muscles in a "warmed-up" state by continuous slight movement. However patients, particularly those with Becker myotonia require long-term medication. The myotonic stiffness responds to class 1 antiarrhythmia drugs, which

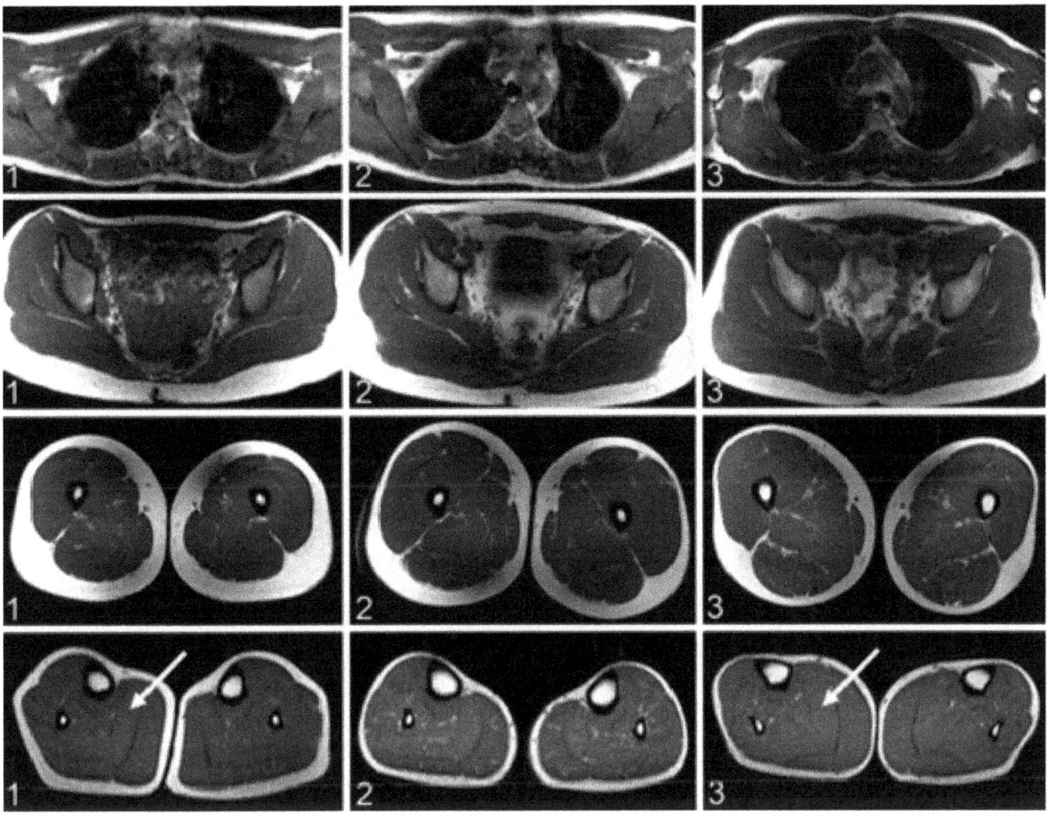

Fig. 13.4 Whole-body magnetic resonance imaging (MRI) findings in three recessive myotonia congenita (RMC) patients corresponding to columns 1–3. Axial sections of T1-weighted turbo spin echo sequences at the level of the shoulder girdle (*top row*), pelvis (*second row*), thighs (*third row*), and calves (*bottom row*). In all patients, shoulder girdle and trunk muscles showed no trophic changes. Patients 1 and 3 had hypertrophy of the thigh and calf muscles (*arrows*). Lower leg muscles of patient 2 were comparatively hypotrophic, with no fatty degeneration or skeletal muscle edema. From Kornblum C et al. Acta Neurol Scand. 2010;121:131–135

inhibit and reduce the repetitive activity. Of the many medications tested that can be administered orally, flecainide and propafenone are the drugs of choice. They preferentially block the noninactivating mutant sodium channels that frequently reopen abnormally. Thus, they have a much greater beneficial effect in PAM than in chloride channel myotonia. Patients with severe myotonia permanens require long-term continuous therapy. The drugs are also highly effective in preventing and reducing the degree of cold-induced stiffness and weakness associated with Paramyotonia congenita (PC, see Sect. 13.3.1). Carbonic anhydrase inhibitors can be an alternative treatment for patients with PAM but may exacerbate chloride channel myotonia.

13.2.7 Differential Diagnosis

For the nondystrophic myotonias PAM, DMC, and RMC the dystrophic myotonias are the most important differential diagnosis. Therefore, given a clinical diagnosis of myotonia by EMG examination, muscle atrophy, cataracts, and tri- and tetranucleotide repeat expansions as in myotonic dystrophies types 1 and 2 (see Chap. 22) must be excluded. The presence of paradoxical myotonia, which is most pronounced during repetitive strong eyelid contractions and eye openings, points to sodium channel myotonia, whereas the warm-up phenomenon of limb muscles may occur in all types of myotonia regardless of the underlying mutated gene. Provocative tests using local cooling are helpful for diagnosing PAM, which can be confirmed by molecular genetics. Na^+ channel myotonia can be easily proven by identifying one of the approximately 30 known *SCN4A* mutations. Because *CLCN1* mutations are distributed over the entire gene, mutational screening requires complete sequencing.

13.3 Adynamia Paramyotonia Complex

13.3.1 Subtypes, Synonyms, Abbreviations

Paramyotonia congenita (PC), Hyperkalemic periodic paralysis (HyperPP).

13.3.2 Genetics and Pathophysiology

Paramyotonia congenita (PC) is caused by mutations in $Na_v1.4$, the voltage-gated Na^+ channel of skeletal muscle, encoded by *SCN4A* on chromosome 17q. The mutations accelerate recovery from the inactivated, refractory state and result in facilitated generation of action potentials. As a consequence, Na^+ inward current is increased, which depolarizes the membrane and thereby activates more Na^+ channels, which generate action potential bursts. This repetitive activity reflects a dominant-positive effect of the mutations that is enhanced by depolarizing factors such as elevated serum K^+ or a cold environment.

Hyperkalemic periodic paralysis (HyperPP) is caused by gain-of-function mutations in the voltage-gated sodium channel $Na_v1.4$ as well. Most mutations destabilize the inactivated state, which causes channel reopening and a persistent current corresponding to a gain-of-function defect. The resulting long-lasting membrane depolarization inactivates wild-type channels whereby the muscle is rendered inexcitable. The membrane depolarization also increases the driving force for K^+, which increases efflux and serum levels of this ion, sustaining the hyperkalemia.

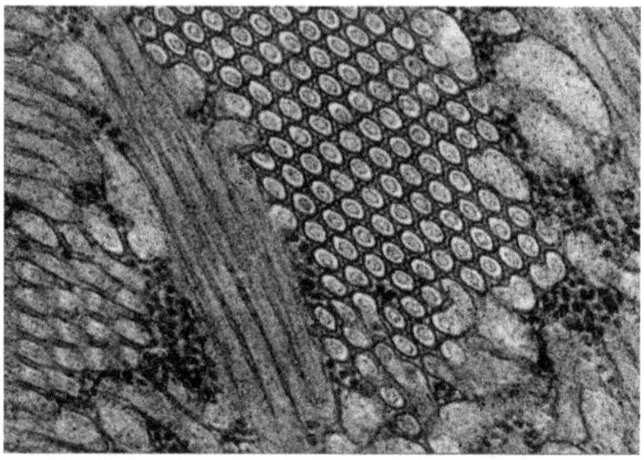

Fig. 13.5 Typical tubular aggregates in a fiber from a periodic paralysis patient. Magnification: ×16,500

13.3.3 Histopathology

In PC, light microscopy may be unremarkable except for nonspecific myopathological changes such as occasional central nuclei, variation of fiber diameter with hypertrophic split, rarely atrophic, and regenerating fibers. ATPase type 2A fibers may be hypertrophied, and the number of type 2B fibers may be decreased as in the Cl^- channelopathies, although areas of normal muscle fiber and distribution of fiber types 1, 2A, and 2B have also been described. In some areas, there may be focal myofibril degeneration with myelin bodies, lipid deposits, tubular aggregates, and occasional subsarcolemmal vacuoles without periodic acid-Schiff (PAS)-positive material. Muscle fiber degeneration followed by phagocyte invasion and fatty replacement may occur, perhaps induced by the cold-induced attacks of weakness.

Muscle fibers of patients with periodic paralysis may show collections of multiple closely packed tubules resulting in a honeycomb appearance, which in cross section are seen mostly on fiber ends. These tubular aggregates are located between longitudinally running myofibrils or underneath the sarcolemma. They may contain an internal circular membrane that is not normally seen in the T-tubule or the sarcoplasmic reticulum from which they originate (Fig. 13.5). Vacuoles resulting from degenerating fibers are also frequently found.

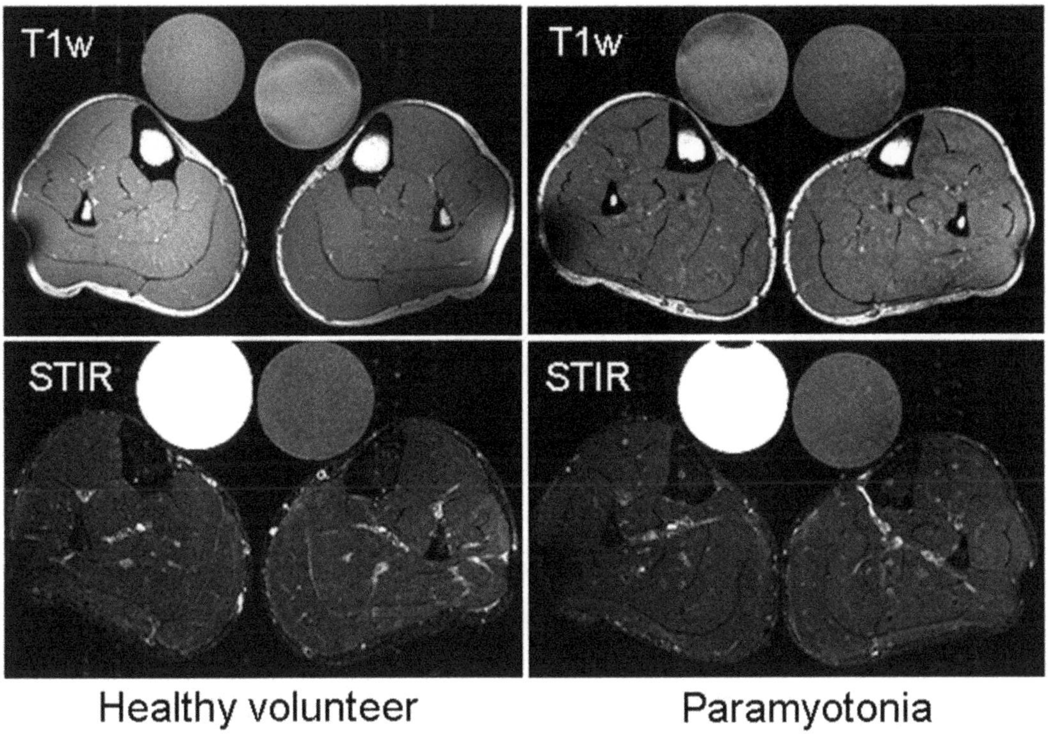

Fig. 13.6 Comparison of lower leg muscles of an adolescent healthy volunteer and an adolescent boy with paramyotonia congenita. Axial T1-weighted 3T MRI scans are in the upper row, and axial STIR MRI scans are in the lower row. No morphological changes are visible in paramyotonia using standard ^{1}H-MRI. Reference tubes filled with 51.3 mM sodium are placed between the lower legs

13.3.4 Clinical Presentation

In contrast to the warm-up phenomenon in MC, PC patients show paradoxical myotonia (i.e., myotonia that worsens with exercise or in the cold). Facial and eyelid muscles are especially sensitive to the cold, so lid paramyotonia may be the most reliable diagnostic sign. During intensive cooling, the stiffness gives way to flaccid weakness or even paralysis. In contrast to cold-induced weakness, potassium-induced weakness is usually of short duration, lasting minutes to hours.

HyperPP patients present with increased serum potassium during episodes of weakness. They may not have any interictal symptoms and are therefore often thought to exhibit a conversion reaction. In this case, the subsequent omission of adequate therapy may cause them to suffer needlessly. Weakness is triggered by a variety of circumstances, including rest after exercise, potassium-rich food, cold environment, emotional stress, fasting, and pregnancy. Between episodes, the disease is often associated with mild myotonia, which does not impede voluntary movements but may be exacerbated at the beginning of weakness.

13.3.5 Imaging Findings

In PC and HyperPP, conventional MRI may be normal (Fig. 13.6). However, in affected patients, the defect of the muscular Na^+ channels leads to a pathological Na^+ influx that is responsible for the symptoms. Therefore, ^{23}Na-MRI is the method of choice. This method enables depiction of an intracellular muscular sodium accumulation simultaneous to development of muscular paresis (Fig. 13.7). The sodium accumulation correlates well with the grade

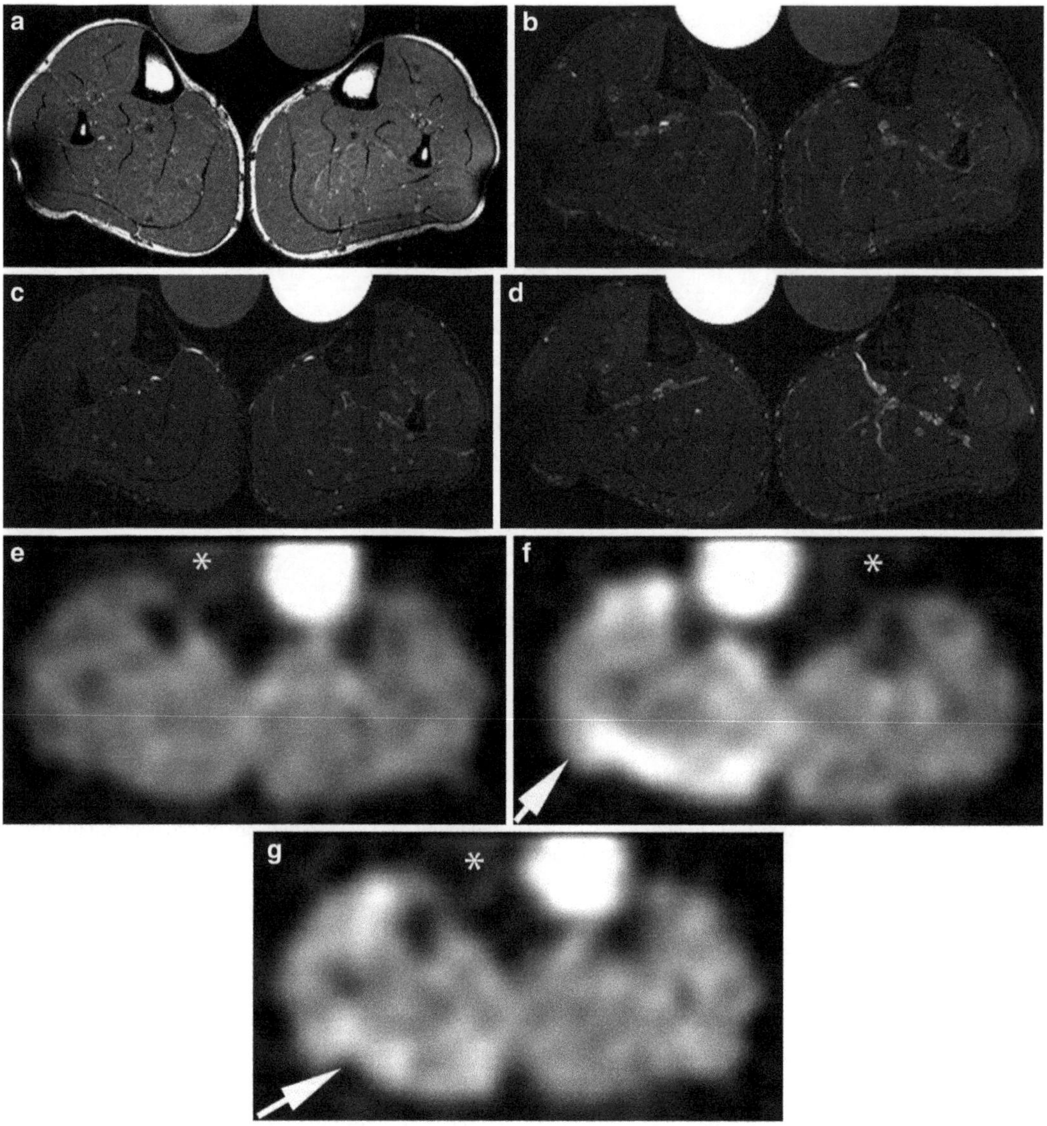

Fig. 13.7 A 22-year-old man with paramyotonia congenita. (**a**) Axial T1-weighted 3T MRI: axial STIR images before (**b**), directly after (**c**), and 2 h after provocation (**d**) of muscle stiffness and paresis by ice bags placed around the right lower leg for 25 min. 3T ^{23}Na-MRI inversion recovery (IR) scans before (**e**), directly after (**f**), and 2 h after provocation (**g**). There is no muscle edema visible after provocation. However, the intracellular sodium concentration is elevated in the right calf muscles both directly after provocation (*arrow*) and 2 h later after re-warming of the lower leg (*arrow*). Note that the signal of the reference tube containing free 0.3 % NaCl solution (*asterisk*) is suppressed in the ^{23}Na-MRI IR sequence, whereas the contralateral reference tube filled with Na^+ in agarose gel is well visible

of paresis and is reproducible. Additionally, ^{23}Na MRI allows noninvasive monitoring of mexiletine (a Na^+ channel blocker) therapy.

Approximately 38 % of PC patients in one study showed normal muscle on T1- and T2-weighted 1.5T MRI examinations of the lower legs. About 12 % of patients had bilaterally symmetrical homogeneous edema before exercise that was confined to the medial head of the gastrocnemius muscle. In another PC cohort, there were edema-like muscular changes in the triceps surae muscles in 10 % of the patients (median age 45 years). Up to 50 % of older patients showed bilaterally symmetrical increased signal intensity of the medial head of the gastrocnemius muscle on T1- and T2-weighted images that was interpreted as fatty infiltration. There was no muscle atrophy in any of the 16 paramyotonia patients studied to date.

In HyperPP, increased ^{1}H signal intensities on T2-weighted ^{1}H-MRI were visible in the triceps surae muscles of 43 % of the patients prior to provocation. In a more recent series using 3T MRI, 8 of 12 HyperPP patients exhibited edema-like changes prior to provocation on short-tau inversion recovery (STIR) images. Seven of the 12 HyperPP patients showed fatty infiltration/degeneration (i.e., high signal intensities in their lower leg muscles) on T1-weighted images. HyperPP patients suffering from permanent weakness present a high degree of lipomatous changes compared to the group without permanent weakness and healthy volunteers. A specific pattern of lipomatous changes was noticeable: The highest degree of fatty atrophy was observed in the triceps surae muscle (gastrocnemius followed by the soleus muscle). The peroneal muscles showed concomitantly the lowest degree of edema-like changes and of fatty atrophy/degeneration.

13.3.6 Therapy

Oral flecainide and propafenone are the drugs of choice for PC. They affect the disease directly by blocking the noninactivating mutant sodium channels. Additionally, reducing serum potassium levels by stimulating the Na^+/K^+ pump (e.g., by continuous mild exercise or carbohydrate ingestion of salbutamol inhalation) helps relieve the attacks of weakness seen with HyperPP. Permanent stabilization of serum K^+ at low levels by thiazide diuretics is also a possibility. Carbonic anhydrase inhibitors are the second choice and may be effective via myoplasmic acidification.

13.3.7 Differential Diagnosis

The main differential diagnosis for PC includes the myotonias, although the sodium channel mutations carriers may be detected by testing for lid paramyotonia after cooling the eye. For primary periodic paralyses, the most important differential diagnoses are secondary periodic paralyses due to kidney malfunction (e.g., Bartter syndrome) or inflammation (e.g., Guillain-Barré syndrome). Therefore, all possibilities of K^+ dysregulation and secondary periodic paralysis should be examined before primary periodic paralyses is considered.

13.4 Hypokalemic Periodic Paralysis

13.4.1 Synonyms, Abbreviations

HypoPP.

13.4.2 Genetics and Pathophysiology

Hypokalemic periodic paralysis is associated with a loss-of-function defect of $Na_v1.4$ or $Ca_v1.1$. The former is the voltage-gated skeletal muscle sodium channel Nav1.4 encoded by *SCN4A* on chromosome 17q, and the latter is the main subunit of the T-tubular voltage-gated L-type Ca^{2+} channel complex encoded by *CACNA1S* on chromosome 1q. The two genetic variants are clinically similar, and in both channel types the mutations are located exclusively in the S4 segments, which convey voltage sensitivity by moving outward during depolarization, enabling channel opening. On the level of the pore current (i.e., the sodium and calcium inward currents, respectively), a loss of function is produced by the mutations: The inactivated state is stabilized in the Na^+ channel mutants, and the channel availability is reduced for the Ca^{2+} channel mutants. However, because the S4 voltage sensors need to move through the membrane field, they are thought to be located in a canaliculus that is interspersed between the intracellular

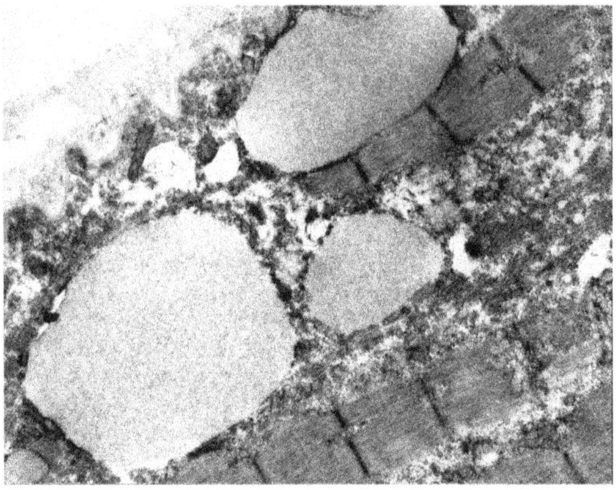

Fig. 13.8 Typical vacuolization in muscle of a hypokalemic periodic paralysis patient. ×400

and extracellular compartments. The HypoPP mutations cause a short circuit of the two compartments—a so-called omega current that depolarizes the membrane and renders the fibers nonexcitable.

13.4.3 Histopathology

In HypoPP, muscle fibers frequently show signs of proliferation, regeneration, and dilation of components of the T-tubular system and the sarcoplasmic reticulum resulting in vacuolization (Fig. 13.8). Contraction of nearby myofibrils and a focal increase of muscle glycogen have also been noted, suggesting that the changes in several organelles account for the permanent myopathy of the disease. Areas with tubular aggregates may also be found.

13.4.4 Clinical Presentation

HypoPP occurs episodically with varying intervals of normal muscle function. Apparently, the underlying ion channel defects are usually well compensated, and an additional trigger is often required for channel malfunction. Weakness episodes in HypoPP are precipitated by glucose-induced hypokalemia and are ameliorated by K^+ intake. Because of the additional uptake of K^+ by muscle in HypoPP, the resulting dyskalemia can be so severe that cardiac complications arise. During an attack, death can occur because of respiratory insufficiency. Independent of the severity and frequency of the paralytic episodes, many patients develop a chronic progressive myopathy during their forties, an age at which the attacks of weakness decrease.

13.4.5 Imaging Findings

There is intramuscular ^{23}Na accumulation in HypoPP. The sodium overload causes muscle edema and weakness in these patients (Fig. 13.9). It can be treated specifically with acetazolamide. Young patients suffer from muscular edema in HypoPP-1, which at this young age may be the only morphological transformation of their muscle tissue (Fig. 13.10). With continued aging and if untreated, lipomatous degeneration of the muscle tissue takes place (Fig. 13.11), and the patient develops permanent muscular weakness. Even this development can be treated with acetazolamide. The muscle edema and weakness disappear under anti-edema treatment, and muscular strength increases (Fig. 13.12).

In a cohort of 25 patients with HypoPP and permanent weakness, 21 displayed fatty muscle degeneration, and 18 exibited edema during ^1H-MRI of the lower legs. The degree of fatty muscle degeneration increased with age. The correlation between water content and Na^+ yielded a linear coefficient of determination (R^2) of 0.63.

13.4.6 Therapy

In patients with HypoPP, all substances that decrease serum K^+ levels—by shifting potassium into the cells or kidney excretion— should be avoided (i.e., high carbohydrate/high salt meals, bicarbonate- and K^+-extruding diuretics, sedentary lifestyle, strenuous physical exercise). Attacks should be treated orally with KCl. Carbonic anhydrase inhibitors are the prophylactic medication of choice. K^+-sparing diuretics (e.g., triamterene, amiloride, spironolactone) may be administered as well.

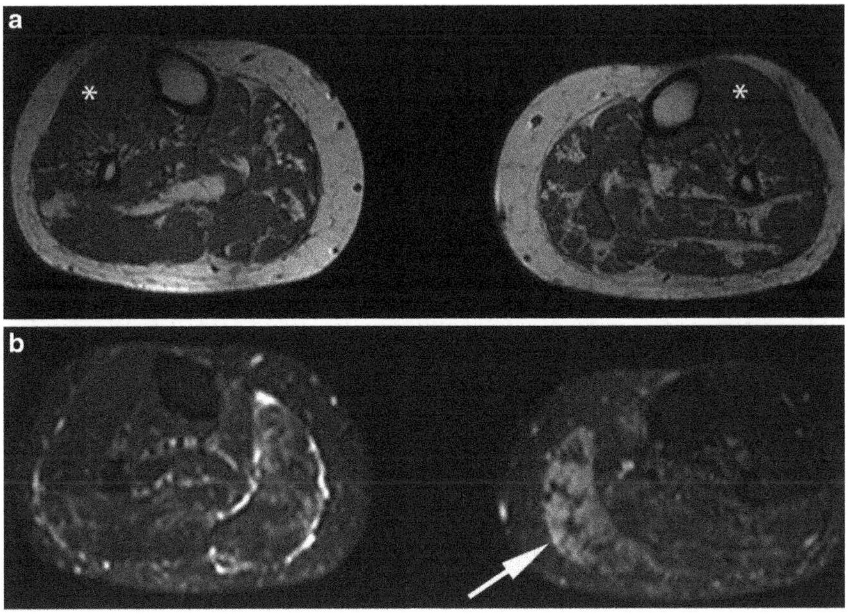

Fig. 13.9 A 44-year-old woman with hypokalemic periodic paralysis type 1 (Cav1.1.R1239H). Axial T1-weighted 3T MRI scans of both calves (TR/TE 700/10 ms) (**a**) and corresponding axial STIR MRI scans (TR/TE 7060/65 ms) (**b**). There are edema-like changes in the medial head of the gastrocnemius muscle, which are pronounced on the left side (*arrow*). Note also the fatty infiltration of the triceps surae muscles and the muscles of the deep posterior compartment. The tibialis anterior compartment is spared (*asterisks*)

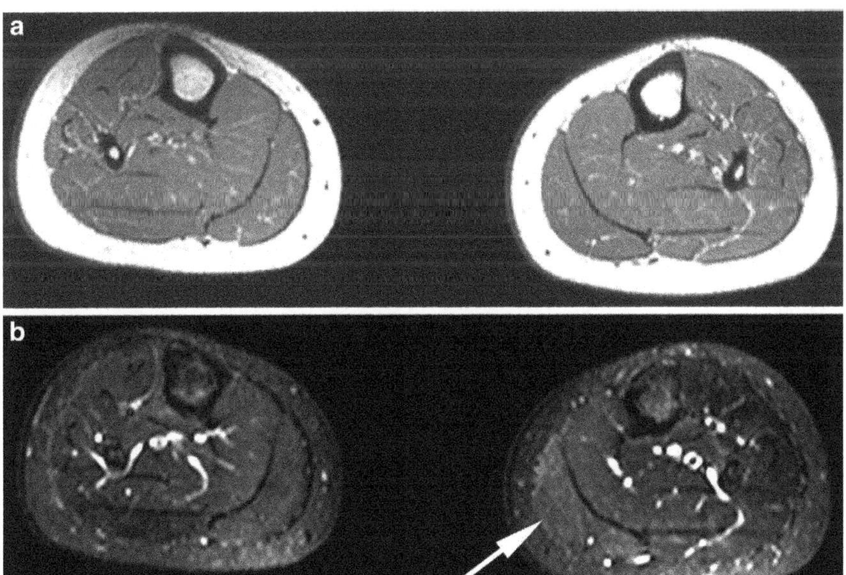

Fig. 13.10 Compared to the moderate muscle degeneration of her mother in Fig. 13.9, the 11-year-old daughter, also diagnosed with hypokalemic periodic paralysis type 1 (Cav1.1.R1239H) has no lipomatous degeneration on T1-weighted MRI (**a**), but shows a slight signal increase on STIR images (**b**) in the medial gastrocnemius muscle on the left side (*arrow*)

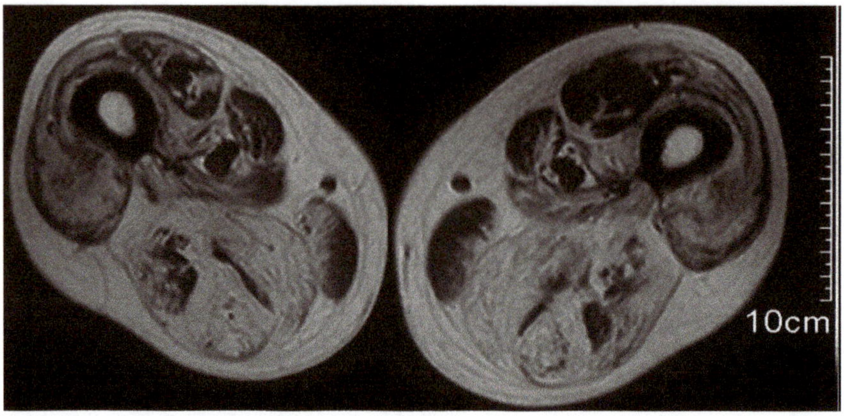

Fig. 13.11 Distinct lipomatous degeneration of both thigh muscles in an elderly HypoPP patient with pronounced fatty changes in the hamstring muscles

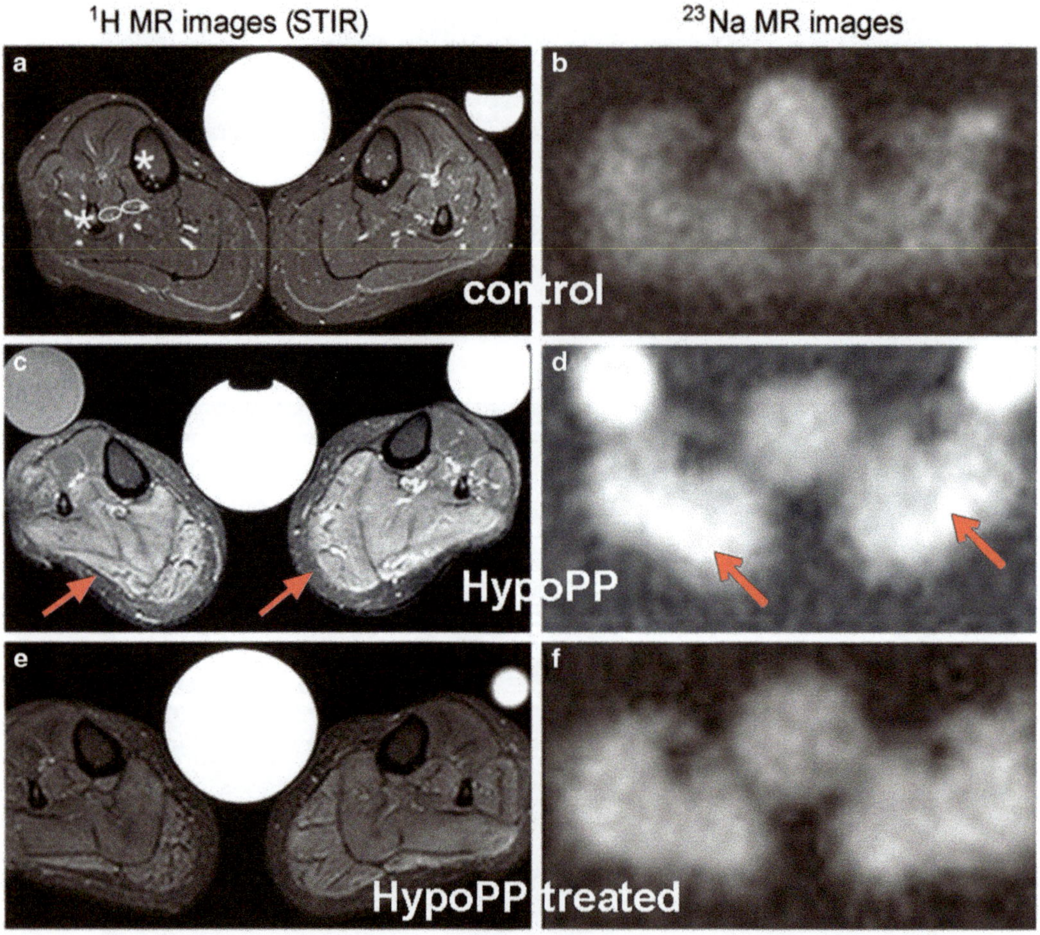

Fig. 13.12 1.5T STIR ^{1}H-MRI (*left column*, **a**, **c**, **e**) and 1.5T ^{23}Na-MRI (right column, **b**, **d**, **f**) from a healthy female control (*top row*) and a female HypoPP patient of similar age before treatment (*center row*) and after treatment with acetazolamide 250 mg/day for 4 weeks (*bottom row*). Note the very high hydrogen intensities in the STIR sequence, representing muscular edema, and the elevated muscular Na^+ concentration before treatment (*arrows* in central row) and their improvement after treatment (*bottom row*). The central reference contains 0.3 % NaCl solution (51.3 mM). Occasional side tubes containing 0.3 % NaCl in agarose gel to the left and 0.6 % NaCl in H_2O to the right were additional standards. The *asterisks* mark the tibial and fibular bone, which have low signal intensity on ^{23}Na-MRI. Modified from Jurkat-Rott K, et al (2009) K^+-dependent paradoxical membrane depolarization and Na^+ overload, major and reversible contributors to weakness by ion channel leaks. Proc Natl Acad Sci U S A. 106(10):4036–41

13.4.7 Differential Diagnosis

For the primary periodic paralyses, the most important differential diagnoses are secondary periodic paralysis due to kidney malfunction (e.g., Bartter syndromes) or inflammation (e.g., Guillain Barré syndrome). Therefore, all possibilites of K^+ dysregulation and secondary periodic paralysis should be examined before primary periodic paralysis is considered. In the past, provocative tests for periodic paralysis were carried out for diagnostic reasons. As they are associated with the risk of inducing a severe attack, they had to be performed by an experienced physician and a stand-by anesthesiologist. Also, serum K^+, glucose, and the electrocardiogram had to be closely monitored. Nowadays, provocative tests should be restricted to patients in whom molecular genetics failed to identify the underlying mutation. Because histological alterations are not specific, a muscle biopsy should be performed only in patients with atypical features or for documentation of a vacuolar myopathy.

13.5 Outlook

Recently, the development of ^{23}Na-MRI at high magnetic field strengths of 3T to 7T allows more precise quantification of intracellular ^{23}Na homeostasis. In addition, ^{23}Na homeostasis may be examined more precisely in healthy volunteers as well as in patients as initial findings indicate the high potential of ^{23}Na-MRI at 7 T (Fig. 13.13) (see Sect. 5.3). In conclusion, we expect a much higher level of acceptance for this new technique in the near future for assessing the pathophysiology of muscular edema-like changes in other muscular dystrophies.

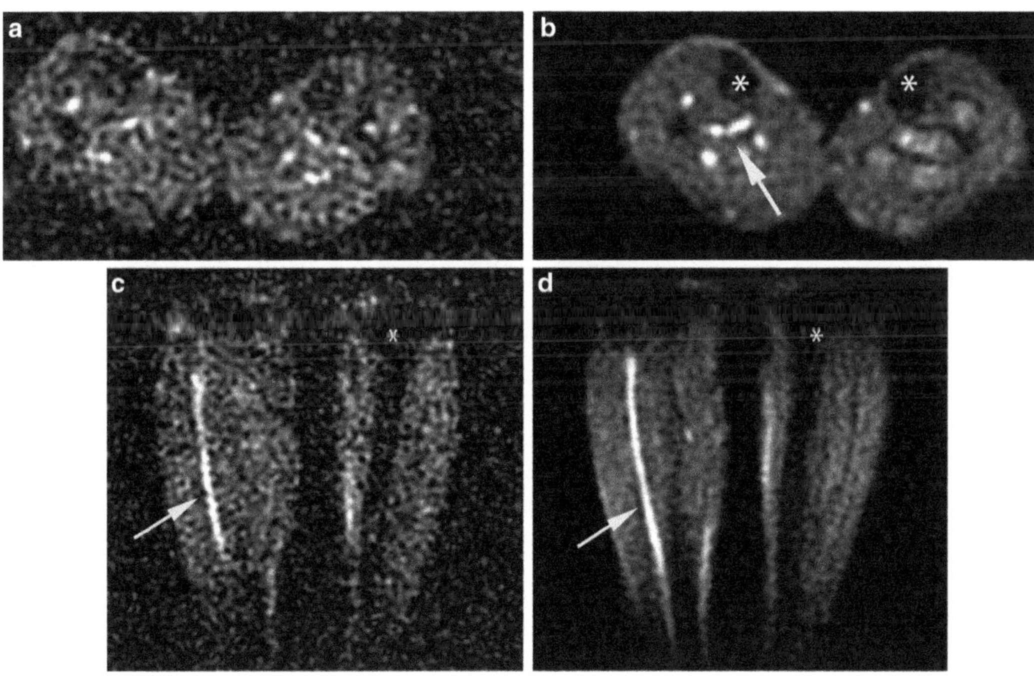

Fig. 13.13 Comparison of axial ^{23}Na-MRI scans of both lower legs of a healthy volunteer acquired with 3T MRI (**a**) and 7T MRI (**b**) as well as the corresponding coronal ^{23}Na-MRI images acquired with 3T MRI (**c**) and 7T MRI (**d**). The *asterisks* mark the tibial bones as structures with low signal intensity. The *arrows* point to vessels with high signal intensity. Clearly visible are the higher signal-to-noise ratio at 7T and the reduced background noise outside the lower legs. Courtesy of Armin Nagel, PhD, Department of Medical Physics in Radiology, German Cancer Research Center, Heidelberg

Channelopathies

Key Points

- Skeletal muscle channelopathies comprise nondystrophic myotonias and periodic paralyses.
- The channelopathies are caused by mutations in chloride, sodium, and calcium channels in skeletal muscle.
- Myotonia is caused by bursts of action potentials and periodic paralysis by the absence thereof.
- Histology frequently shows unspecific myopathic signs. However, it may show an absence of type 2B fibers in myotonia congenita and the presence of vacuoles and tubular aggregates in periodic paralysis.
- Conventional MRI is frequently normal. Hypertrophy is found only in myotonia congenita.
- ^{23}Na-MRI is able to depict intracellular muscular sodium accumulation in correlation with the development of muscular paresis in paramyotonia and Hyperkalemic and Hypokalemic periodic paralysis.
- The sodium accumulation correlates well with the grade of paresis and is reproducible.
- Treatment of myotonia and paramyotonia aims to block repetitive firing of action potentials using the sodium channel blockers flecainide and propafenone.
- Treatment of periodic paralysis by diuretics such as carbonic anhydrase inhibitors aims to rectify the serum potassium level and alleviate the muscular edema and weakness.

Suggestions for Further Reading

Amarteifio E, Nagel AM, Weber MA, et al. Hyperkalemic periodic paralysis and permanent weakness: 3-T MR imaging depicts intracellular 23Na overload-initial results. Radiology. 2012;264:154–63.

Jurkat-Rott K, Weber MA, Fauler M, et al. K^+-dependent paradoxical membrane depolarization and Na^+ overload, major and reversible contributors to weakness by ion channel leaks. Proc Natl Acad Sci U S A. 2009; 106:4036–41.

Kornblum C, Lutterbey GG, Czermin B, et al. Whole-body high-field MRI shows no skeletal muscle degeneration in young patients with recessive myotonia congenita. Acta Neurol Scand. 2010;121:131–5.

Lehmann-Horn F, Jurkat-Rott K, Rüdel R. Nondystrophic myotonias and periodic paralyses. In: Rimoin DL, Connor JM, Pyeritz RE, Korf BR, editors. Emery and Rimoin's principles and practice of medical genetics. Fifth edition, Vol. II, Chap. 138. Philadelphia: Churchill Livingstone, Elsevier; 2007. p. 3024–46.

Lehmann-Horn F, Jurkat-Rott K, Rüdel R. Diagnostics and therapy of muscle channelopathies – guidelines of the Ulm Muscle Centre. Acta Myologica. 2008;27: 98–113.

Nagel AM, Laun FB, Weber MA, et al. Sodium-MRI using a density adapted 3D radial acquisition technique. Magn Reson Med. 2009;62:1565–73.

Nagel AM, Amarteifio E, Lehmann-Horn F, et al. 3 Tesla sodium inversion recovery magnetic resonance imaging allows for improved visualization of intracellular sodium content changes in muscular channelopathies. Invest Radiol. 2011;46:759–66.

Ryan AM, Matthews E, Hanna MG. Skeletal-muscle channelopathies: periodic paralysis and nondystrophic myotonias. Curr Opin Neurol. 2007;20:558–63.

Weber MA, Nielles-Vallespin S, Huttner HB, et al. Evaluation of patients with paramyotonia at ^{23}Na MR imaging during cold induced weakness. Radiology. 2006a;240:489–500.

Weber MA, Nielles-Vallespin S, Essig M, et al. Muscle Na^+ channelopathies – MRI detects intracellular ^{23}Na accumulation during episodic weakness. Neurology. 2006b;67:1151–8.

Weber MA, Nagel AM, Jurkat-Rott K, et al. Sodium (^{23}Na) MRI detects elevated muscular sodium concentration in Duchenne muscular dystrophy. Neurology. 2011;77:2017–24.

Metabolic Myopathies

14

Anna Pichiecchio and Eleonora Tavazzi

14.1 Introduction and Classification

Various metabolic pathways are involved in producing energy in skeletal muscles, but the level of activation varies according to the type of muscle fiber, the intensity and duration of the exercise, and the nutritional status of the individual.

The principal sources of energy are lipids (fatty acids and derivatives) and carbohydrates (glycogen). Under starvation conditions, amino acids are the main fuel.

Under physiological conditions, acyl groups derived from fatty acids are transported to mitochondria by carnitine, where they are further processed (β-oxidation) to produce acetyl-coenzyme A (CoA). Glycogen metabolism starts in the sarcoplasm. Here, through glycolysis, glycogen is converted to pyruvate, which enters the mitochondria and is transformed to acetyl-CoA. Acetyl-CoA is thus derived from both lipids and carbohydrates. It generates energy (adenosine triphosphate, ATP) by oxidation via the Krebs (tricarboxylic acid) cycle and the respiratory chain.

There are two main muscle fiber types that use different metabolic pathways and are activated in diverse conditions. Type 1 fibers are characterized by high endurance and a large number of mitochondria. These fibers generate ATP by oxidative, aerobic metabolism. Type 2 fibers have low mitochondrial density and are involved in short-term anaerobic activity. Their preferred fuel is glycogen.

Metabolic myopathies derive from one or more defects in any step of the aforementioned metabolic pathways. They might be classified according to multiple criteria, such as the substrate involved (fatty acids, glycogen, blood glucose), the metabolic pathway affected, or the predominant clinical picture (exercise intolerance with rhabomyolysis or progressive muscle weakness). Here we describe the most common metabolic disorders, divided into three principal subgroups: glycogen storage diseases (GSDs), mitochondrial disorders, and lipid storage diseases.

A. Pichiecchio (✉) • E. Tavazzi
Department of Neuroradiology,
C. Mondino National Institute of Neurology Foundation, IRCCS, Via Mondino, 2, 27100 Pavia, Italy
e-mail: anna.pichiecchio@mondino.it

14.2 Pompe Disease and Other Glycogen Storage Diseases

Although several unique GSDs are discussed in the literature, there are only four related to clinically significant muscle weakness: Pompe disease (GSD type II), GSD type III, GSD type V, and GSD type VII. The overall frequency of GSDs is 1:20,000 births. GSDs II and III are the most common forms seen during infancy and type V during adulthood.

M.P. Wattjes and D. Fischer (eds.), *Neuromuscular Imaging*, DOI 10.1007/978-1-4614-6552-2_14,

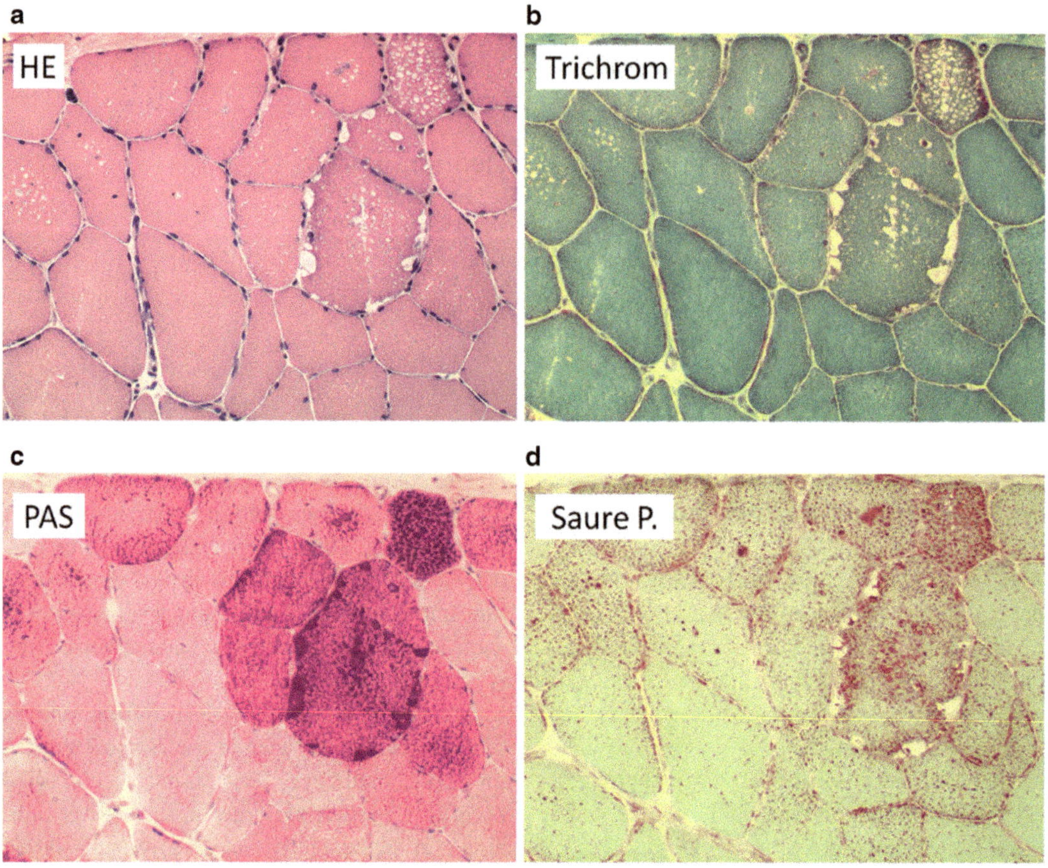

Fig. 14.1 Characteristic pathological features of glycogen storage disease II (GSDII). Several fibers contain cytoplasmic or subsarcolemmal vacuoles (*arrow*) (**a**: H&E; **b**: Gomori trichrome), which are periodic acid-Schiff (PAS)-positive (**c**, *arrow*), indicating glycogen, and acid phosphatase-positive (**d**, *arrow*), indicating that the glycogen is deposited in lysosomes. Courtesy of Cornelia Kornblum, Bonn, Germany

14.2.1 Pompe Disease

14.2.1.1 Synonyms, Abbreviations

Acid maltase deficiency (AMD), glycogenosis type II (GlyII, GSDII)

14.2.1.2 Genetics and Pathophysiology

Pompe disease is a rare autosomal recessive lysosomal storage disorder caused by mutations in the acid α-glucosidase (GAA) gene on chromosome 17. Almost 200 mutations have been identified. The gene encodes for the lysosomal GAA, which catalyzes the hydrolysis of α-1,4 and 1,6 links of lysosomal glycogen to release glucose when energy is needed. The enzyme might be absent, not functioning, or partially active depending on the genetic mutation. However, the genotype only rarely relates to the clinical phenotype.

It is still unclear how the defective enzyme promotes the disease. It could be due to mechanical interruption of the contractile apparatus related to an autophagic process promoted by ruptured lysosomes or to altered myofibrillar morphology.

14.2.1.3 Histopathology

Increased muscle fiber vacuolization and autophagy are the histopathological hallmarks of the disease (Fig. 14.1). The vacuoles have high glycogen content, vary in size and shape, show

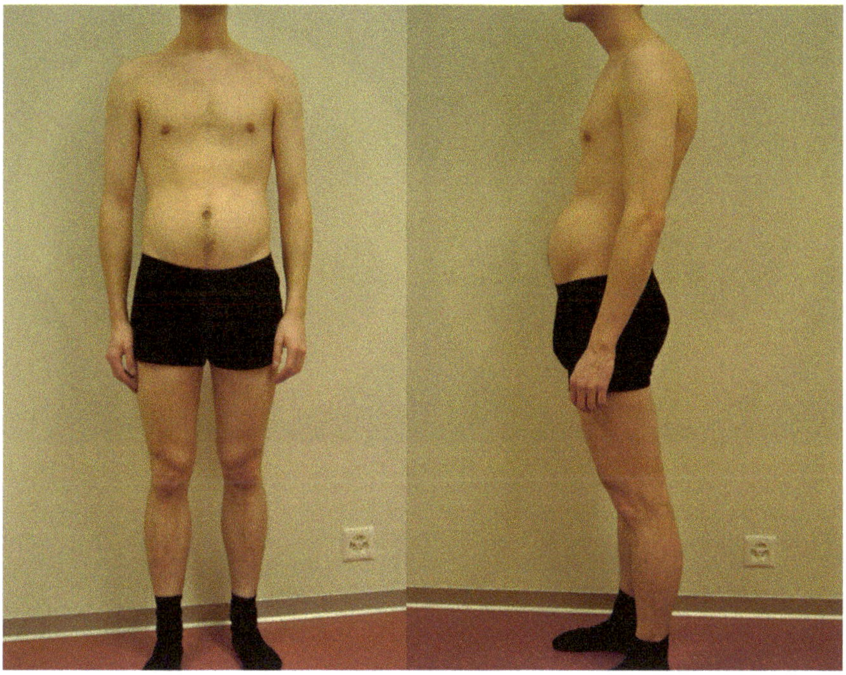

Fig. 14.2 Adult Pompe (GSD II) patient with marked axial weakness. Note the hyperlordosis and abdominal muscle weakness. Courtesy of Dirk Fischer, Basel, Switzerland

periodic acid-Schiff (PAS) positivity (a glycogen marker), and react strongly for acid phosphatase (a specific marker for lysosomes).

In the infantile form, the muscle fiber structure is severely compromised and shows no residual GAA activity. The degree of vacuolization and residual GAA activity are extremely variable in late onset patients and do not depend on the age of onset, disease duration, or clinical features. In the adult manifestation of Pompe disease, muscle biopsies may demonstrate only nonspecific changes or be normal.

To confirm the clinical diagnosis of Pompe disease, GAA enzyme activity should be measured in a tissue specimen (e.g., skin fibroblasts, muscle tissue, leukocytes). If the mutations are known, Pompe disease can also be diagnosed by genetic testing.

14.2.1.4 Clinical Presentation

GSDII is classified into infantile, juvenile, and adult forms. The classic infantile phenotype is characterized by a very early onset (< 6 months) with severe myopathy, cardiomyopathy, and respiratory failure, leading to death by the age of 2 years. In contrast, late-onset phenotypes (second to sixth decade) are extremely heterogeneous. The usual clinical picture is a slowly progressive proximal myopathy, often with respiratory involvement secondary to diaphragm and accessory respiratory muscle weakness (Fig. 14.2). Atrophy of the paraspinal muscles may lead to scoliosis, scapular winging, and low back pain. The heart is usually spared.

14.2.1.5 Imaging Findings

Clinical and muscle biopsy findings are rather unspecific in GSD II. Therefore, muscular imaging can be a helpful diagnostic tool. Computed tomography (CT) and magnetic resonance imaging (MRI) have proven to assess reliably the muscle involvement pattern of the disease. There is a positive correlation between muscular strength and the degree of muscle involvement detected with MRI.

CT studies in adult patients have shown that the disease spreads from trunk to extremities over the years, with paraspinal and thigh muscles being

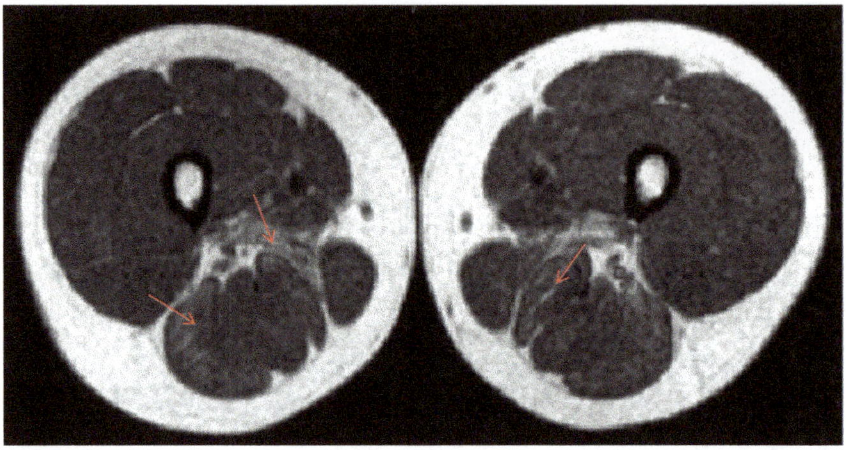

Fig. 14.3 Axial T1-weighted magnetic resonance imaging (MRI) scan at the level of the thigh in an adult patient affected by GSDII during the initial phase of Pompe disease (GSDII). Note the early involvement of the adductor magnus (*arrows*) and mild substitution of the semimembranosus and long head of the biceps muscles (*arrows*)

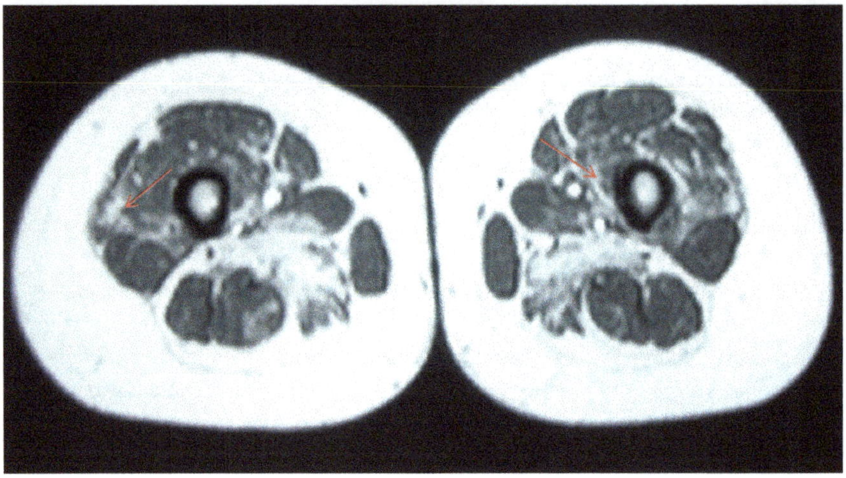

Fig. 14.4 Axial T1-weighted MRI scan at the level of the thigh in an adult patient affected by GSDII during the intermediate phase of Pompe disease (GSD II). Note the fatty replacement of the posterior compartment (see Fig. 14.2) plus involvement of the vastus intermedius, vastus medialis, and partially of the vastus lateralis muscles (*arrows*)

more severely affected than lower leg and shoulder girdle muscles.

Severe involvement of the thigh muscles, with selective sparing of the short head of the biceps femoris, gracilis, and sartorius muscles has been demonstrated. Some authors described an involvement pattern related to the clinical stage, with initial fatty infiltration of the adductor magnus, semimembranosus (Fig. 14.3), and variably semitendinosus muscles followed by fatty infiltration of the long head of the biceps femoris, vastus intermedius, and vastus medialis (and, to a lesser extent, the vastus lateralis) (Fig. 14.4). The short head of the biceps, lateral portions of the vastus lateralis (Fig. 14.5), and leg muscles (Fig. 14.6) are usually spared. The sartorius, rectus femoris, and gracilis tend to be spared or even hypertrophic even during late disease stages (Fig. 14.5).

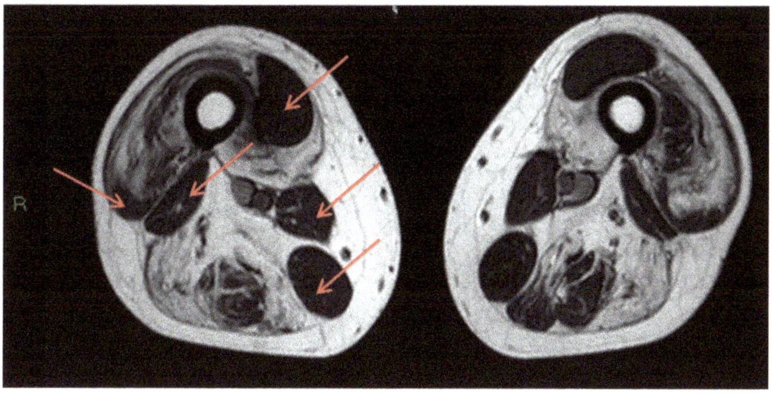

Fig. 14.5 Axial T1-weighted MRI scan at the level of the thigh in an adult patient affected by Pompe disease (GSDII) in the advanced phase of the disease. Note the selective sparing of the short head of the biceps, sartorius, rectus femoris, gracilis, and peripheral portions of the vastus lateralis muscles (*arrows*). The sartorius, rectus femoris, and gracilis are hypertrophic

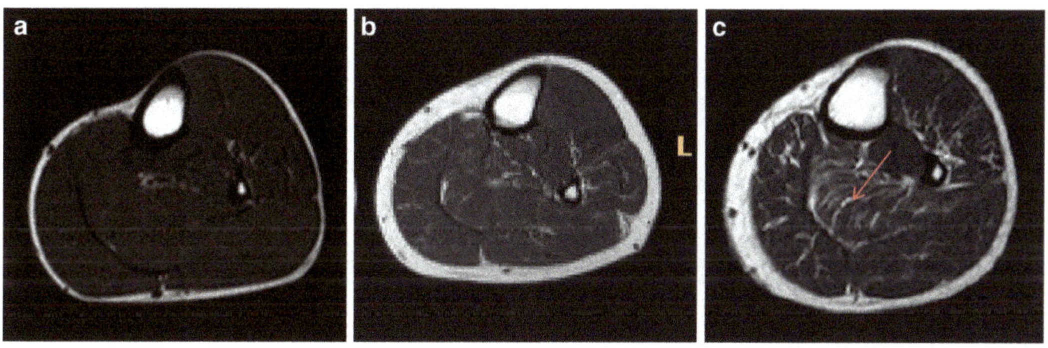

Fig. 14.6 Axial T1-weighted MRI scans at the level of the leg in adult patients affected by GSDII. The leg muscles are usually spared (**a**) or only mildly affected, or they exhibit diffuse, very mild fat replacement (**b**). In the advanced phases, more prominent involvement of the soleus can be detected (**c**) (*arrow*)

Paraspinal muscles can also be involved, particularly the posterior paraspinal and psoas muscles, which become severely atrophied. Based on our own experience, this pattern is more evident during the intermediate and advanced phases of the disease (Fig. 14.7). GSDII must always be considered in any case of unexplained paraspinal muscle atrophy. Trunk muscle atrophy can also be an unspecific finding and may also be seen in association with oxidative energy defects, such as mitochondrial myopathies (i.e., NADH-CoQ reductase deficiency), or in patients with low back pain.

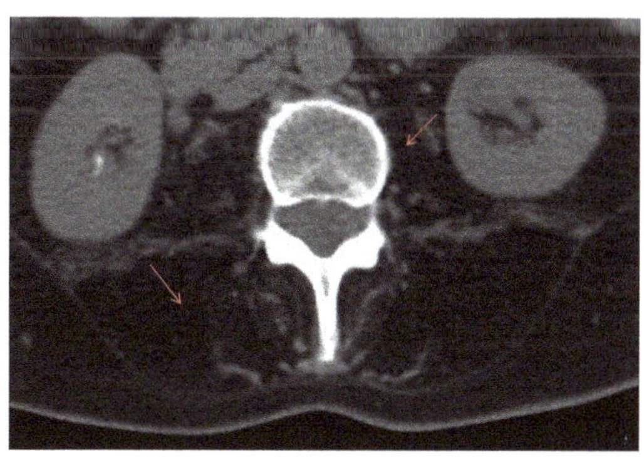

Fig. 14.7 Axial computed tomography (CT) image at the lumbar level for the evaluation of the paraspinal muscles in an adult patient affected by GSDII: atrophy and fat substitution of both paraspinal (multifidus, erector spinae) and ileo-psoas muscles are evident (*arrows*). Unexplained atrophy of the paraspinal muscles is not a specific finding for GSD II, but can be suggestive in adult patients both asymptomatic or with low back pain

Other authors, using whole-body MRI, have detected subtle neck and shoulder girdle muscle involvement and prominent involvement of the subscapularis muscles (Fig. 14.8). Facial and masticatory muscles are well preserved.

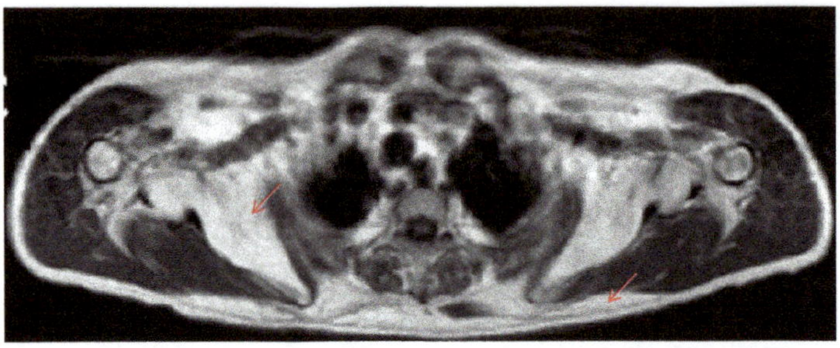

Fig. 14.8 Axial T1-weighted MRI scan obtained during a 1.5T whole-body MRI examination of a 40-year-old GSDII patient who was involved in intensive sports. Note the severe fatty infiltration at the shoulder girdle level (subscapularis and trapezius muscles). From Carlier et al (2011) Whole-body muscle MRI in 20 patients suffering from late onset Pompe disease: involvement patterns. Neuromuscul Disord. 21:791–9. Reprinted with permission from Elsevier Limited

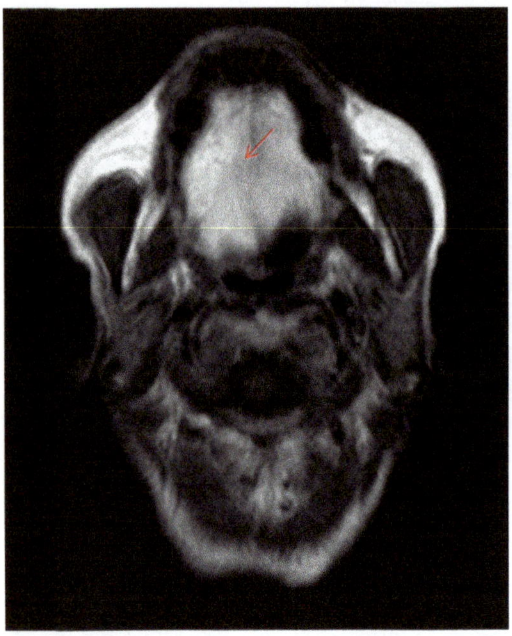

Fig. 14.9 Axial T1-weighted image of the head and neck region of a GSDII patient shows hyperintensity (*arrow*), indicating massive fat replacement in the tongue

Frequently, there is adipose substitution of the tongue (Fig. 14.9), which might be the only sign in mildly affected patients. Tongue involvement is usually proportional to the severity of clinical impairment (Fig. 14.10).

Mildly increased signal intensities on T2-weighted images can be detected mainly in leg muscles in a small percentage of patients (Fig. 14.11). The underlying pathological mechanism is still uncertain. It is unlikely to be due to muscle edema because of the lack of concomitant increases in T1 relaxation times. It might be related to the high glycogen content as proven by muscle biopsies and described in other GSDs (III, V, VII).

Regarding the juvenile form of GSDII, MRI data suggest that adductor magnus involvement is the earliest manifestation of the disease in siblings carrying the same GAA substitutions, emphasizing consistent radiological expression of the same genetic background.

In childhood-onset Pompe disease, the anterior compartment of thigh muscles is preferentially involved, but on CT scans the distinctive pattern manifests as striking high-density areas involving the rectus femoris (Fig. 14.12a), adductor magnus, and tibialis anterior. This pattern is not seen in adult forms of GSDII, nor has it been documented in other myopathic disorders. It is related to the accumulation of calcium in dense globular bodies formed by a chronic degenerative process affecting autophagic vacuoles. The pathogenetic mechanism is still unknown. The high-density areas increase over time, resulting in a marbled pattern (Fig. 14.12b), but neither moth-eaten nor washed-out changes develop as is seen in the affected muscles of adult patients. Interestingly, the high CT densities slightly decrease, paralleling clinical improvement, after enzyme replacement therapy (ERT). In the adult form, the distribution of fatty replacement does not change.

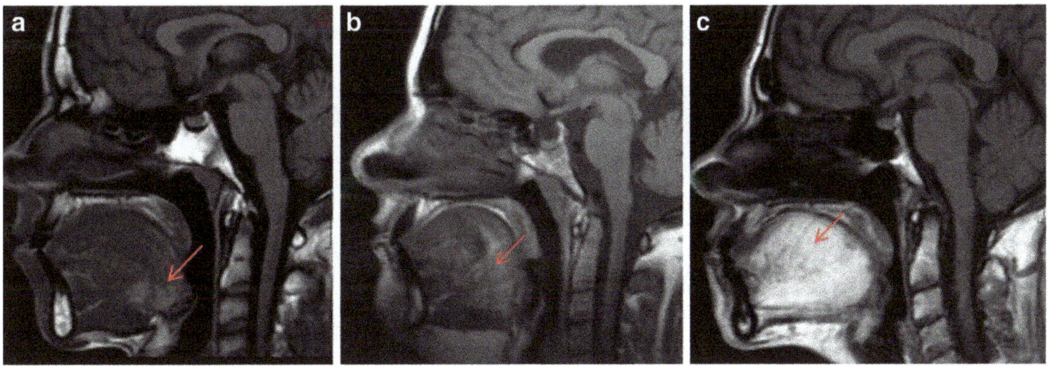

Fig. 14.10 Sagittal T1-weighted images of the head, focusing at the level of the tongue in adult GSDII patients. Note the areas of hyperintensity (*arrows*), indicating progressive, increasing fat replacement of the tongue, related to mild (**a**), moderate (**b**) and severe (**c**) functional stages. Complete involvement becomes evident in the more advanced stages of the disease

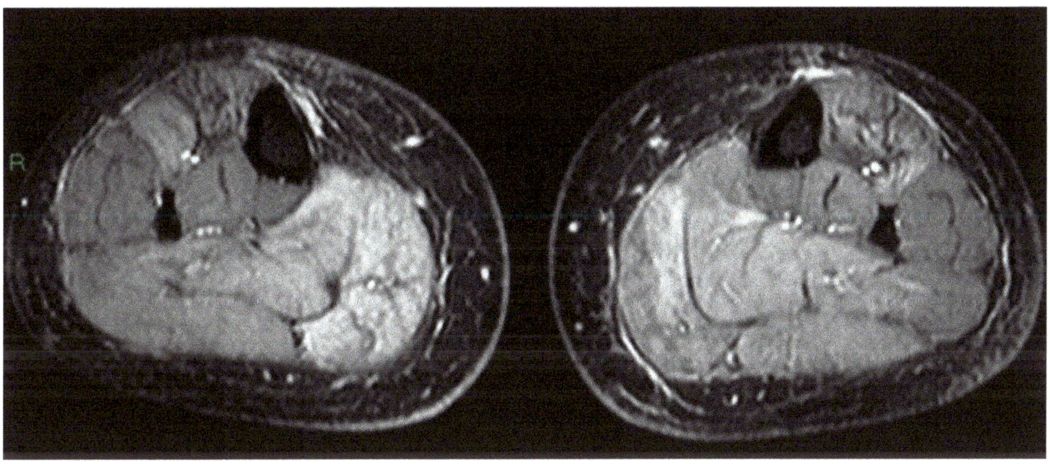

Fig. 14.11 Axial short tau inversion recovery (STIR) MRI with fat suppression at the level of the leg in an adult patient affected by GSDII. Note the areas of mild hyperintensity involving the posterior compartment, predominantly the medial gemini, and to a lesser extent the tibialis anterior. The meaning of this finding is still uncertain, but it is likely due to glycogen accumulation

There are only a few reports of ultrasonography findings in infantile forms of Pompe disease. They describe normal echo intensities and muscle hypertrophy, which was confirmed by MRI studies.

Visual assessment of muscle involvement using grading scales ("qualitative assessment") and quantitative analysis of muscle structure—in particular intramuscular fat and muscle volumes ("quantitative assessement")—is suitable for assessing the rate of disease progression and monitoring treatment response in GSDII patients. Qualitative MRI assessment performed 6 and 24 months after the beginning of ERT in adult patients shows that the pattern of distribution of intramuscular adipose substitution in already affected muscles remains unaltered. Both clinical assessment and quantitative MRI reveal definite improvement in the anterior spared thigh muscles. However, progression of intramuscular fat accumulation and the limited responsiveness

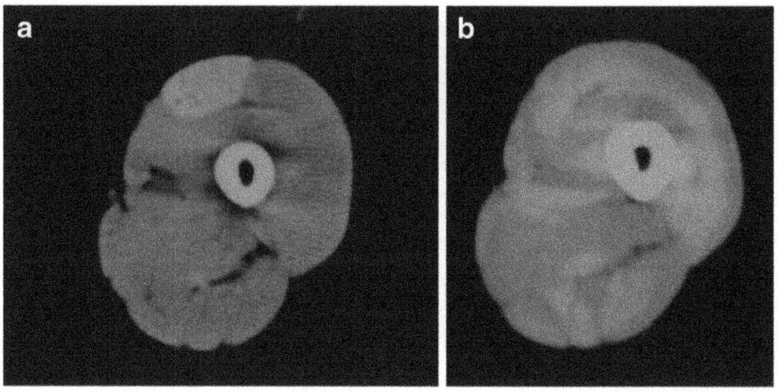

Fig. 14.12 Axial skeletal muscle CT image from a patient with childhood-onset Pompe disease at 13 years (**a**) and 22 years (**b**) of age. The rectus femoris is significantly affected, with a high density area (*arrow*), but the posterior compartment of the thigh is relatively spared (**a**). As the thigh density areas become more diffuse, a diffuse marble pattern appeared (**b**). Courtesy of Keiko Ishigaki, Tokyo, Japan

of posterior, more compromised thigh muscles confirms the necessity of early treatment intervention.

14.2.1.6 Therapy

Patient management consists of multidisciplinary supportive care modalities, including genetic counseling and respiratory, physical (aerobic submaximum exercise), and dietary therapies (high-protein, low carbohydrates, L-alanine). ERT with alglucosidase alfa (Myozyme), a recombinant human GAA (rh-GAA), has recently been introduced. For infantile Pompe disease, ERT shows major benefits regarding survival and cardiomyopathy evolution. In infants, the presence or absence of cross-reactive immunological material (CRIM) may affect prognosis. CRIM-negative patients are completely unable to form any precursor form of native enzyme and have a poorer clinical outcome. The therapeutic benefit for juvenile- and adult-onset cases is less significant, but improvement in motor and respiratory function has been shown. The response to ERT may be less robust in those with more advanced phases of the disease, underscoring the need for early diagnosis and treatment initiation.

14.2.1.7 Differential Diagnosis

- Limb-girdle muscular dystrophy (LGMD) (see Chap. 19). It has a similar pattern of muscle involvement and disease course. Muscle MRI in LGMD, though, usually shows (in contrast to GSDII) fatty replacement of leg muscles.
- Polymyositis (see Chap. 26). T2-weighted images clearly depict high signal intensity of muscles related to inflammation (Fig. 14.13). This finding might lead to some confusion only when is focal, as high muscle glycogen content can cause increased signal intensity on T2-weighted images as well.
- Congenital muscular dystrophy with rigid spine syndrome (SEPN1) (see Sect. 15.3). The sartorius (spared in GSDII) is a hallmark of the muscle pattern on MRI. Tongue involvement is typical for GSDII, even in mild forms.

Metabolic Myopathies: Pompe Disease

Key Points

- GSDII is an autosomal recessive myopathy caused by deficiency of GAA, an enzyme involved in the degradation of lysosomal glycogen.
- Infantile, juvenile, and adult forms of GSDII are recognized. The fatal infantile phenotype is characterized by early onset with severe myopathy, cardiomyopathy, and respiratory failure. Late-onset phenotypes show slowly progressive proximal muscle weakness and respiratory involvement.
- There is a characteristic MRI pattern of thigh muscle involvement with prominent fat

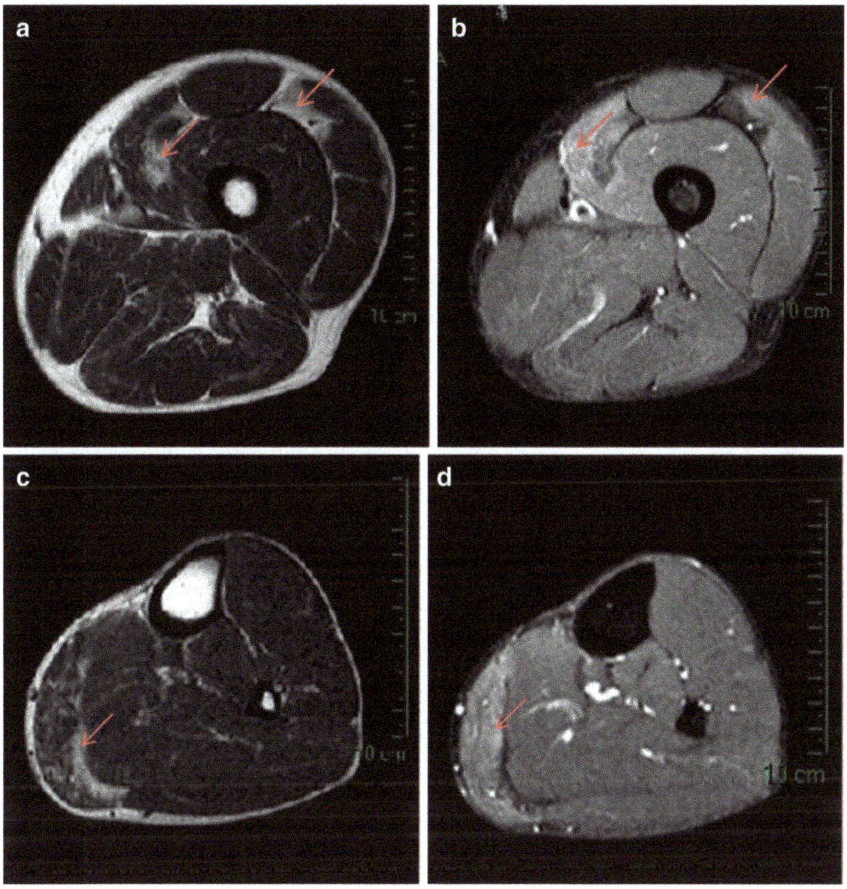

Fig. 14.13 Axial T1-weighted and STIR MRI scans at the level of the thigh (**a**, **b**) and leg (**c**, **d**) of a patient affected by dystrophic inflammatory myopathy. Diffuse mild fat replacement is evident on T1-weighted images, more focal in the vastus lateralis and medialis muscles (*arrows*) (**a**) and in the medial gastrocnemius muscle (*arrow*) (**c**). STIR sequences with fat suppression reveal increased water content in the same muscles due to muscle edema from the inflammation (**b**, **d**) (*arrows*). The exception is the vastus lateralis, where the dystrophic process is predominant

replacement of the posterior compartment. It is related to the clinical stage. Leg muscles are usually spared. Subscapular and paraspinal muscles are involved as well. The tongue is selectively infiltrated even in mildly affected patients.

- A promising novel therapeutic advance is rh-GAA, which so far has proved to have major clinical benefits in infants. It has not been shown to reverse muscle imaging findings in adults, underscoring the need for prompt early diagnosis and treatment initiation.

Suggestions for Further Reading

Angelini C, Semplicini C. Metabolic myopathies: the challenge of new treatments. Curr Opin Pharmacol. 2010;10:338–45.

Cinnamon J, Slonim AE, Black KS, et al. Evaluation of the lumbar spine in patients with glycogen storage disease: CT demonstration of patterns of paraspinal muscle atrophy. Am J Neuroradiol. 1991;12:1099–103.

de Jager AEJ, van der Vilet TM, van der Ree TC, et al. Muscle computed tomography in adult-onset acid maltase deficiency. Muscle Nerve. 1998;21:398–400.

Del Gaizo A, Banerjee S, Terk M. Adult onset glycogen storage disease type II (adult onset Pompe disease): report and magnetic resonance images of two cases. Skeletal Radiol. 2009;38:1205–8.

Dlamini N, Jan W, Norwood F, et al. Muscle MR findings in siblings with juvenile-onset acid maltase deficiency (Pompe disease). Neuromuscul Disord. 2008; 18:408–9.

Fleckenstein JL, Crues III JV, Haller RG. Inherited defects of muscle energy metabolism: radiologic evaluation. In: Fleckenstein JL, Crues III JV, Reimers CD, editors. Muscle imaging in health and disease. New York: Springer-Verlag; 1996. p. 253–67.

Ishigaki K, Mitsuhashi S, Kuwatsuru R, et al. High-density areas on muscle CT in childhood-onset Pompe disease are caused by excess calcium accumulation. Acta Neuropathol. 2010;120:537–43.

Katzin LW, Amato AA. Pompe disease: a review of the current diagnosis and treatment recommendations in the era of enzyme replacement therapy. J Clin Neuromuscul Dis. 2008;9:421–31.

Pichiecchio A, Uggetti C, Ravaglia S, et al. Muscle MR in adult-onset acid maltase deficiency. Neuromuscul Disord. 2004;14:51–5.

Ravaglia S, Pichiecchio A, Ponzio M, et al. Changes in skeletal muscle qualities during enzyme replacement therapy in late-onset type II glycogenosis: temporal and spatial pattern of mass vs. strength response. J Inherit Metab Dis. 2010;33:737–45.

14.2.2 Other Glycogen Storage Diseases

14.2.2.1 Glycogenosis Type III

Synonyms, Abbreviations

GSDIII, GlyIII, Cori-Forbes disease, Debranching enzyme deficiency

Genetics and Pathophysiology

GSDIII is a rare autosomal recessive disorder characterized by debranching enzyme (DE) deficiency (localized on chromosome 1p21). DE facilitates the breakdown of intracellular glycogen, a source of energy during high-intensity aerobic and/or anaerobic exercise, with two independent catalytic activities (oligo-1,4-1,4-glucantransferase and amylo-1,6-glucosidase).

Histopathology

The enzymatic activity is usually deficient in both muscle and liver (subtype IIIa). In 15 % of patients, it involves only the liver (IIIb). Muscle biopsy shows glycogen accumulation underneath the sarcolemma and within myofibrils. A definitive diagnosis is made measuring enzyme activity in muscle or liver tissue or by direct genetic analysis.

Clinical Presentation

The global incidence of GSDIII is 1/400,000, but it is much higher in non-Ashkenazi Jewish communities, where it affects 1/5400 subjects. GSDIII patients usually suffer during childhood from liver dysfunction and hypoglycemia. Neuromuscular involvement in GSDIII is variable, only rarely being the dominant feature of the disease. Compared to clinical manifestations of other defects in the glycogenolytic pathway, muscle weakness is relatively more common in GSDIII patients than exercise intolerance, muscle cramps, and myoglobinuria, The age of first clinical presentation in adult cases is the third to sixth decade.

Imaging Findings

Localized fatty infiltration is already evident in early disease stages, especially at the level of the soleus (Fig. 14.14), and it is more pronounced at the muscle insertion. Pseudo-hypertrophy of the quadriceps is characteristic at the intermediate stage of the disease, disappearing during the advanced stages. A mild diffuse increased signal intensity on T2-weighted images can be observed in leg muscles. The possible underlying pathophysiological concept was discussed earlier in this chapter (see Sect. 14.2.1 GSDII).

Whereas fatty accumulation clearly marks disease progression, as in GSDII, metabolic abnormalities observed by MR spectroscopy (MRS) precede visible muscle damage. The results of multiparametric functional/advanced MRI (^{31}P-,^{1}H-, and ^{13}C-MRS and arterial spin labeling) not only suggest that impaired glycogenolysis causes inadequate substrate supply to the mitochondria, but also that altered perfusion might be responsible for impaired postexercise phosphocreatine recovery, contributing to exercise intolerance.

Therapy

No specific therapy is available.

Differential Diagnosis

GSDV and GSDVII. MRI of muscle is not useful in the differential diagnosis, which is mainly based on clinical and histopathology findings. That is, muscle weakness and hypotonia are more frequent in GSDIII than exercise intolerance, muscle cramps with myoglobinuria, or hemolytic

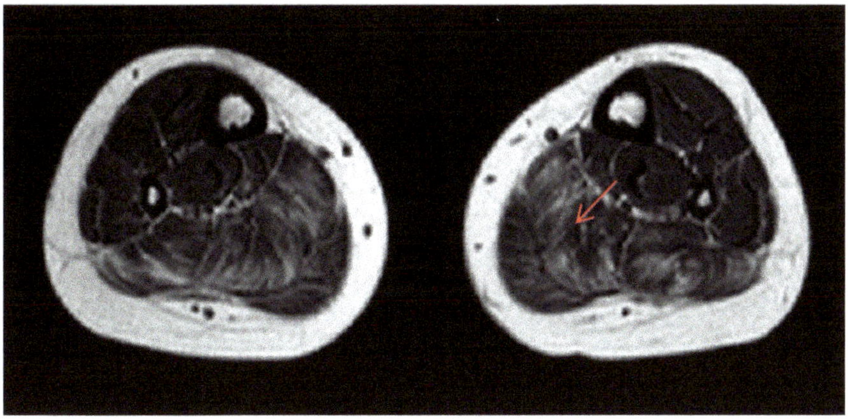

Fig. 14.14 Axial T1-weighted MRI scan at the level of the leg in an adult patient affected by GSDIII. No obvious atrophy is evident. Fat infiltration is present diffusely in the posterior compartment, primarily in the soleus (*arrow*)

anemia as are seen in GSDV (Sect. 14.2.2.2) and GSDVII (Sect. 14.2.2.3); reduced or absent phosphorylase activity, as in GSDV; and phosphofructokinase deficiency, as in GSDVII.

14.2.2.2 Glycogenosis Type V

Synonyms, Abbreviations

GSDV, GlyV, McArdle disease, myophosphorylase deficiency

Genetics and Pathophysiology

McArdle disease is a rare autosomal recessive metabolic myopathy caused by deficiency of the glycogenolytic enzyme myophosphorylase. Myophosphorylase initiates glycogen breakdown, converting glycogen to lactate by disrupting the 1,4 linkages between glycosyl units. The gene for myophosphorylase is localized on chromosome 11(q12-13.2), and more than 65 mutations have been identified so far.

Histopathology

Muscle tissue usually shows increased glycogen content but to a lesser extent than in other GSDs. Also, there is an absence or, more rarely, a decrease in myophosphorylase activity (Fig. 14.15). Phosphorylase activity is lost in muscle fibers as they mature, whereas it is normal in liver and smooth muscle. It is worth mentioning that whereas in inflammatory myopathies the biopsy target is the edematous muscle in GSDV relatively normal-appearing muscle is favored as the biopsy site. In fact, in GSDV edematous necrotic injured muscle may produce a small amount of fetal phosphorylase, which can cause a false-negative histopathological result.

Clinical Presentation

GSDV is a rare disease; its incidence is reported as 1/100,000. The usual age of onset is during the first 10–15 years. The typical clinical symptoms of GSDV are myalgia and muscle cramps triggered by exercise, both isometric and aerobic, such as weight lifting and jogging. The exercise intolerance is due to the inability to break down stored muscle glycogen for muscle contraction. The muscle recovers with rest. Rhabdomyolysis and myoglobinuria occur in about 33 % patients following intense exercise. After a short period of rest, most patients experience a "second wind" phenomenon and can continue exercising without difficulty. This phenomenon is based on the metabolic shift to fatty acid oxidation.

Imaging Findings

Unlike GSDII and VII, McArdle's patients rarely develop severe muscular fatty deterioration, and MRI results are frequently normal. Paraspinal muscles can show adipose substitution as in GSDII, but psoas muscles are usually spared (Fig. 14.16).

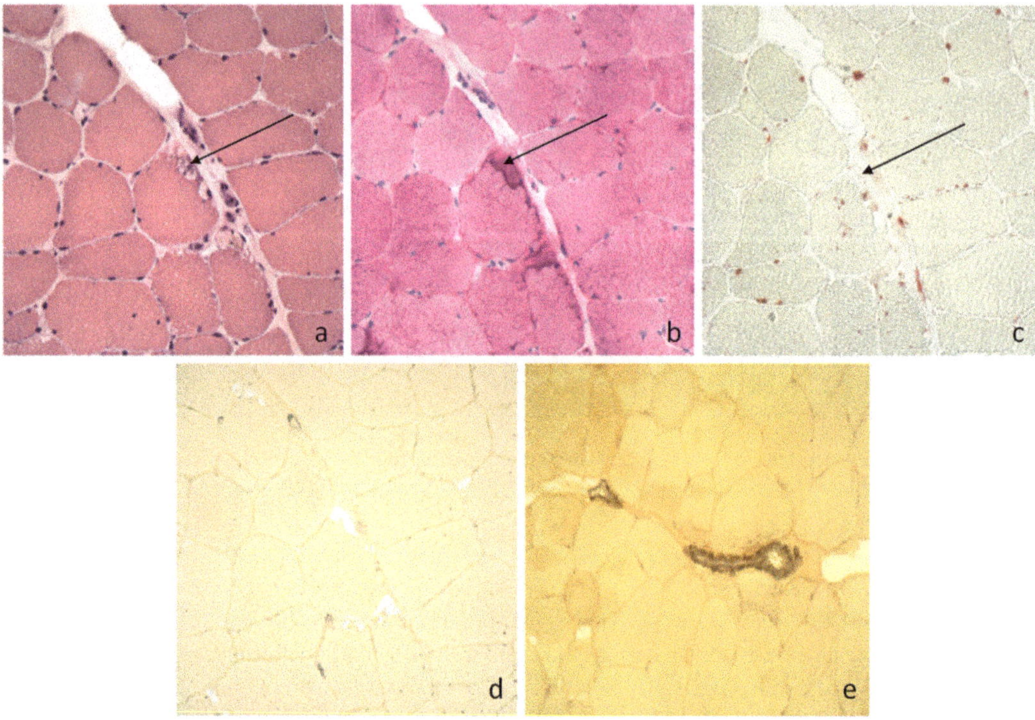

Fig. 14.15 Characteristic pathological features in GSDV. Several fibers contain subsarcolemmal vacuoles (*arrows*) (H&E) (**a**). The vacuoles contain glycogen (PAS-positive) (**b**) but are not located in lysosomes (acid phosphatase-negative) (**c**). Cytoplasmic phosphorylase staining: negative (**d**) compared to the normal control (**e**). Courtesy of Cornelia Kornblum, Bonn, Germany

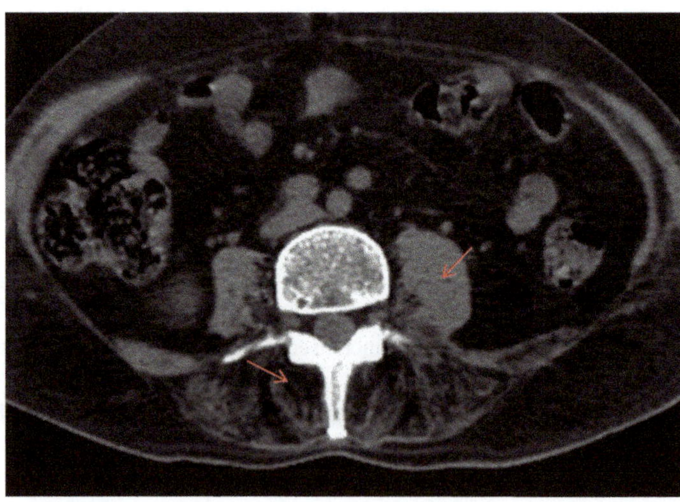

Fig. 14.16 Axial CT image at the lumbar level for evaluating paraspinal muscles in an adult GSDIII patient. Note that the paraspinal muscles are substituted with fat (*arrow*), whereas the psoas muscles maintain their trophism (*arrow*)

Contrary to what usually happens in healthy subjects, GSDV muscles do not show edema-like changes during the early postexercise phase, a typical but not specific imaging feature of the disease. These data are based on quantitative analysis of variations in T2 relaxation times from MRI images, which reflect pH variations and which are lower in McArdle's patients than in healthy subjects. The usefulness of these findings might reside in preliminary screening of patients with exercise intolerance due to myalgias.

On the other hand, muscle MRI performed 24 h after exercise shows edematous changes of the thigh muscles, beginning at the muscle–tendon junction. This elevation on T1 and T2 relaxation times is likely related to concomitant muscle necrosis, which is completely reversible as demonstrated by follow-up MRI.

In GSDV, ^{31}P-MRS fails to show any cytosolic acidification or phosphor monoester (PME) accumulation. PME accumulation is not observed during exercise, in contrast to GSD VII, because of the inability to cleave glucosyl units from glycogen. Moreover, calf muscles show a decreased PCr/Pi ratio at rest and a low rate of PCr resynthesis during recovery from aerobic exercise, confirming that mitochondrial respiratory chain impairment plays an additional role in conditioning the energy supply to contracting muscle.

Therapy

Several drugs have been tested in GSDV, mostly with insignificant results. Pyridoxyne has been found to be reduced in patients with GSDV, but pyridoxine implementation did not improve the clinical picture or alleviate symptoms. Angiotensin-converting enzyme (ACE) inhibitors (e.g., ramipril) have been tested in the so-called ACE phenotype—characterized by high ACE activity—with unsatisfactory results. Aminoglycosides, which might be able to facilitate the synthesis of full-length proteins, have been tested in several inherited diseases and in GSDV but did not produce any significant clinical amelioration. Oral sucrose seems to alleviate muscular symptoms during exercise. Intravenous administration of sucrose has been tried, but side effects limit its efficacy.

Differential Diagnosis

- GSDVII (Sect. 14.2.2.3). The clinical picture is similar, but muscle MRI is not useful. ^{31}P-MRS can be of some help (see above).
- GSDII (Sect. 14.2.1). Paraspinal muscle imaging can be of some help as mentioned.
- Carnitine palmitoyl deficiency (CPT) (Sect. 14.4.1). CPT can cause recurrent rhabdomyolysis and myoglobinuria, but the differential diagnosis is based on histopathology (i.e., reduced CPT activity in specific essays).

14.2.2.3 Glycogenosis Type VII

Synonyms, Abbreviations

GSDVII, GlyVII, Tauri's disease, Phosphofructokinase (PFK) deficiency

Genetics and Pathophysiology

GSDVII is an autosomal recessive disease caused by alteration of genes encoding for phosphofructokinase (PFK) (chromosome 12q13.3) PFK is a regulatory enzyme that acts on the initial steps of the glycolytic pathway, phosphorylating fructose-6 phosphate.

Histopathology

Muscle biopsy is characterized by glycogen accumulation similar to that seen in GSDV, complete absence of enzyme activity in muscles, and decreased activity in erythrocytes.

Clinical Presentation

GSDVII is clinically similar to McArdle disease, manifesting with exercise intolerance during childhood, early fatigability, and exertional muscle cramps. Unlike GSDV, patients suffer from hemolytic anemia caused by reduced PFK activity in erythrocytes. A subtype of "late-onset" PFK deficiency with fixed muscle weakness was described in four patients and may represent a genetically distinct disorder.

Imaging Findings

No specific pattern of muscle involvement has been described for this disease. ^{31}P-MRS demonstrates PME accumulation in muscles during exercise, although there is no abnormal accumulation of PME during ischemic exercise. Also, a partial glycolytic block has been reported in an adult patient affected by late-onset PFK, with residual glycolytic flow shown by a slow decrease of intracellular pH during anaerobic exercise. The combination of this finding with the presence of late-onset myopathy suggest that this form may depend on a partial lack of the enzyme and on a distinct pathogenetic mechanism.

Therapy

No treatment is currently available.

Differential Diagnosis

- ^{31}P-MRS can be helpful distinguishing GSDVII from GSDV (see above) but not from other enzyme defects in which glycolysis is blocked distal to phosphorylase.
- The only other disease with clinical features and MRS findings similar to GSDVII is phosphoglycerate kinase deficiency, which has X-linked recessive inheritance.

Metabolic Myopathies: Other Glycogen Storage Diseases

Key Points

- GSDIII, GSDV, and GSDVII are rare metaoblic disorders with enzyme defects in converting glycogen to fructose-6-phosphate (III, V) or fructose-6-phosphate to lactate (VII).
- Muscle weakness and hypotonia are common muscle symptoms in GSDIII, and exercise intolerance and muscle cramps predominate in GSDV and GSDVII.
- Muscle biopsy usually shows increased glycogen content.
- Fatty infiltration parallels disease progression in GSDIII. Calf muscles are most often affected, primarily the soleus. No abnormal muscle structures or selective patterns of muscle involvement are seen in GSDV and GSDVII. Spectroscopic and perfusion MRI have been used to investigate metabolic muscle dysfunction with the aim of finding supplementary indices of disease characterization. ^{31}P-MRS can be helpful distinguishing GSDVII from GSDV.
- Therapy is not currently available. Some attempts have been undertaken to treat GSDV, but most of them failed to produce significant amelioration or they were not well tolerated.

Suggestions for Further Reading

Angelini C, Semplicini C. Metabolic myopathies: the challenge of new treatments. Curr Opin Pharmacol. 2010;10:338–45.

Fleckenstein JL, Crues III JV, Haller RG. Inherited defects of muscle energy metabolism: radiologic evaluation. In: Fleckenstein JL, Crues III JV, Reimers CD, editors. Muscle imaging in health and disease. New York: Springer-Verlag; 1996. p. 253–67.

Jehenson P, Leroy Willig, A, de Kerviler E, et al. MR imaging as a potential diagnostic test for metabolic myopathies: importance of variations in the T2 of muscle with exercise. AJR Am J Roentgenol. 1993;161:347–51.

Marbini A, Gemignani F,Saccardi F, et al. Debrancher deficiency neuromuscular disorder with pseudohypertrophy in two brothers. J Neurol. 1989;236:418–20.

Massa R, Lodi R, Barbiroli B, et al. Partial block of glycolysis in late-onset phosphofructokinase deficiency myopathy. Acta Neuropathol. 1996;91:322–9.

Siciliano G, Rossi B, Martini A, et al. Myophosphorylase deficiency affects muscle mitochondrial respiration as shown by ^{31}P-MR spectroscopy in a case with associated multifocal encephalopathy. J Neurol Sci. 1995;128:84–91.

Sivakumar K, Vasconcelos O, Goldfarb L, et al. Late-onset muscle weakness in partial phosphofructokinase deficiency: a unique myopathy with vacuoles, abnormal mitochondria, and absence of the common exon 5/intron 5 junction point mutation. Neurology 1996;46:1337–42.

Wary C, Nadaj-Pakleza A, Laforêt P, et al. Investigating glycogenosis type III patients with multi-parametric functional NMR imaging and spectroscopy. Neuromuscul Disord. 2010;20:548–58.

14.3 Mitochondrial Diseases

14.3.1 Synonyms, Abbreviations

MELAS (mitochondrial encephalomyopathy, lactic acidosis, stroke-like episodes); MERFF (myoclonic epilepsy, ragged red fibers); chronic progressive external ophthalmoplegia (CPEO) (ptosis, external ophthalmoplegia, mitochondrial myopathy); Kearns–Sayre syndrome (external ophthalmoplegia, pigmentary retinopathy, heart block, ataxia, muscle weakness with occasional fatigue on exertion)

14.3.2 Genetics and Pathophysiology

Mitochondria are small intracellular organelles with several important functions, including a key role in energy production via the electron-transport chain and respiratory chain. The spectrum of diseases caused by impaired mitochondrial structure and/or function is broad and in dynamic evolution. They can be related to defects of mitochondrial DNA, be maternally inherited, or related to defects of nuclear genes required for mitochondrial functions. In the latter condition, diseases are transmitted to offspring according to mendelian rules of inheritance (autosomal dominant, autosomal recessive, or X-linked).

14.3.3 Histopathology

The muscular histopathological hallmark of mitochondrial disorders is clusters of mitochondria accumulating in the subsarcolemmal region of muscle fibers, the so-called ragged red fibers (RRFs), as seen with Gomori trichrome staining (Fig. 14.17a). Mitochondrial proliferation is another typical feature of mitochondrial disorders, as showed by increased staining of muscle fibers with succinate dehydrogenase. Reduced COX staining is seen in some mitochondrial disorders characterized by reduced COX activity (Fig. 14.17b).

14.3.4 Clinical Presentation

The severity and type of clinical symptoms related to mitochondrial dysfunction depends on the percentage of mitochondrial DNA (mtDNA) mutated and on the amount of energy required by the tissue to function properly. Therefore, tissues with high energy demand—e.g., muscles, heart, brain—are more frequently affected. The description of each disease is beyond the scope of this chapter. However, the clinical presentation of muscle impairment in these disorders is almost invariably characterized by exercise intolerance and early fatigue. Rest promptly alleviates the symptoms, which, however, may

a b

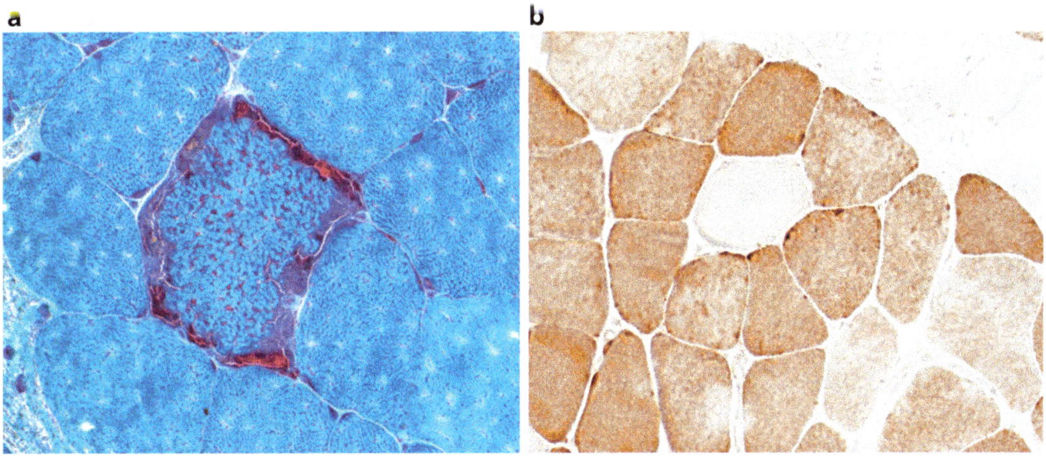

Fig. 14.17 Characteristic pathological features of mitochondrial myopathies. Typical "ragged red fiber" (*arrow*) (Gomori trichrome stain) (**a**). COX-negative fiber (*arrow*) (cytochrome oxidase stain) (**b**). Courtesy of Cornelia Kornblum, Bonn, Germany

recur with activity resumption. Exercise intolerance is generally associated with rhabdomyolysis, with consequent release of myoglobin and lactate into the bloodstream. Sometimes fixed muscle weakness is present with various patterns of muscle involvement. Multisystemic involvement is frequently associated with muscle impairment, such as in the most common mitochondrial phenotypes.

1. Mitochondrial encephalomyopathy, lactic acidosis, and stroke-like episodes (MELAS)
2. Chronic progressive external ophthalmoplegia (CPEO), with ptosis, external ophthalmoplegia, and mitochondrial myopathy
3. Myoclonus epilepsy with ragged red fibers (MERRF)
4. Kearns–Sayre syndrome (external ophthalmoplegia, pigmentary retinopathy, heart block, ataxia, and muscle weakness with occasional fatigue on exertion)

The diagnostic assessment of mitochondrial disorders with muscular symptoms includes the measurement of lactate at rest and after mild physical exertion. Usually a diagnostic muscle biopsy is necessary to confirm the diagnosis. RRFs and COX-negative fibers are classic findings but might be absent. Therefore, in addition to light microscopy, biochemical assessment of the respiratory chain complexes is often done to prove it is a mitochondrial myopathy. The usefulness of any further test depends on the clinical suspicion. These tests might include assessment of specific enzyme activity, brain MRI, and/or clinical and instrumental cardiac evaluation.

14.3.5 Imaging Findings

To date, only mitochondrial myopathy associated with progressive external ophthalmoplegia has been studied by muscle MRI. Atrophy and a fine, diffuse, fatty infiltration (i.e., "marbling") of thigh muscles are usual. Selective prominent fatty infiltration of the sartorius and gracilis muscles is particularly common, although selective involvement of other limbs is not seen in this form. T2-weighted sequences reveal little associated edema-like changes. The paucity of edematous changes correlates with minimal histopathological evidence of myonecrosis or inflammation.

The severity of ophthalmoplegia is not necessarily correlated with the degree of extraocular muscle (EOM) volume, which can be clearly atrophic (Fig. 14.18) or nearly normal. In this latter case, the presence of a bright signal in EOMs on T1-weighted images may be useful in the differential diagnosis (Fig. 14.19).

These findings suggest a selective vulnerability of EOMs in CPEO and the sartorius and gracilis muscles, raising the possibility that some feature shared by these muscles might account for their deterioration.

A description of brain MRI scans from patients with mitochondrial myopathy is beyond the scope of this chapter. By themselves, these findings do not provide high sensitivity or specificity for the diagnosis of mitochondrial diseases. It is useful to remember that cerebral and cerebellar atrophy are quite common features in childhood and adults and that several disorders present with widespread leukodystrophy. MELAS classically demonstrates hyperintense T2 lesions that do not follow vascular territories predominantly in gray and subcortical white matter in the temporal, parietal, and occipital lobes. Spectroscopy may show increased lactic acid levels in the brain parenchyma during the acute phase of this disease and in chronic lesions. Focal, bilateral symmetrical basal ganglia and periaqueductal gray matter lesions are typical of Leigh syndrome.

14.3.6 Therapy

Therapeutic strategies comprise both dietary supplementation and a nonpharmaceutical approach. Coenzyme Q10, L-arginine, and nucleotide supplementation show efficacy in terms of alleviating symptoms related to exercise intolerance. Based on the notion that ketogenic bodies stimulate mitochondrial biogenesis, a ketogenic diet has been tested with promising results.

With respect to the nonpharmaceutical approach, both resistance and endurance training seems to improve muscle strength and exercise

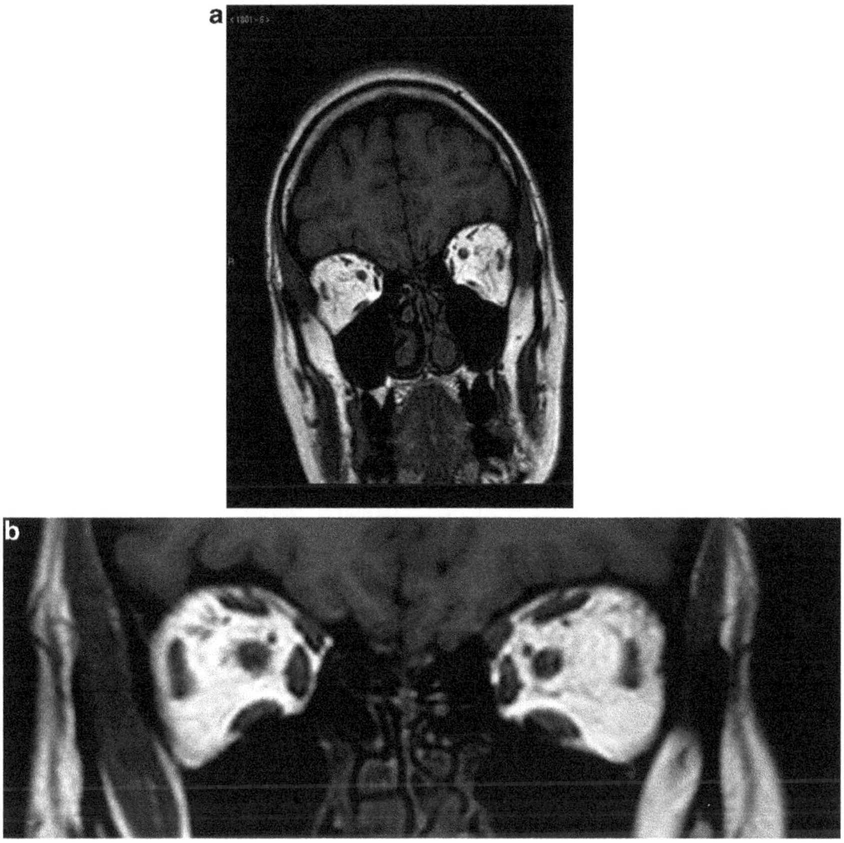

Fig. 14.18 Patient with chronic progressive external ophthalmoplegia (CPEO). (**a**) Coronal T1-SE weighted orbital image, note the small, thread-like extraocular muscles bilaterally. (**b**) Healthy control subject. Coronal T1-SE weighted orbital image. Note the normal extraocular muscles

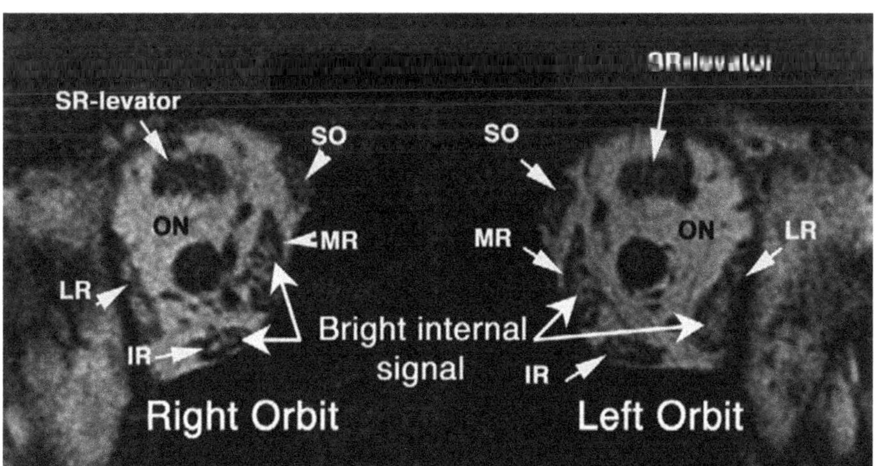

Fig. 14.19 Coronal T1-weighted MRI shows abnormal bright internal signal in multiple extraocular muscles (*right* MR, *right* IR, *left* MR, *left* LR muscle) in the deep orbit of a patient with CPEO. *ON* optic nerve. From Ortube et al (2006) Orbital magnetic resonance imaging of extraocular muscles in chronic progressive external ophthalmoplegia: specific diagnostic findings. J AAPOS. 10(5):414–8. Reprinted with permission from Elsevier Limited

resistance by stimulating mitochondrial biogenesis and activation of quiescent satellite cells containing nonmutant mtDNA.

14.3.7 Differential Diagnosis

– GSDV (Sect. 14.2.2.2), GSDVII (Sect. 14.2.2.3), CPT II (Sect. 14.4.1) deficiency. They are all characterized by episodes of rhabdomyolysis triggered by exercise and the presence of some recessive mitochondrial disorder. The differential diagnosis is based on (1) the presence of clinical symptoms suggestive of multisystemic involvement in mitochondrial disorders, usually absent in the other disorders, and (2) histopathological findings.

Metabolic Myopathies: Mitochondrial Diseases

Key Points

- Impairment of mitochondrial structure or function has severe consequences in terms of energy supply to several organs, with high-energy demand organs such as brain, heart, and muscles more significantly affected.
- Mitochondrial disorders are usually characterized by multisystemic involvement. Clinical symptoms related to muscle impairment are commonly represented by early fatigability during exercise and myoglobinuria. Sometimes muscle weakness is present.
- The diagnostic assessment includes measurement of lactate at rest and after light physical exertion and a muscle biopsy that typically shows ragged red fibers.
- Any further test depends on the clinical suspicion. Muscle MRI has not been proven to be useful.
- The therapeutic approach includes dietary supplementation and exercise.

Suggestions for Further Reading

Berardo A, DiMauro S, Hirano M. A diagnostic algorithm for metabolic myopathies. Curr Neurol Neurosci Rep. 2010;10:118–26.

Carlow TJ, Depper MH, Orrison WW. MR of extraocular muscles in CPEO. AJNR Am J Neuroradiol. 1998;19:95–99.

DiMauro S. Pathogenesis and treatment of mitochondrial myopathies: recent advances. Acta Myol. 2010;29:333–8.

Fleckenstein JL, Haller RG, Girson MS, et al. Focal muscle lesions in mitochondrial myopathy: MR imaging evaluation. Magn Reson Imaging. 1992;2 Suppl:121.

Friedman SD, Shaw DW, Ishak G, et al. The use of neuroimaging in the diagnosis of mitochondrial disease. Dev Disabil Res Rev. 2010;16:129–35.

Hassani H, Horvath R, Chinnery PF. Mitochondrial myopathies: developments in treatment. Curr Opin Neurol. 2010;23(5):459–65.

Ortube MC, Bhola R, Demer JL. Orbital magnetic resonance imaging of extraocular muscles in chronic progressive external ophtalmoplegia: specific diagnostic findings. J AAPOS. 2006;10:414–8.

Van Adel BA, Tarnopolsky MA. Metabolic myopathies: update 2009. J Clin Neuromuscul Dis. 2009; 10:97–121.

14.4 Lipid Storage Diseases

Lipid storage myopathies are related to disorders of lipid metabolism, such as defects of long-chain fatty acid or carnitine transport, endogenous triglyceride metabolism, or β-oxidation. Among the diseases included in this group, so far only four disease entities have been characterized genetically: primary carnitine deficiency, multiple acyl-CoA dehydrogenase deficiency, and two neutral lipid storage diseases (with ichthyosis and myopathy, respectively). As there are no muscle imaging data available for any of them, they are not described further here. The only lipid storage disease in which muscle MRI has been applied is carnitine palmitoyl transferase II deficiency.

14.4.1 Carnitine Palmitoyl Deficiency II

14.4.1.1 Synonyms, Abbreviations

CPT II

14.4.1.2 Genetics and Pathophysiology

Carnitine palmitoyl deficiency II is a rare recessive, semi-dominant disorder (chromosome 1p32). It is caused by a defect in the gene encoding for carnitin-palmitoyl transferase II (CPT II), one of the enzymes that transfer long-chain fatty acylcoenzyme A across the barrier of the mitochondrial membrane to gain access to the enzymes of β-oxidation.

14.4.1.3 Histopathology

In about 20 % of the muscle biopsies for CPT II, there is a slight-to-moderate increase in lipid content. Specific assays showing reduced CPT activity are required for the diagnosis.

14.4.1.4 Clinical Presentation

Neonatal, infantile, and adult forms have been reported. The neonatal and the infantile forms are severe, usually lethal, generally because of paroxysmal cardiac arrhythmias. A few hundred CPT II patients have been described. The adult form, characterized by muscle involvement, is most common and least severe.

The most common symptoms of the adult form are myalgias and muscle stiffness after long exercise. This form is the most common cause of myoglobinuria in young adults. The heart is not affected. The central nervous system may be involved in neonatal and infantile cases, manifesting as hepatic leukoencephalopathy.

14.4.1.5 Imaging Findings

^{1}H-MRS is helpful diagnostically and for monitoring the disease and the response to treatment. It can detect the deficiency of total carnitine and estimate the high acylcarnitine conjugation fraction via measurement of muscle carnitine T2 relaxation. The presence of this late peak initially and its disappearance after dietary therapy because of an increase in the free carnitine fraction, are consistent with high fat intolerance.

14.4.1.6 Therapy

Intravenous glucose administration shows some efficacy. A promising compound is bezafibrate, which upregulates CPT2 mRNA and improves enzyme activity in cultured fibroblasts and myoblasts. A small study of six patients showed alleviation of the clinical symptoms with reduced frequency of rhabdomyolysis and significantly improved fatty acid oxidation.

14.4.1.7 Differential Diagnosis

- GSDV (Sect. 14.2.2.1), GSDVII (Sect. 14.2.2.3), CPT II (Sect. 14.4.1) deficiency. They are all characterized by episodes of rhabdomyolysis triggered by exercise. The differential diagnosis is based on (1) the presence of clinical symptoms suggesting a multisystemic involvement in mitochondrial disorders, usually absent in the other disorders and (2) histopathological findings.

> **Metabolic Myopathies: Lipid Storage Diseases**
>
> **Key Points**
>
> - Lipid storage disorders are related to disordered lipid metabolism, such as defects of long-chain fatty acid or carnitine transport, endogenous triglyceride metabolism, or β-oxidation.
> - Only four of the disorders have been characterized genetically: primary carnitine deficiency, Multiple acyl-CoA dehydrogenase deficiency, and two Neutral lipid storage diseases (with ichthyosis and myopathy, respectively).
> - Muscle MRI (^{1}H-MRS), applied only to CPT II, shows the absence of total carnitine and the high acylcarnitine conjugation fraction via measurement of muscle carnitine T2.
> - Bezafibrate showed promising results on a small sample of patients, with clinical improvement and normalization of fatty acid oxidation.

Suggestions for Further Reading

Angelini C, Semplicini C. Metabolic myopathies: the challenge of new treatments. Curr Opin Pharmacol. 2010;10:338–45.

Bruno C, Dimauro S. Lipid storage myopathies. Curr Opin Neurol. 2008;21(5):601–6.

Laforêt P, Vianey-Saban C. Disorders of muscle lipid metabolism: diagnostic and therapeutic challenges. Neuromuscul Disord. 2010;20:693–700.

Liang WC, Nishino I. Lipid storage myopathy. Curr Neurol Neurosci Rep. 2011;11:97–103.

Ohkuma A, Noguchi S, Sugie H, et al. Clinical and genetic analysis of lipid storage myopathies. Muscle Nerve. 2009;39:333–42.

Videen JS, Haseler LJ, Karpinski NC, et al. Noninvasive evaluation of adult onset myopathy from carnitine palmitoyl transferase II deficiency using proton magnetic resonance spectroscopy. J Rheumatol. 1999;26:1757–63.

15 Congenital Myopathies

Susana Quijano-Roy, Daniela Avila-Smirnow, Robert-Yves Carlier, Jorge A. Bevilacqua, Norma Beatriz Romero, and Dirk Fischer

15.1 Introduction

Susana Quijano-Roy and Dirk Fischer

Congenital myopathies (CMs) are a clinically and genetically heterogeneous group of early-onset myopathies that are classified according to the predominant histopathological findings in skeletal muscle. CMs usually exhibit distinctive morphological abnormalities such as rods, an increased number of central nuclei or central or multiple cores. In most patients, the clinical presentation with weakness and hypotonia is "congenital" or appears during the first years of life with delayed motor milestones. In most patients, the classic histopathological findings guide one to the correct genetic diagnosis. Classic central core disease (CCD) is related to *RYR1* mutations (see Sect. 15.2), and multi-minicore disease (MmD) is most often related to *SEPN1* mutations (see Sect. 15.3). Disorders with an increased number of central nuclei may be inherited as an X-linked trait (myotubular myopathy) (see Sect. 15.4), or more often they are autosomal dominant (DNM2 related) (see Sect. 15.5). CM with protein aggregates, such as nemaline myopathy and cap disease, are described in Sections 15.6 (ACTA1) and 15.7 (TPM2). Some pathological overlap between genetic distinct disorders has been described, making a genetic diagnosis sometimes difficult. Recently, different involvement patterns for CM have been identified based on muscle imaging. They can help to

S. Quijano-Roy (✉)
Garches Neuromuscular Center (GNMH), Raymond Poincare Hospital, Paris Ile de France Ouest University Hospitals (APHP), Versailles Saint-Quentin-en-Yvelines University (UVSQ), 104 boulevard R. Poincare, 92380 Garches, France
e-mail: susana.quijano-roy@rpc.aphp.fr

D. Avila-Smirnow
Servicio de Pediatría, Unidad de Neurología, Complejo Asistencial Dr. Sótero del Río, Red de Salud UC, Lira 85, 6° piso, Santiago, Chile
e-mail: avidaniela@gmail.com

R.-Y. Carlier
Pôle neuro-locomoteur, Service d'imagerie médicale, Hopital Raymond Poincare, 104 Boulevard R. Poincaré, 92380 Garches, France
e-mail: robert.carlier@rpc.aphp.fr

J.A. Bevilacqua
Department of Neurology and Neurosurgery, Hospital Clinico Universidad de Chile, Santiago, Chile
email: jbevilac@med.uchile.cl

N.B. Romero
Morphology Neuromuscular Unit of the Myology Institute, Pitie-Salpetriere University Hospital, UPMC, Paris, France
email: nb.romero@institut-myologie.org

D. Fischer
Department of Neuropaediatrics, University Children's Hospital Basel, Spitalstrasse 33, Basel 4056, Switzerland

Department of Neurology, University Hospital Basel, 4031 Basel, Switzerland
email: Dirk.Fischer@ukbb.ch

M.P. Wattjes and D. Fischer (eds.), *Neuromuscular Imaging*, DOI 10.1007/978-1-4614-6552-2_15,

narrow the differential diagnosis. Presently, there is no curative therapy for any of the congenital myopathies. Supportive care, including early respiratory and scoliosis management, and the clinical management of symptoms and complications is still the only available therapy.

Suggestions for Further Reading

North KN. Congenital myopathies. In: Engel AG, Franzini-Armstrong C, editors. Myology, 3rd ed. New York: McGraw Hill; p. 1473–533.

Quijano-Roy S, Carlier RY, Fischer D, et al. Muscle imaging in congenital myopathies. Semin Pediatr Neurol. 2011;18:221–9.

15.2 RYR1-Related Myopathies

Daniela Avila-Smirnow, Robert-Yves Carlier, Susana Quijano-Roy

15.2.1 Synonyms, Abbreviations

Central core disease (CCD); Central core myopathy; Malignant hyperthermia (MH); Multi-minicore/minicore/multicore disease (MmD); Ryanodine receptor type 1 (RYR1)-related myopathy.

15.2.2 Genetics and Pathophysiology

Ryanodine receptor type 1 (*RYR1*) gene mutations (19q13.2, OMIM #18090) have been associated with a variety of CMs and with malignant hyperthermia (MH). CMs related to *RYR1* include CCD, MmD, congenital fiber-type disproportion (CFTD), core-rod myopathy, and CMs with nuclear internalization and structure disorganization. In particular, in CCD, *RYR1* mutations are usually dominant but autosomal recessive mutations have been also described. RYRs represent a family of mammalian calcium channels located in the endoplasmic/sarcoplasmic reticulum (ER/SR). Three isoforms are recognized: RYR1, first described in skeletal muscle; RYR2 in cardiac muscle; RYR3 in the brain. *RYR1* gene is located in chromosome 19q13.2 and spans 104 exons. The RYR1 protein is composed of 5037 amino acids. It is responsible for the release of calcium from the SR that is required for excitation contraction coupling in skeletal and cardiac muscle. CCD is probably the most common CM, but the exact incidence is not known. Because of the lack of typical histopathological findings at an early age, this condition might be underdiagnosed.

15.2.3 Histopathology

Muscle biopsies of patients with *RYR1* mutations vary widely even within families and in the same patient over time. The typical finding of CCD on light microscopy is the "central core," which is located in type I fibers (Fig. 15.1). These structures correspond to central areas of muscle fiber devoid of enzymatic oxidative activity due to an absence of mitochondria. Central cores run along all or most of the longitudinal axis of the fiber. In contrast, in MmD cores span only a portion of the long axis of the fiber. In CCD, cores might be single or multiple and centrally or laterally located. Type I fiber predominance and atrophy are frequently observed and may be the only abnormality in young children. Some cases of fatty tissue replacement and fibrosis have been described. Immunohistochemistry shows desmin, plectin, γ-filamin, and αB-crystallin accumulation in cores. Electron microscopically, cores appear as well-defined areas devoid of mitochondria and with structural disorganization. Mitochondrial accumulation has been described at the periphery of some cores and in the subsarcolemmal region. Z-line disruption might be present.

15.2.4 Clinical Presentation

The clinical features and severity of CCD are extremely variable (Fig. 15.2). Most affected patients have clinical manifestations during infancy with hypotonia, muscle weakness, delayed motor milestones, hyporeflexia, and orthopedic deformities. Weakness is mostly axial and proximal, especially in the pelvic girdle. Facial weakness may be present, and even ptosis and ophthalmoparesis have been reported in a small proportion of cases, mimicking myasthenia. Orthopedic deformities include congenital hip dislocation, scoliosis, and lumbar hyperlordosis. Global hyperlaxity is frequent, but it is not associated with significant limb joint contractures. The clinical course is usually mild and

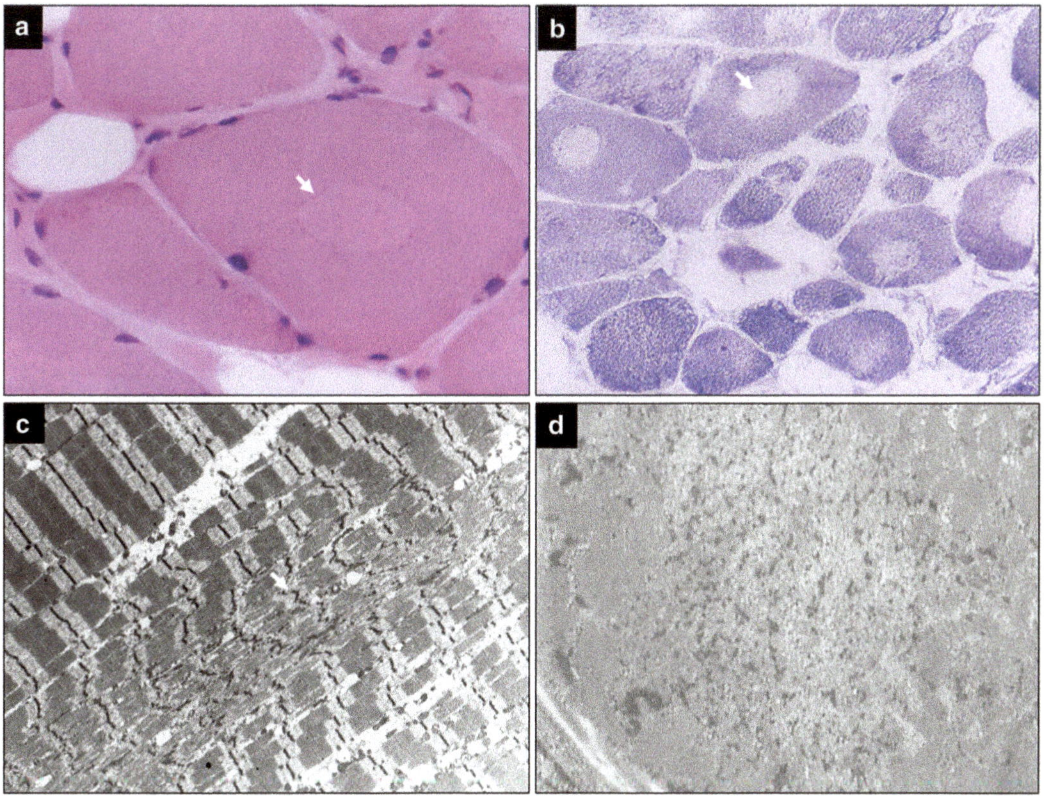

Fig. 15.1 Histological findings in ryanodine receptor type 1 (RYR1)-related myopathy. (**a, b**) Light microscopy of central core disease with typical central core lesions (*white arrows*) as seen by H&E (**a**) and NADH (**b**) staining. Courtesy M. Olivé, Barcelona, Spain. (**c, d**) Electron microscopy of a patient with typical disruption of sarcomeres and streaming of (*dark*) Z lines (*white arrows*) (**c**) and severe sarcomere disorganization (**d**) in a patient with fetal akinesia syndrome. Courtesy of N.B. Romero, Paris, France

nonprogressive, although severe cases have been reported that included the fetal akinesia syndrome or severe congenital phenotypes with hypotonia and progressive scoliosis. These patients require mechanical ventilation. Apart from these severe presentations, most other patients achieve walking. There is no evidence of abnormal cardiac function. Creatine kinase (CK) levels are usually in the normal range, but phenotypes with high CK levels and signs of rhabdomyolysis have been recently reported.

15.2.5 Imaging Findings

Muscle imaging has revealed a characteristic distribution pattern in the thighs and lower legs in RYR1-related myopathies (Fig. 15.3). In the pelvic girdle, the gluteus maximus muscle is predominantly affected. In the thigh, the vasti, adductor magnus, biceps femoris, and often sartorius muscles are selectively involved, whereas the rectus femoris, gracilis, adductor longus, and semitendinosus muscles are spared. In the legs, the soleus muscle is markedly affected and, to a lesser extent, the peroneal group, with relative sparing of the gastrocnemii and the anterior compartment muscles. A number of patients do not display this typical pattern, particularly those with recessive forms or in cases associated with ophthalmoplegia. In patients with *RYR1* mutations, whole-body imaging techniques (Fig. 15.4) often reveal involvement of masticator muscles and of neck extensor muscles. In the pelvic girdle, arm, and lumbar trunk muscles, the degree of fatty infiltration is moderate. The glutei, biceps brachii, and lumbar paravertebral muscles are particularly affected. Milder involvement is observed in the forearm and shoulder, with the subscapularis muscle predominantly affected.

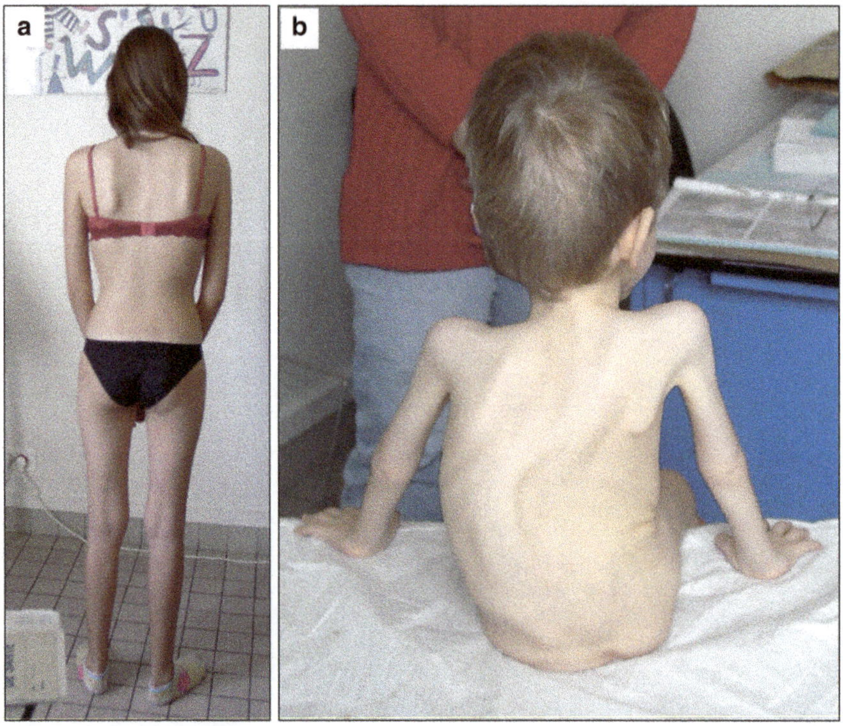

Fig. 15.2 Clinical variability in RYR1-related myopathies. (**a**) A 13-year-old girl with mild proximal weakness and fatigability. (**b**) A 3-year-old non-ambulatory boy with severe early scoliosis, and respiratory insufficiency

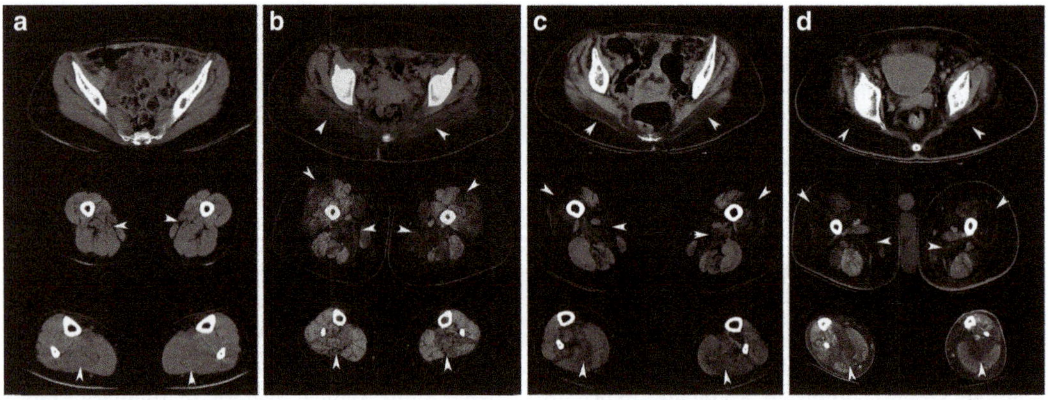

Fig. 15.3 Muscular imaging in four RYR1-CCD patients ranging from a mild to a severe clinical phenotype shows characteristic patterns of muscle involvement. The first mild changes appear in the medial thigh compartment and soleus muscles (**a**, *arrowheads*). In more severely affected patients, involvement of the gluteus maximus muscle, quadriceps, and lateral gastrocnemius are observed (**b**, **c**), whereas the gluteus minimus, the hamstrings, and the tibialis anterior muscles are relatively preserved (**d**). From Fischer D, et al (2006) Muscle imaging in dominant core myopathies linked or unlinked to the ryanodine receptor 1 gene. Neurology;67(12):2217–20). Reprinted with permission from Wolters Kluwer Health

15.2.6 Differential Diagnosis

Overlapping features are observed in the various forms of congenital myopathies and congenital muscular dystrophies (see Chap. 16). In particular, patients with mutations in *SEPN1* (see Sect. 15.3), *DNM2* (Sect. 15.5), or *COL6*

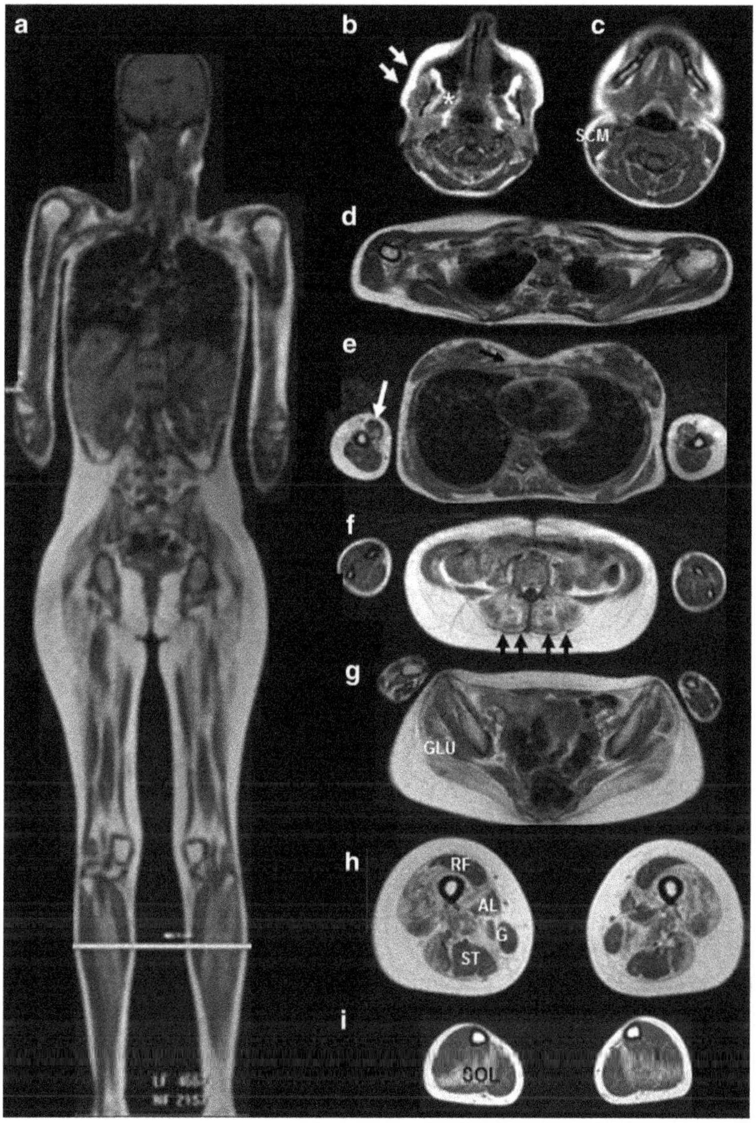

Fig. 15.4 Whole-body T1-weighted turbo spin echo magnetic resonance imaging (MRI) frontal (**a**) and axial views (**b–i**) in a 13-year-old girl with a *RYR1* dominant mutation and mild weakness. Frontal whole-body view shows moderate to severe involvement predominantly in the pelvic girdle and lower limbs. (**b–i**) Head axial views with mild to moderate involvement of the masticator muscles in the head: masseter (*arrows* in **b**) and pterygoids (*white star* in **b**). In contrast, neck muscles are well preserved (sternocleidomastoid, SCM in **c**). Shoulder muscles are thin, but there is no abnormal signal (**d**). Upper trunk and upper limbs show involvement of the biceps brachii muscles (*white arrow* in **e**). Lumbar paravertebral muscles are severely affected (*black arrows* in **f**). Pelvic girdle shows moderate to severe involvement of gluteal muscles (*GLU*). In the thigh, severe abnormalities of muscles are observed, with selective sparing of the rectus femoris (*RF*), gracilis (*G*), adductor longus (*AL*), and semitendinosus (*ST*) muscles. (**h**) In the lower leg, the soleus muscle (*SOL*) is markedly affected, with preservation of the other muscles. (**i**) From Quijano-Roy S, et al (2012) Whole body muscle MRI protocol: pattern recognition in early onset NM disorders. Neuromuscul Disord. 22:S68–84. Reprinted with permission from Elsevier

(see Sect. 16.4) genes may mimic the CCD phenotype. Biopsy, clinical features, and imaging findings can help narrow the differential diagnosis. External ophthalmoplegia, ptosis, and facial and bulbar involvement are more typical for centronuclear myopathy due to *DNM2* mutations (see Sect. 15.5) or myasthenic syndromes. The need for nocturnal ventilation in an ambulatory patient is highly suggestive of *SEPN1*-related myopathy (see Sect. 15.3). Distal striking hyperlaxity associated with proximal joint contractures is characteristic for Ullrich syndrome due to *COL6* gene mutations (see Sect. 16.4). Other conditions not associated with myopathies—e.g., denervation, malignant hyperthermia, *MYH7*-associated-hypertrophic cardiomyopathy (see Sect. 21.2.3)—may also show cores. Concerning involvement patterns on muscle imaging, the typical *RYR1* profile in lower limbs may overlap with that of severe *SEPN1*-mutation cases. However, in those cases, whole-body imaging (MRI) offers additional information, allowing a straightforward differential diagnosis. Whereas with whole-body MRI the *RYR1*-mutation patients may show quite diffuse involvement of masticator and upper arm muscles, those with the *SEPN1* mutation have more limited abnormalities (sternocleidomastoid muscle atrophy and selective marked infiltration of paravertebral muscles). A flow chart demonstrating how muscle imaging findings can be used for differentiating congenital myopathies is provided in Chap. 25 (see Sect. 25.2).

Congenital Myopathies: RYR1 Related Myopathies

Key Points

- Most patients with *RYR1*-associated CCD display signs of the disease during infancy, manifesting as hypotonia, slowly progressive axial and proximal muscle weakness, delayed motor milestones, hyporeflexia, and orthopedic deformities.
- Muscle biopsies of patients with *RYR1* mutations typically show the presence of "central cores" devoid of enzymatic oxidation in type I fibers.
- The majority of patients with identified *RYR1* mutations show a typical MRI pattern of leg muscle involvement, with the vasti, adductor magnus, and sartorius muscles predominantly affected and the rectus femoris, adductor longus, and gracilis muscles spared. In the lower legs, the soleus, gastrocnemius, and peronal group muscles are affected, and the tibialis anterior is usually preserved.
- Whole-body MRI reveals additional moderate involvement of the biceps brachii, subscapularis, lumbar paravertebral, and glutei muscles and milder involvement of the masticator, neck extensor, and forearm muscles.

Suggestions for Further Reading

Bevilacqua JA, Monnier N, Bitoun M, et al. Recessive RYR1 mutations cause unusual congenital myopathy with prominent nuclear internalization and large areas of myofibrillar disorganization. Neuropathol Appl Neurobiol. 2011;37:271–84.

Fischer D, Herasse M, Ferreiro A, et al. Muscle imaging in dominant core myopathies linked or unlinked to the ryanodine receptor 1 gene. Neurology 2006;67: 2217–20.

Jungbluth H, Davis MR, Müller C, et al. Magnetic resonance imaging of muscle in congenital myopathies associated with RYR1 mutations. Neuromuscul Disord. 2004;14:785–90.

Jungbluth H, Dowling JJ, Ferreiro A, et al. 182nd ENMC International Workshop: RYR1-related myopathies, 15–17th April 2011, Naarden, The Netherlands. Neuromuscul Disord. 2012; 22:453–62.

Klein A, Jungbluth H, Clement E, et al. Muscle magnetic resonance imaging in congenital myopathies due to ryanodine receptor type 1 gene mutations. Arch Neurol. 2011;68:1171–9.

Malicdan MCV, Nishino I. Central Core Disease. Gene Reviews. 2010. (http://www.ncbi.nlm.nih.gov/books/NBK1391/) Last Update: 11 May 2010.

Quijano-Roy S, Avila-Smirnow D, Carlier Y. Whole body muscle MRI protocol: pattern recognition in early-onset neuromuscular disorders. Neuromuscul Disord. 2012; 22 Suppl 2:S68–84.

Sewry CA, Jimenez-Mallebrera C, Muntoni F. Congenital myopathies. Curr Opin Neurol. 2008;21:569–75.

Treves S, Jungbluth H, Muntoni F, et al. Congenital muscle disorders with cores: the ryanodine receptor calcium channel paradigm. Curr Opin Pharmacol 2008;8:319–26.

15.3 Selenoproteinopathies

Susana Quijano-Roy, Daniela Avila-Smirnow, Robert-Yves Carlier

15.3.1 Synonyms and Abbreviations

SEPN1-related myopathy (*SEPN1*-RM); congenital muscular dystrophy (CMD) with rigid spine syndrome; rigid spine syndrome type 1 (RSMD1); multi-minicore disease (MMD); multi-minicore myopathy

15.3.2 Genetics and Pathophysiology

Selenium is an essential trace element, and selenoprotein N (SelN) was the first selenium-containing protein shown to be directly involved in inherited human diseases. Mutations in the *SEPN1* gene (1p35-36), encoding SelN, cause a group of muscular disorders (OMIM# 606210) characterized predominantly by affected axial paraspinal muscles. SelN, a glycoprotein localized in the endoplasmic reticulum, is involved in various antioxidant defense systems and several metabolic pathways, including redox-regulated calcium homeostasis. SelN is highly expressed from mid-gestation, suggesting an important role in embryogenesis. Although its pathophysiological role in skeletal muscle remains unclear, data indicate that SelN might be a key regulator of satellite cells' function in skeletal muscle tissue.

15.3.3 Histopathology

SEPN1 mutations were initially described in patients with CMD who presented with selective spinal rigidity and normal expression of the protein merosin (RSMD1). Histopathological findings included nonspecific dystrophic changes, including variation in fiber size, increased central nuclei, fiber degeneration and regeneration, and increased endomysial connective tissue. Later, *SEPN1* mutations were also reported in the classic form of multi-minicore myopathy (MMD), in congenital fiber disproportion myopathy (CFTD), and in a desminopathy with Mallory body-like inclusions. Histopathological findings of *SEPN1*-related MMD include multiple small areas of sarcomeric disorganization and/or diminished oxidative activity ("minicores"). In contrast to the typical central cores seen in *RYR1*-CCD (see Sect. 15.2), minicores may be observed in type I and type II fibers. In addition, minicores are short and span only a few sarcomeres in the longitudinal fiber axis. *SEPN1*-related myopathy behaves as a dystrophic process in paraspinal axial muscles, whereas the muscle pathology in limb girdle muscles is closer to that seen in other congenital myopathies, often lacking necrosis, regeneration, or marked endomysial fibrosis (Fig. 15.5).

15.3.4 Clinical Presentation

Clinical features in patients with *SEPN1* mutations are strikingly homogeneous in contrast to the histopathological findings, which are rather heterogeneous. The clinical manifestation is characterized by selective weakness of cervicoaxial muscles that becomes evident early in life. It is often associated with a delay in motor milestones. Later, weakness and hypotonia are replaced by cervicoaxial spinal stiffness, often associated with thoracic spinal lordotic deformity and characteristic "S"-shaped thoracic translation of the spine (Fig. 15.6). No major joint contractures are observed in the limbs. The voice is typically nasal. Concerning motor performances, these patients complain characteristically of fatigability and to a lesser extend of weakness. Many patients, however, are able to run and climb stairs. A major clinical complication is the restrictive respiratory insufficiency that occurs during the first years of life. These symptoms are aggravated by diaphragmatic dysfunction, leading to nocturnal hypoventilation. Mechanical ventilation is required in most children before they reach adulthood. A patient affected with a myopathy who is still ambulatory but requires mechanical ventilation at night is highly suspected to have *SEPN1*-RM, particularly if these symptoms are accompanied by rigid spine syndrome not associated with major joint contractures. Most patients remain ambulatory through adulthood. Respiratory insufficiency seems to stabilize during the third to fourth decades of life if there is adequate ventilation and the scoliosis is treated.

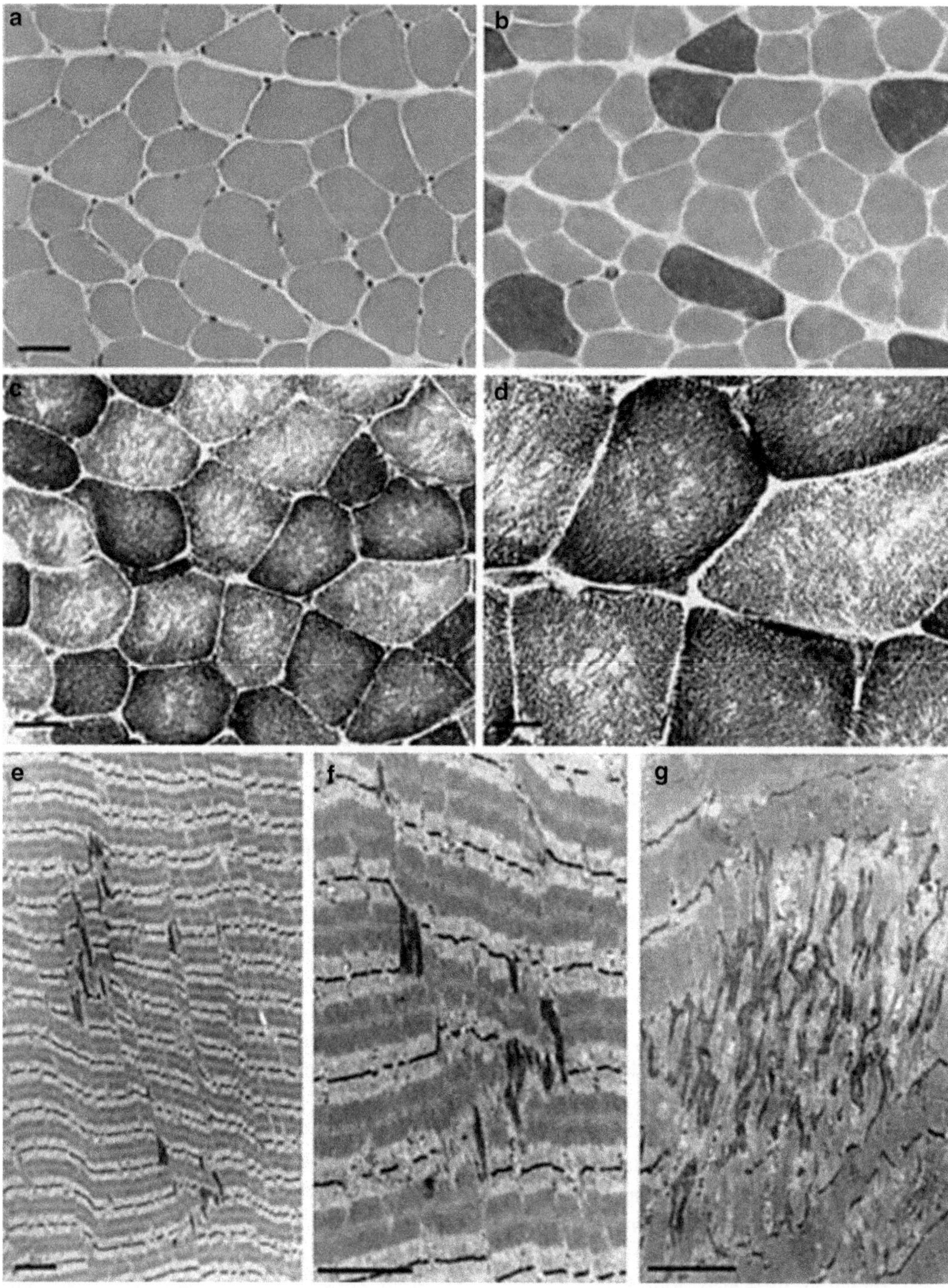

Fig. 15.5 Histochemical and ultrastructural features of SEPN1-related multi-minicore-disease: **a–d**, Serial transverse cryostat sections. (**a**, **c**) 5 years old patient. Left deltoid stained with H&E (**a**) and myosin adenosine triphosphatase pH 9.4 (**b**). Note the variable fiber sizes and predominance of type 1 (lighter) fibers. Although all the type 2 fibers have large diameters, both large and small type 1 fibers are observed, which produces a smaller mean diameter ("type 1 relative hypotrophy"). (**c**, **d**) 14 years old patient. Right deltoid stained with nicotinamide

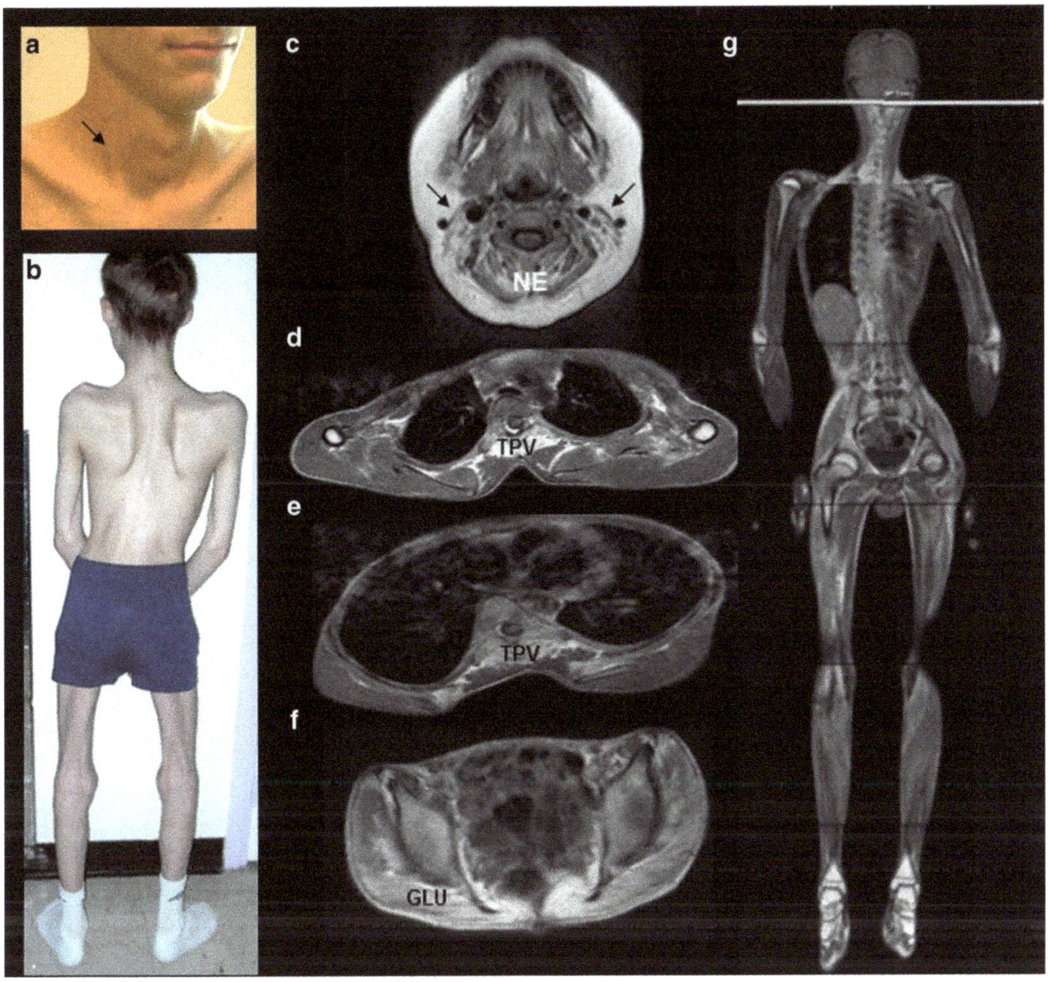

Fig. 15.6 Typical features in *SEPN1* patients: severe hypotrophy of sternocleidomastoid muscle (*SCM*), which is observed clinically (*arrow* in **a**) and on whole body MRI (*arrows* in **c**). Clinical picture (**b**) and frontal whole-body MRI view (**g**) reveal the characteristic translation of the dorsal spine, thoracic lordosis, and hypotrophy of the internal thigh leading to a "brackets" aspect of the lower limbs. Fatty infiltration of neck and upper limb muscles with selective affection of neck extensors (*NE* in **c**), thoracic paravertebral (*TPV* in **d** and **e**), and gluteus muscles (*GLU*) (**f**). Note the diffusely reduced subcutaneous tissue (lipoatrophy in **d–f**) and the severe thoracic lordosis (**e**, **f**). (**c–g**) From Quijano-Roy S, et al (2012) Whole body muscle MRI protocol: pattern recognition in early-onset NM disorders. Neuromuscul Disord. 22:S68–84. Reprinted with permission from Elsevier

Fig. 15.5 (continued) adenine dinucleotide–tetrazolium reductase (NADH-TR) (**c**) and succinate dehydrogenase (**d**). Multiple focal areas lacking oxidative activity are present in most type 1 (darker) and type 2 fibers. As shown here, in two different biopsy specimens, there was no significant increase in endomysial connective tissue. (**e–g**) Longitudinal electron micrography sections from two different patients (**e**, **f**) and (**g**). Left quadriceps and left deltoid at 23 and 5 years of age, respectively. (**e**, **f**) Mild, early-stage minicore lesions. The sarcomeres appear out of register. Z-line streaming is limited to one sarcomere in length and three to four myofibrils in width. The longitudinal myofilament array is still recognizable. (**g**) Electron-dense material of Z-line origin forming irregular zones with severe focal disorganization of the myofibrillar structure. Bars = 40 μm in **a** and **b**, 25 μm in **c**, 12.5 μm in **d**, and 2.5 μm in **e–g**. From Ferreiro A, et al (2002) Mutations of the selenoprotein N gene, which is implicated in rigid spine muscular dystrophy, cause the classical phenotype of multiminicore disease: reassessing the nosology of early-onset myopathies. Am J Hum Genet. 71:739–49. Reprinted with permission from The American Society of Human Genetics

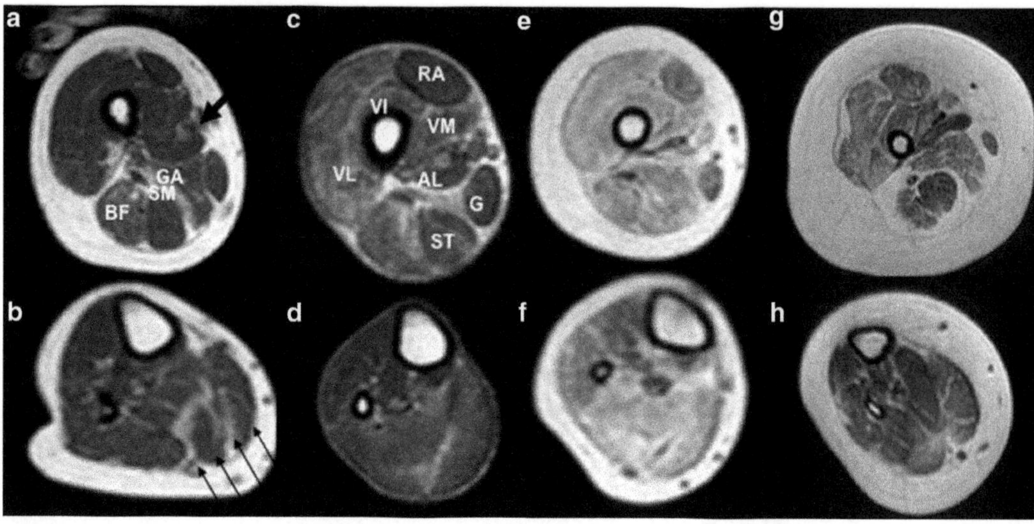

Fig. 15.7 Thigh and lower leg MRI features in four *SEPN1* patients with different degrees of severity. The patient with the mildest case shows in the thigh (**a**), atrophy of the sartorius muscle (*thick black arrow*) and selective fatty infiltration of the (great) adductor magnus (*GA*), semimembranosus (*SM*), and biceps femoris (*BF*). In patients with moderate severity (**c**, **d**), there is a similar distribution of abnormalities in the thigh (**c**) with additional involvement of the vastii (VV). In the lower leg, there is mild abnormal involvement of the posterior compartment (**b**, *arrows*). The most severe cases (**e**–**f** and **g**–**h**) show the same pattern of abnormalities, with severe fatty infiltration of the thigh (**e**, **g**) and better preservation of the rectus femoris (*RF*), adductor longus, gracilis (*G*), and semitendinosus muscles (*ST*). In the lower leg (**b**, **d**, **f**, **h**), the posterior compartment is always predominantly affected (*thin black arrows in b*)

15.3.5 Imaging Findings

The distribution pattern on whole-body MRI is characterized by striking axial involvement with severe involvement of the paraspinal, intercostal, abdominal, and gluteal muscles. In the neck, severe selective atrophy of the sternocleidomastoid muscle and fatty infiltration of neck extensors can be observed. Muscles of the head, shoulder, and upper extremities are often preserved, particularly the tongue (Fig. 15.6). Sparing of the tongue is helpful for distinguishing this profile from Pompe disease (see Sect. 14.2.1). In the lower limbs, there is often predominant involvement of the sartorius, which typically is associated with fatty infiltration of the biceps femoris, semimembranosus, and adductor magnus muscles. In more advanced stages, the vastus lateralis may also be involved, leading to overlapping features to the *RYR1* (see Sect. 15.2) pattern in the thigh. The lower leg is often not affected during early stages, but if there is fatty infiltration, it is often more severe in the posterior compartment (Fig. 15.7).

15.3.6 Differential Diagnosis

SEPN1-RM is difficult to diagnose during the first years of life in the absence of specific clinical or pathological features. With advancing age, however, the clinical features become highly suggestive. Because of the risk of "hidden" life-threatening respiratory complications, it is important always to consider this entity in the clinical differential diagnosis of a floppy infant. Neuromuscular imaging, particularly using whole-body muscle MRI, is a helpful tool for distinguishing patients with *SEPN1* mutations from other patients with similar clinical findings (e.g., progressive scoliosis, spinal stiffness). This phenotype is observed not only in *SEPN1*-RM but also in patients with mutations in other genes that are difficult to analyze or with poor muscle tissue-specific markers such as *RYR1* (see Sect. 15.2), *COL6* genes (see Sect. 16.4), lamin A/C (*LMNA*) (see Sect. 16.3 and Chap. 18), and acid α-glucosidase (*GAA*) (see Sect. 14.2.1). Whole-body MRI shows distinct profiles of muscle involvement in all these entities. A flow chart demonstrating how muscle imaging findings may be used for the differentiation of congenital myopathies is provided in Sect. 25.2.

Interestingly, findings similar to those of *SEPN1*-RM have been described in the thigh in patients with mutations in the *SECISBP2* gene (selenocysteine insertion sequence-binding protein 2). It is a multisystem disorder with defective biosynthesis of many selenoproteins. This disease results in a complex phenotype (azoospermia, axial muscular dystrophy, photosensitivity, enhanced systemic and cellular insulin sensitivity). In contrast to *SEPN1*-RM, more severe involvement of the adductor magnus was observed than that in sartorius muscle.

Congenital Myopathies: Selenoproteinopathies

Key Points

- *SEPN1*-related myopathy is histologically heterogeneous (CMD, MMD, congenital fiber-type disproportion) but clinically homogeneous.
- Weakness is predominantly axial, with relatively preserved limb girdle motor function. Affected children develop scoliosis and require nocturnal mechanical ventilation before adulthood.
- Patients usually remain ambulatory most of their lives.
- Muscle MRI in the lower limbs may help distinguish *SEPN1* from *COL6* and *LMNA* profiles because of the selective involvement of the sartorius muscle. However, the thigh involvement pattern may not be informative enough in patients with similar phenotypes (Pompe's disease, *RYR1*-RM). In those cases whole-body MRI allows a straightforward diagnosis by showing atrophy of the sternocleidomastoid muscle and fatty infiltration of the paravertebral muscles, whereas tongue, shoulder, and arm muscles are well preserved.

Suggestions for Further Reading

Arbogast S, Beuvin M, Fraysse B, et al. Oxidative stress in SEPN1-related myopathy: from pathophysiology to treatment. Ann Neurol. 2009;65:677–86.

Ferreiro A, Estournet B, Chateau D, et al. Multi-minicore disease—searching for boundaries: phenotype analysis of 38 cases. Ann Neurol. 2000;48:745–57.

Jungbluth H, Muntoni F, Ferreiro A, et al. 150th ENMC international workshop: core myopathies, 9–11th March 2007, Naarden, The Netherlands. Neuromuscul Disord. 2008;18:989–96.

Jungbluth H, Sewry CA, Muntoni F. Core myopathies. Semin Pediatr Neurol. 2011;18:239–49.

Mercuri E, Clements E, Offiah A, et al. Muscle magnetic resonance imaging involvement in muscular dystrophies with rigidity of the spine. Ann Neurol. 2010;67:201–8.

Scoto M, Cirak S, Mein R, et al. SEPN1-related myopathies: clinical course in a large cohort of patients. Neurology 2011;76:2073–8.

15.4 X-linked Myotubular Myopathy

Jorge A. Bevilacqua, and Norma Beatriz Romero

15.4.1 Synonyms, Abbreviations

X-linked myotubular myopathy (XLMTM); severe neonatal Centronuclear myopathy (CNM); "Necklace fiber" myopathy

15.4.2 Introduction and Classification

Myotubular myopathy is seen in a group of centronuclear myopathies (CNMs) comprising a series of congenital disorders, mainly characterized by the presence of centrally located nuclei in biopsied muscle fibers. Three forms of CNM are recognized according to the mode of inheritance: X-linked recessive myotubular myopathy caused by mutations in the myotubularin 1 gene (*MTM1*, OMIM 300400) (addressed in this chapter); an autosomal dominant CNM caused by mutations in the *DNM2* gene encoding dynamin 2 (DNM2) (OMIM 160150) (see Sect. 15.5); an autosomal recessive form due to mutations in the *BIN1* gene encoding amphiphysin 2 (OMIM 255200).

In XLMTM, affected males most frequently present with severe hypotonia and respiratory

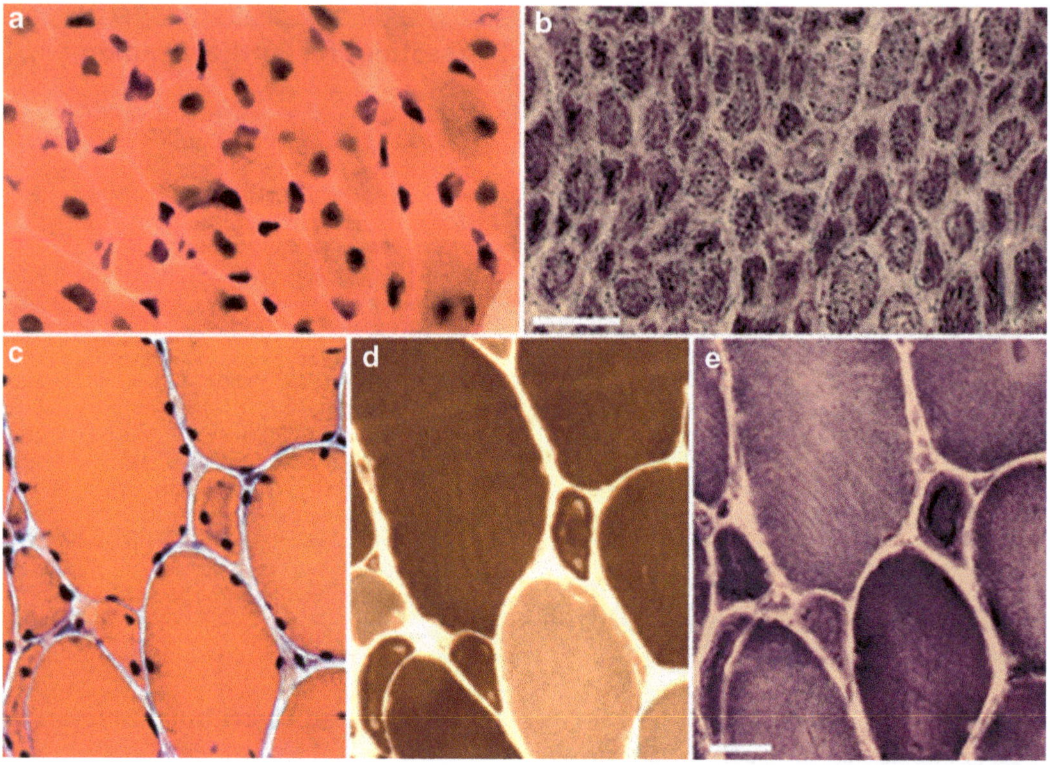

Fig. 15.8 Histological findings in a muscle biopsy from a neonate with XLMTM (**a**, **b**), and his asymptomatic mother (**c**, **d**, **e**) show "necklace" fibers. From Bevilacqua et al (2009) "Necklace" fibers, a new histological marker of late-onset MTM1-related centronuclear myopathy. Acta Neuropathol. 117:283–9). Reprinted with permission from Springer

insufficiency at birth, often leading to early postnatal death. Mutations in *MTM1* have been increasingly recognized as the underlying cause of "atypical" forms of XLMTM in male newborns, female infants, carrier women, and adult men with a mild form of the myopathy who lead normal lives. A less severe form of myopathy linked to *MTM1* mutations has now been described in female carriers and adult men. It is called "Necklace fiber myopathy" based on the histological appearance of the muscle fibers (Fig. 15.8).

15.4.3 Genetics and Pathophysiology

Myotubular myopathy is an X-linked recessive myopathy caused by mutations in the myotubularin gene (*MTM1*) on chromosome Xq28 encoding the 3′ phosphoinositide-phosphatase myotubularin 1. Mutations in the myotubularin (*MTM1*) gene have now been identified in the majority of affected males. Disease-causing sequence changes include deletions/insertions, nonsense, missense, and splice mutations (approximately 25 % each). *MTM1* mutations are distributed throughout the entire coding sequence, localizing most commonly to exons 12, 4, 11, 8, and 9. The maternal carrier state of *MTM1* mutations is estimated at 85 %; maternal mosaicism has been reported in a few families.

A clear genotype–phenotype correlation has been difficult to establish. It has been shown, however, that some nontruncating mutations are associated with a more favorable prognosis, although most mutations are associated with severe phenotypes.

The pathogenesis of myotubularin-related myopathy is not yet fully elucidated. Myotubularin belongs to a large family of dual-specificity

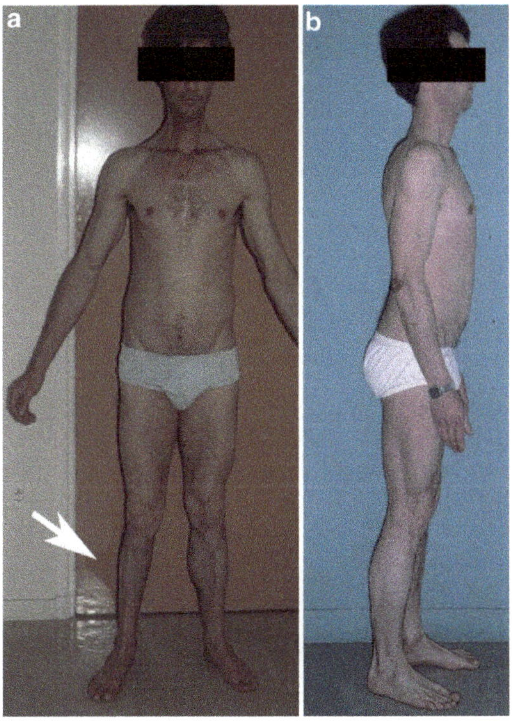

Fig. 15.9 Clinical appearance of a male patient with late-onset XLMTM. This case is a patient from the series by Bevilacqua et al. (2009). (**a**, **b**) Note the athletic appearance of the patient. Patient showing marked asymmetry of the calves with right calf atrophy (white arrow in a), also seen in Figs. 15.10c, 15.11a. From Bevilacqua et al (2009) "Necklace" fibers, a new histological marker of late-onset MTM1-related centronuclear myopathy. Acta Neuropathol. 117:283–9). Reprinted with permission from Springer

phosphatases involved in the epigenetic regulation of signaling pathways interrelated with cellular growth and differentiation. A specific function has been proposed for myotubularin in regulating phosphoinositide-derived second messengers with crucial roles in membrane trafficking. To date, however, no skeletal muscle protein interactors of MTM1 have been identified. Thus, either disruption of the MTM1 structure or loss of enzymatic activity may underlie the deleterious effects of specific *MTM1* mutations, but it is not possible to exclude the role of unidentified protein–protein interactions in the muscle tissue. Observations in animal and cellular models indicate that myotubularin plays a role in muscle fiber maintenance but not in myogenesis. These data suggest that disturbed remodeling of cytoskeletal and extracellular architecture plays a role in the pathophysiology of XLMTM.

15.4.4 Histopathology

Biopsy findings in neonatal XLMTM patients show a fiber population with a typical myotube-like appearance characterized by central nuclei surrounded by a clear halo. Fibers are predominantly type I, usually smaller than those in age-matched controls, and with oxidative and ATPase reactions the appearance is characteristic (Fig. 15.8). In the milder juvenile or adult form of *MTM1*-linked myopathy, the biopsy shows fiber size variability with a predominance of type I fibers, increased endomysial tissue, and adipose replacement. Nuclear centralization or internalization is present in about one-fourth of the fibers. In these cases, the histological hallmark is the presence of small, atrophic fibers underneath the sarcolemma in a basophilic ring or "necklace" following the contour of the cell ("necklace fibers") (Fig. 15.8).

15.4.5 Clinical Presentation

The X-linked form due to mutations in the *MTM1* gene has been clinically well characterized. The classic neonatal form shows severe hypotonia and generalized muscle weakness at birth. Most affected boys die during the first year of life from respiratory insufficiency. The onset of milder forms is during early childhood, with delayed motor milestones followed by insidious muscle weakness beginning in the proximal lower limbs and spreading later to the shoulder girdle, neck, and trunk. Contractures are frequent. Cardiac function is usually preserved. CK values are normal or slightly increased. One remarkable feature observed in these cases is asymmetrical calf atrophy (Fig. 15.9). The majority of carriers of the X-linked form are asymptomatic, but a few patients show signs of mild muscle weakness, especially if additional genetic abnormalities are present (e.g., skewed X inactivation, structural X-chromosomal abnormalities). As for other centronuclear myopathies, management of *MTM1*-related myopathy is mainly supportive based on a multidisciplinary approach. The neonatal form of the disease is often fatal during infancy.

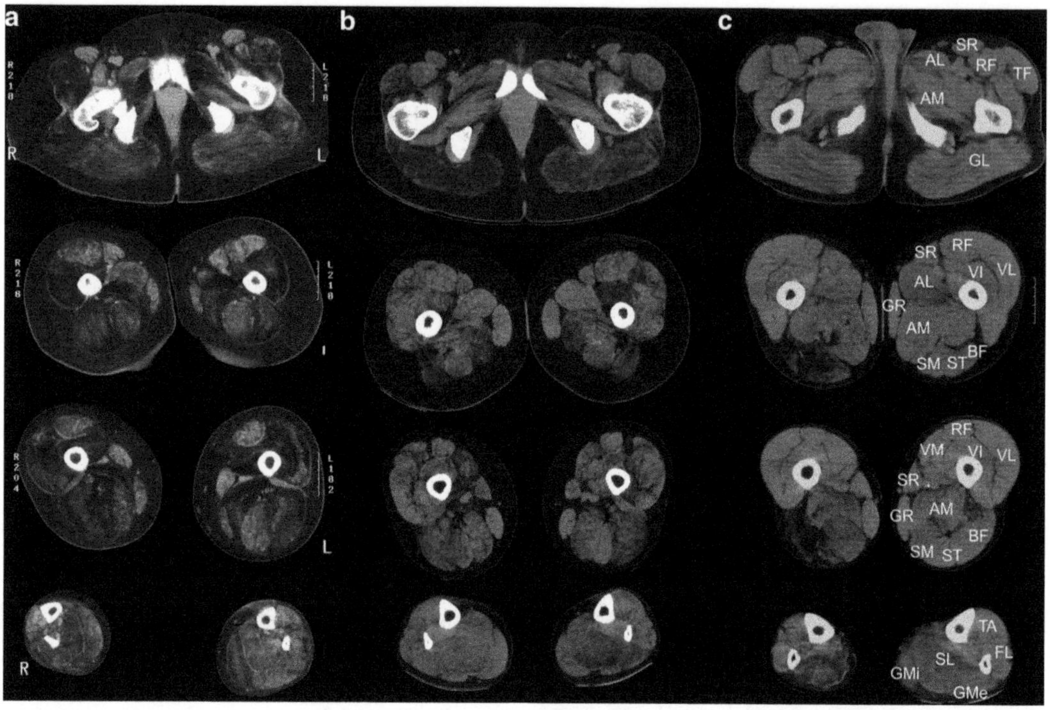

Fig. 15.10 Comparative lower limb computed tomography (CT) imaging from three patients with the adult form of XLMTM ("Necklace myopathy"). Lower limb CT scans from patients 1 (**a**), 2 (**b**), and 4 (**c**), obtained at 43, 26, and 49 years of age, respectively. Muscle involvement was observed in the soleus (*SL*), biceps femoris (*BF*), semimembranosus (*SM*), semitendinosus (*ST*), adductor magnus (*AM*), vastus intemedius (*VI*), lateralis (*VL*), and gluteus maximus (*GL*) muscles. In contrast, the rectus femoris (*RF*), gracilis (*GR*), and sartorius (*SAR*) muscles in the thigh and the gastrocnemii (*GM*) and anterior compartment muscles of the lower leg were relatively spared. Note the marked asymmetry of the calves in **a** and **c**. In this patient, muscle involvement was limited to the right posterior leg and thigh compartments (**c**). From Bevilacqua et al (2009) "Necklace" fibers, a new histological marker of late-onset MTM1-related centronuclear myopathy. Acta Neuropathol. 117:283–9). Reprinted with permission from Springer

15.4.6 Imaging Findings

Imaging findings of *MTM1*-related myopathy have been mainly described for Necklace fiber myopathy. Lower-limbs CT imaging and MRI of patients with Necklace myopathy showed moderate to severe abnormalities in the pelvic girdle, particularly in the gluteus (i.e., minimus, medius, maximus) muscles. The most severe changes were observed in the posterior compartment of the thigh (Figs. 15.10 and 15.11), where the biceps femoris, semimembranosus, and to a lesser extent the semitendinosus were consistently affected at onset. In the middle thigh, the adductor magnus was involved, whereas the adductor longus, sartorius, and gracilis were relatively preserved. Signal abnormalities in the anterior compartment of the thigh touched the vasti intermedius and medialis, in contrast to the relatively normal appearances of the rectus femoris and vastus lateralis. Two of the patients reported in the series had markedly asymmetrical calves, both having atrophy on the right calf and pseudo-hypertrophy on the left (Figs. 15.10 and 15.11). The soleus was always the most affected muscle in the lower legs and showed moderate to severe changes in the three studied patients. The medial and lateral gastrocnemii and the muscles of the anterior compartment of the leg were comparatively less involved or unaffected.

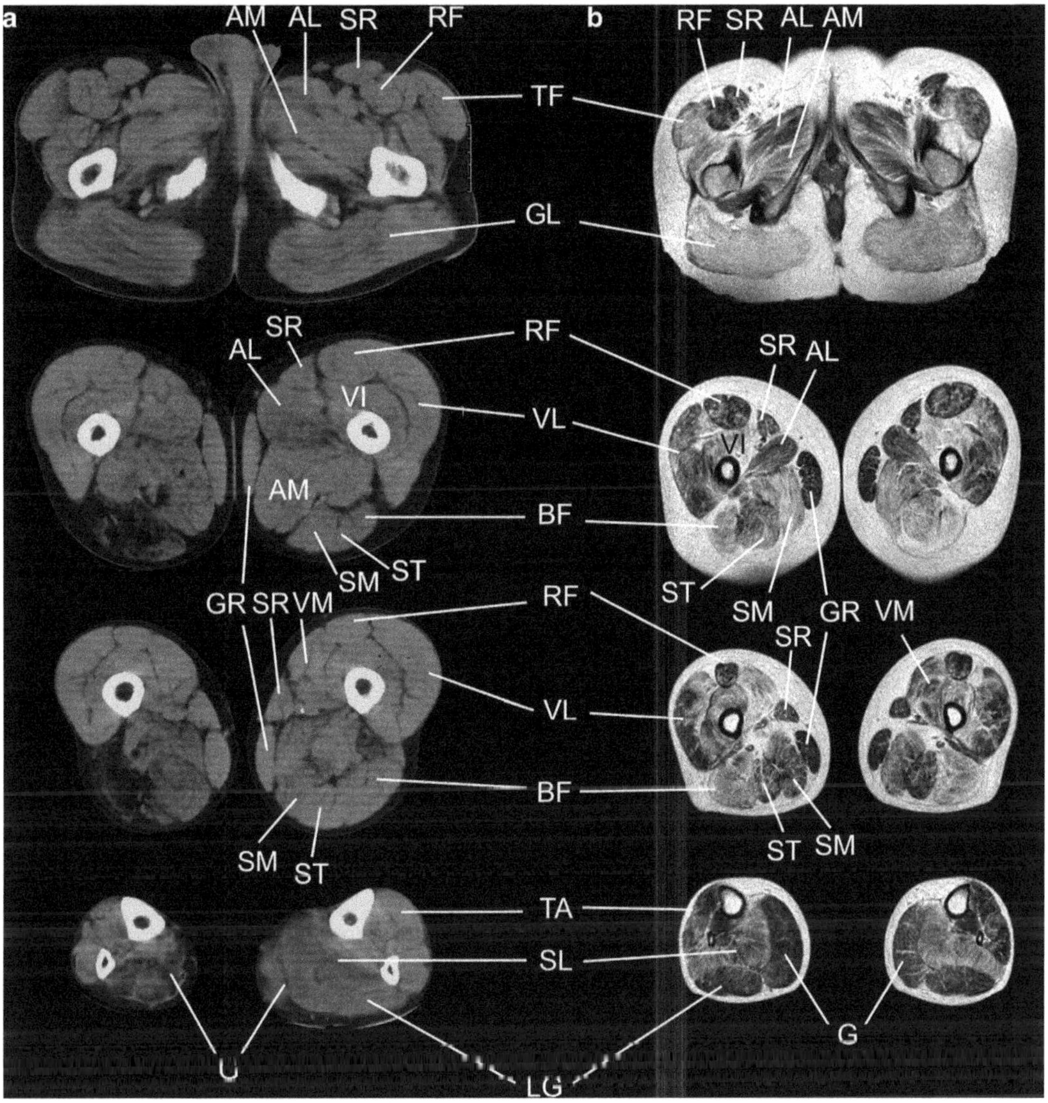

Fig. 15.11 Comparative CT and MRI lower limb imaging of two patients. Patient 4: CT scan (**a**) obtained at 49 years of age shows asymmetry of the calves and selective alteration of the right biceps femoris and posterior leg muscles. Patient 2: MRI (**b**) obtained at 32 years of age shows marked involvement of the gluteus (*GL*), posterior thigh muscles, and vastus intermedius (*VI*) and lateralis (*VL*) muscles. Rectus femoris (*RF*), sartorius (*SR*), gracilis (*GR*) and adductor longus (*AL*) muscles were relatively spared. In the leg, the soleus (*SL*) was consistently affected, whereas the gastrocnemii (*GM*) and anterior leg compartment muscles (*TA*) were less affected or unaffected. From Bevilacqua et al (2009) "Necklace" fibers, a new histological marker of late-onset MTM1-related centronuclear myopathy. Acta Neuropathol. 2117:283–9). Reprinted with permission from Springer

In a case of an early severe form of XLMTM in a girl with skewed X-inactivation, lower-limbs MRI showed diffuse involvement of the pelvic girdle with relative sparing of the adductor longus in the thigh and the tibialis anterior, extensor digitorum longus, and both gastrocnemii muscles in the lower legs. There are no published imaging findings of the severe neonatal forms in boys. In the case of the oldest known clinically affected female carrier of myotubular myopathy, lower limb muscle CT scans of the 77-year-old woman showed marked fatty replacement in the glutei, posterior thigh muscles (except sartorius and gracilis), and gastrocnemii. There was also asymmetrical right soleus involvement in the legs. Asymmetry has also been shown on chest radiographs from patients affected by myotubular myopathy, who presented with an elevated right hemi-diaphragm.

15.4.7 Differential Diagnosis

The differential diagnosis for myotubular myopathy varies according to the age of onset. In the neonatal form, the differential diagnosis should consider other CMs including congenital myotonic dystrophy (see Chap. 22) in which the histological appearance of the muscle of both entities is similar. Presentation in juvenile and adult patients requires that XLMTM be distinguished from other CMs, particularly those due to *DNM2* (see Sect. 15.4) and *BIN1* mutations. A flow chart demonstrating how muscle imaging results can be used for differentiating congenital myopathies is provided in Chap. 25 (see Sect. 25.2).

Congenital Myopathies: (X-linked) Myotubular Myopathy

Key Points

- XLMTM is a severe, usually fatal, neonatal-onset congenital myopathy that rarely present with atypical juvenile and adult onset.
- Screening for the *MTM1* gene should be considered in female patients with suggestive clinical and histopathological features.
- Clinical onset at birth is frequently fatal because of severe respiratory impairment and should be distinguished from other congenital myopathies.
- In juvenile patients, adult men. and carriers, XLMTM may lead to a milder, or subsymptomatic, myopathy.
- Muscle biopsy is indispensable for diagnosis and allows identification of the various phenotypical forms of the disease (i.e., neonatal, "necklace"). Congenital forms of myotonic dystrophy (DM-I) should be always ruled out.
- Imaging in milder affected patients show diffuse involvement of the thigh and posterior leg with relative sparing of the rectus femoris, gracilis, sartorius, and gastrocnemius muscles.

Suggestions for Further Reading

Bevilacqua JA, Bitoun M, Biancalana V, et al. "Necklace" fibers, a new histological marker of late-onset MTM1-related centronuclear myopathy. Acta Neuropathol. 2009;117:283–91.

Biancalana V, Caron O, Gallati S, et al. Characterisation of mutations in 77 patients with X-linked myotubular myopathy, including a family with a very mild phenotype. Hum Genet. 2003;112:135–42.

Grogan PM, Tanner SM, Ørstavik KH, et al. Myopathy with skeletal asymmetry and hemidiaphragm elevation is caused by myotubularin mutations. Neurology 2005;64:1638–40.

Hammans SR, Robinson DO, Moutou C, et al. A clinical and genetic study of a manifesting heterozygote with X-linked myotubular myopathy. Neuromuscul Disord. 2000;10:133–37.

Jungbluth H, Wallgren-Pettersson C, Laporte J. Centronuclear (myotubular) myopathy. Orphanet J Rare Dis. 2008;3:26.

Romero NB. Centronuclear myopathies: a widening concept. Neuromuscul Disord. 2010;20:223–22.

Sutton IJ, Winer JB, Norman AN, et al. Limb girdle and facial weakness in female carriers of X-linked myotubular myopathy mutations. Neurology 2001;57: 900–2.

15.5 Dynamin 2-Related Centronuclear Myopathy

Daniela Avila-Smirnow, Robert-Yves Carlier, Susana Quijano-Roy

15.5.1 Synonyms and Abbreviations

Autosomal dominant centronuclear myopathy (CNM); dynamin 2 (DNM2); DNM2-related CNM (DNM2-CNM)

15.5.2 Genetics and Pathophysiology

Centronuclear myopathy (CNM) is related to three genes according to mode of inheritance. Autosomal dominant CNM is related to dynamin 2 (*DNM2*), autosomal recessive CNM to amphiphysin (*BIN*), and X-linked CNM to myotubularin (*MTM1*) (see Sect. 15.4) mutations. However, no genetic defect can be identified in 30 % of CNM cases.

The majority of CNMs are caused by dominant *DNM2* mutations, including sporadic cases, which are due to dominant de novo mutations. *DNM2* is located in chromosome 19p13.2 (OMIM 160150) and is composed of 22 exons. It codes for dynamin 2 (DNM2) a 98-kDA protein. Dynamins are a superfamily of large GTPases involved in membrane trafficking. They act as scaffolding molecules. Hydrolization of GTP involves the formation and release of vesicles from biological membranes. In particular, DNM2 participates in endocytosis, exocitosis, intracellular membrane trafficking, actin assembly, and centrosome cohesion. DNM2, though ubiquitously expressed, is more abundant in cardiac and skeletal muscle.

Various pathophysiological hypotheses have been exposed in *DNM2*-related CNM. Alteration of membrane trafficking and signaling pathway is one of the hypotheses. Excitation-contraction coupling impairment due to T-tubule dysfunction has also been suggested. Finally, abnormal centrosome function due to an alteration of DNM2 transport to the centrosome or a change of its interaction with centrosomal components has been hypothesized. Genotype–phenotype correlation hypotheses have started to merge and allow an efficient screening strategy for molecular diagnosis (e.g., heterozygous de novo mutations in the PH domain, associated with early, severe onset). In addition to CNM, dissimilar *DNM2* mutations are associated with Charcot–Marie–Tooth (CMT) peripheral neuropathy (CMTD1B and CMT2M), suggesting a tissue-specific impact of the mutations.

15.5.3 Histopathology

In *DNM2*-related CNM, light microscopy shows significant nuclear centralization and internalization, radiating sarcoplasmic strands (RSSs), and type I fiber predominance and atrophy (Fig. 15.12c–f). In young children (< 5 years of age), this triad might be incomplete or absent. In contrast, at the severe end of the spectrum, infants with marked congenital myopathy and respiratory failure may have severe abnormalities on muscle biopsy indistinguishable from those of myotubular myopathy due to *MTM1* mutations (Fig. 15.13d). Centralization is defined as the presence of one nucleus in the center of the muscle fiber and internalization as the presence of one or more nuclei anywhere in the sarcoplasm. Nuclear centralization is more common than nuclear internalization in CNM because of the *DNM2* mutations. Dystrophic features such as increased connective tissue, fatty replacement, and even regenerating fibers may be observed as well. RSSs radiating from the central nucleus are seen with NADH-TR, SDH, and COX stains. Electron microscopy shows centralized nuclei, and RSSs (Fig. 15.12f). Mitochondria, Golgi complex, sarcoplasmic reticulum, and glycogen particles accumulate between central nuclei and between myofibrils. The radiating appearance is due to the deceasing diameter of myofibrils from the periphery to the center of the muscle fiber. Necklace fibers or clear dystrophic changes including fibrosis, fatty infiltration, and degenerating fibers are features observed in a number of cases.

15.5.4 Clinical Presentation

Severity ranges from severe neonatal forms to mild late-onset forms. Also, there are interfamilial and intrafamilial variations in age of onset and severity. Muscle weakness is more pronounced in the distal limb, trunk, and neck extensor muscles. Facial weakness, ptosis, and ophthalmoparesis are often associated or appear during the course of the disease (Fig. 15.13e, f). Neonatal onset may mimic Myotubular myopathy due to *MTM1* mutations. Patients may have a history of decreased fetal movements and at birth or early in infancy present with generalized hypotonia, ptosis, ophthalmoparesis, and facial and bulbar weakness. Nasogastric tube feeding or gastrostomy and ventilator support are often required at least during the early ages. In contrast to *MTM1* patients, symptoms associated with severe *DNM2*-related CMN tend to diminish during the

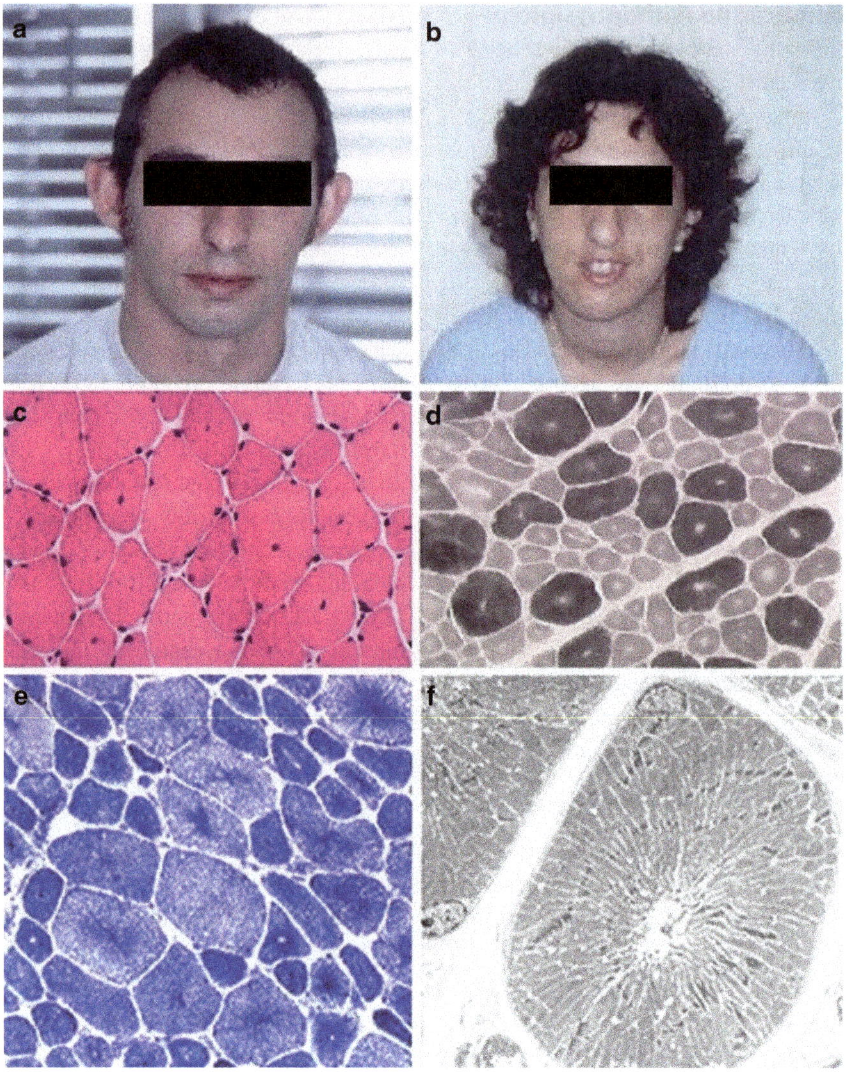

Fig. 15.12 Clinical and pathological findings observed in early adult-onset *DYN2*-CNM. Patients present with mild facial weakness and bilateral ptosis (**a**, **b**). Characteristic histopathological findings are myotube-like fibers that show an increased number of centralized nuclei (H&E, ×20) (**c**); presence of fiber type 1 predominance and atrophy (ATP 9.4) (**d**); radial distribution of sarcoplasmic strands seen by NADH (**e**) and electron microscopy (**f**). Courtesy of Norma Romero, Paris, France. From Fischer et al (2006) Characterization of the muscle involvement in dynamin 2-elated centronuclear myopathy. Brain. 129:1463. Reprinted with permission from Oxford University Press

first years. These children may be weaned from the ventilator, can eat orally, and achieve walking. Later, there is slowly progressive impairment of motor bulbar and respiratory function, and the patients may become wheelchair-bound or require mechanical ventilation. Mid-face hypoplasia has been reported in several patients, particularly those with noninvasive nasal mask ventilation.

The majority of reported patients with *DNM2*-related CNM show a milder phenotype, with normal or subnormal motor development and weakness starting during childhood or early adulthood. Deep tendon reflexes are weak or absent. Ptosis, ophthalmoparesis, and distal involvement are typical findings but are rare in other congenital myopathies (Fig. 15.12a, b).

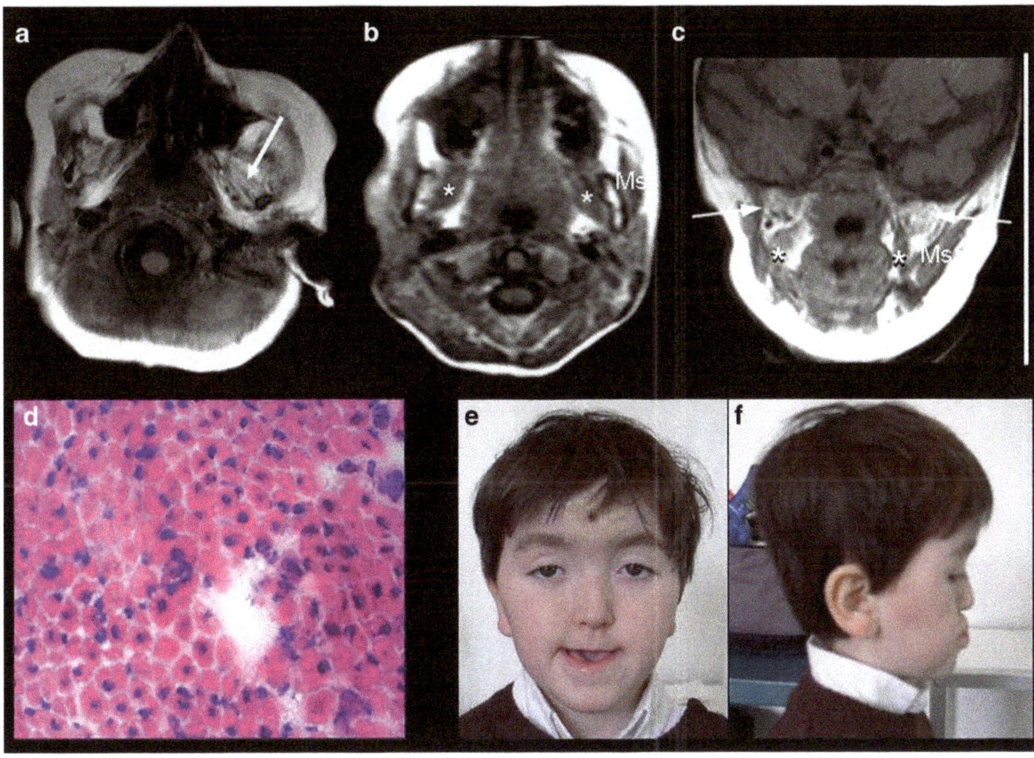

Fig. 15.13 Head MRI, histology, and clinical findings in a 5-year-old boy with *DNM2* mutation. (**a–c**) MRI findings in head muscles: axial (**a**, **b**) and frontal (**c**) views. There is relatively selective involvement of the lateral pterygoid muscles (*white arrow*), with other masticator muscles, such as the masseter (*Ms*) and medial pterygoid muscles (*white stars*) preserved. (**d**) A quadriceps muscle biopsy, obtained at age 6 months showed type 1 fibers. Note the predominant and abundant central nuclei. (**e**, **f**) Clinical features in frontal (**e**) and lateral (**f**) views. Note the myopathic facies and ptosis. The patient showed ophthalmoparesis. In the lateral view, there is hypoplasia of the mid-face and prognatism. Of note, the patient used a nasal mask for night ventilation. (**c**) From Susman RD, et al (2010) Expanding the clinical, pathological and MRI phenotype of DNM2-related centronuclear myopathy. Neuromuscul Disord. 20:229–37. Reprinted with permission from Elsevier

Many patients show pes cavus, wasting of calf and thenar muscles, or contractures of long finger flexor and Achilles tendons. Reduced jaw opening and elbow contractures are also reported. Spinal stiffness and scoliosis may develop as the disease progresses (Fig. 15.14b, c). Cryptorchidia, pectum excavatum, and high-arched palate have been reported in a number of cases. CK levels are usually normal or only mildly increased, although there are reports of patients with moderate CK elevation—up to 10 times normal. Other abnormalities reported sporadically are cataracts, neutropenia, mild white matter changes, cognitive impairment or speech retardation, muscle pseudohypertrophy, insulin-dependent diabetes, and biventricular dilated cardiomyopathy. Needle electromyography shows the usual myogenic changes. It also reveals, in some patients, spontaneous activity and signs of an axonal motor neuropathy.

15.5.5 Imaging Findings

Whole-body MRI in muscle performed in a few children with early symptoms defines a distinct profile. The most abnormal findings are observed in masticator muscles of the head and in axial and distal limb compartments. Limb girdle and proximal muscles are less severely involved. There is selective, severe involvement of lateral pterygoid muscles in the head with sparing of other masticator muscles such as the medial pterygoid and masseter muscles, and the tongue. The temporal muscle may also be abnormal but to a lesser degree (Fig. 15.13a–c). Poor muscle bulk is

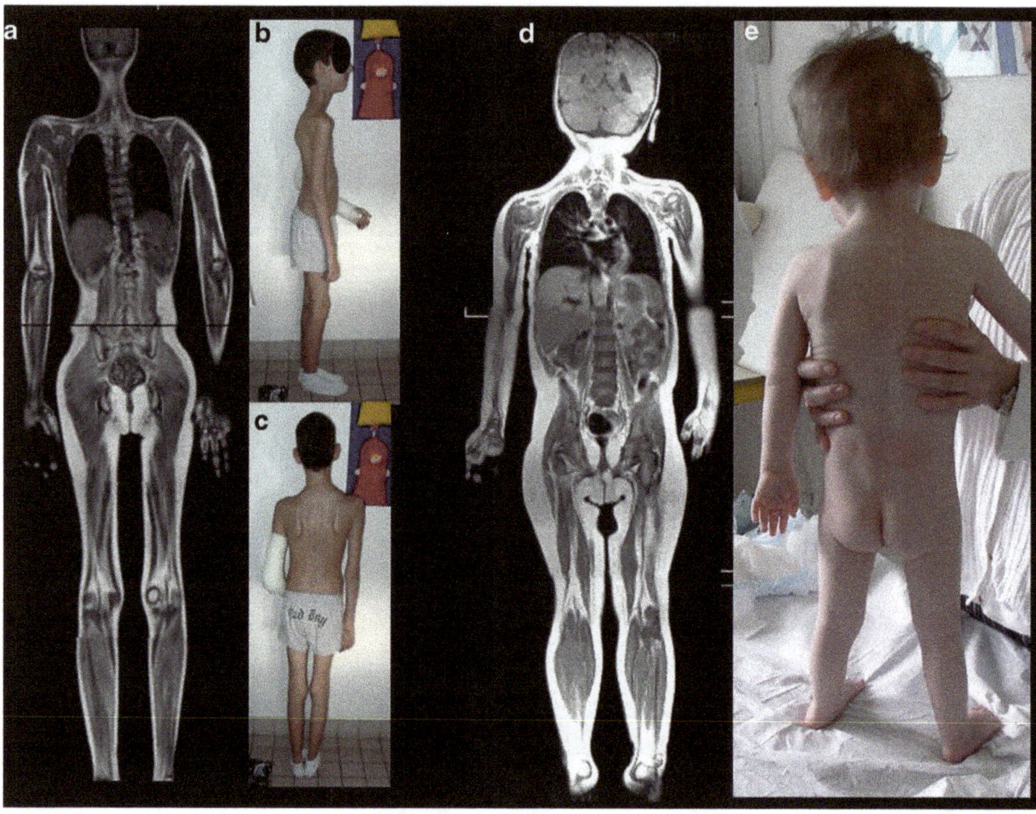

Fig. 15.14 (**a–c**) A 12-year-old *DNM2* patient. Frontal whole-body MRI (**a**) reveals abnormalities of the gluteus maximus and thigh and lower leg muscles, with relative sparing of shoulder and arms. Clinically (**b**), there is mild spinal asymmetry and marked amyotrophy in the lower limb. Whole-body MRI (**d**) and clinical features (**e**) of a 3-year-old boy with diffuse hypotonia and weakness (unable to stand without support). (**d**) From Susman RD, et al (2010) Expanding the clinical, pathological and MRI phenotype of DNM2-related centronuclear myopathy. Neuromuscul Disord. 20:229–37. Reprinted with permission from Elsevier

observed in the sternocleidomastoid muscle. A markedly abnormal signal is seen in the neck extensor and lumbar spinal extensors, deep forearm compartment, and gluteus minimus muscle. The gluteus maximus is less abnormal or may show only reduced volume. In the lower limbs, the leg shows much more severe changes than the thigh, with soleus, medial gastrocnemius peroneus, and tibialis anterior muscles predominantly affected. Tibialis posterior, popliteal, and lateral gastrocnemius muscles are particularly spared. The thigh is often relatively preserved and may show only selective involvement of the semimembranosus, adductor longus, and biceps femoris, with less severe changes in the semitendinosus, adductor magnus, and vastus lateralis and intermedius muscles. The gracilis, sartorius, and rectus femoris muscles are particularly spared. Progressive involvement of muscles of the lower limbs has been described in adults by sequential MRI and CT of pelvic region and lower limbs (Figs. 15.14a, d, 15.15, and 15.16). The earliest changes are seen in distal muscles followed by the posterior compartment of the thigh and the gluteus minimus muscle. In the lower leg, the soleus and tibialis anterior are the first muscles affected. Later in the disease course, the peroneus and gastrocnemius medialis also become involved. In the thigh, the semimembranosus and biceps femoris in the posterior compartment are the first muscles to show signs of fatty infiltration. The anterior compartment may also be affected, but later and to a lesser degree, with the abnormalities more restricted to the

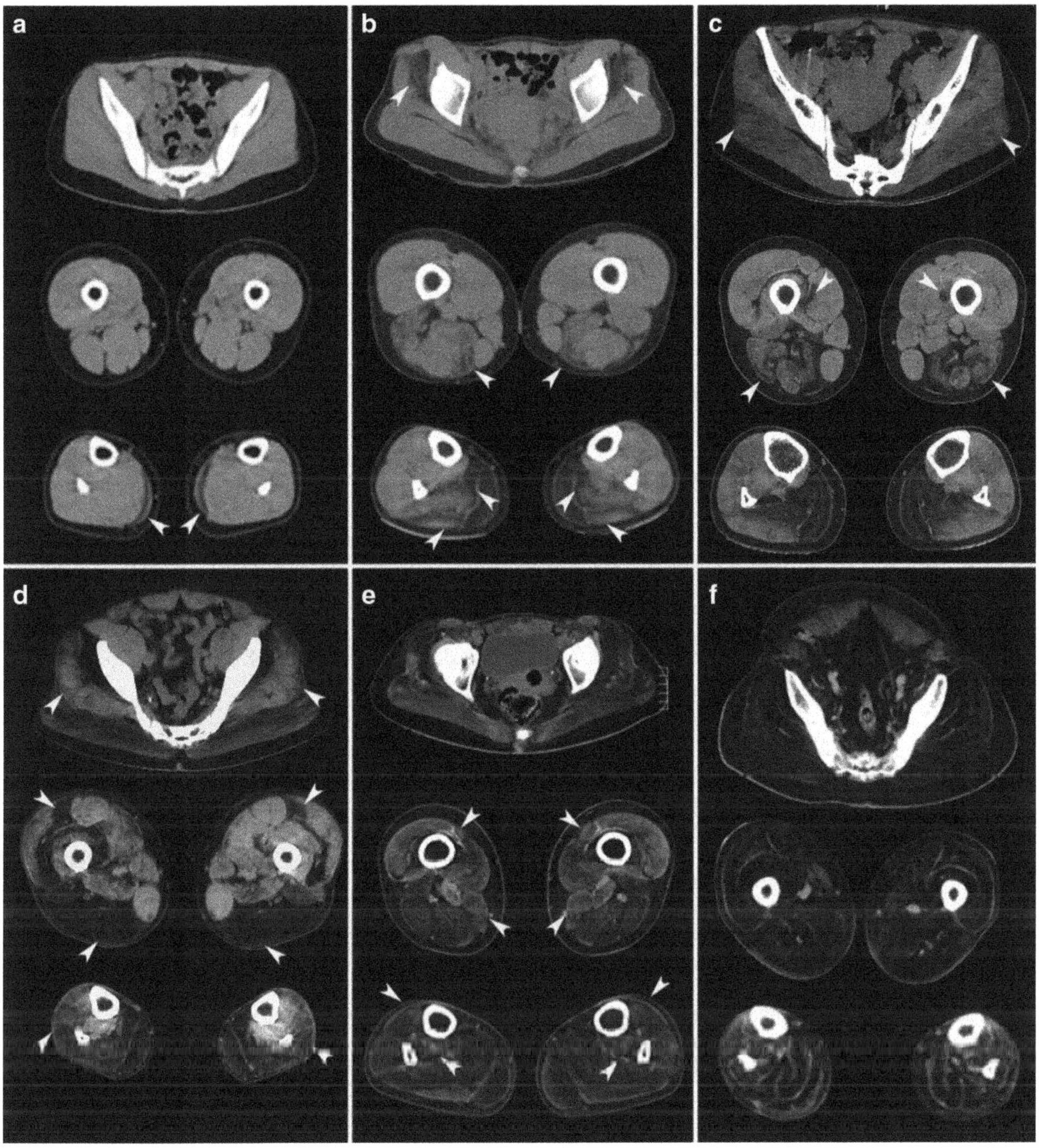

Fig. 15.15 Muscular imaging of six *DNM2*-CNM patients ranging from a mild (**a**, 12 years old) to a very severe clinical phenotype (**f**, 74 years old) shows a characteristic temporal pattern of early, predominantly distal muscle involvement. The first changes appear in the distal lower leg muscles (medial gastrocnemius (*arrowheads*)) (**a**), followed by involvement of the soleus, lateral gastrocnemius, and thigh biceps femoris and gluteus minimus muscles (**b**). Later, the remaining posterior thigh compartment muscles are affected, with mild quadriceps changes and gluteus maximus muscle involvement (**c**). These changes precede degenerative changes in the anterior lower leg and the gluteus medius muscles (**d**). Sartorius, gracilis, and rectus femoris are relatively preserved for a long time (**d**) and are the last affected muscles (**e**). Courtesy of Dirk Fischer, Basel, Switzerland. From Fischer et al (2006) Characterization of the muscle involvement in dynamin 2-elated centronuclear myopathy. Brain. 129:1463. Reprinted with permission from Oxford University Press

rectus femoris and vastus intermedius muscles. The vastus lateralis and medialis muscles are relatively spared. The medial compartment of the thigh is usually preserved, showing selective impairment of the long adductor muscle.

15.5.6 Differential Diagnosis

BIN1- and *MTM1*-related CNMs (see Sect. 15.4) are distinguished from *DNM2*-related CNMs by mode of inheritance, although there are clinical and histopathological overlaps. CNMs due to

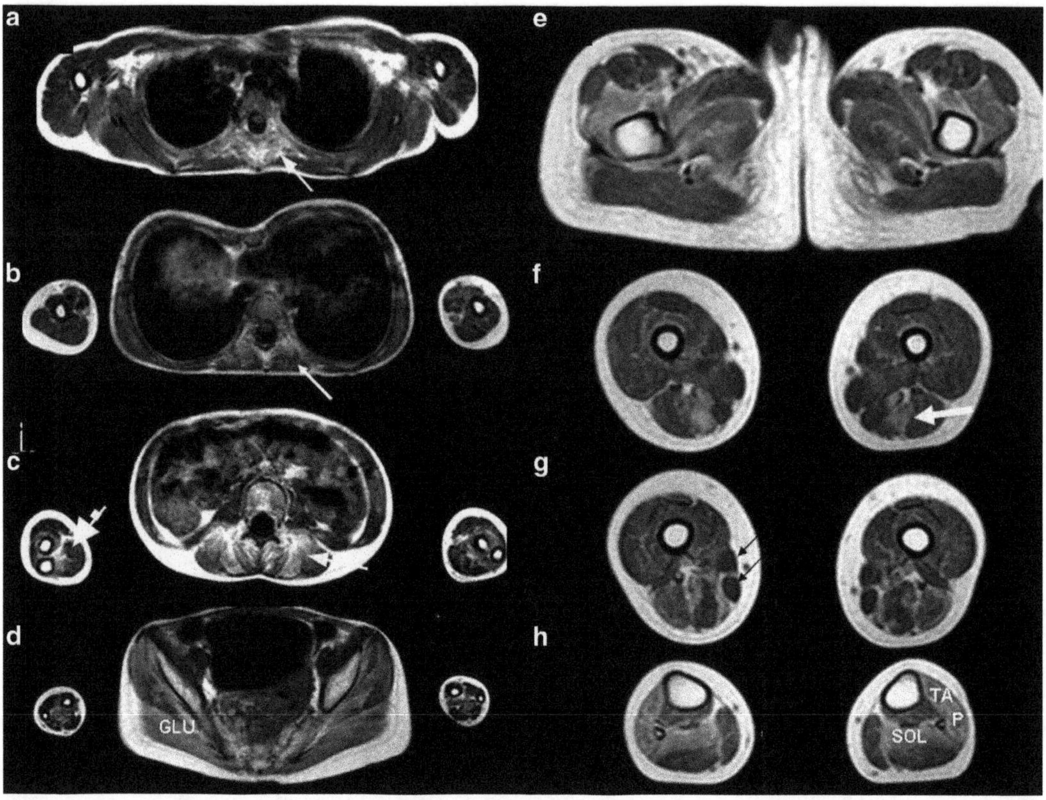

Fig. 15.16 Axial views of whole-body T1-weighted tubo spin echo MRI sequences of *DNM2*-CNM. The most affected muscles in the axial skeleton are the thoracic and lumbar extensors (*thin arrows* in **a**, **b**, and **c**). Muscles in the shoulders and arms are preserved, but there is abnormal signal of the deep compartment of the forearm (*thick arrow* in **c**). In the pelvic girdle (**d**, **e**), signal changes are observed in the gluteus maximus muscle (*GLU*). In the thigh (**f**, **g**), the most involved muscles are in the posterior compartment, particularly the hamstring muscles (*thick white arrow* in **f**). Note particular sparing of gracilis and sartorius muscles (*thin black arrows* in **c**). The lower leg has the most prominent abnormalities in the tibialis anterior (*TA*), peroneus (*P*), and soleus (*SOL*) muscles. (**a**, **c**, **g**, **h**) From Susman RD, et al (2010) Expanding the clinical, pathological and MRI phenotype of DNM2-related centronuclear myopathy. Neuromuscul Disord. 20:229–37. Reprinted with permission from Elsevier

BIN1 and *DNM2* mutations are often characterized by early-onset proximal and facial weakness, ptosis, and motor developmental delay. Patients achieve walking but later in life often experience a slowly progressive course. In both entities, muscle biopsy reveals round fibers with nuclear centralization and type I fiber predominance. In contrast, X-linked CNMs caused by *MTM1* gene mutations typically have a severe onset and poor prognosis with generalized muscle hypotonia at birth associated with ptosis, ophthalmoparesis, swallowing, and severe breathing dysfunction. Biopsy shows muscle fibers with central nuclei similar to myotubes. NADH-TR staining shows a dark central area with a lighter peripheral ring. As dominant de novo mutations are possible with the *DNM2* gene, sporadic cases may be difficult to distinguish from *BIN1*- and *MTM1*-related cases prior to molecular investigations. In severe infants, particularly males, overlap of clinical and pathological features may be observed between *MTM1*- and *DNM2*-related CNMs. Because of the very different prognoses of the two forms, rapid genetic diagnosis is crucial for distinguishing and managing this two entities. A flow chart demonstrating how muscle imaging findings may be used for differentiating congenital myopathies is provided in Chap. 25 (see Sect. 25.2).

Congenital Myopathies: Dynamin 2-Related Centronuclear Myopathy

Key Points

- *DNM2*-CNM phenotypes range from severe neonatal to mild late-onset. Distinct clinical features are facial and bulbar hypotonia, ptosis, marked distal involvement, and Achilles tendon and long finger flexor contractures.
- Most patients initially improve and are able to walk, although later the disease course is usually slowly progressive. The main complications are respiratory and feeding dysfunction, distal joint contractures, and scoliosis.
- MRI of the lower limbs is characterized by early involvement of the distal lower leg muscles and later thigh involvement. The soleus, medial gastrocnemius peroneus, and tibialis anterior muscles are predominantly affected in the lower legs. The semimembranosus and biceps femoris muscles in the posterior compartment are the most affected thigh muscles.
- Whole body MRI in *DNM2*-related CNM shows selective involvement of muscles in the head, axis, pelvic girdle, and distal limbs. *Head*: There is severe involvement of the lateral pterygoid muscle; the temporal muscle may be mildly affected. *Axis*: Neck extensors and thoracic and lumbar paraspinal muscles are the most affected muscles. *Upper limbs*: The deep compartment of the forearm shows the most severe changes. *Pelvic girdle*: The gluteus minimus muscle is preferentially affected. The gluteus maximus shows less involvement but may be atrophic.

Suggestions for Further Reading

Böhm J, Biancalana V, Dechene ET, et al. Mutation spectrum in the large GTPase dynamin 2, and genotype–phenotype correlation in autosomal dominant centronuclear myopathy. Hum Mutat. 2012;33:949–59

Fischer D, Herasse M, Bitoun M, et al. Characterization of the muscle involvement in dynamin 2-related centronuclear myopathy. Brain 2006;129:1463–9.

Quijano-Roy S, Avila-Smirnow D, Carlier RY. Whole body muscle MRI protocol: pattern recognition in early-onset neuromuscular disorders. Neuromuscul Disord. 2012; 22 Suppl 2:S68–84.

Romero NB. Centronuclear myopathies: a widening concept. Neuromuscul Disord. 2010;20:223–22

Schessl J, Medne L, Hu Y, et al. MRI in DNM2-related centronuclear myopathy: evidence for highly selective muscle involvement. Neuromuscul Disord. 2007;17:28–32.

Susman RD, Quijano-Roy S, Yang N, et al. Expanding the clinical, pathological and MRI phenotype of DNM2-related centronuclear myopathy. Neuromuscul Disord. 2010;20:229–37.

15.6 *ACTA1*-Related Myopathies

Dirk Fischer

15.6.1 Synonyms, Abbreviations

Actin myopathy (AM); intranuclear rod myopathy (IRM); actinopathy, actin filament aggregate myopathy (AFAM); *ACTA1*-related nemaline myopathy (NM); cap myopathy; *ACTA1*-related congenital fiber type disproportion (CFTD)

15.6.2 Genetics and Pathophysiology

Actin monomers are expressed in all human cells. The polymerized form of actin is called F-actin, which is a major part of the intracellular cytoskeleton. Actin forms the core of the thin filament in skeletal muscle fibers, where it interacts with myosin (the major component of thick filaments) and many other associated proteins to form the contractile apparatus, which is also known as the sarcomere. The sarcomere is the key element in muscle fibers that produces the force for muscle contraction. Skeletal muscle-specific α-actin—the principal actin isoform in adult skeletal muscle—is encoded by the *ACTA1* gene located on chromosome 1q42.1. The *ACTA1* gene (OMIM 102610) contains seven exons. Many patients with actin-related myopathies have no family history (de novo dominant mutations).

15.6.3 Histopathology

Muscle biopsies in patients with *ACTA1* mutations show a wide range of abnormalities. In general, *ACTA1* mutations have been described in various congenital pathological abnormalities ranging from relatively discrete signs of altered fiber type size disproportion (CFTD) to protein aggregate deposition found in Nemaline myopathy, Intranuclear rod myopathy (IRM), Actin filament aggregate myopathy, and Cap myopathy. Mixtures of these histopathological phenotypes may be seen in a single biopsy. CFTD is characterized by the presence of (at least 12 %) smaller type 1 fibers than type 2 fibers, sometimes with type 1 fiber predominance. In addition to these more subtle changes, *ACTA1* mutations may manifest with intramuscular protein aggregate deposition such as typical nemaline bodies (NBs), which are characterized by rod-like inclusions in skeletal muscle sarcoplasm. NBs are barely visible on H&E staining but stain reddish or purple using the modified Gomori trichrome stain (Fig. 15.17). Other patients show only intranuclear rods, which are the hallmark of IRM. Another type of protein aggregates observed in relation to *ACTA1* mutations are so-called cap structures.

15.6.4 Clinical Presentation

The clinical phenotypes of actin-related myopathies are variable. The most severe phenotype is severe, neonatal-onset with hypotonia and facial, respiratory, axial, and proximal limb weakness. These patients often die from respiratory failure during the first year of life. Facial weakness and a high-arched palate are often observed, but ophthalmoplegia seems not to be a typical finding in actinopathies. Onset during infancy or early childhood ("typical congenital myopathy") with weakness mostly in facial, bulbar, respiratory, and limb muscles seems the most common presentation. Motor milestones are often delayed but finally obtained. Proximal, more than distal, limb girdle weakness has been reported. The clinical course usually is slowly progressive or nonprogressive. Survival to adulthood is common (Fig. 15.18). A remarkable variation in age of onset and clinical severity was observed in

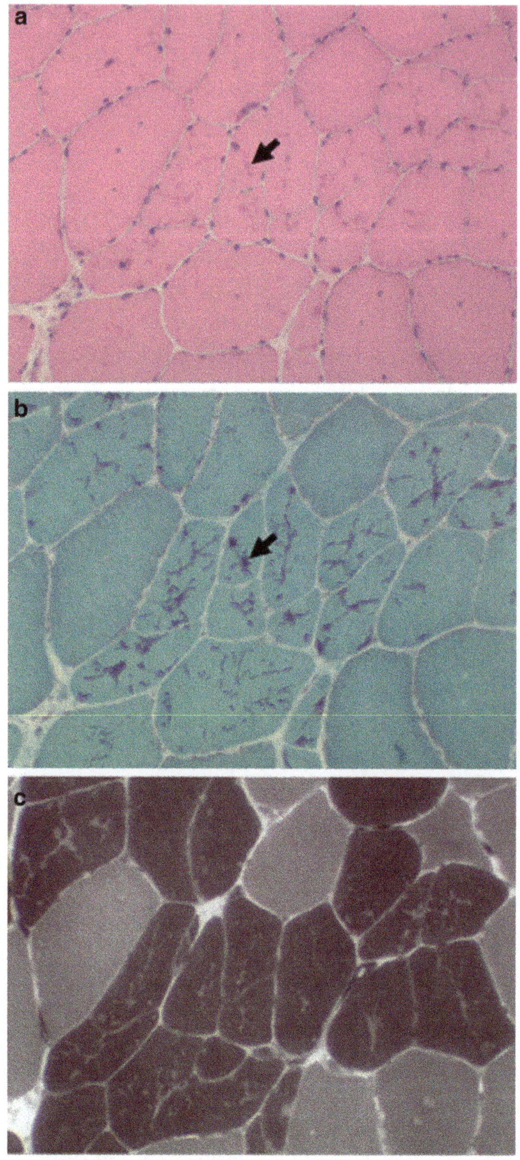

Fig. 15.17 Histopathological findings in *ACTA1*-related nemaline myopathy. Note the presence of protein aggregate deposits (*black arrow*, nemaline bodies), which are characterized by rod-like inclusions scattered throughout the skeletal muscle sarcoplasm. Nemaline bodies are often hardly visible on H&E staining (**a**) but stain reddish or purple using the modified Gomori trichrome stain (**b**). They may occur in both type I and type II (dark) fibers, as demonstrated on ATPase pH 9.4 staining (**c**). Courtesy of Cornelia Kornblum, Bonn, Germany

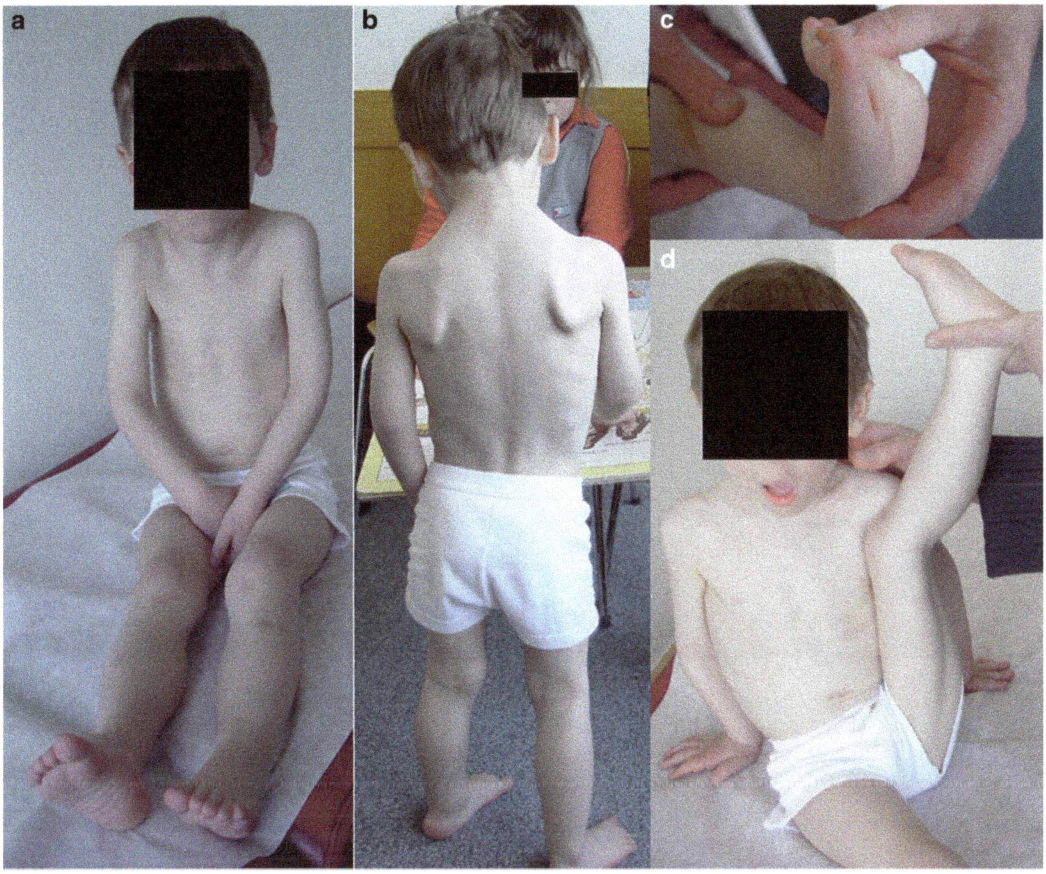

Fig. 15.18 Clinical findings in a patient with *ACTA1*-related nemaline myopathy with mild proximal weakness, discrete scapular winging, and fatigability (**a**, **b**). Of note is the presence of hyperlaxity in the fingers (**c**) and hips (**d**)

three affected members of the same family, suggesting additional modifying factors.

15.6.5 Imaging Findings

Data on muscle imaging in *ACTA1*-related myopathies are limited. The few published data and anecdotal reports suggest that the most affected regions are the adductor magnus, posterior thigh compartment, and tibialis anterior and soleus muscles (Fig. 15.19).

15.6.6 Differential Diagnosis

Newborns present with hypotonia with or without respiratory distress. They exhibit delayed acquisition of motor milestones. During early childhood there is facial and limb girdle weakness. Serum CK levels are often normal or only slightly elevated. Diagnosis is difficult during the first years of life in the absence of specific clinical or pathological features. In the presence of NBs, there is clinical and histopathological overlap with other nemaline myopathies due to mutations in the tropomyosin 2 (see Sect. 15.7), tropomyosin 3, and nebuline (see Sect. 21.3.3) genes. In the absence of specific histopathological findings, the diagnosis is even more complicated. Distinguishing *ACTA1*-related myopathy from other congenital disorders (other congenital myopathies, congenital myasthenic syndromes) is challenging. The value of muscle imaging has yet to be determined as the published data for this entity are sparse.

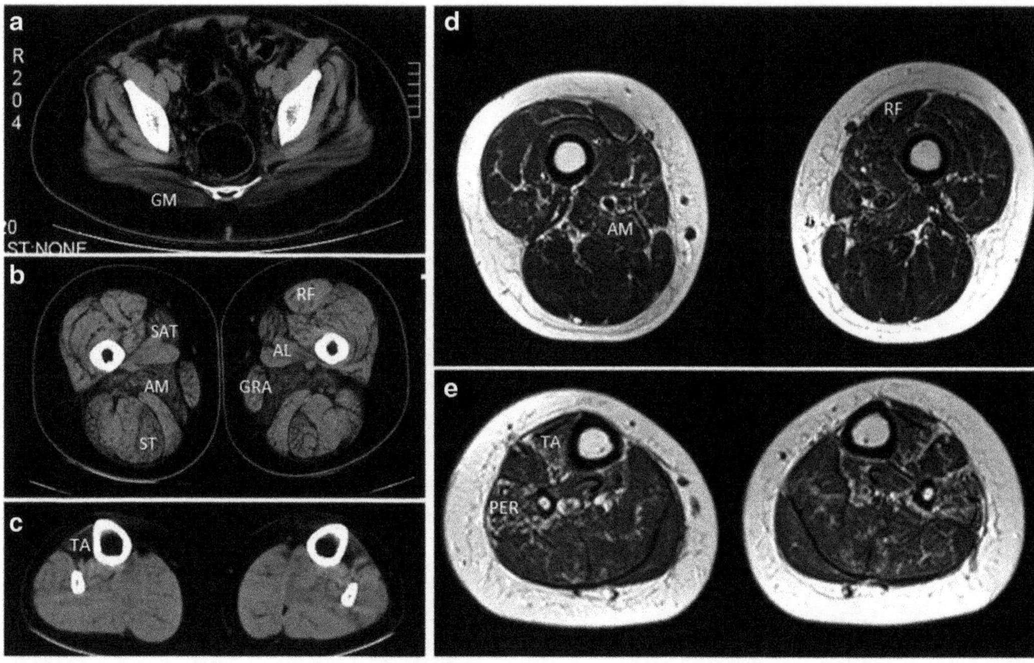

Fig. 15.19 Muscle imaging of patients with mutations in the *ACTA1* gene. CT of the pelvis (**a**), thigh (**b**), and lower legs (**c**) and MRI of the thigh (**d**) and lower legs (**e**) are shown. There is prominent involvement of the gluteus maximus (*GM*), with medial and posterior thigh involvement affecting the sartorius (*SAT*), adductor magnus (*AM*), and semimembranosus (*ST*) and sparing the adductor longus (*AL*), rectus femoris (*RF*), and gracilis (*GRA*) muscles. In the lower legs, the tibial anterior (*TA*), and peroneal (*PER*) muscles are affected. From Quijano-Roy S, et al (2011) Muscle imaging in congenital myopathies. Semin Pediatr Neurol. 18:221–9. Reprinted with permission from Elsevier Limited

Congenital Myopathies: ACTA1-Related Myopathies

Key Points

- The clinical phenotypes in *ACTA1*-related myopathies are variable, ranging from late-childhood-onset slowly progressive proximal weakness to severe, neonatal-onset with facial, respiratory, axial, and limb weakness, resulting in early death.
- *ACTA1* mutations may manifest histologically as Nemaline myopathy, Intranuclear rod myopathy, Actin filament aggregate myopathy, Cap myopathy, Myopathy with core-like areas, or CFTD.
- Imaging in a few milder affected patients showed diffuse involvement of the thigh (mainly the adductor magnus and vastii) and leg (tibialis anterior and soleus) with relative sparing of the rectus femoris, gracilis, and gastrocnemius muscles.

Suggestion for Further Reading

Jungbluth H, Sewry CA, Counsell S, et al. Magnetic resonance imaging of muscle in nemaline myopathy. Neuromuscul Disord. 2004;14:779–84.

Laing NG, Dye DE, Wallgren-Pettersson C, et al. Mutations and polymorphisms of the skeletal muscle alpha-actin gene (ACTA1). Hum Mutat. 2009;30:1267–77.

North KN, Laing NG. Skeletal muscle alpha-actin diseases. Adv Exp Med Biol. 2008;642:15–27.

Ryan MM, Schnell C, Strickland CD, et al. Nemaline myopathy: a clinical study of 143 cases. Ann Neurol. 2001;50:312–20.

Sparrow JC, Nowak KJ, Durling HJ, et al. Muscle disease caused by mutations in the skeletal muscle alpha-actin gene (ACTA1). Neuromuscul Disord. 2003;13:519–31.

15.7 *TPM2*-Related Myopathies

Daniela Avila-Smirnow, Robert-Yves Carlier, Susana Quijano-Roy, Dirk Fischer

15.7.1 Synonyms, Abbreviations

β-Tropomyosin 2 (*TPM2*)-related myopathy; β-tropomyosin 2 (*TPM2*)-related nemaline myopathy (NM); β-tropomyosin 2 (*TPM2*)-related cap myopathy (CM); cap disease; β-tropomyosin 2 (*TPM2*)-related congenital fiber-type disproportion (CFTD); *TPM2*-related arthrogryposis multiplex congenita

15.7.2 Genetics and Pathophysiology

The *TPM2* gene is localized in chromosome 9p13.2-p13.1 (OMIM *190990) and contains nine exons. The coded protein β-tropomyosin (β-Tm) is 284 amino acid residues in length. Mutations in the *TPM2* gene are usually de novo and heterozygous. They have been described in patients with variable clinical and histological presentations, mostly in the context of nemaline myopathy, cap disease, congenital fiber-type disproportion (CFTD), or arthrogryposis syndromes. The majority of the reported patients are diagnosed as having nemaline myopathy. However, this form of congenital myopathy is more often due to mutations in other genes, particularly those coding for skeletal α-actin (see Sect. 15.6) and nebulin (see Sect. 21.3.3). In contrast, *TPM2* mutations are the most frequent genetic cause of Cap myopathy Cap disease.

Tropomyosines (Tm) are a family of actin-binding proteins widely expressed in all cell types. Three types of Tm are found in human skeletal muscle: α-Tm (αTm-fast), β-Tm, and γ-Tm (αTm-slow) coded by the *TPM1*, *TPM2*, and *TPM3* genes. Tm dimers are made up of two coiled-coil alpha helical chains. Dimers then form a continuous polymer, lying in each of the two grooves of F-actin, which is located in the thin filament of the sarcomere. It is supposed that β-Tm has an important role in the regulation of calcium sensibility during muscle contraction. β-Tm is important for stabilizing the sarcomere structure. The exact mechanisms by which *TPM2* mutations lead to impaired muscle contraction and to disease are not fully known.

15.7.3 Histopathology

Muscle biopsies in patients with *TPM2* mutations show results similar to those seen with *ACTA1* mutations. There are a wide range of abnormalities, ranging from relative discrete signs of fiber type size disproportion to the protein deposits seen in Nemaline myopathy (Fig. 15.17). Cap myopathy, a recently described entity, is considered a variant of nemaline myopathy. It owes its name to the shape of the peripheral protein accumulation in the muscle fibers that mimics a cap. Caps consist of protein inclusions seen as peripheral accumulations in type 1 fibers using ATPase, H&E, Gomori's trichrome, and nicotinamide adenine dinucleotide–tetrazolium reductase (NADH-TR) stains. They show a partly irregular and abnormally coarse-meshed pattern (Fig. 15.20). Caps are immunohistochemically positive for actin, actinin, tropomyosin, and troponin; in some cases, desmin positivity has been reported. On electron microscopy, the sarcomeric structure is normal, but there is some disorganization of thin filaments and partial loss of thick filaments.

15.7.4 Clinical Presentation

Clinically, most patients acquire walking ability, but a large spectrum of phenotypes has been observed. The clinical phenotypes range from a severe presentation (with weakness and respiratory failure requiring invasive mechanical ventilation) to mild muscle weakness without joint contractures. Milder forms with hypotonia, delayed motor milestone development, and slow running are more common (Fig. 15.21). Generalized muscle wasting and weakness, particularly in the proximal and axial muscles, thoracic scoliosis, mild facial weakness, nasal voice, high-arched palate, long thin face, and mild micrognathia has been described. CK levels are normal. Heart function is usually normal, although rarely reduced systolic function has

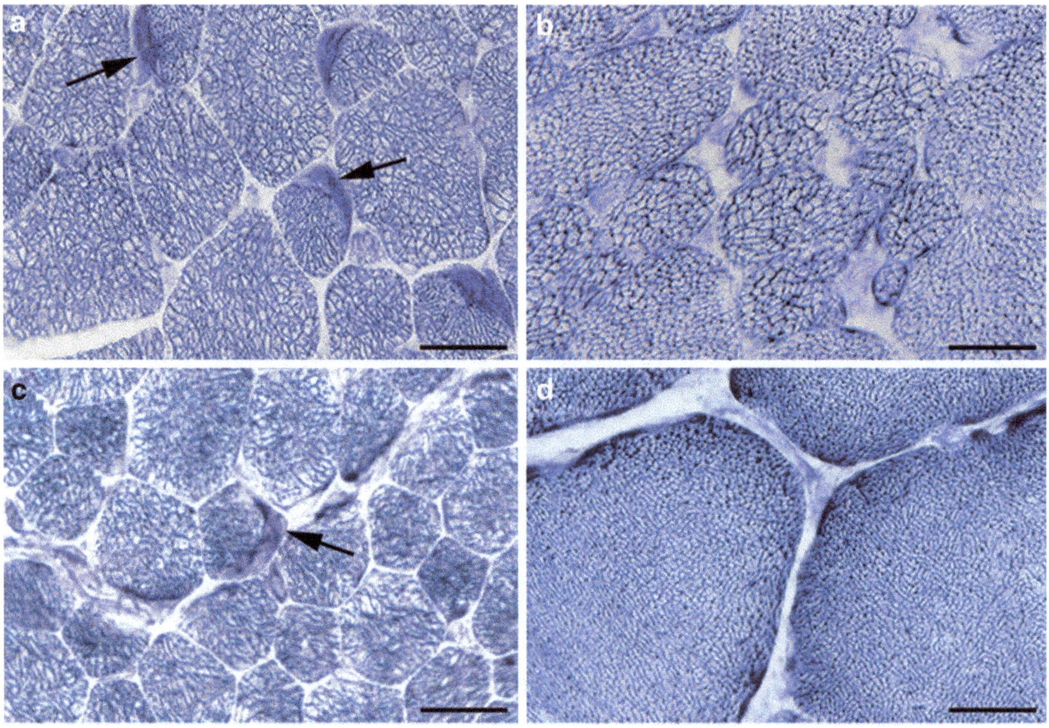

Fig. 15.20 (**a**, **b**, **c**) Muscle biopsy of cap disease and *TPM2* mutations stained for nicotinamide adenine dinucleotide–tetrazolium reductase. There is increased variability of fiber size, near uniformity of type 1 fibers, and a irregular, coarse-meshed intermyofibrillar network. There are fibers with cap structures (*arrows*) (**a**, **c**). Type 1 fibers of normal adult controls for comparison (**d**). Bars = 20 μm. From Ohlsson M, et al (2008) New morphologic and genetic findings in cap disease associated with [β]-tropomyosin (TPM2) mutations. Neurology. 71:1896–901). Reprinted with permission from Wolters Kluwer Health

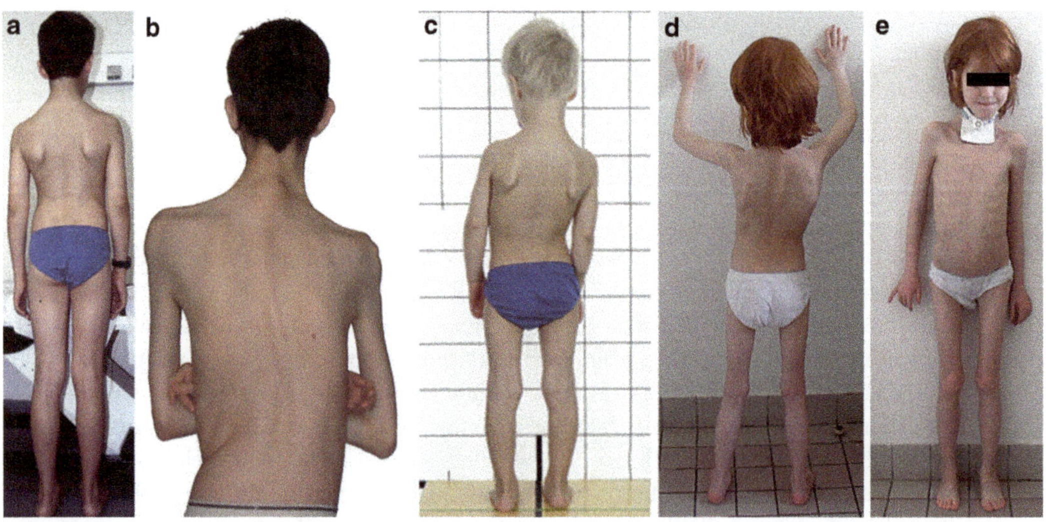

Fig. 15.21 Patients with cap disease and *TPM2* mutations. A 15-year-old patient (**a**) had winging of the scapulae and increased lumbar lordosis. The same patient at age 42 years (**b**) exhibits muscular atrophy and scoliosis. A 3-year-old patient (**c**) with winging of the scapulae, increased lumbar lordosis, mild scoliosis, and pes planovalgus. A 7-year-old patient (**d, e**) with reduced muscle bulk, lumbar hyperlordosis, mild thoracic scoliosis, valgus feet, and bilateral ptosis. From Ohlsson M, et al (2008) New morphologic and genetic findings in cap disease associated with [β]-tropomyosin (TPM2) mutations. Neurology 271:1896–901. Reprinted with permission from Wolters Kluwer Health

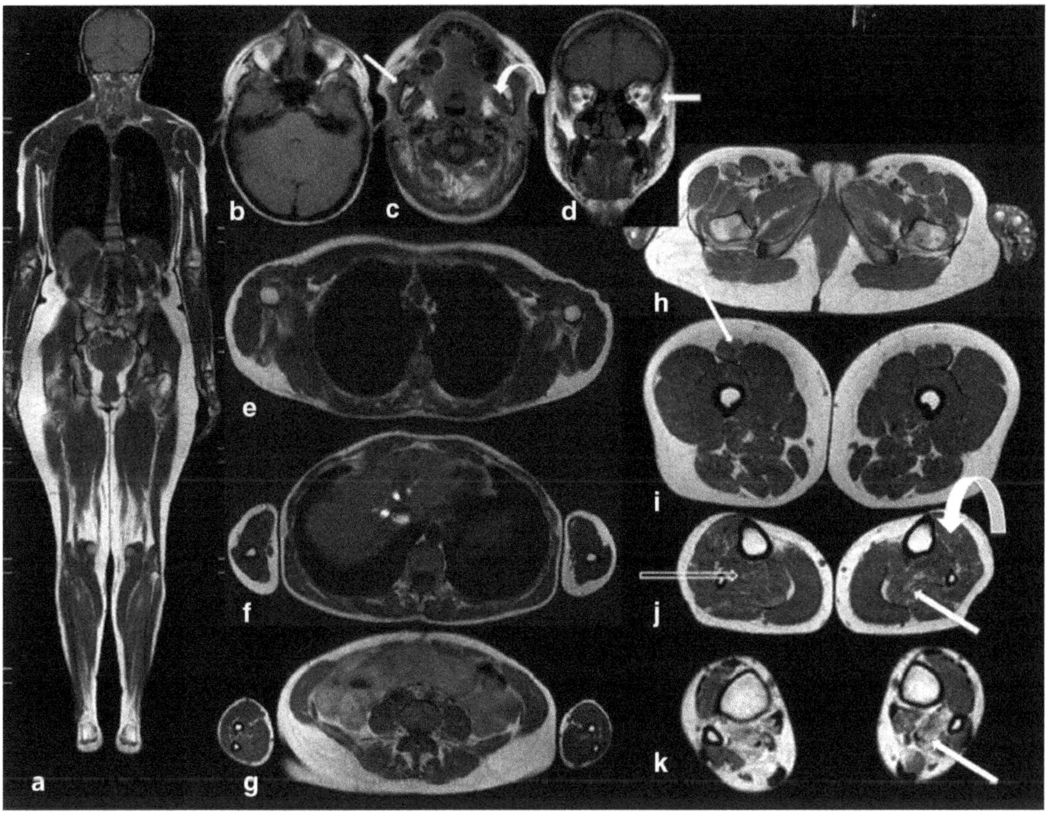

Fig. 15.22 Whole-body T1-weighted MRI of a patient with *TPM2* mutation. (**a**) Frontal fusioned image. (**b**, **c**) Axial images of the head show mild fatty infiltration of the temporal (*empty curved arrow*), masseter (*oblique arrow*), and lateral pterygoid (*thick curved arrow*) muscles. (**d**) Coronal image of the head displays mild fatty infiltration of the temporal muscle (*horizontal arrow*). (**e**, **f**, **g**) Axial images of the chest/shoulder, upper arms, and abdomen show no significant abnormalities. (**h**, **i**) Axial images of the pelvic girdle and thigh show mild fatty changes of the rectus femoris (*arrow*). (**j**) Axial image of the upper lower leg displays mild fatty infiltration of the soleus (*arrow*), tibialis anterior (*curved arrow*), and tibialis posterior (*empty arrow*) muscles. (**k**) Axial image of the distal lower leg shows moderate fatty replacement of the flexor digitorum (*arrow*). From Jarraya M, et al (2012) Whole-body muscle MRI in a series of patients with congenital myopathy related to TPM2 gene mutations. Neuromuscul Disord 22:S137–147. Reprinted with permission from Elsevier Limited

been reported. Also, phenotypes without major weakness but marked joint contractures have been observed. In this group, patients born with congenital joint malformation show predominant axial and distal involvement. Most of these cases are classified as distal arthrogryposis syndrome and less often as multiple pterygium syndrome (then called Escobar syndrome).

15.7.5 Imaging Findings

A recent study on whole-body MRI in six *TPM2* patients revealed a number of common features. All had involvement of facial and distal lower leg muscles. In the head, mainly temporal, medial, and lateral pterygoid muscles were most affected. The temporal muscle is the most severely affected cranial muscle. Shoulder, arm, and forearm muscles are relatively spared, with minor changes occasionally seen in the deltoid, subscapularis, and anterior and posterior arm compartment muscles. In the thighs, the rectus femoris, vastus lateralis, and semimembranosus muscles were most involved. The gracilis and sartorius muscles also showed mild involvement. Otherwise, the thigh was relatively spared. In the distal lower legs, the most frequently affected muscles were the soleus and the flexor digitorum muscles, followed by the gastrocnemii muscles, peroneal, and tibialis anterior muscles (Fig. 15.22).

15.7.6 Differential Diagnosis

Newborns with hypotonia, delayed motor milestone acquisition, or onset during early childhood with facial and distal lower leg weakness may have a primary *TPM2* deficiency. Serum CK levels are often normal or only slightly elevated. Diagnosis is difficult during the first years of life in the absence of specific clinical or pathological features. In the presence of NBs, mutations in the *ACTA1* (see Sect. 15.6), and nebuline (see Sect. 21.3.3) genes are more common. In addition, nemaline myopathy is occasionally caused by mutations in α-tropomyosin (*TPM3*), troponin T1 (*TNNT1*), cofilin-2 (*CFL2*), and *KBTBD13* genes. In the presence of cap structures, *TPM2* mutations are most common. In the absence of specific histopathological findings, the diagnosis may be complicated. The recently observed pattern of muscle imaging with temporal and distal lower leg involvement may be of help in the differential diagnosis. A flow chart demonstrating how muscle imaging findings can be used for differentiating congenital myopathies is provided in Chap. 25 (see Sect. 25.2).

Congenital Myopathies: TPM2-Related Myopathies

Key Points

- The clinical phenotypes in *TPM2*-related myopathies are variable, ranging from severe neonatal onset (with facial, respiratory, axial, and limb weakness) late-childhood onset of slowly progressive weakness with or without joint contractures and arthrogryposis syndromes.
- *TPM2* mutations have been described in various pathological conditions: Nemaline myopathy, Cap disease, and congenital fiber-type disproportion.
- Whole-body MRI show involvement of masticator muscles (in particular the temporal and pterygoid muscles) as well as marked distal lower leg involvement affecting the soleus, flexor digitorum, and tibial anterior muscles. Apart from the rectus femoris, vastus lateralis, and semimembranosus muscles, thigh muscles are relatively spared.

Suggestions for Further Reading

Clarke NF, Domazetovska A, Waddell L, et al. Cap disease due to mutation of the beta-tropomyosin gene (TPM2). Neuromuscul Disord. 2009;19:348–51.

Donner K, Ollikainen M, Ridanpaa M, et al. Mutations in the beta-tropomyosin (TPM2) gene—a rare cause of nemaline myopathy. Neuromuscul Disord. 2002;12:151–8.

Jarraya M, Quijano-Roy S, Monnier N, et al. Whole-body muscle MRI in a series of patients with congenital myopathy related to TPM2 gene mutations. Neuromuscul Disord. 2012;22 Suppl 2:S137–47.

Lehtokari VL, Ceruterick-de Groote C, de Jonghe P, et al. Cap disease caused by heterozygous deletion of the beta-tropomyosin gene TPM2. Neuromuscul Disord. 2007;17:433–42.

Ohlsson M, Quijano-Roy S, Darin N, et al. New morphologic and genetic findings in cap disease associated with beta-tropomyosin (TPM2) mutations. Neurology. 2008;71:1896–901.

Congenital Muscular Dystrophies

16

Susana Quijano-Roy, Daniela Avila-Smirnow, Robert-Yves Carlier, Tracey A Willis, and Volker Straub

16.1 Introduction and Classification

Susana Quijano-Roy, Daniela Avila-Smirnow, Robert-Yves Carlier

Congenital muscular dystrophies (CMDs) comprise a group of heterogeneous disorders. Dystrophic features of the striated muscle, hypotonia, muscle weakness, motor delay and symptom onset at birth or during the first months of life are the key features. Certain types of CMD are associated with central nervous system (CNS) and eye involvement. There are many genes responsible for these diseases and an overlap exists with other hereditary myopathies including congenital myopathies (see Chap. 15) and limb-girdle muscular dystrophies (see Chap. 18). Together with the congenital myopathies, CMDs are the most frequent hereditary myopathies during early childhood. Their incidence has been estimated at 1/21,500 with a prevalence of 1/125,000 in Northeastern Italy and an incidence of 1/16,000 in Western Sweden. However, frequency is difficult to document precisely because of the overlapping phenotypes, the lack of defined nosological frontiers, underestimation of mild forms, and geographic differences. In large cohorts of individuals with CMD, causative mutations can be identified in 25–50 % of cases. In occidental countries the most frequent forms are merosin and collagen VI deficient forms.

Clinical onset is at birth or during the first months of life, and is characterized by muscular hypotonia and poor spontaneous movements. Children with later clinical onset may present with gross motor developmental delay or arrest, as well as joint and/or spinal rigidity. The clinical course is variable, initially allowing achievement of motor milestones in many patients before the onset of progressive weakness. Joint contractures, spinal deformities, and respiratory impairment affect quality of life and life-span. Several clinical markers are useful in that they point to diagnose, such as muscle hypertrophy in dystroglycanopathies (see Sect. 16.5). A cutaneous syndrome with distal

S. Quijano-Roy, M.D., Ph.D. (✉)
Pediatric Department Garches Neuromuscular Center (GNMH), Raymond Poincare Hospital, Paris Ile-de-France Ouest University Hospitals (APHP), Versailles Saint-Quentin-en-Yvelines University (UVSQ), 104 Boulevard R. Poincare, 92380 Garches, France
e-mail: susana.quijano-roy@rpc.aphp.fr

D. Avila-Smirnow
Servicio de Pediatría, Unidad de Neurología, Complejo Asistencial Dr. Sótero del Río. Red de Salud UC, Lira 85, 6° piso., Santiago, Chile
e-mail: avidaniela@gmail.com

R.-Y. Carlier
Pole Neuro-Locomoteur, Service d'imagerie Medicale, Hopital Raymond Poincare, Garches, France
e-mail: robert.carlier@rpc.aphp.fr

T.A. Willis
Neuromuscular Department, The Robert Jones and Agnes Hunt Orthopaedic Hospital, NHS Foundation Trust, Oswestry Shropshire, UK

V. Straub
Neurology, The Harold Macmillan Chair of Medicine, Institute of Genetic Medicine, University of Newcastle upon Tyne, International Centre for Life, Central Parkway, Newcastle upon Tyne NE1 2BZ, UK
e-mail: volker.straub@newcastle.ac.uk

M.P. Wattjes and D. Fischer (eds.), *Neuromuscular Imaging*, DOI 10.1007/978-1-4614-6552-2_16,

hyperlaxity and proximal contractures is found in patients with collagen VI deficiency (see Sect. 16.4). The need for night mechanical ventilation in ambulatory patients is observed in SEPN1-related myopathy (see Sect. 15.3). Spinal rigidity is observed in any form of CMD and is typical of SEPN1- related disease when isolated. Spinal rigidity associated with other limb joint contractures is more likely observed in LMNA- (Sect. 16.3), COL6- (see Sect. 16.4), and merosin-deficient (see Sect. 16.2) CMD. Dystroglycanopathies account for the largest clinical spectrum with CNS and eye malformation syndromes such as Walker–Warburg syndrome (WWS) and Muscle–eye–brain disease (MEB). Milder phenotypes include mild cognitive impairment or even isolated muscle symptoms. Striking white matter abnormalities but otherwise normal brain structure are typical of merosin deficiency. Creatine kinase (CK) levels are often markedly increased in dystroglycanopathies and merosin deficiency. Moderate CK elevations can be found in LMNA-related CMD (L-CMD). Histopathological analyses of muscle biopsies in CMD patients often show dystrophic changes but may be only mildly myopathic. Muscle computed tomography (CT) and MRI reveal abnormal patterns in several CMDs. Whole-body muscle MRI allows simultaneous CNS examination, which is helpful in the diagnostic workup of CMD associated with high CK levels (merosin deficient CMD and dystroglycanopathies). Muscle MRI may have an important diagnostic impact with those diseases without mental retardation but with associated spinal stiffness, joint contractures and/or hyperlaxity, and normal CK. There are important clinical overlaps of some congenital myopathy forms, and identification of their different muscle imaging patterns often helps to guide one to the correct molecular studies. The best known muscle MRI patterns are those in patients with *COL6* (see Sect. 16.4), *LMNA* (see Sect. 16.3), *SEPN1* (see Sect. 15.3), *RYR1* (see Sect. 15.2), and *DNM2* (see Sect. 15.5) gene mutations, and with Pompe disease (see Sect. 14.2.1).

Diagnosis of the CMDs relies on clinical findings, brain and muscle imaging, muscle biopsy histology, muscle and/or skin immunohistochemical staining, and molecular genetic testing. CMDs may be classified with respect to various aspects: physiopathological, clinicopathological, syndromic, molecular. Historically, classifications began to appear during the second part of the 20th century with the description of syndromic forms with brain malformations observed in discrete geographic populations (Fukuyama/FCMD in Japan, MEB disease in Finland, and a contrasting contracture phenotype with normal intelligence, initially labeled classic or occidental CMD). During the 1990s, a major step forward came from the observation of differential merosin protein expression separating "merosin positive" from "merosin-negative" classic CMD forms. At present, at least 20 genes have been found to account for the most frequent forms of CMD. The main CMD subtypes, grouped by the involved protein function and gene in which causative mutations occur, are: laminin α2 (merosin) deficiency caused by *LAMA2* gene mutations; collagen VI deficient CMD or Ullrich CMD (UCMD) caused by *COL6A1*, *COL6A2* or *COL6A3* genes; the dystroglycanopathies, caused by mutations in *POMT1*, *POMT2*, *FKTN*, *FKRP*, *LARGE*, *POMGNT1*, *ADG*, B3GALNT2, DPM2, DPM3, DOLK, ISPD, GTDC2, TMEM5; the SEPN1-related myopathy/CMD (previously known as rigid spine syndrome, RSMD1) due to mutations in *SEPN1* gene; and finally a laminopathy or LMNA-related CMD (L-CMD) caused by mutations in the *LMNA* gene. Several less well known CMD subtypes have been reported. Because of the great genetic heterogeneity and growing complexity of nosology in CMDs and other hereditary myopathies, there is a trend to name the disorders by the gene, adding "related myopathies" or "related dystrophies (-RM/RD). A classification of CMD according to CNS abnormalities, intelligence, immunohistochemistry (IHC) and clinical findings is presented in Fig. 16.1.

Suggestions for Further Reading

Mercuri E, Muntoni F. The ever expanding spectrum of congenital muscular dystrophies. Ann Neurol. 2012;72(1):9–17.

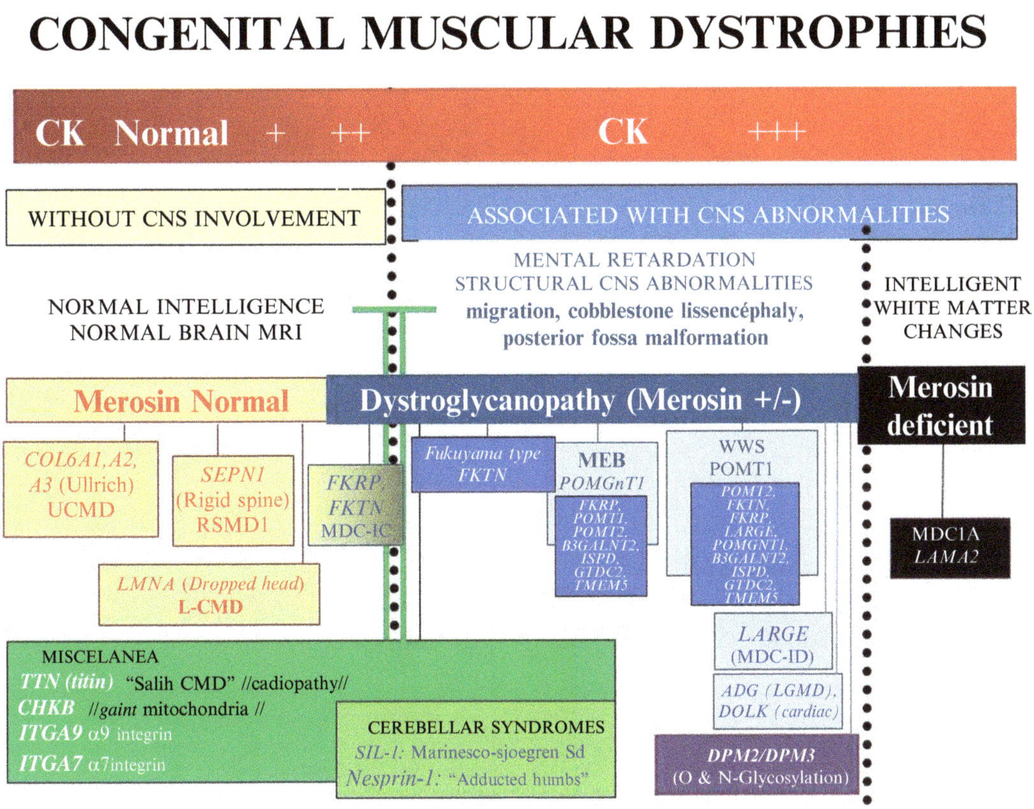

Fig. 16.1 Overview and algorithm for diagnosis of CMD. CK levels, brain MRI, cognitive status, inmunohistochemical characteristics and clinical features allow in most patients to address the molecular diagnosis. Three major subsets of CMDs can be distinguished most frequently (from right to left): (*right*) patients with high CK levels, isolated brain white matter changes, normal intelligence, with abnormal merosin staining (*merosin deficient CMD, type MDC1A, LAMA2 mutations*); (*middle*) patients with high CK levels, mental retardation, often abnormal brain MRI (MEB disease, Walker–Warburg syndrome, Fukuyama CMD, incomplete forms), abnormal alpha dystroglycan staining, merosin can be reduced secondarily (*dystroglycanopathies*); (*left*) normal brain and cognitive status and normal merosin staining (*merosin positive CMDs*); they may show *normal CK levels* (mutations in *SEPN1* or *COL6* genes), moderately increased CK (*LMNA*) or increased (*FKRP, FKTN*). Below the frequent forms, a number of entities recently described or less frequent are indicated, either associating mental retardation (*middle zone*) or with normal intelligence (*left side*)

Quijano-Roy S, Avila-Smirnow D, Carlier RY. Whole body muscle MRI protocol: pattern recognition in early-onset neuromuscular disorders. Neuromuscul Disord. 2012;22:S68–84.

Sparks S, Quijano-Roy S, Harper A, et al. Congenital muscular dystrophy overview. In: Pagon RA, Bird TD, Dolan CR, et al. editors. *Gene Reviews* [Internet]. 1993–2001; updated 2011.

Wang CH, Bonnemann CG, Rutkowski A, et al. International Standard of Care Committee for Congenital Muscular Dystrophy. Consensus statement on standard of care for congenital muscular dystrophies. J Child Neurol. 2010;25:1559–81.

16.2 Merosin Deficient CMD

Susana Quijano-Roy, Daniela Avila-Smirnow, Robert-Yves Carlier

16.2.1 Synonyms and Abbreviations

Merosinopathy or (primary) Lamininopathy; (primary) Merosin deficiency; α2 laminin/Merosin-deficient CMD; α2 laminin/merosin

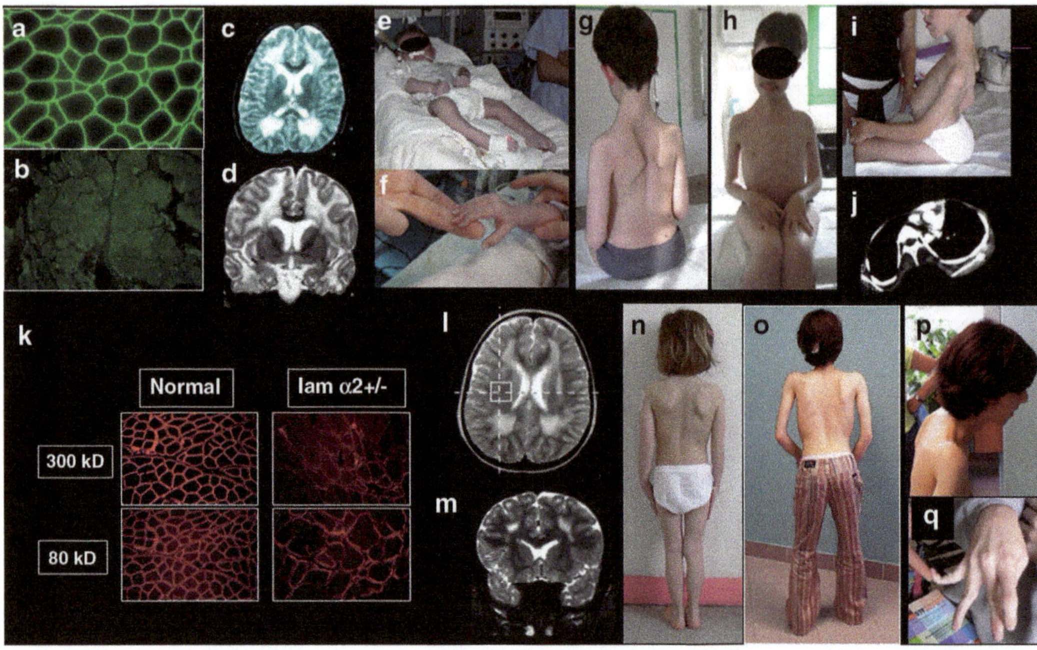

Fig. 16.2 Immunohistochemical and clinical features in merosin deficient patients (complete deficiency (**a–j**) and partial deficiency (**k–p**). (**a, b**) Muscle biopsy with normal (**a**) and complete absence of α2 chain of merosin (**b**), courtesy of N.B. Romero; (**c, d**) brain MRI T2 sequences axial (**c**) and frontal views (**d**) showing diffuse abnormal white matter signal, with spared corpus callosum and capsula interna. (**e–f**) Patient with severe onset, requiring mechanical ventilation from birth. Note diffuse proximal and distal joint contractures in upper and lower extremities. (**g–i**) Nonambulatory patients with typical findings of complete merosin deficiency: relative macrocephaly, diffuse joint contractures, spinal stiffness. Patient treated by brace from early age (**g–h**) and after development of lordoscoliosis (**i**), with progressive respiratory and orthopaedic complications due to thoracic lordosis with bronchial compression by vertebral bodies. (**k–q**) Partial merosin deficiency: (**k**) immunohistochemical results using two antibodies in an ambulatory patient: absence of one (300 kDa) and partial staining of the other (80 kDa), Courtesy of N. B. Romero Paris, France. (**l–m**) Brain MRI T2 sequences, axial (**l**) and frontal views (**m**) showing milder white matter abnormalities than nonambulatory patients. (**n–q**) Clinical features of three patients with mild merosin deficiency. Note the spinal stiffness and elbow contractures (**o, p**) and the distal hyperlaxity in fingers (**q**)

negative CMD; Muscular dystrophy congenital type 1 A (MDC1A); LAMA2-related dystrophy (LAMA2-RD).

16.2.2 Genetics and Pathophysiology

Merosin is a laminin protein (laminin 2) and constitutes a key ligand in the extracellular matrix, interacting with the dystroglycan-dystrophin glycoprotein complex (DGC). Merosin has a heterotrimeric structure composed by three laminin chains. One of them, the laminin α2 chain, is coded by the *LAMA2* gene localized in 6q22–23 (OMIM #607855). Biallelic mutations of *LAMA2* gene are responsible for primary merosin deficiency. Merosin is part of the extracellular DGC, thereby linking the intracellular cytoskeleton to the extracellular matrix. Mutations of the merosin gene result in disruption of the normal stability of the DGC, resulting in increased susceptibility to cytoskeletal and sarcolemmal damage. This structural defect may cause further increase the calcium ion influx and finally increase the production of reactive oxygen species (ROS), which can cause more muscle protein and membrane damage.

16.2.3 Histopathology

Muscle biopsy shows a classic dystrophic picture. Deficiency of α2 laminin may be detected by IHC tests on muscle or skin tissues. Antibodies are directed against different fragments of the laminin α2 chain including 80 kDa Chemicon (prepared against the 80-kDa fragment of the carboxy-terminal LG region); 300-kDa or Novocastra directed at the 300-kDa fragment; or Alexis, an antibody for the entire laminin α2 chain (Fig. 16.2a, b, k). Merosin/laminin α2 deficiency is easier to detect with antibodies that recognize the 300-Da fragment. Overexpression of laminin α4 and α5 may also be useful, leading to the suspicion of mild laminin α2 deficiency. Secondary reduction of laminin α2 can also be found in other forms of CMD, particularly the Dystroglycanopathies.

Laminin α2 is also present in Schwann cells, which accounts for a progressive sensorimotor polyneuropathy with signs of dysmyelination. Post mortem CNS analysis revealed pale, spongiform white matter with astrocytosis and demyelination.

16.2.4 Clinical Presentation

Merosin deficiency is marked by a wide spectrum of clinical manifestations, ranging from severe, early-onset CMD to milder later childhood-onset Limb-girdle-type muscular dystrophy. Additional findings include high serum CK concentrations. Children with early-onset disease have profound hypotonia with muscle weakness at birth or infancy, poor spontaneous movements with contractures of the large joints, and a weak cry often associated with respiratory failure; most of the affected children do not achieve independent ambulation (Fig. 16.2e–i). The intellect is usually normal but some patients have epileptic seizures that are generally easy to control with standard drugs. Feeding difficulties with failure to thrive, aspiration, and recurrent chest infections are typical. Progressive respiratory insufficiency and scoliosis develop regularly, leading to severe orthopaedic complications and the need of mechanical ventilation in many patients later in the disease course. Scoliosis associated with thoracic lordosis is common and can further impair respiratory function owing to bronchial obstruction by the anterior parts of the thoracic vertebral bodies (Fig. 16.2j). Primary cardiac involvement is not a typical feature. Patients with later-onset disease have proximal muscle weakness. They remain ambulatory but typically have delayed motor milestones and may develop muscle pseudo-hypertrophy and rigid spine syndrome with joint contractures (Fig. 16.2n–q).

16.2.5 Imaging Findings

16.2.5.1 CNS

All affected individuals have diffuse white matter changes in the periventricular and subcortical white matter (hypointense on T1-weighted imaging and hyperintense on T2-weighted/FLAIR sequences). Although these abnormalities in myelination may be detected earlier, they are progressive and are consistently detected at 1 year of age persisting over time (Fig. 16.2c, d, l, m). There is striking sparing of some areas, such as the corpus callosum, the internal capsule and the cerebellum. Studies using both proton magnetic resonance spectroscopy (^{1}H-MRS) and diffusion-weight imaging (DWI) have identified abnormal water content thought to be related to leaky basal membrane connections rather than hypomyelination. In particular, brain ^{1}H-MRS reveals very low *N*-acetylaspartate (NAA) and creatinine concentrations, suggesting axonal damage in addition to an increased water signal with possible edema in the white matter. These findings are hypothesized to result from increased permeability of the blood–brain barrier caused by the absence of laminin α2 in the basal lamina of the cells of the cerebral blood vessels. In a small proportion of patients, cognitive impairment and epilepsy are associated with dysplastic cortical changes on brain MRI predominantly localized in the occipital and temporal region.

16.2.5.2 Muscle Imaging

Data on muscle imaging in this entity is limited. Unpublished preliminary data and anecdotal reports suggest that the most affected regions and muscles are the posterior thigh, medial thigh (adductor magnus), and soleus muscle in the lower leg (Fig. 16.3).

16.2.6 Differential Diagnosis

Newborns and/or infants presenting with hypotonia with or without respiratory distress and delayed acquisition of motor milestones as well as children with weakness of the limb-girdle type may have a primary merosin deficiency. High serum CK concentrations, merosin deficiency detected by immunohistochemical staining of muscle or skin biopsy samples, and white matter

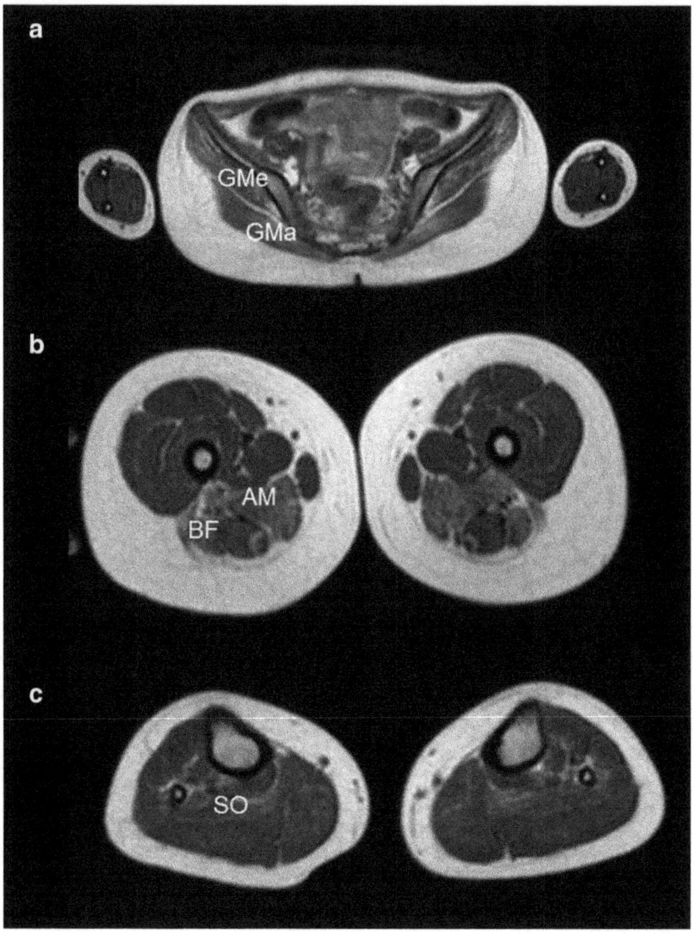

Fig. 16.3 WBMRI T1-TSE in a 8-year-old ambulatory patient with mutations in the *LAMA2* gene. (**a**) The forearm is spared. The involvement is most important in the gluteus medius (GMe) and less severe in the gluteus maximus muscle. (**b**, **c**) The legs have predominant fatty infiltration in the posterior thigh compartment, in particular the adductor magnus muscle (AM) and biceps femoris (BF), and less severe in the lower leg, with involvement of the soleus (SO) muscle

changes on brain MRI distinguish this entity from other disorders. These features should separate Merosin deficiency from other CMD, congenital myopathies (Chap. 15), metabolic myopathies (Chap. 14), Myotonic dystrophy (Chap. 22), Congenital myasthenic syndromes, and Spinal muscular atrophy (see Chap. 29).

Congenital Muscular Dystrophies: Merosin Deficient CMD

Key Points

- Primary merosin deficiency is a recessive form of CMD presenting usually with a severe, quite homogeneous clinical and pathologic phenotype.
- The diagnosis is based on clinical findings (diffuse hypotonia and weakness, multiple joint contractures); elevated serum CK concentration; and an abnormal white matter signal in the absence of mental retardation
- Immunohistochemical staining of muscle and/or skin sections shows complete or partial laminin $\alpha 2$ deficiency, which may be evident only in partially deficient patients by using several commercial antibodies.
- The definitive diagnosis is based on identifying mutations of *LAMA2*, the gene encoding the protein laminin subunit $\alpha 2$.
- MRI is particularly important for detecting the white matter changes in the brain. Data dealing with muscle imaging is still limited.

Suggestions for Further Reading

Allamand V, Guicheney P. Merosin-deficient congenital muscular dystrophy, autosomal recessive (MDC1A, MIM #156225, LAMA2 gene coding for alpha2 chain of laminin). Eur J Hum Genet. 2002;10:91–4.

Geranmayeh F, Clement E, Feng LH, et al. Genotype–phenotype correlation in a large population of muscular dystrophy patients with LAMA2 mutations. Neuromuscul Disord. 2010;20:241–50.

Meinen LS, Ruegg MA. Treatment approaches in laminin-α2-deficient congenital muscular dystrophy (MDC1A). Neuromuscul Disord. 2009;19:543.

Vainzof M, Richard P, Herrmann R, et al. Prenatal diagnosis in laminin alpha2 chain (merosin)-deficient congenital muscular dystrophy: a collective experience of five international centers. Neuromuscul Disord. 2005; 15:588–94.

16.3 Lamin A/C-Related CMD

Susana Quijano-Roy, Daniela Avila-Smirnow, Robert-Yves Carlier

16.3.1 Synonyms and Abbreviations

Lamin A/C-related congenital muscular dystrophy (L-CMD); congenital laminopathy, congenital Emery-Dreifuss muscular dystophy (EDMD); LMNA-related myopathy (LMNA-RM).

16.3.2 Genetics and Pathophysiology

Nuclear envelopathies are a group of hereditary diseases caused by mutations of genes that encode proteins of the nuclear envelope such as lamins and emerin (see Chap. 18). The nuclear lamina is a network of lamin polymers. Lamins A and C are A-type lamins both of which are derived by alternative splicing from the same gene, *LMNA* (chromosome 1q22, OMIM #613205). Mutations in the *LMNA* gene may have dominant or recessive autosomal transmission, being often a de novo mutation and have been reported to be associated with a number of phenotypes. Among them there is a spectrum of muscle disorders with onset from birth (L-CMD) to adult age (EDMD, LGMD1B). For more details, see Chap. 18.

16.3.3 Histopathology

The muscle histopathology shows nonspecific myopathic or dystrophic changes, including variation in fiber size, increased number of internal nuclei, increased endomysial connective tissue, and necrotic fibers. Muscle biopsy is not helpful for diagnostic purposes in Lamin A/C related CMD because of the lack of specificity and the absence of immunostaining abnormalities for lamins A/C. Routine immunostaining of the markers of α-2 laminin and collagen VI are normal. However, there may be irregular staining of α-DG and abnormal calpain-3 bands have been observed in a few patients.

16.3.4 Clinical Presentation

The recently described form of L-CMD is at the severe end of the clinical spectrum of the striated muscle laminopathies. In fact, the clinical features and the disease course are so distinct that diagnosis is often based mainly on clinical findings, even the absence of specific biochemical markers. The serum CK levels are often increased but rarely higher than four to five fold the normal values. There are two levels of severity. One subgroup of patients have early, severe onset characterized by poor spontaneous movement and motor achievements (Fig. 16.4). The second subgroup includes patients who present initially with a milder disease course. These patients acquire head support, sitting and even walking abilities but present during the first or second year of life with striking, progressive neck weakness (dropped head syndrome) (Fig. 16.5). These infants are unable to hold up their heads and crawl, although they can walk independently and sit. The initial rapid decline in their cervical/axial strength is followed by a period of milder progression or stasis of progression. Progressive restrictive respiratory insufficiency and a flat thorax is observed. All children require continuous mechanical ventilation. In the most severe, early form, ventilation is needed by the second year of life. For those with the dropped head phenotype, ventilation has to be provided during the first to second decade of

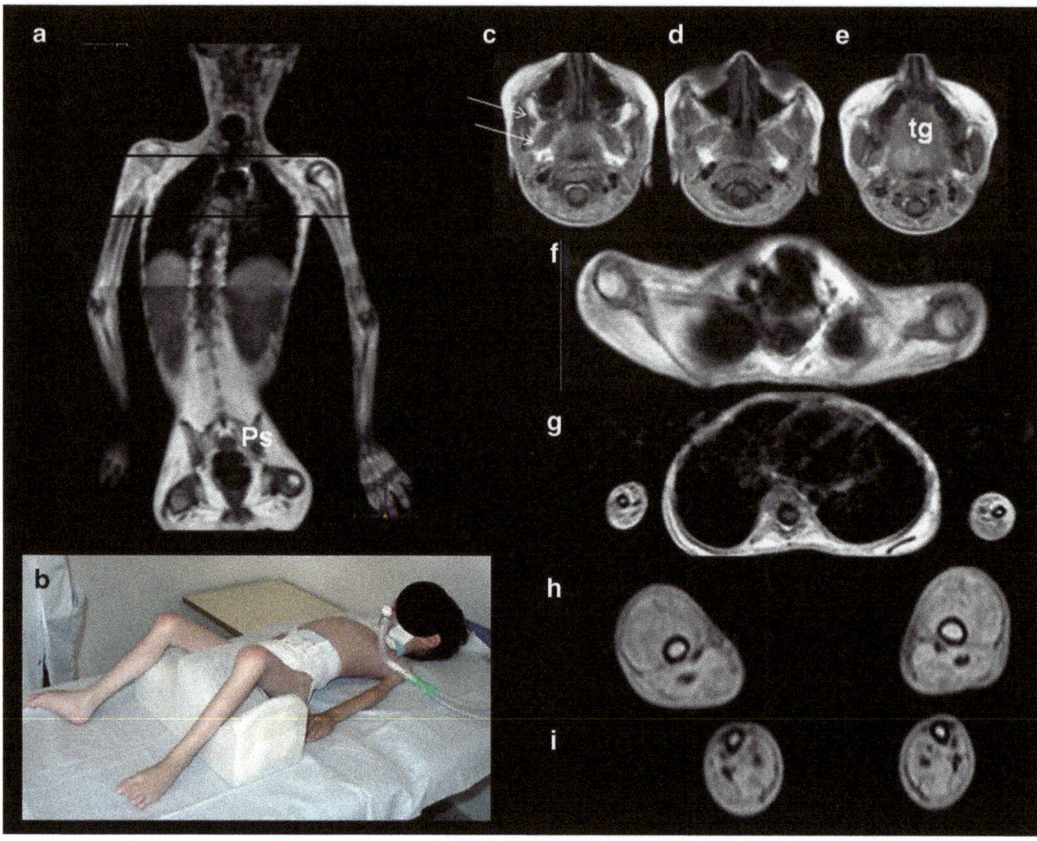

Fig. 16.4 Clinical and WBMRI findings in a patient with severe congenital laminopathy (L-CMD). (**b**) A 8-year-old boy who never acquired trunk or head control, tracheotomized at age 2 years, developing stiff dorsal lumbar hyperlordosis and diffuse severe amyotrophy. No antigravitatory movements are possible but facial muscles are preserved. Joint contractures are localized in lower extremities (hip, knee, ankles) but not in the elbows. (**a**, **c–i**) muscle WBMRI T1-TSE sequences: diffuse severe involvement. Only head muscles (masticator muscles, arrows in C; tongue, tg in **e**) and psoas (Ps in **a**) are relatively preserved. Figure **b** from Quijano-Roy S. et al. (2008) De novo LMNA mutations cause a new form of congenital muscular dystrophy. Ann Neurol. 64(2):177–86. Reprinted with permission from John Wiley and Sons. All remaining from Quijano-Roy S et al. (2012) Whole body muscle MRI protocol: pattern recognition in early onset NM disorders. Neuromuscul Disord. 22:S68–84. Reprinted with permission from Elsevier Limited

life. Spinal stiffness with dorsal and lumbar hyperlordosis and joint contractures develop during the first decade. There is a distal predominance in lower limbs (talipes), but, in contrast to classic Emery Dreifuss muscular dystrophy (EDMD) there are usually no contractures at the elbow level (Fig. 16.6n, o). The widespread absence of subcutaneous tissue is also a frequent finding. Cardiac involvement is rarely observed during the first years. However, severely affected non ambulatory patients may show cardiac affection similar to those seen with other laminopathies (LGMD2B, AD-EDMD), and sudden death has been reported early in life. Recent research has identified that decreased levels of glutathione in the blood may be a possible early marker of cardiomyopathy in LMNA-mutated patients with still preserved left ventricle function. Inhibitors of ERK1/2 signalling, a therapeutic approach from cancer treatment, have shown improvement of cardiac involvement and prolonged survival in LMNA-mutated mouse model.

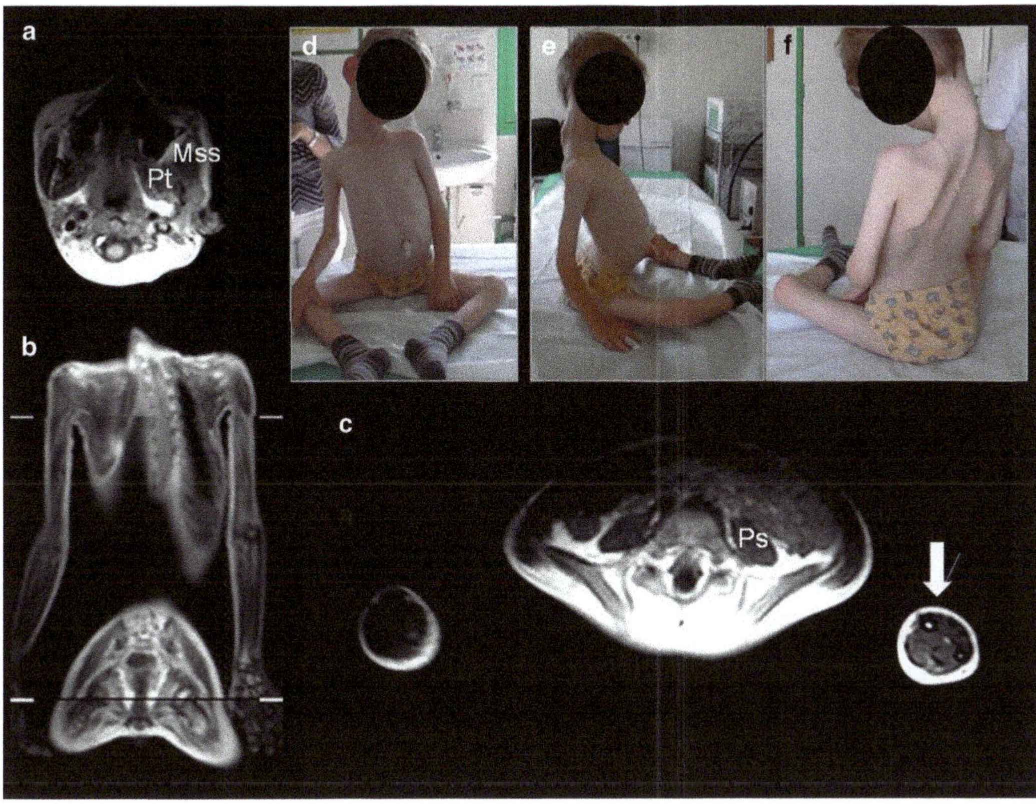

Fig. 16.5 Clinical and MRI findings in a patient with dropped head syndrome. (**a**–**c**) WBMRI T1-TSE sequence: severe diffuse involvement sparing masticator muscles (Pterygoid, *Pt*; masseter, *Mss*), forearm (*arrows*) and psoas muscles (Ps). (**d**–**f**) Patient with dropped head syndrome at age 7 years. Note the severe atrophy of lower limbs with talipes, and of the arms compared to forearms, the stiff hyperextension of the spine in a dorsolumbar hyperlordosis, the loss of head support. Figures **d** and **f** from Quijano-Roy S. et al. (2008) De novo LMNA mutations cause a new form of congenital muscular dystrophy. Ann Neurol. 64(2):177–86. Reprinted with permission from John Wiley and Sons

16.3.5 Imaging Findings

Most patients with striated laminopathies who have been examined with muscle MRI were found to have late-onset phenotypes (AD-EDMD, LGMD1B) and most of the studies were limited to lower limbs. Patients show predominant involvement of vastus lateralis in the thigh and medial gastrocnemius in the lower leg. Other muscles involved are the glutei, vasti, adductor longus and magnus, semimembranosus, the long head of the biceps femoris and the soleus muscles (Fig. 16.6a–m). Interestingly, in patients with isolated cardiac symptoms, lipodystrophy or peripheral neuropathy, leg muscle imaging may reveal a similar pattern with varying degrees of alteration in the soleus and the medial head of the gastrocnemius (see Chap. 18). These findings support the concept of a continuum of skeletal muscle involvement among phenotypes of LMNA-gene-mutation-related skeletal myopathy and cardiomyopathy.

Whole-body MRI studies in young children with the severe congenital phenotype documented diffuse fatty infiltration and atrophy sparing the psoas, forearm muscles, and muscles of the head and neck region. In particular, masticator and tongue muscles are normal even during advanced stages when patients lack trunk or head control (Fig. 16.4c–e). This involvement leads to a recognizable "negative" pattern. Of note, subcutaneous fat is also diffusely reduced, suggesting

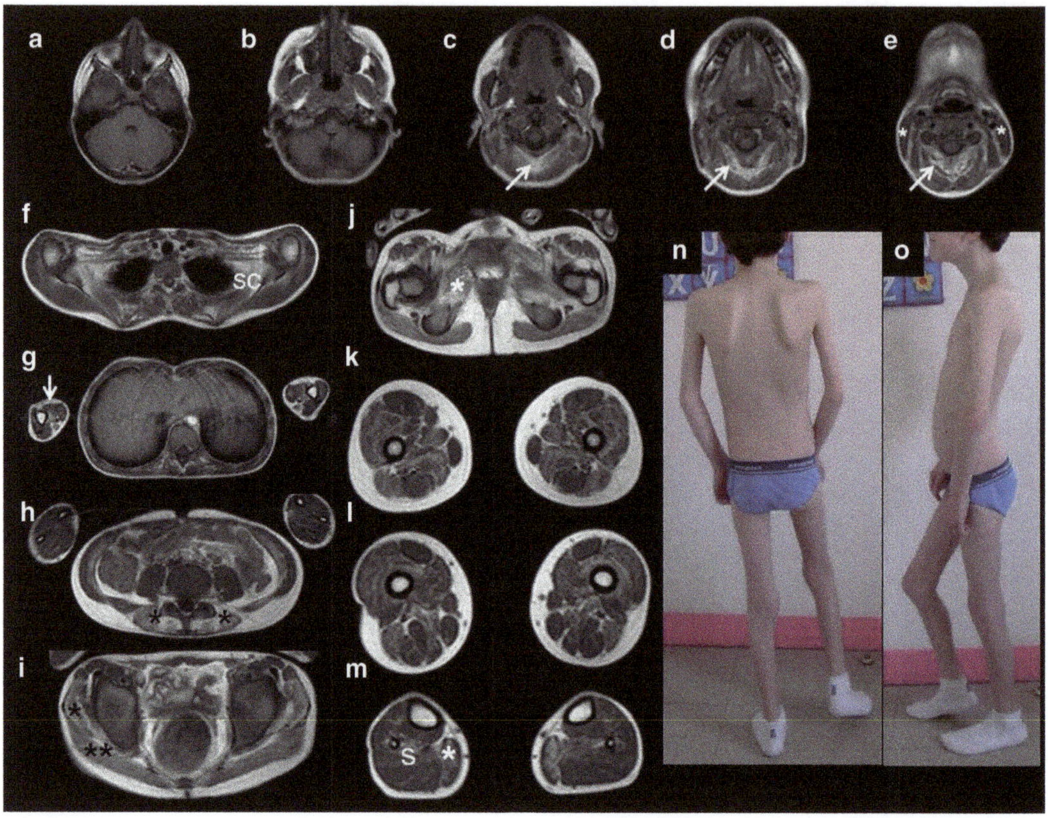

Fig. 16.6 WBMRI and clinical features of a 10-year-old boy with EDMD (**a–m**). Muscle WBMRI T1-TSE sequences showing spared head muscles (**a–d**), while neck extensors are affected (white arrows in (**c–e**)). Note the sparing of the sternocleidomastoid muscle (*white stars* in **e**). Other affected muscles are: subscapular in shoulders (SC), biceps in arm (*white arrow* in **g**), lumbar paraspinals (*black stars* in **h**), gluteus maximus (*double star* in **i**) and medius (*black star* in **i**), pelvic muscles (*white star* in **j**). In the thigh, involvement is diffuse with relative sparing of rectus femoris, sartorius, gracilis and semitendinosus muscles (**k–l**). The lower legs show selective involvement of the posterior compartment, in particular of the medial gastrocnemius muscle (*white star* in **m**) and less severe of the soleus muscle (S). (**n–o**) Clinical findings in the patient, showing spinal stiffness, scapula alata, elbow and asymmetric ankle contractures. Predominant wasting is seen in humero-peroneal muscles. Figures **f**, **l**, **m** from Quijano-Roy S et al. (2012) Whole body muscle MRI protocol: pattern recognition in early onset NM disorders. Neuromuscul Disord. 22:S68–84. Reprinted with permission from Elsevier Limited

lipoatrophy. Although these patients are not cognitively impaired, a recent MRI description reported a focal abnormality with high signal intensity in the white matter.

16.3.6 Differential Diagnosis

Overlapping clinical symptoms are observed with the other CMDs and myopathies associated with a severe or progressive course, particularly those with a rigid spine syndrome, joint contractures or respiratory or cardiac complications. COL6-related myopathies show a typical muscle MRI pattern. Primary merosin deficiency (Sect. 16.1) can be diagnosed by the marked white matter changes and the absence of merosin in the muscle biopsy. Dystroglycanopathies (Sect. 16.5) without mental retardation (due to *FKRP* or *FKTN* mutations) often have very high CK levels and abnormal α-dystroglycan immunohistochemistry. SEPN1-RM (Sect. 15.3) can show multi-minicores in the muscle biopsy, and Pompe disease (Sect. 14.2.1) is associated with abnormal glycogen deposition in muscle tissue on a biopsy.

Congenital Muscular Dystrophies: Lamin A/C-Related CMD

Key Points

- Congenital muscular dystrophy due to *LMNA* mutations is a recently described entity.
- Clinically, this entity represents the most severe clinical manifestation of all striated laminopathies. Progressive weakness and respiratory and cardiac complications lead to a severe phenotype. Cardiac involvement is not an early symptom but may, as in other laminopathies be life-threatening.
- Characteristic clinical features are absence of motor milestones or loss of acquired tonus in cervico-axial muscles (dropped head syndrome), predominant weakness in the proximal upper and distal lower limbs, stiff and hyperextended spine, and slightly increased CK levels.
- In severe cases, muscle imaging shows diffuse involvement, sparing the muscles of head and neck, forearm, and psoas. In patients with milder disease, lower limb features are similar to those observed in late-onset laminopathies (e.g., EDMD) with involvement predominantly of the vastus lateralis, soleus, and medial gastrocnemius muscles.

Suggestions for Further Reading

A mutation database of LMNA mutations is available and constantly updated (www.umd.be/LMNA).

Deconinck N, Dion E, Ben Yaou R, et al. Differentiating Emery–Dreifuss muscular dystrophy and collagen VI-related myopathies using a specific CT scanner pattern. Neuromuscul Disord. 2010;20:517–23.

Mercuri E, Clements E, Offiah A, et al. Muscle magnetic resonance imaging involvement in muscular dystrophies with rigidity of the spine. Ann Neurol. 2010;67:201–8.

Quijano-Roy S, Mbieleu B, Bönnemann CG, et al. De novo LMNA mutations cause a new form of congenital muscular dystrophy. Ann Neurol 2008;64(2):177–86.

Worman HJ. Nuclear lamins and laminopathies. J Pathol 2012;226:316–25.

16.4 Collagenopathies

16.4.1 Synonyms and Abbreviations

Collagenopathies; Ullrich CMD (UCMD), scleroatonic Ullrich CMD, Ullrich/Bethlem myopathy; COL6-related myopathy (COL6-RM).

16.4.2 Genetics and Pathophysiology

Three genes coding for collagen VI α chains (*COL6A1*, *COL6A2* and *COL6A3*) have been found to be responsible for two disorders initially described separately: Ullrich congenital muscular dystrophy (UCMD, OMIM #254090), described in 1930 as "congenital atonic-sclerotic muscular dystrophy" and Bethlem myopathy (BM, OMIM #158810). Collagens are major constituents of extracellular matrices (ECM), and are found in most connective tissues. They provide structural and mechanical stability to tissues, but they also play crucial roles in cell–ECM interactions. Collagen type VI (ColVI) is a hetero-trimeric molecule composed of three individual α(VI) chains. The α1(VI), α2(VI), and α3(VI) chains assemble intracellularly as monomers and subsequently form dimers and tetramers that are then secreted and form microfibrils in the extracellular space. ColVI plays a number of biological roles, notably in maintaining tissue integrity by providing a structural link between different components of connective tissues basement membranes. In addition to its structural role, ColVI supports adhesion, spreading and migration of cells as well as cell survival. *COL6A1* gene is localized in 21q22.3 while *COL6A2* and *COL6A3* are both in chromosome 2 (2q37). Inheritance may be dominant or recessive, with most patients having de novo mutations which exert dominant negative effects. Genotype–phenotype correlations

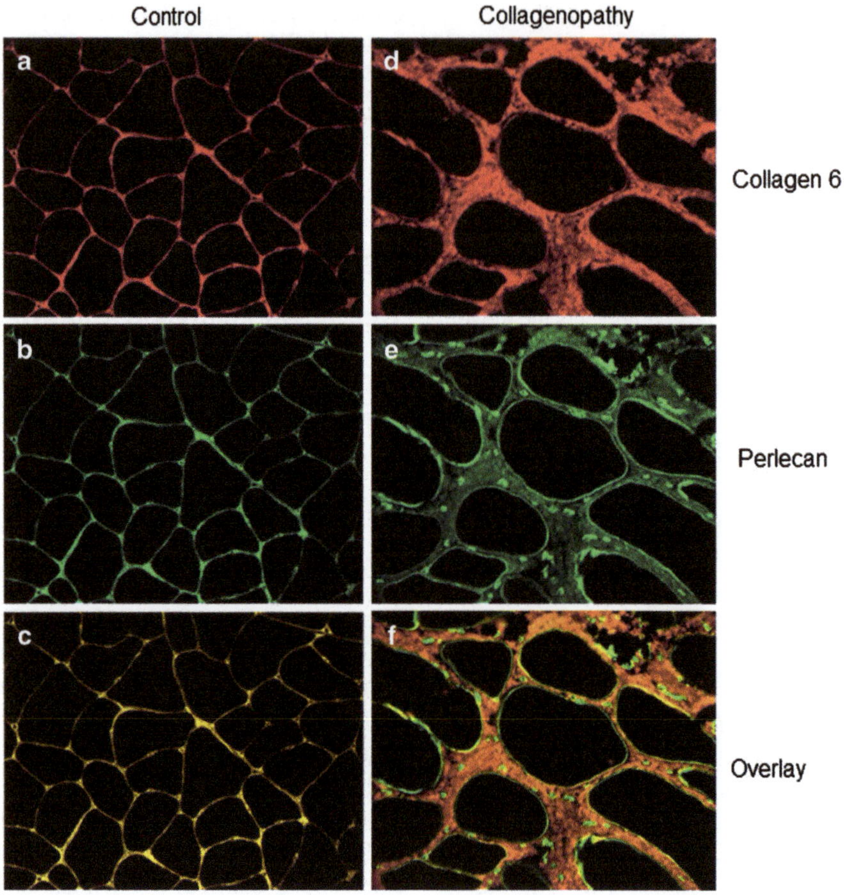

Fig. 16.7 Immunohistochemical features in a patient with collagenopathy. (**a–c**) Muscle biopsy with normal collagen 6 (**a**, *red*) and perlecan (**b**, *green*) staining. Both are located at the basal membrane which therefore stains in yellow when overlaying both stainings (**c**, *yellow*). Abnormal findings in a patient with collagenopathy (**d–f**). The absent location of collagen 6 at the basal membrane is only visible when overlaying both stainings (**f**), where the increased connective tissue overlays in yellow, while the basal lamina only stains for perlecan (*green*). Courtesy of Norma Romero, Paris, France

have also started to emerge. Dominant de novo exon splicing mutations that enable the synthesis and secretion of altered tetramers show a later or milder presentation than homozygous nonsense mutations leading to premature termination of translation and complete loss of function. The past decade has provided significant advances in terms of the identification of altered cellular functions in animal models of ColVI-myopathies and patients' samples. In particular, mitochondrial dysfunction leading to apoptosis via the permeability transition pore (PTP) and a defect in the autophagic clearance system of skeletal muscle have recently been reported, thereby opening potential therapeutic pathways.

16.4.3 Histopathology

Muscle biopsy pathology consists of myopathic to markedly dystrophic changes. Abnormal expression of ColVI may be detected in muscle tissue using antibodies that recognize human ColVI. However, this technique is not very sensitive unless there is marked deficiency. In these cases, particularly when there is no interstitial deposition of the protein, double labelling with perlecan or collagen V may allow detection of subtle abnormalities of collagen VI expression in the basal lamina (Fig. 16.7). Immunolabeling on skin fibroblast cultures is also used to study collagen VI expression and secretion patterns and

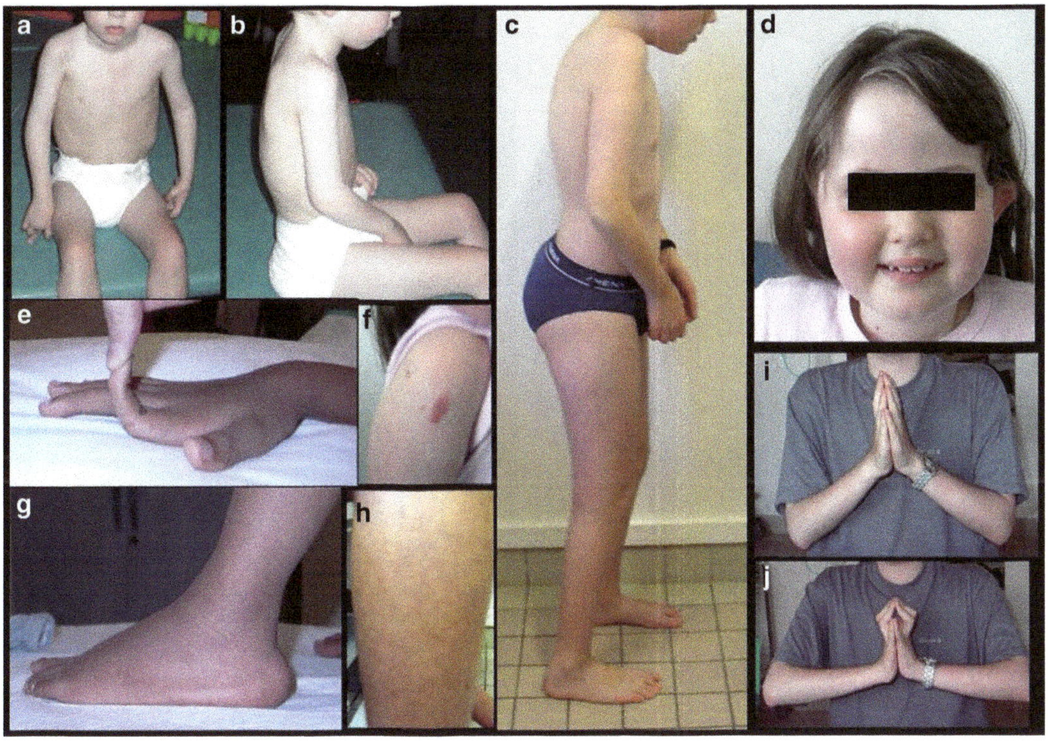

Fig. 16.8 Clinical features of patients with Ullrich syndrome. (**a**–**b**) Boy who did not acquired walking (early-severe UCMD). There is stiff dorsal kyphosis and elbow and lower limb joint contractures. (**c**) Moderate severe form (walking acquired) with similar features in a milder severity. (**d**–**j**) Typical phenotypical markers including round facies and thin neck (**d**), distal finger hyperlaxity (**e**), scar hypertrophy (**f**), calcaneum protrusion (**g**), granulous skin (**h**), and finger contractures revealed in the praying posture of hands with maximal extension of wrist (**j** compared to **i**)

flow cytometry techniques are reported to offer objective quantification.

16.4.4 Clinical Presentation

There is a clinical continuum in myopathies associated with collagen VI defects. It ranges from the congenital form (UCMD) to the less severe phenotype, Bethlem myopathy (BM), with less well defined intermediate phenotypes in between (mild Ullrich to severe Bethlem forms). Bethlem myopathy is characterized mainly by a retractile phenotype (fingers, wrist, elbows and ankles) with patients remaining ambulatory and not requiring ventilation. The Ullrich syndrome (UCMD, OMIM #254090) shows early-onset of hypotonia and weakness as well as prominent proximal joint contractures associated with a striking distal hyperlaxity. These abnormalities may result in severe orthopedic and respiratory complications. Congenital hip luxation is frequent in UCMD and skin features such as follicular hyperkeratosis and hypertrophic scars or keloid formation are commonly observed (Figs. 16.8 and 16.9d–f). Patients do not show intellectual impairment or cardiac affection. Muscle enzymes may be slightly increased. Motor and respiratory functions are quite correlated and are often aggravated by orthopaedic complications of joints (contractures) and spine (kyphoscoliosis). Although a proportion of children never walk and require mechanical ventilation before the end of the first decade (early severe group), most patients acquire the ability to walk. Among them, many lose it during the first

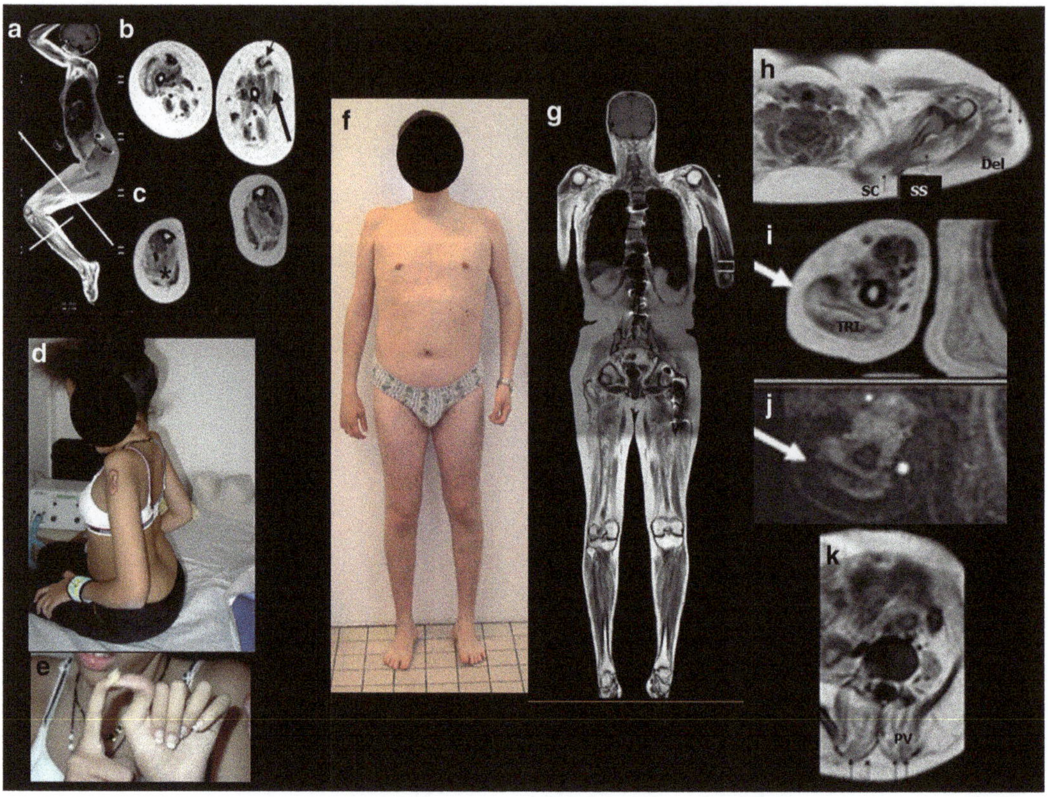

Fig. 16.9 Clinical and MRI findings in patients with COL6 related myopathy (**a**–**e**): Ullrich moderate progressive form (**f**–**k**: intermediary Ullrich/Bethlem). (**a**–**c**) WBMRI (T1-TSE) in a 12-year-old girl with UCMD, who lost walking at age 10 years. (**a**) Due to severe knee and hip contractures, a specific setting is required to get views of thigh and leg perpendicular to the axe of the limbs. Note the typical findings of COL6 myopathy in lower limbs. (**b**) Thigh showing vastus lateralis *rolled-cake*-like bands (*thick black arrow*) and rectus anterior vertical knotch (*thin arrows*). (**c**) Lower leg shows the hyperintense rim between soleus and gastrocnemii muscles (*black stars*). (**d**, **e**) Clinical features of the patient, with elbow contractures and hypertrophic scar (**d**), and striking finger hyperlaxity (**e**). (**f**–**k**) Clinical and radiological features of a 21-year-old patient with intermediary phenotype Ullrich/Bethlem. (**f**) Onset of symptoms in infancy (with motor delay, hyperlaxity), a slowly progressive course and development of elbow and mild ankle contractures in late childhood. (**h**–**k**) WBMRI shows typical "tigroid" pattern, with alternant bands of hyper- and hypointensity (*arrows*) in different regions: (**h**) shoulder: radial bands in Deltoid (Del), perpendicular in subscapular (SC) and supraspinatus (SS) muscles. (**i**–**j**) Arm using T1-TSE sequence (**i**) or STIR sequence (**j**): horizontal band in triceps brachii (TRI). (**k**) Severe fatty infiltration and vertical bands in the lumbar paravertebral (PV) muscles. Figures **a**, **b**, **c** and **g** from Quijano-Roy S, et al. (2012) Whole body muscle MRI protocol: pattern recognition in early onset NM disorders. Neuromuscul Disord. 22:S68–84. Reprinted with permission from Elsevier Limited

or second decade and develop severe respiratory insufficiency during the following years (moderate progressive group). Finally, there are children who acquire walking ability and remain ambulatory into adulthood without major respiratory dysfunction (mild Ullrich or intermediary Ullrich–Bethlem group). This simple clinical classification has recently allowed to make genotype–phenotype correlations.

16.4.5 Imaging Findings

Most patients show distinct abnormalities in multiple muscles all over the body, sparing the head. Alternating bands of increased and decreased signal intensity corresponding to preserved and to fatty infiltrated muscle are observed using T1-weighted turbo spin echo sequences, giving a striped (*tigroid*) pattern. These bands invariably follow the same distribution in each muscle. It can be identified as a "*rolled cake*"-like shape in the vastus lateralis muscle, a vertical bright shadow in the rectus anterior, and a fatty infiltrated rim between the gastrocnemius and soleus muscles (Fig. 16.9b, c). In addition, similar horizontal bands in triceps brachii, multiple radial lines in deltoid and lumbar extensor muscles, bands across glutei (in frontal views), and large perpendicular stripes in small muscles such as the subscapular and supraspinatus, are present (Fig. 16.9h–k). Frontal views are helpful to detect vertical bands in certain muscles, such as the gluteus maximus (Fig. 16.9g). In mildly affected or young patients, bands may not be so clearly defined and therefore muscle MRI profile may not be very distinct. Still, fatty infiltration is quite selective. The lumbar, gluteus maximus, thigh and leg muscles are predominantly affected. The most preserved muscles in the thigh are rectus anterior, sartorius and gracilis muscles, which help recognizing the profile in a patient clinically suggestive for collagenopathy (Fig. 16.9d–f). It is important to remark that in these patients the diagnostic bands may only be evident in a limited number of muscles (thigh, leg and arm are particularly sensitive). Therefore, in our experience, whole-body MRI very much improves the diagnostic impact in those patients without specific findings in thigh or lower leg by revealing the quasi-patognomonic diffuse tigroid pattern out of lower limbs.

16.4.6 Differential Diagnosis

Muscle weakness and contractures, associated with variable degrees of hyperlaxity are observed in many other early-onset myopathies, including other CMDs and congenital myopathies (in particular due to *SEPN1*, *LAMA2* and *RYR1* mutations, Chap. 15) but also the Limb-girdle muscular dystrophies and other diseases of connective tissues such as Ehlers–Danlos (EDS)-like syndromes. In patients with marked spinal stiffness and elbow contractures, the phenotype overlaps with Emery–Dreifuss muscular dystrophy (due to *LMNA*, *EDM* or *FHL-1* gene mutations, Chap. 18). The absence of markedly elevated CK levels, the lack of a cardiac phenotype and the presence of the distinct tigroid MRI pattern are highly suggestive of a COL6-related myopathy. Abnormalities observed in vastus lateralis in other muscular dystrophies (dysferlin, calpain-3, Chap. 19) may resemble the "*rolled cake* COLVI sign" but the bands are not observed at other levels, again enhancing the importance of whole-body MRI.

Congenital Muscular Dystrophies: Collagenopathies

Key Points

- Clinically, COL6-related myopathies are a continuum of phenotypes from the severe non ambulatory Ullrich syndrome to the mild Bethlem myopathy.
- Although diagnosis is often oriented by particular clinical markers (striking distal hyperlaxity together with axial and proximal joint contractures, skin hyperkeratosis, kyphoscoliosis), it may be difficult to distinguish from other myopathies and connective tissue disorders.
- Identification of (partial) collagen VI deficiency by IHC staining on muscle is often difficult and may require studies on skin fibroblast to analyze collagen VI secretion and chains quantification.
- Muscle imaging shows in most *COL6* mutated patients a very recognizable "tigroid" pattern. Characteristic bands or hyperintense rims of fatty infiltration are observed in many different muscles, in particular in lower limbs (rectus anterior, vastus lateralis, rim between soleus and gastrocnemius) but also in arms (triceps, deltoid), axial-trunk (subscapular, paravertebral) and limb girdles (gluteus in frontal views).
- When lower limb findings are not enough informative whole-body MRI is required to search for distinct features in other regions.

Suggestions for Further Reading

Allamand V, Briñas L, Richard P, et al. ColVI myopathies: where do we stand, where do we go? Skelet Muscle. 2011;23;1:30.

Allamand V, Merlini L, Bushby K. 166th ENMC International Workshop on Collagen type VI-related Myopathies, 22–24 May 2009, Naarden, The Netherlands. Neuromuscul Disord. 2010;20:346–54.

Briñas L, Richard P, Quijano-Roy S, et al. Early onset collagen VI myopathies: genetic and clinical correlations. Ann Neurol. 2010;68:511–20.

Mercuri E, Lampe A, Allsop J, et al. Muscle MRI in Ullrich congenital muscular dystrophy and Bethlem myopathy. Neuromuscul Disord. 2005;15:303–10.

Nadeau A, Kinali M, Main M, et al. Natural history of Ullrich congenital muscular dystrophy. Neurology 2009;73:25–31.

16.5 Dystroglycanopathies

Tracey A. Willis, Volker Straub

16.5.1 Synonyms and Abbreviations

WWS, MEB, Fukuyama congenital muscular dystrophy (FCMD), congenital muscular dystrophy 1C (MDC1C/CMD1C), congenital muscular dystrophy 1D (MDC1D/CMD1D), LGMD2I, LGMD2K, LGMD2M, LGMD2N, LGMD2O, POMT1 related muscular dystrophy, POMT2 related muscular dystrophy, POMGnT1 related muscular dystrophy, LARGE related muscular dystrophy, Fukutin related muscular dystrophy, FKRP related muscular dystrophy, DAG1 related muscular dystrophy.

16.5.2 Introduction and Classification

α- and β-dystroglycan, integral components of the DGC, derive from post translational cleavage of a precursor polypeptide encoded by the DAG1 gene. The basement membrane receptor α-dystroglycan (ADG) and the transmembrane β-dystroglycan protein (BDG) are integral to maintaining the stability of the sarcolemma by connecting components of the extracellular matrix to the internal cytoskeleton of the muscle fibre. Correct expression and glycosylation of ADG is essential to maintain DGC function and integrity. Several proteins have shown to be involved in the posttranslational modification of this key component of the DGC. POMT1 (protein-O-mannosyltransferase 1), POMT2 (protein-O-mannosyltransferase 2) and POMGnT1 (protein O-linked mannose β1,2-*N*-acetylglucosaminyltransferase) have been shown to catalyze specific steps of O-linked glycosylation of ADG. LARGE (like-acetylglucosaminyltransferase) has recently been suggested to act as a bifunctional glycosyltransferase, with both xylosyltransferase and glucuronyltransferase activities that are important for ADG function. The function of the proteins fukutin and FKRP (fukutin related protein) has not been fully explained. Aberrant glycosylation of ADG has been associated with a number of CMDs and limb girdle muscular dystrophies (LGMDs). Unlike congenital disorders of glycosylation involving the N-linked pathway, these O-linked disorders possess distinctive muscle, eye, and brain phenotypes and are collectively referred to as dystroglycanopathies.

16.5.3 Genetics and Pathophysiology

Mutations in at least seven genes have so far been identified in patients with dystroglycanopathies. These include *POMT1* (located on chromosome9q34, OMIM #236670), *POMT2* (14q24, OMIM #613150), POMGNT1 (1p34, OMIM #253280), *LARGE* (22q12, OMIM #613154), *FKTN* encoding fukutin (1q31, OMIM #253800), FKRP encoding fukutin related protein (19q13, *OMIM* #606612), and *DAG1* encoding the dystroglycan gene (3p21, OMIM #613818). Dolichyl-phosphate mannosyltransferase 2 (DPM2 [MIM 603564]), Dolichyl-phosphate mannosyltransferase 3 (DPM3 [MIM605951]), Dolichol Kinase (DOLK [OMIM 610746]), Isoprenoid Synthase Domain Containing (ISPD [OMIM 614631]), Glycosyltransferase-like domain containing 2 (GTDC2 [OMIM 147730]), and Transmembrane protein 5 (TMEM5 [OMIM 605862]). They cause a spectrum of diseases from severe CMDs, usually associated with structural brain malformations and eye involvement to milder forms of limb girdle muscular dystrophy (LGMD). WWS, MEB, and Fukuyama congenital muscular dystrophy (FCMD) represent the more severe end of the spectrum, whilst MDC1C and LGMD are milder and do not have any associated brain involvement. The various forms of

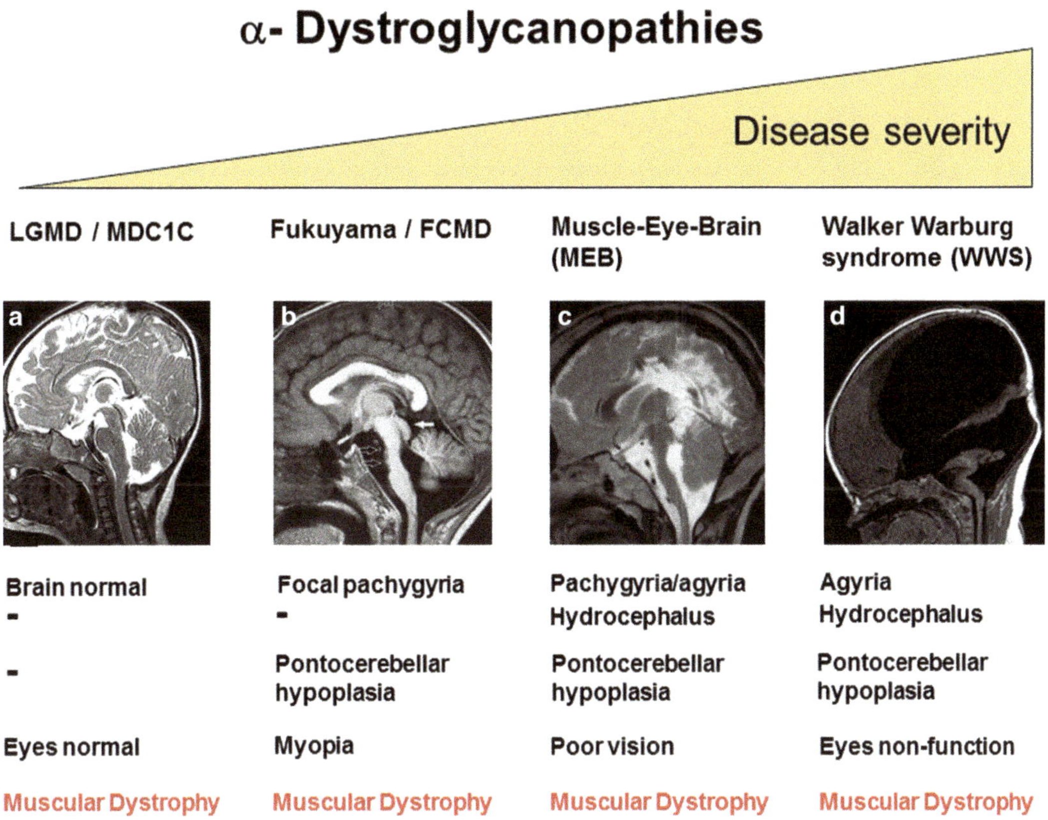

Fig. 16.10 Overview of clinical phenotypes in α-dystroglycanopathies and disease severity ranging from isolated late onset limb girdle muscular dystrophy (LGMD) and early onset congenital muscular dystrophy (CMD). In addition to muscular dystrophy, patients with Fukuyama congenital muscular dystrophy (FCMD) also have mild ocular abnormalities (myopia) and central nervous system involvement with focal pachygyria and pontocerebellar hypoplasia. Muscle eye brain (MEB) disease presents with more severe eye and brain affection including generalized cortical gyration anomalies (pachygyria, polymicrogyria and agyria), while Walker–Warburg Syndrome (WWS) have lissencephaly type II, other brain abnormalities and are usually blind to different abnormalities in the eyes. Modified after T. Voit and F. Tomé (2004) in Engel AE, Franzini-Armstrong C. Myology. 3rd ed. 1203–1238. (**a**) with courtesy of Dirk Fischer, Basel, Switzerland; (**b**) taken from Jakkani RK et al. (2012) MRI findings in Fukuyama congenital muscular dystrophy: a rare case report. Acta Neurol Belg. 2012;112:401–3. Reprinted with permission from Springer. (**c**) taken from Hehr et al. (2007) Novel POMGnT1 mutations define broader phenotypic spectrum of muscle-eye-brain disease. Neurogenetics. 8:279–88, reprinted with permission from Springer; (**d**) with courtesy of Mike Wattjes, Amsterdam, The Netherlands

LGMD associated with abnormal ADG expression also do not show any brain involvement but can present with severe respiratory and cardiac muscle involvement (Fig. 16.10). Some of the dystroglycanopathies have higher regional prevalence rates due to founder mutations. In Japan e.g. FCMD is the most common form of CMD due to a retrotransposal insertion in the 3' noncoding region of the fukutin gene, whereas a founder mutation in the *FKRP* gene that originates from Northern Europe is the main cause for LGMD2I, the single most common dystroglycanopathy.

FKRP is thought to be a tissue specific glycosyltransferase involved in the O-mannosylation of ADG. It is expressed in many tissues including skeletal muscle, placenta and heart and more weakly in lung, liver, kidney, pancreas and brain. Mutations in *FKRP* show the most striking heterogeneity and have been found in patients with prenatal WWS with cobblestone lissencephaly and eye abnormalities, MEB, MDC1C and

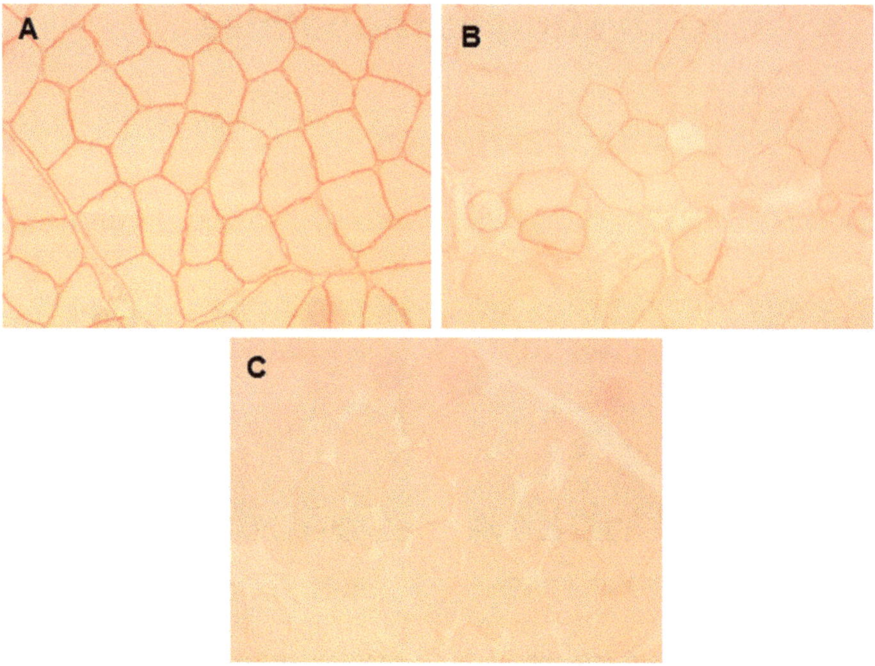

Fig. 16.11 α-Dystroglycan immunhistochemistry on frozen muscle sections. Normal labelling of the basal lamina in a control (**a**), partially mosaic, (**b**) and completely absent reaction (**c**) in patients with LGMD2I due to *FKRP* gene mutations. Courtesy of Dirk Fischer, Basel, Switzerland

LGMD2I. It has been suggested that the wide phenotypical variation seen could be partly explained by the specific point mutation. Patients with the milder LGMD2I phenotype are in most cases homozygous for the common C826A/Leu279Ile *FKRP* mutation. *DAG1*, *POMT1*, *POMT2*, *POMGNT1*, *LARGE* and fukutin mutations occur less commonly than *FKRP* mutations. However, there is a broad phenotypic spectrum in most of the dystroglycanopathies.

16.5.4 Histopathology

Typically muscle biopsies of patients with dystroglycanopathies show features of a muscular dystrophy. There can be variable degrees of fibre atrophy and hypertrophy, fibrosis, adipose tissue, necrosis, increased number of internal nuclei and regeneration. There appears to be no correlation between the pattern of histopathology and a specific gene defect.

Immunolabelling of ADG on skeletal muscle cryosection with the monoclonal antibody IIH6 represent a good screening marker of dystroglycanopathies (Fig. 16.11). The amount of depleted glycosylated epitopes seems to correlate with the severity of the phenotype and therefore complete absence on immunostaining is associated with the most severe cases, such as WWS. α-dystroglycan glycosylation is important for binding to basement membrane components like laminin 211. Abnormalities in the basal lamina have been demonstrated in the muscle and brain of both animal models and patients with various forms of dystroglycanopathy.

16.5.5 Clinical Presentation

Dystroglycanopathies constitute a broad and continuous spectrum of disease severity, from congenital muscular dystrophy syndromes associated with structural brain and eye malformations (compare Figs. 16.1 and 16.10) to mild limb girdle phenotypes. All known dystroglycanopathies are inherited in an autosomal recessive fashion.

Walker–Warburg Syndrome

Clinical features depend on the severity of involvement in muscle, eye, and brain. Generally these patients are severely affected with a muscular dystrophy and the majority of patients die before the age of 3 years (mean age of survival

0.8 year). Affected children generally do not reach any motor or cognitive milestones, commonly have seizures and need gastric tube feeding. The brain malformations typically include a lissencephaly type II, in which an impaired neuronal migration causes a cobblestone cortex. Other brain abnormalities include obstructive hydrocephalus, cerebral hypoplasia, corpus callosum agenesis, neuronal heterotopias, fusion of the hemispheres, pontocerebellar hypoplasia with fourth ventricle dilatation and occasionally an occipital encephalocele and Dandy–Walker cyst. Eye abnormalities show also a broad variation and can result from both anterior and posterior chamber abnormalities including retinal detachment resulting in blindness, cataracts, colobomas and other iris malformations, microphthalmia, persistent hyperplastic primary vitreous and Peters anomaly. Although WWS tends to be clinically homogenous, it is genetically heterogeneous. In 40 % of WWS patients, a mutation is found in either *POMT1* or *POMT2*, however mutations have been found in *POMGNT1*, fukutin, *FKRP* and *LARGE*. There is no clinical distinction within these patients depending on their genotype.

Muscle–Eye–Brain Disease

MEB is characterised by CMD, structural eye abnormalities and brain anomalies. The phenotype of MEB is similar to WWS but less severe. The central nervous system involvement is variable including the whole spectrum of cortical gyration anomalies (pachygyria, polymicrogyria and agyria) particularly located in the posterior fossa in addition to white matter abnormalities. Some patients are severely affected with motor and cognitive delay and autistic features, whereas other patients are able to walk and develop speech. Mutations in the POMGNT1 gene seem to be more frequently associated with MEB than mutations in the other dystroglycanopathy genes. Initially this condition was thought to be exclusively found in a Finnish population, however advances in molecular diagnoses have identified non-Finnish MEB patients and patients with atypical phenotypes, such as preserved vision.

Fukuyama Congenital Muscular Dystrophy

In FCMD, the protein fukutin is proposed to be a glycosyltranferase involved in the biosynthesis of the O-mannosylglycan. Patients may present very similar to WWS and MEB with generalized hypotonia, cognitive delay and seizures. The clinical presentation can be very variable even within the same family. Some patients show severe cognitive impairment and refractory seizures, others are able to walk and have obtained seizure control. The brain anomalies are also similar to those seen in WWS and MEB, although hydrocephalus is rare. The eye involvement is more variable and tends to affect the retina predominantly ranging from simple myopia, retinal detachment, to persistent hyaloid artery and microphthalmia. Patients with mutations in *FKTN* gene have been identified in non-Asiatic populations, with a broad spectrum of phenotypes overlapping that of *FKRP* ranging, from severe phenotypes with brain malformation to hyper-CKemia without major muscle weakness and normal cognitive function.

Congenital Muscular Dystrophy 1C and 1D

Patients with MDC1C caused by mutations in the *FKRP* gene present early in life, usually before the age of 6 months, with hypotonia and weakness, predominantly affecting limb girdle muscles. It is usually associated with severe wasting in these muscle groups. Patients are usually unable to walk and also develop severe restrictive respiratory insufficiency progressing to respiratory failure in the second decade. The brain is usually spared, except for severe mutations which can lead to more extensive changes as seen in WWS and MEB. MDC1C is much more common than MDC1D, which has been described in a patient with compound heterozygous mutations in the LARGE gene. The patient was hypotonic at birth and had severe cognitive delay due to a neuronal migration disorder.

Limb Girdle Muscular Dystrophy Variants

The LGMD type 2 variants caused by mutations in the dystroglycanopathy genes include LGMD2I, LGMD2K and LGMD2M-O. The most prevalent of these LGMDs is LGMD2I

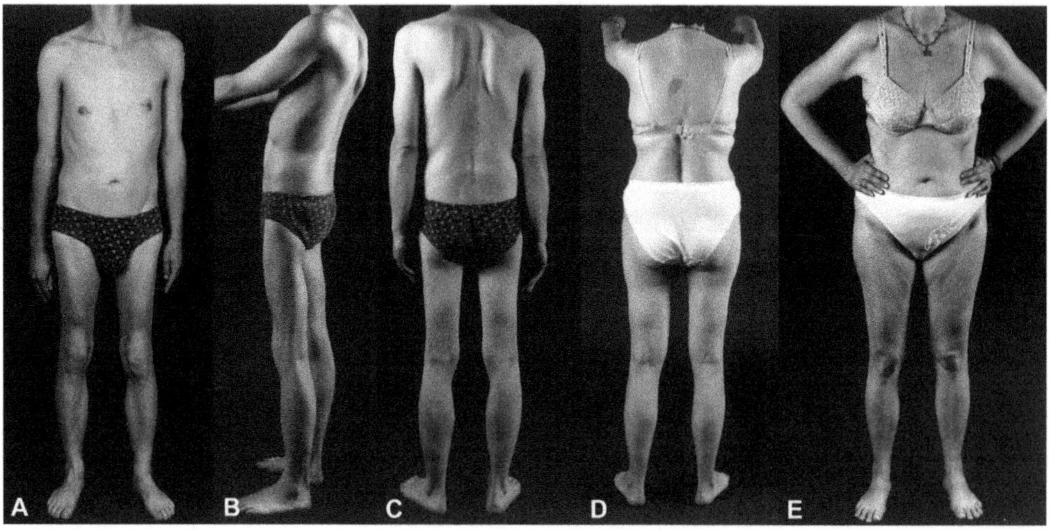

Fig. 16.12 Clinical phenotype of two siblings with LGMD2I: patient 2 (**a–c**) with scapular winging, severe atrophy of the gluteus maximus and the posterior thigh muscles as well as calf hypertrophy, whereas his sister (patient 1; **d**, **e**) with a similar degree of severity had no weakness of the scapular fixator muscles. From Fischer D, et al. (2005) Diagnostic value of muscle MRI in differentiating LGMD2I from other LGMDs. J Neurol. 252:538–47. Courtesy of Dirk Fischer, Basel, Switzerland. Reprinted with permission from Springer

caused by mutations in the *FKRP* gene. Mutations in fukutin (LGMD2N), *POMT1* (LGMD2K), *POMT2* (LGMD2N) and *POMGNT1* (LGMD2O) as well as in *DAG1* and *LARGE* seem to be very rare causes of a LGMD.

In LGMD2I, the phenotype can range from asymptomatic carriers to an early onset DMD like phenotype with an associated cardiomyopathy and respiratory failure. Patients present with progressive proximal weakness predominantly affecting the pelvic girdle and as the condition progresses, the shoulder girdle. These patients do not present brain or eye abnormalities (Fig. 16.12).

16.5.6 Imaging Findings

The pattern of skeletal muscle pathology has not been systematically reviewed in any of the dystroglycanopathies apart from LGMD2I. The main reason for this is the low prevalence of the other dystroglycanopathies and the fact that muscle MRI, in contrast to brain MRI, does not play a role in the diagnostic workup of patients with WWS, MEB or FCMD. Structural brain abnormalities detected by MRI are not discussed in this chapter.

In LGMD2I MRI has shown that changes occur predominantly in the posterior compartments of both the thighs and the lower legs (Figs. 16.13 and 16.14), with more marked changes occurring in the biceps femoris long head muscle, adductor magnus muscle, semitendinosus muscle, and semimembranosus muscle with the gracilis muscle, sartorius muscle, vastus lateralis muscle, and the rectus femoris muscle being relatively spared until later (Fig. 16.13). Even at a stage where all the muscles in the thigh are almost completely replaced by fat tissue (Fig. 16.13), including the gracilis and the sartorius muscle, some patients can still manage to walk. In the lower legs predominant involvement is seen in the gastrocnemii muscles and the soleus muscle with the tibialis anterior muscle and peroneus longus muscle being spared until the late stages of the disease (Fig. 16.14).

16.5.7 Therapy

Presently there is no curative therapy for the treatment of the dystroglycanopathies. There have been advances in the supportive care given to patients with both CMD and LGMD including timely respiratory support, cardio protective therapy and the treatment of seizures secondary to the brain abnormalities associated. Anecdotal reports have also suggested that glucocorticosteroids may have a beneficial effect on the muscle

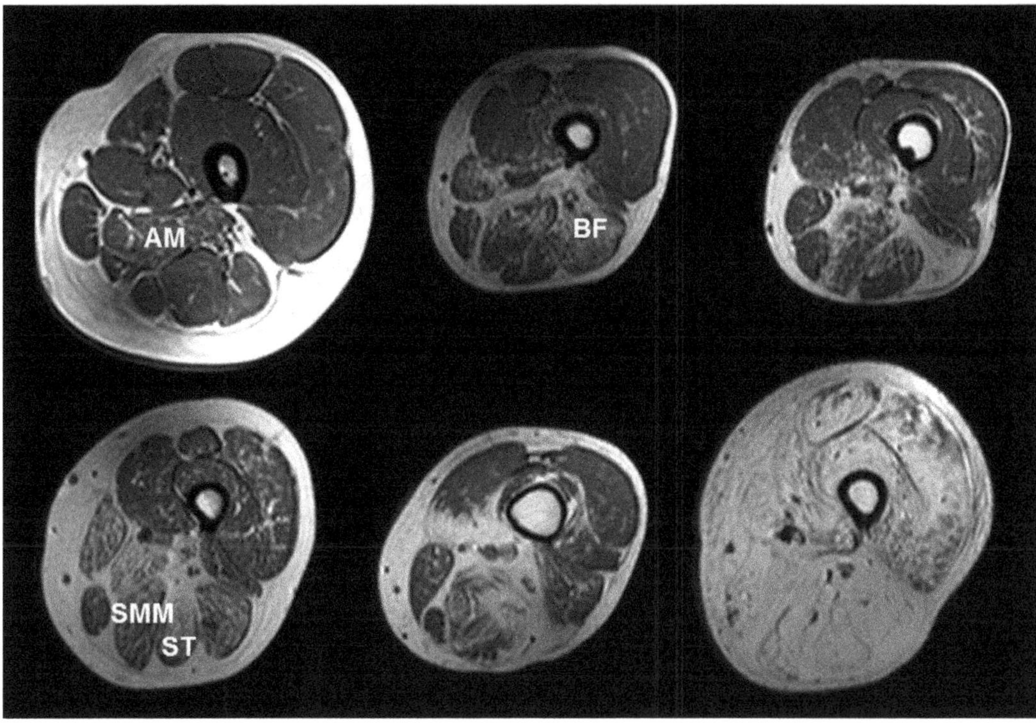

Fig. 16.13 The panel shows T1-weighted axial images through the thighs of six ambulant patients with a genetically confirmed diagnosis of LGMD2I. All patients were homozygous for the C826A/Leu279Ile founder mutation in the *FKRP* gene. The MRI scans show an increase in pathology with the muscles in the posterior compartment being more severely affected than the muscles in the anterior compartment. The most severe changes are seen in the adductor magnus (AM) and biceps femoris (BF), and to a lesser extent in the semimembranosus (SMM) and semitendinosus (ST) muscles. Patients can still be ambulant even if on MRI all thigh muscles seem to be completely replaced by fat

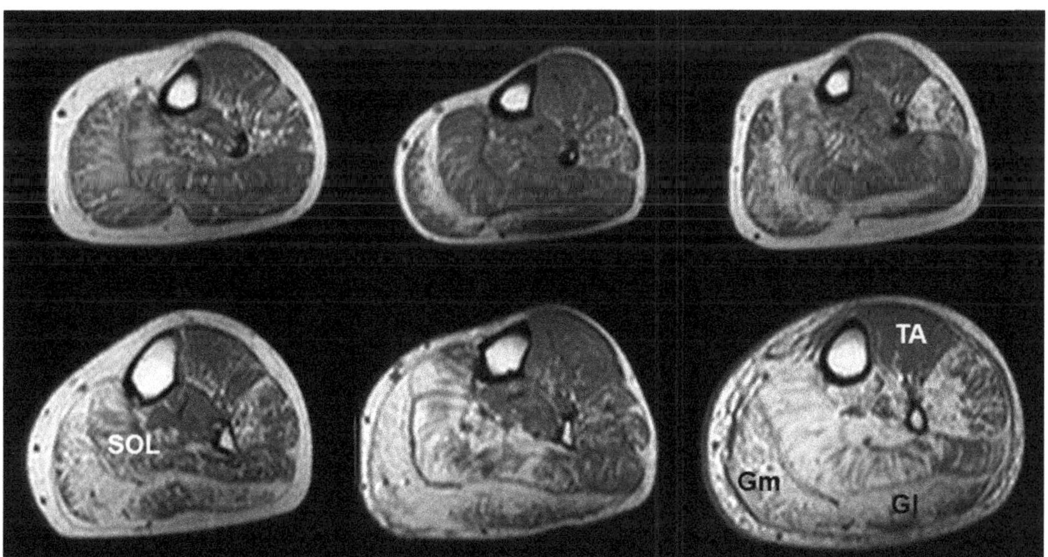

Fig. 16.14 The panel shows T1-weighted axial images through the calves of six ambulant patients with a genetically confirmed diagnosis of LGMD2I. All patients were homozygous for the C826A/Leu279Ile founder mutation in the *FKRP* gene. The MRI scans show an increase in pathology with the muscles in the posterior compartment being more severely affected than the muscles in the anterior compartment. The most severe changes are seen in the medial (Gm) and lateral (Gl) gastrocnemius muscles, and to a lesser extent in the soleus (SOL) muscles. The tibialis anterior (TA) muscle is the best preserved muscle in the lower leg of LGMD2I patients

function in patients with dystroglycanopathies, but more systematic studies will be necessary to support this treatment.

16.5.8 Differential Diagnosis

Other CMDs and LGMDs obviously come into the differential diagnosis of the dystroglycanopathies. The most common form of CMD, MDC1A (Sect. 16.2), is caused by mutations in the laminin α-2 gene (*LAMA2*) and presents with marked muscle weakness and atrophy, joint contractures, inability to achieve independent ambulation, raised CK levels, and white matter changes on MRI of the brain. These patients can have learning disabilities, epileptic seizures and neuronal migration disorders as described in the dystroglycanopathies.

When it comes to the differential diagnosis of LGMD2I, skeletal muscle MRI may indeed be a helpful diagnostic tool to distinguish patients with LGMD2I from other forms of LGMD (Chap. 19), from Becker muscular dystrophy (Chap. 17), the myofibrillar myopathies (Chap. 20) or late onset Pompe disease (Sect. 14.2.1). The differential diagnostic spectrum of late onset limb girdle weakness is very broad and includes both genetic and acquired diseases. A flow chart demonstrating how muscle imaging may be used for the differentiation of LGMD2I from other LGMD is provided in Chap. 25.

Congenital Muscular Dystrophies: Dystroglycanopathies

Key Points

- Dystroglycanopathies is a collective term for the CMDs and LGMDs caused by aberrant glycosylation of α-dystroglycan (ADG).
- The CMDs include WWS, MEB, FCMD, MDC1C and MDC1D. The LGMDs include LGMD2K, LGMD2I and LGMD2M-O.
- Mutations in at least seven genes have so far been identified in patients with dystroglycanopathies. These include *DAG1, POMT1, POMT2, POMGnT1, LARGE, fukutin* and *FKRP.*
- Muscle biopsies show variable levels of ADG expression, not clearly correlated with the clinical phenotype.
- Skeletal muscle imaging does not play an important role in the diagnostic workup of patients with dystroglycanopathies, but maybe helpful to distinguish LGMD2I from other diseases with predominant limb girdle weakness.

Suggestions for Further Reading

Brown SC, Winder SJ. Dystroglycan and dystroglycanopathies: Report of the 187th ENMC Workshop 11–13 November 2011, Naarden, The Netherlands. Neuromuscul Disord. Mar 19. 2012.

Fischer D, Walter MC, Kesper K, et al. 2005. Diagnostic value of muscle MRI in differentiating LGMD2I from other LGMDs. J Neurol 252, 538–47.

Godfrey C, Clement E, Mein R, et al. 2007. Refining genotype phenotype correlations in muscular dystrophies with defective glycosylation of dystroglycan. Brain 130, 2725–35.

Hewitt JE, 2009. Abnormal glycosylation of dystroglycan in human genetic disease. Biochim Biophys Acta 1792, 853–61

Mercuri E, Messina S, Bruno C, et al. 2009. Congenital muscular dystrophies with defective glycosylation. Neurology 72, 1802–9.

Muntoni F, Torelli S, Wells DJ, et al. 2011. Muscular dystrophies due to glycosylation defects: diagnosis and therapeutic strategies. Curr Opin Neurol 24, 437–42.

17 Dystrophinopathies

Tracey A. Willis and Volker Straub

17.1 Introduction and Classification

Duchenne muscular dystrophy (DMD, OMIM #310200) and Becker muscular dystrophy (BMD, OMIM #300376) are also referred to as the dystrophinopathies and are among the most common and best characterized forms of muscular dystrophy worldwide, with DMD affecting one in 3,500 newborn males.

17.1.1 Synonyms, Abbreviations

Duchenne muscular dystrophy (DMD), Becker muscular dystrophy (BMD).

17.2 Genetics and Pathophysiology

Dystrophinopathies have an X-linked recessive mode of inheritance, distinguishing them from the large group of autosomal recessive and dominant limb girdle muscular dystrophies (LGMDs), which also present with progressive weakness and wasting of the pelvic and shoulder girdle muscles. Although the majority of DMD and BMD cases are transmitted in an X-linked manner, with a positive family history or a known carrier status in the mother, approximately 30 % result from a de novo mutation. The dystrophin protein is encoded by the largest gene described to date, spanning 2.5 million bp of genomic sequence on the X chromosome (Xp21.2-p21.1). Mutations that result in the absence or severe reduction of the dystrophin protein generally manifest as DMD, whereas a less severe reduction and/or expression of an internally truncated, semifunctional protein generally manifests as BMD. The size of the mutation is not the determining factor in severity, but the type of mutation and location can be. Deletions, duplications and missense mutations that interrupt the reading frame generally lead to DMD, whereas in-frame mutations generally lead to the less severe BMD phenotype. There are exceptions to these rules, however, and further research is ongoing to identify possible modifier genes. Dystrophin is organized into four domains: amino-terminal actin-binding domain; central rod domain; cysteine-rich domain; carboxyl-terminal domain. The localization of the deletions has shown that the amino-terminal, cysteine-rich and carboxyl terminal domains are essential for dystrophin function, whereas the central rod domain can accommodate large in-frame deletions.

Approximately 65 % of the mutations in the dystrophin gene are caused by intragenic deletions and

T.A. Willis
Neuromuscular Department, The Robert Jones and Agnes Hunt Orthopaedic Hospital, NHS Foundation Trust, Oswestry Shropshire, UK

V. Straub (✉)
Neurology, The Harold Macmillan Chair of Medicine, Institute of Genetic Medicine, University of Newcastle upon Tyne, International Centre for Life, Central Parkway, Newcastle upon Tyne NE1 2BZ, UK
e-mail: volker.straub@newcastle.ac.uk

M.P. Wattjes and D. Fischer (eds.), *Neuromuscular Imaging*, DOI 10.1007/978-1-4614-6552-2_17,

the remaining 35 % of the mutations are caused by duplications and point mutations. Although deletions can occur anywhere in the dystrophin gene, deletion hotspots are located in the central part of the 79 exons comprising the gene.

In skeletal muscle tissue, the dystrophin protein is integral to the stability of the myofibers. Dystrophin is expressed as a 427-kDa protein that consists of two apposed globular heads with a flexible rod- shaped center. It forms part of the dystrophin glycoprotein complex (DGC), which works as a transmembrane linkage between the extracellular matrix and the cytoskeleton. Mutations of the dystrophin gene result in disruption of the normal stability of the DGC, resulting in increased susceptibility to loss of cytoskeletal and sarcolemmal integrity. It is believed that this structural defect gives rise to a further misregulation of mainly calcium ionsand increased production of reactive oxygen species (ROS), which can cause further protein and membrane damage. Increased ROS is also a sign of altered mitochondrial function which leads to reduced muscular energy production.

17.3 Clinical Presentation

Patients with DMD tend to show their first symptoms at 3–5 years of age (Fig. 17.1). The initial presentation may include signs of delayed motor milestones or even a global developmental delay, isolated speech delay, a waddling gait, calf hypertrophy and increased frequency of falling. Boys tend to run more slowly than their peers. Sometimes elevated liver enzymes are a first misleading finding. Hence the serum creatine kinase (CK) activity and the γ-glutamyl transferase level should therefore always be checked prior to a liver biopsy in a boy with developmental delay.

Generally young boys with DMD develop a waddling gait often accompanied by toe walking and tight Achilles tendons. Hypertrophy of the calf and other muscles can also be seen, including forearm muscles and less commonly the tongue. At first presentation, the serum CK is often elevated 10–100 times of the normal upper limit. As the disease progresses weakness increases in the proximal muscles, initially the lower limb muscles but eventually involving the neck flexors, shoulders and arms. Difficulty climbing stairs is often seen at 8–10 years of age, and loss of ambulation occurs between 10 and 15 years. The clinical course has become more variable since steroid treatment was introduced. Once ambulation has been lost there is often a steady decline in respiratory function with many of these boys requiring nocturnal ventilation in their late teens/early twenties. Scoliosis or kyphoscoliosis may progress or develop once a boy is non-ambulant and wheelchair-bound. This situation, in turn, contributes to further decline in respiratory function and compromised gastrointestinal function. Cardiomyopathy develops later in

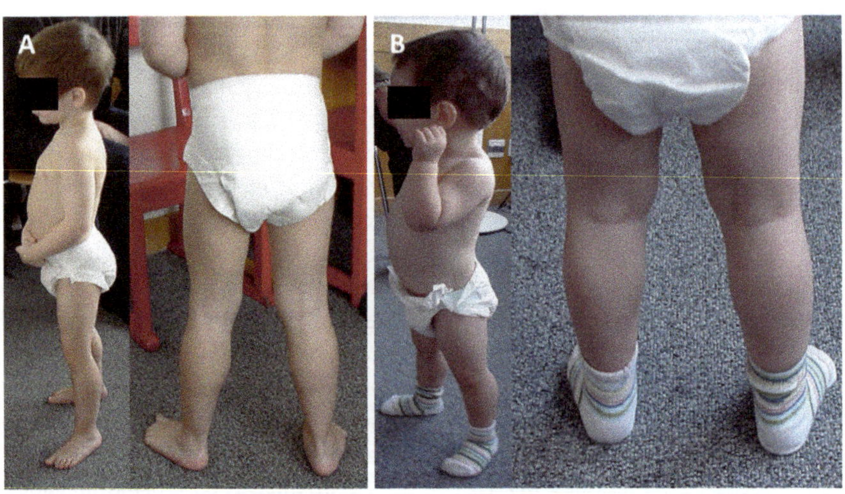

Fig. 17.1 Clinical findings in Duchenne muscular dystrophy. (**a**) DMD patient at disease onset (age of 3.5 years) already showing slight hyperlordosis, a broad based stance, and pseudohypertrophy of calves. (**b**) similar findings in a patient in whom diagnosis was made at the age of 2 years. Courtesy of Dirk Fischer, Basel, Switzerland

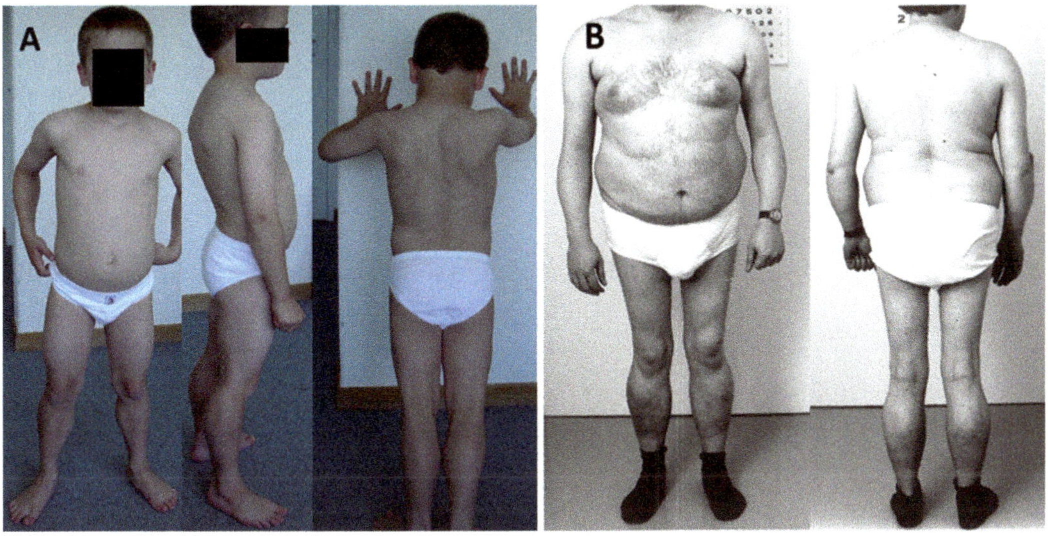

Fig. 17.2 Clinical findings in BMD. The clinical presentation is often similar as in DMD with predominant limb girdle weakness, but age of onset is later. (**a**) BMD patient (9 years) at onset, and (**b**) BMD patient, 25 years (about 10 years after onset) with thigh atrophy, pseudohypertrophy of calves, but no scapular winging. Courtesy of Dirk Fischer, Basel, Switzerland. B with permission from Springer (Fischer D, et al. (2005) J Neurol. 252;538–547)

the disease course with the majority of the patients developing signs of cardiomyopathy in their late teens and early twenties. Nutrition plays a major role in the late stages of DMD, and poor nutrition can be a serious complication exacerbating weakness and respiratory function.

Approximately 30 % of patients with DMD and some with BMD have a low level of intellect and present with cognitive impairment involving several domains (e.g., learning difficulties). Children with DMD or BMD perform poorly at tests, particularly on verbal skills, but also have challenges processing complex verbal information. In addition, patients frequently present with an attention deficit hyperactivity disorder, autistic spectrum disorder, or obsessive-compulsive disorder.

The BMD phenotype manifests more slowly and evolves over a longer period of time. Patients typically present during late childhood or even adulthood (Fig. 17.2). In contrast to DMD patients who are wheelchair bound by their mid-teens, BMD patients are able to ambulate for a longer time, often into their fourth decade and in sometimes up to their seventh decade. Life expectancy in mild BMD, although diminished compared to that of the general population, may be into their seventh or eighth decade.

17.4 Histopathology

Histopathological changes in muscle biopsies of dystrophinopathy patients show dystrophic changes similar to those seen in other muscular dystrophies. Findings include increased variation in fiber size, fibrosis, degenerating fibers, regeneration, and in later stages variable replacement of muscle tissue by fat and connective tissue. Specific immunhistochemical (IHS) markers facilitate the diagnosis, using commercial antibodies directed toward three domains of the dystrophin protein usually allowing a reliable diagnosis of DMD and BMD. IHS is sometimes successful in identifying symptomatic female carriers (Fig. 17.3).

17.5 Imaging Findings

17.5.1 Skeletal Ultrasonography

Muscle US can be highly predictive for detecting a neuromuscular disorder in children from birth through their teenage years. The sensitivity of 78 % and specificity of 91 % reported is increased to a sensitivity of 81 % and a specificity of 96 % in

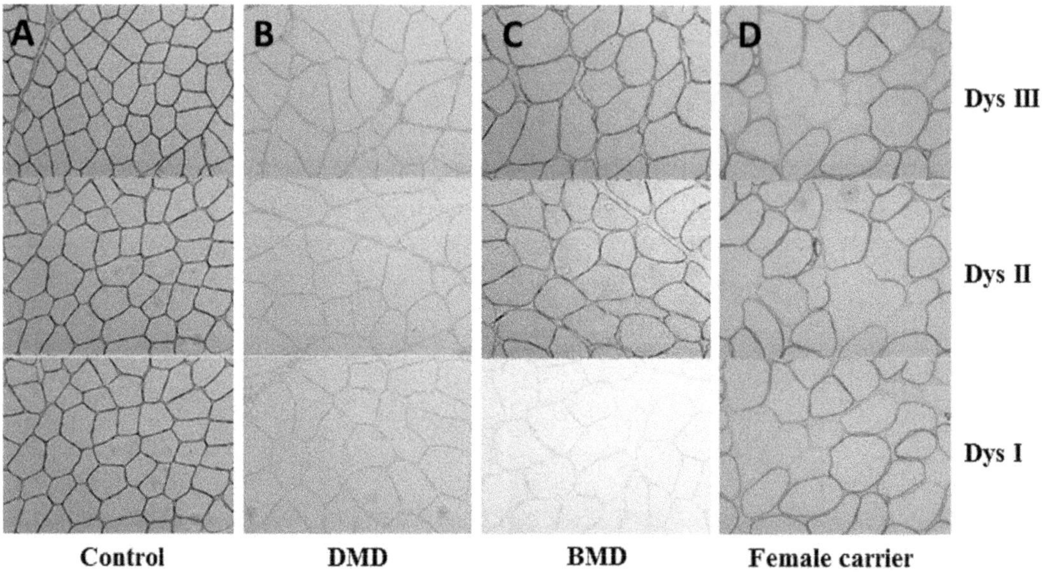

Fig. 17.3 Immunhistochemistry using commercial antibodies (DYS I, DYS II, and DYS III) against three differential domains of the dystrophin protein: (**a**) normal sarcolemmal dystrophin staining in a control. (**b**) completely absent dystrophin staining using all three antibodies in a DMD patients. (**c**) normal sarcolemmal dystrophin staining using DYS III and DYSII antibody, but absent dystrophin staining using DYS I in a BMD patient indicating the presence of a partially present (shortened) dystrophin protein. (**d**) partially (mosaic) absent reaction in a female DMD carrier using all three antibodies. Courtesy of Dirk Fischer, Basel, Switzerland

children > 3 years of age. In children < 3 years, the sensitivity decreases because of structural changes in the muscle usually being minor at this early age. If an abnormality is detected, more-invasive tests are required. Muscle US is a suitable screening tool for detecting a neuromuscular condition in children (see Chap. 2). These sensitivities are different for specific neuromuscular diseases, approaching 100 % for clinically affected patients with DMD, but only 25–45 % for those with mitochondrial myopathies. Its diagnostic value for other specific neuromuscular diseases has not been studied, and only small series have been reported.

The pattern of muscle involvement can also be described with US. As with magnetic resonance imaging (MRI) and computed tomography (CT), US can help with the differential diagnosis. Muscle US can also detect suitable muscles to biopsy, thereby preventing biopsy of severely affected muscles. Those with pronounced fibrosis and atrophy may provide specimens that are not interpretable.

Changes in muscle in muscular dystrophies seen with US were first described for DMD. Preclinical cases of DMD can appear normal on US scans, unlike the changes seen by MRI. Once the first clinical signs manifest, however, muscle US reveals abnormalities in almost every patient. The proximal muscles have the highest echo intensities, and within the muscle there is a homogeneous, fine granular appearance.

The pattern of infiltration in the muscles in DMD shows sparing of the gracilis and sartorius muscles, even in patients with severe pathology. The selective involvement in "mid-stage" DMD has demonstrated sparing of the gracilis and sartorius muscles, the peroneus and tibialis anterior muscles, and the posterior muscles in the lower leg. The same pattern of sparing was also observed In BMD.

17.5.2 Skeletal CT

The use of CT in early-DMD patients has documented changes that are reflected in both US and MRI scans and are pattern-specific for DMD. In a recent study, DMD patients aged 6 months to 12 years, who were reported to be preclinical, with motor skills still continuing to develop, were

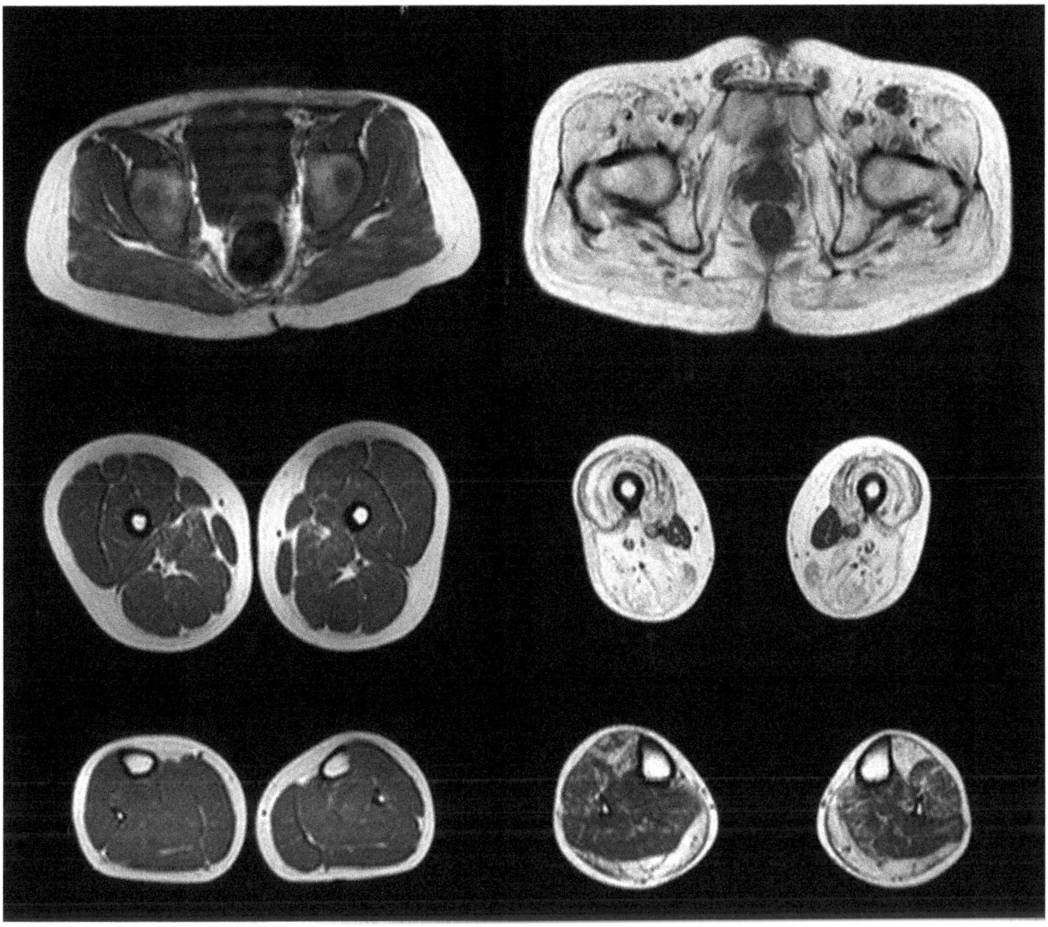

Fig. 17.4 The T1-weighted axial MR images through the pelvic girdle and leg muscles of two ambulant patients with dystrophinopathies show the broad spectrum of muscle pathology. The images on the left are from an 8-year-old boy with DMD who clinically showed the typical symptoms of the disease, despite the fact that hardly any muscle pathology was detectable on MRI. The images on the right are from a 43-year-old patient with BMD, who despite severe muscle pathology in his thigh muscles was still ambulant

imaged using quantitative CT. Hounsfield units (HU) were used and correlated with the age of the patient. The HU refer to the density of the muscle seen on CT imaging. Changes in HU in individual muscles were demonstrated, particularly those that visually did not appear to be affected. Less-affected muscles that were generally well preserved, such as the anterior and posterior tibialis muscles, showed higher HUs. A slow, gradual regression rate was reported for the gracilis muscle, reflecting the so-called selective pattern of involvement seen in DMD even during the preclinical stage. This regression rate was analyzed cross sectionally, correlating the degree of disease severity seen in the boys clinically with the HU value obtained from the CT scans of the gracilis muscle. Although this study was important from a quantitative perspective and identified that gross visual inspection alone is insufficient, there were no longitudinal data and no age-matched controls.

17.5.3 Skeletal Muscle MRI

Because of the progressive nature of DMD, there has been a need to develop an objective, noninvasive measurement of disease progression. Muscle MRI allows evaluation of the muscles over time. Standard T1-weighted images are often normal during the early stages of DMD (Figs. 17.4, 17.5,

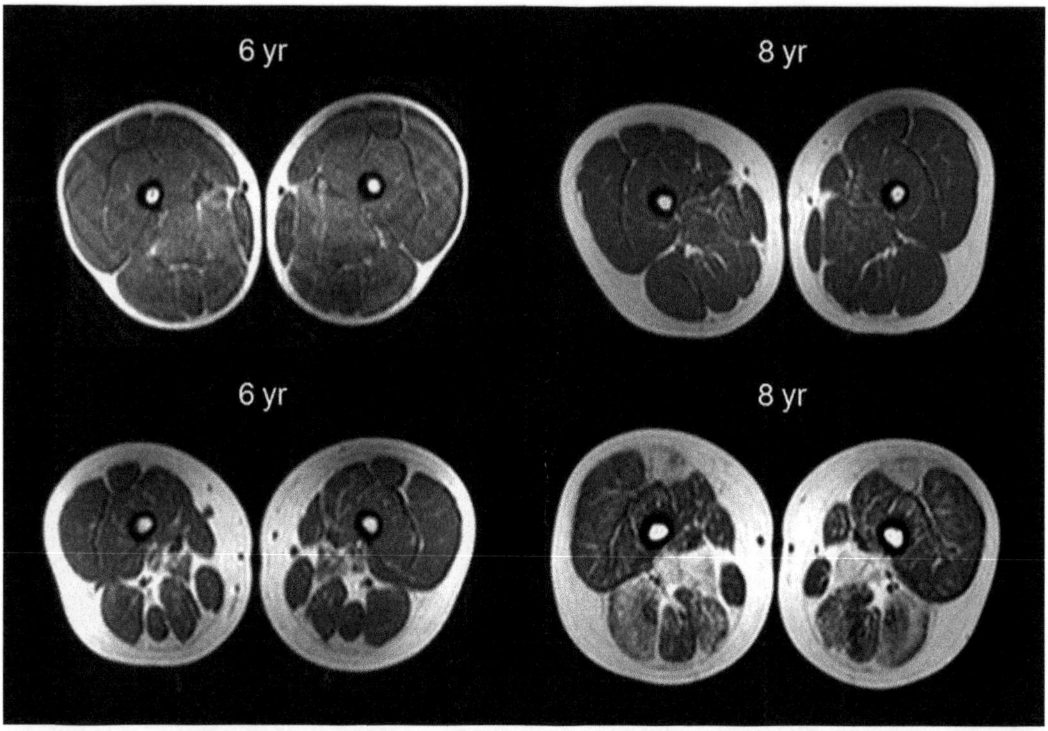

Fig. 17.5 The panel shows axial T1-weighted MR images through the thighs of four different boys with a genetically confirmed diagnosis of DMD. The images illustrate that there can be differences in the degree of pathology and the amount of muscle mass between patients of the same age. The images also illustrate that boys of different ages and therefore different levels of clinical severity can show similar MRI features

and 17.6), but after 6–7 years progressive involvement is usually evident (Figs. 17.5 and 17.6). The degree of muscle pathology may vary among DMD boys of a specific age despite the fact that the overall pattern of involvement is fairly consistent in all patients (Figs. 17.5 and 17.6). Single muscles, such as the rectus femoris, are more severely affected in some patients, and the overall muscle mass also shows interindividual variation (Figs. 17.5 and 17.6).

The abnormal signals are initially confined to the gluteus maximus and adductor magnus, followed by involvement of the quadriceps, rectus femoris and biceps femoris (Figs. 17.5 and 17.6). There is relative sparing of the sartorius, gracilis, semimembranosus and semitendinosus muscles (Figs. 17.5 and 17.6). In the lower legs, the gastrocnemius muscles are affected earlier than the other muscle groups (Figs. 17.5 and 17.6), however on fat suppressed T2-weighted images (e.g. STIR), oedematous changes and possible signs of inflammation can be seen in the muscles not thought to be affected on the standard T1-weighted images. These findings are interesting as they do suggest an inflammatory element, or phase of necrosis associated with oedema, pre-dating the fibrotic/dystrophic change seen later (see Chap. 4).

The abnormal signals are initially confined to the gluteus maximus and adductor magnus, followed by involvement of the quadriceps, rectus femoris, and biceps femoris (Figs. 17.5 and 17.6). There is relative sparing of the sartorius, gracilis, semimembranosus, and semitendinosus muscles (Figs. 17.5 and 17.6). In the lower legs, the gastrocnemius muscles are affected earlier than the other muscle groups (Figs. 17.5 and 17.6). On fat-suppressed T2-weighted images [e.g., STIR images], edematous changes and possible signs of inflammation can be seen in the muscles

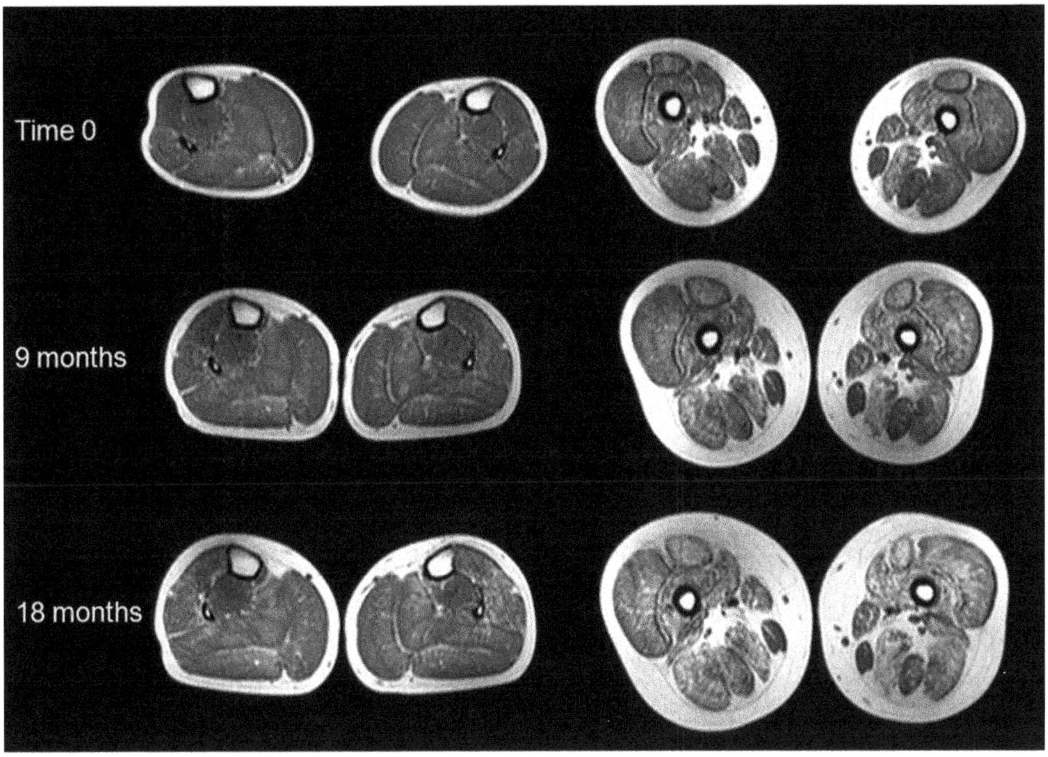

Fig. 17.6 The axial T1-weighted MR images through the calves and thighs of a 6 years old (a) and an 8 years old (b) boy (age at time 0) with DMD show the progression of muscle pathology by MRI over a period of 18 months. The proximal muscles are much more severely affected than the lower leg muscles. In the thigh, the gracilis and the sartorius muscles were best preserved

thought not to be affected based on the standard T1-weighted images. These findings are interesting as they suggest an inflammatory element, or phase of necrosis associated with edema, predating the fibrotic/dystrophic changes seen later (see Chap. 4). Many studies have assessed the pattern of pathology and temporal changes in DMD using subjective, qualitative scoring or semi-quantitative rating scales (see Chap. 4). More recently, techniques such as the three-point Dixon imaging technique have been used to quantify the changes. The results can also be used on a longitudinal basis (see Chap. 5). Strong correlations with both the fat fractions on quantitative MRI and disease progression as indicated on functional testing have been documented. Manual muscle testing and myometry did not demonstrate the same strong correlation with the fat fractions analyzed with quantitative MRI. Quantitative MRI using the three-point Dixon technique is a potentially useful objective, noninvasive tool that correlates strongly with disease progression and particularly functional testing. It is not reliant on patient effort, which in a pediatric situaton is vitally important. The muscle involvement in patients with BMD overall shows a pattern similar to that described for patients with DMD. The sartorius and gracilis are often the most well preserved muscles. Even at a stage where muscles in the thigh are almost completely replaced by fat tissue, patients with BMD are still able to walk (Fig. 17.4).

17.6 Therapy

Currently no curative treatment is available for these conditions. However, the standards of care have been improving steadily over the last few decades and have been disseminated world-wide, prolonging survival, improving quality of life and limiting morbidity from the complications associated with DMD and BMD. The only treatments we have currently are steroids and, cardiac, respiratory and scoliosis management offered in a timely fashion and the clinical management of symptoms and complications.

There have been a number of clinical trials testing new therapeutic strategies, which in itself is a positive development. One of the most promising approaches based on pre-clinical studies and proof of principal studies in humans is the application of antisense oligonucleotides (AONs) for DMD. Trials are ongoing based on AON-induced exon skipping of exon 51 using two different chemical backbones, 2-*0*-methyl AONs (PRO051) and morpholino AONs (AVI-4658).

17.7 Differential Diagnosis

A dystrophinopathy should always be considered in the differential diagnosis of male patients with progressive limb-girdle weakness and elevated serum CK activity. Patients with BMD or a female carrier of a dystrophin mutation may also present with dilated cardiomyopathy with or without muscle weakness as a first symptom.

As both DMD and BMD patients present with limb-girdle weakness, many of the LGMDs (see Chap. 19) fall into the differential diagnosis. Sarcoglycanopathies (see Sect. 19.4) can closely mimic DMD, although inheritance patterns and immunostaining of muscle tissue obtained by biopsy should point to the correct diagnosis. LGMD2I (see Sect. 16.5) may also present with features resembling DMD or BMD, including calf hypertrophy, markedly elevated CK levels, and respiratory and cardiac complications. Genetic analysis can confirm the diagnosis. The various forms of Emery–Dreifuss muscular dystrophy (see Chap. 18) and Pompe disease (see Sect. 14.2.1) are other genetic muscle diseases that can present with progressive limb-girdle weakness. They need to be included in the differential diagnoses of dystrophinopathies. Milder forms of congenital muscular dystrophies (see Chap. 16), particularly the dystroglycanopathies (see Sect. 16.5) and MDC1A (see Sect. 16.2), can also present with predominantly limb-girdle weakness and elevated serum CK and need to be distinguished from the dystrophinopathies. A flow chart demonstrating how muscle imaging and clinical findings may be used to differentiate the dystrophinopathies from other LGMDs is provided in Chap 25.

Dystrophinopathies

Key Points

- The dystrophinopathies DMD and BMD are caused by mutations in the dystrophin gene.
- The dystrophin gene is located on the X chromosome and is the largest known gene to date.
- DMD presents with delayed motor milestones, calf hypertrophy and a raised CK from around 3 years of age, whereas onset of BMD is later and much more variable in childhood through to adulthood. BMD can also present with isolated cardiomyopathy and only minor muscle weakness.
- There is no cure for DMD; however supportive treatment is available including steroid treatment, scoliosis surgery, non-invasive ventilation and treatment of cardiomyopathy.
- Muscle imaging is less important for diagnostic purposes in the dystrophinopathies but might help to define objective measures of muscle pathology.

Suggestions for Further Reading

Arai Y, Osawa M, Fukuyama Y. Muscle CT scans in preclinical cases of Duchenne and Becker muscular dystrophy. Brain Develop. 1995;17:95–103.

Bushby K, Finkel R, Birnkrant DJ, et al. Diagnosis and management of Duchennemuscular dystrophy, part 1: diagnosis, and pharmacological and psychosocial management. Lancet Neurol. 2010a;9:77–93.

Bushby K, Finkel R, Birnkrant DJ, et al. Diagnosis and management of Duchenne muscular dystrophy, part 2: implementation of multidisciplinary care. Lancet Neurol. 2010b;9:177–89.

Engel AE, Franzini-Armstrong C. Myology. In: Chapter 1: Muscular Dystrophies, 3rd ed. Dystrophinopathies 2004;2:961–1025.

Finanger EL, Russman B, Forbes SC, et al. Use of skeletal muscle MRI in diagnosis and monitoring disease progression in Duchenne muscular dystrophy. Phys Med Rehabil Clin N Am. 2012;23:1–10.

Jansen M, van Alfen N, Nijhuis van der Sanden MW, et al. Quantitative muscle ultrasound is a promising longitudinal follow-up tool in Duchenne muscular dystrophy. Neuromuscul Disord. 2012;22:306–17.

Mercuri E, Pichiecchio A, Allsop J, et al. Muscle MRI in inherited neuromuscular disorders: past, present and future. J Mag Res Imag. 2007;25:433–40.

Torriani M, Townsend E, Thomas BJ, et al. Lower leg muscle involvement in Duchenne muscular dystrophy: an MR imaging and spectroscopy study. Skeletal Radiol. 2012;41:437–45.

Wren T, Bluml S, Tseng-Ong L, et al. Three point technique of fat quantification of muscle tissue as a marker of disease progression in Duchenne muscular dystrophy: preliminary study. AJR Am J Roentgenol. 2008;190:W8–12.

18 Emerinopathies and Laminopathies

Nicola Carboni and Marco Mura

18.1 Introduction and Classification

Emerinopathies and laminopathies are disorders caused by alterations in genes coding for ubiquitous proteins of the nuclear envelope.

The nuclear envelope is a complex membrane structure that separates the nucleus from the cytoplasm in eukaryotic cells. It consists of an outer nuclear membrane (ONM), an inner nuclear membrane (INM), nuclear pore complexes, and the nuclear lamina, a fibrous meshwork located immediately underneath the INM.

The inner and ONMs are joined at nuclear pore complexes, essential aqueous channels that mediate bidirectional transport of proteins, RNAs, and ribonucleoprotein complexes across the nuclear envelope, from the nucleus to the cytoplasm and vice versa (Fig. 18.1).

The structural elements of the nuclear envelope have different physical and biochemical properties. The outer membrane is particularly rich in Klarsicht/ANC-1/Syne homology (KASH) domain proteins. These molecules bind to Sad1p/UNC-84 (SUN) domains proteins of the INM within the periplasmic space of the nuclear envelope. Other proteins highly expressed in the ONM are nesprins, which bind to actin. The nuclear pore complex is composed mainly of proteins known as nucleoporins. Integral membrane proteins of the INM include emerin, lamina-associated polypeptide (LAP) 1, LAP2, MAN1, lamin B receptor, and nurim. The majority of these proteins interact with lamins, chromatin, and other proteins located within the nucleus. The nuclear lamina is an intermediate filament network composed mainly of proteins called lamins.

The most common disorders of the nuclear envelope are emerinopathies and laminopathies, respectively caused by mutations in the emerin gene (*STA*), also known as *EMD* gene, and the lamin A/C gene (*LMNA*). Alterations of the *EMD* gene cause the X-recessive form of Emery–Dreifuss muscular dystrophy. Mutations of the *LMNA* gene are associated with different clinical entities.

The variety of clinical entities associated with alterations of the *LMNA* gene can be divided broadly into two groups based on organ system compromise. The first group of disorders, affecting skeletal and cardiac muscle and peripheral nerves, includes the autosomal dominant and recessive forms of Emery–Dreifuss muscular dystrophy (EDMD2 and EDMD3), limb-girdle muscular dystrophy 1B (LGMD1B), dilated cardiomyopathy with conduction defects (DCM1A), the autosomal recessive form of sensorimotor peripheral axonal neuropathy CMT2B1. The second group comprises lipodystrophies, premature

N. Carboni (✉)
Neuromuscular Unit, Multiple Sclerosis Center, University of Cagliari, Cagliari, Italy
e-mail: nikola.carboni@tiscali.it

M. Mura
Complex Operative Unit of Radiology, AOU Cagliari, Policlinico di Monserrato, Cagliari, Sardinia, Italy

M.P. Wattjes and D. Fischer (eds.), *Neuromuscular Imaging*, DOI 10.1007/978-1-4614-6552-2_18,

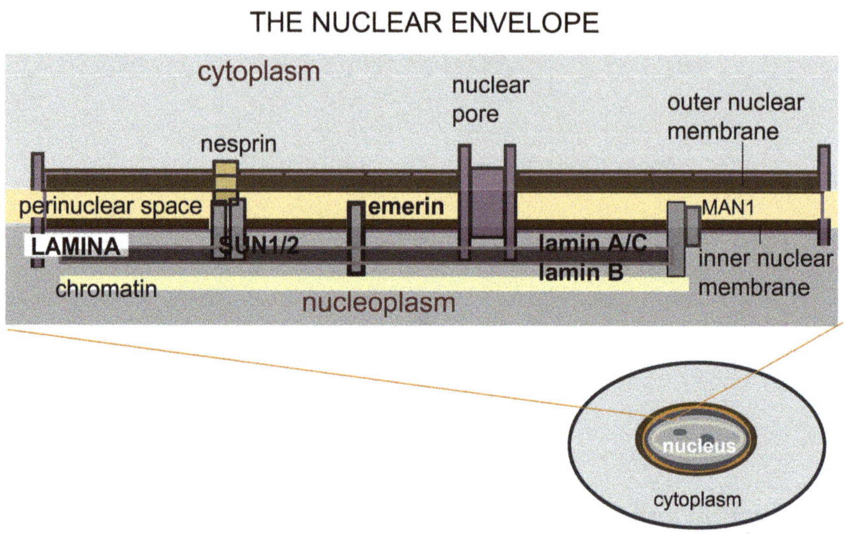

Fig. 18.1 Nuclear envelope. See outer and inner nuclear membranes, nuclear pore complexes, and nuclear lamina. Courtesy of Dr. Giovanna Lattanzi, CNR, Bologna

aging syndrome, and mandibuloacral dysplasia. Finally, numerous heterogeneous situations with overlapping syndromes have been reported, forming a group of disorders characterized by the concomitant presence of two or more clinical entities.

As yet, exact estimates of the prevalence and incidence of disorders due to *LMNA* and *STA* gene mutations are unavailable. Some authors report an incidence of 1/1,000,000 for the X-recessive form of EDMD and an incidence between 1/100,000 and 3/100,000 for the autosomal dominant form of EDMD. There are no reports on the incidence and prevalence of either LGMD1B or lipodystrophy due to *LMNA* gene mutations. The incidence of dilated cardiomyopathy with conduction defects due to alterations of the gene coding for A-type lamins is between 5/100,000 and 8/100,000.

18.2 X-Linked Emery–Dreifuss Muscular Dystrophy

18.2.1 Synonyms, Abbreviations

Emery–Dreifuss muscular dystrophy (EDMD), X-linked Emery–Dreifuss muscular dystrophy (X-EDMD, EDMD1)

18.2.2 Genetics and Pathophysiology

The X-linked form of Emery–Dreifuss muscular dystrophy is a clinical entity caused by alterations of the gene coding for emerin.

Emerin is encoded by the *EMD/STA* gene, located on chromosome Xq28. This small nuclear envelope protein contributes to the structural integrity of the INM, where it interacts with nesprin 1α, lamins, actin, barrier-to-autointegration factor (BAF), and molecules involved in gene expression, the regulation of transcription, and RNA splicing. All of these interactions lead to the hypothesis that emerin has a role in nuclear assembly, maintenance of nuclear envelope stability, and gene regulation. Mutations in the *STA* gene are responsible for the X-linked recessive form of Emery–Dreifuss muscular dystrophy (X-EDMD) (OMIM#310300). The pathogenetic variations so far identified include deletions, insertions, duplications, missense, and nonsense mutations.

18.2.3 Histopathology

The histopathological findings of muscle biopsies from subjects with X-EDMD may include mild to moderate changes in fiber size and shape, atrophic fibers, internal muscle nucleation, mild

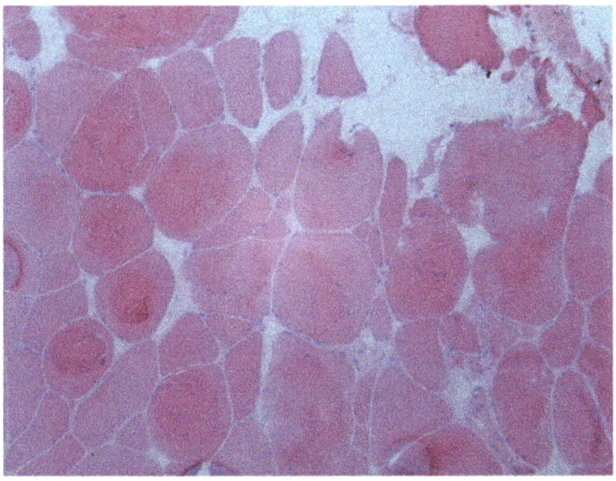

Fig. 18.2 Severe dystrophic alterations in an adult patient with the X-linked form of Emery–Dreifuss muscular dystrophy. note the marked variation in fiber size and shape, the increased connective and adipose tissue, internal nucleation, splitting, and necrosis

Fig. 18.3 Immunohistochemistry. Absence of emerin labeling in a patient with the X-linked recessive form of Emery–Dreifuss muscular dystrophy

increase of adipose and connective tissue, and more rarely the presence of necrotizing and regenerating fibers. Other structural abnormalities include decreased size of type 1 fibers and core formation.

In rare cases, muscular dystrophies related to *STA* gene mutations may present markedly severe histological alterations on muscle biopsy (Fig. 18.2). Histopathology may reveal overt dystrophic changes such as marked fiber size variability, increased connective tissue, and abundant necrotic/regenerating fibers; cellular infiltrates may also be present.

Immunohistochemistry studies clearly show the absence of emerin but normal labeling of lamins and all sarcolemmal membrane-associated proteins (Figs. 18.3 and 18.4).

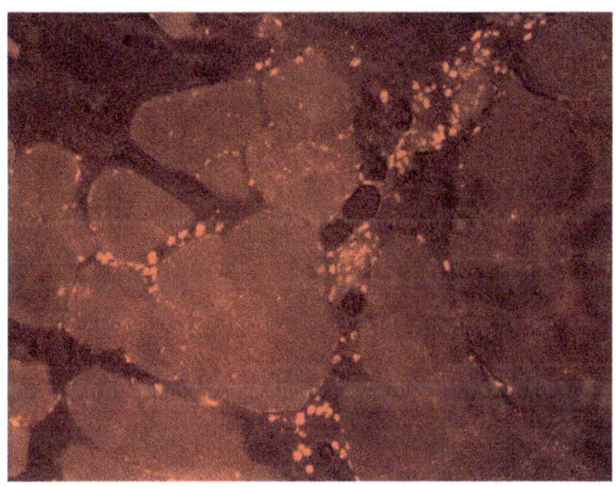

Fig. 18.4 Immunohistochemistry. Normal lamin A/C labeling in a patient with the X-linked recessive form of Emery–Dreifuss muscular dystrophy

18.2.4 Clinical Presentation

The clinical features of EDMD include early contractures of the elbows and Achilles tendons, weakness of humeroperoneal muscles, rigidity of the spine, and cardiac abnormalities. In classic X-linked inheritance, males have full clinical manifestations of the disease, whereas females are carriers and are usually asymptomatic (Fig. 18.5). However, females may develop cardiac alterations including conduction defects, supraventricular tachycardia, dilated cardiomyopathy, and even heart failure. Although rare, males can also present with a limb girdle-like phenotype associated with alterations in the *STA* gene. Patients almost invariably develop symptoms of cardiac impairment during the third decade of life.

Cardiac disease usually presents with conduction defects or other onset modalities, including supraventricular arrhythmias.

With time, patients may develop dilatation of atria and ventricles—up to overt dilated cardiomyopathy. Individuals with *STA* gene mutations are at high risk of sudden cardiac death, generally due to severe bradyarrhythmias.

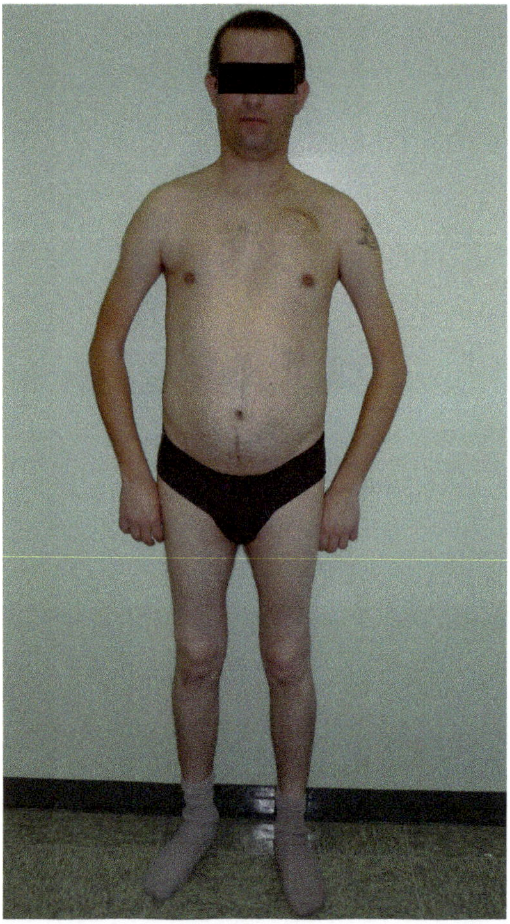

Fig. 18.5 Clinical features of an adult male with the X-linked recessive form of Emery–Dreifuss muscular dystrophy. Note the humeral-peroneal distribution of hypotrophy, contractures of the elbows and Achilles tendons, and rigidity of the spine

In EDMD1 patients, the risk of sudden death due to cardiac arrest can be dramatically reduced by pacemaker implantation. However, recent reports of sustained ventricular tachycardia episodes in young males with the X-EDMD have shown that *STA* gene alterations potentially determine the development of lethal ventricular arrhythmias.

18.2.5 Imaging Findings

To date, there have been few imaging studies of skeletal muscle impairment in EDMD1 patients. Two patients with involvement predominantly of the lower leg soleus muscles and minor changes in thigh muscles have been described. Recently, a muscle imaging study conducted on a large family demonstrated possible compromise of the medial head of the gastrocnemius in adult patients and variable compromise of thigh muscles. The thigh muscles affected were the semimembranosus, vastii, adductor magnus, and the long head of the biceps femoris (Figs. 18.6, 18.7, and 18.8).

18.2.6 Therapy

There is currently no treatment available to cure patients with EDMD1. Symptomatic treatment is the only treatment strategy available. In particular, correct management of cardiac and respiratory complications may increase the quality of life and life expectancy of these patients.

18.2.7 Differential Diagnosis

The clinical entities that may mimic X-EDMD are the forms of EDMD due to other genes, including *LMNA* (see Sects. 18.2 and 18.3), *FHL1*, *SYNE1*, and *SYNE2*. These variants of EDMD have the same clinical features as EDMD1, being characterized by a humeroperoneal pattern of muscular weakness, contractures of the elbows and Achilles tendons, rigid spine, and cardiac compromise. Other disorders to be ruled out in the differential diagnosis of X-EDMD are Bethlem myopathy (see Sect. 16.4), rigid spine muscular dystrophy 1 (RSMD1) related to *SEPN1* mutations (see Sect. 15.3), and limb-girdle muscular dystrophy 2A (LGMD2A) (see Sect. 19.2). The clinical phenotype for subjects suffering from these disorders is similar to that of patients with EDMD1. Imaging findings of EDMD due to *LMNA* gene alterations are dealt with in the next section and are not be discussed here. So far, there are no descriptions of skeletal muscle imaging studies in subjects with *FHL1*, *SYNE1*, or *SYNE2* gene alterations.

Bethlem myopathy (see Sect. 16.4) is a relatively benign disorder caused by alterations in

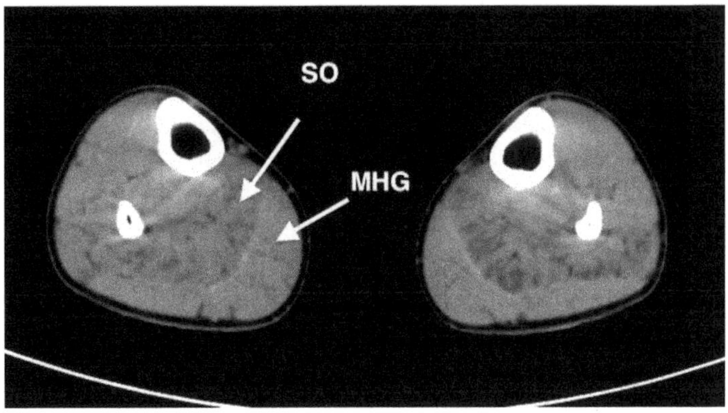

Fig. 18.6 Computed tomography (CT) scans of leg muscles in a young patient with the X-linked form of Emery–Dreifuss muscular dystrophy. Note the severe bilateral alterations in the soleus (*SO*) muscles

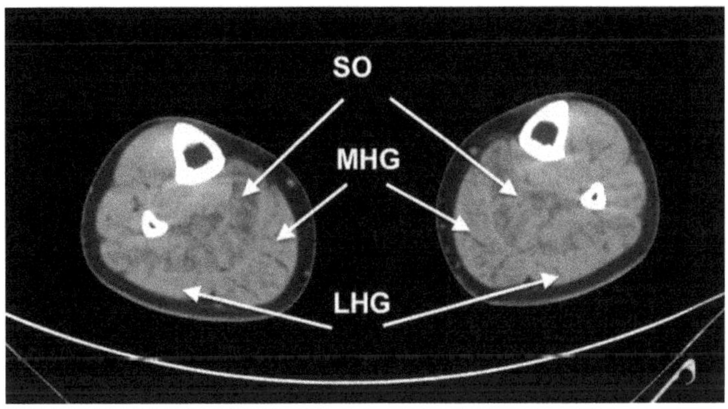

Fig. 18.7 CT scans of leg muscles in a patient with the X-linked form of Emery–Dreifuss muscular dystrophy. Note the alterations in the soleus (*SO*) and medial head of the gastrocnemius (*MHG*)

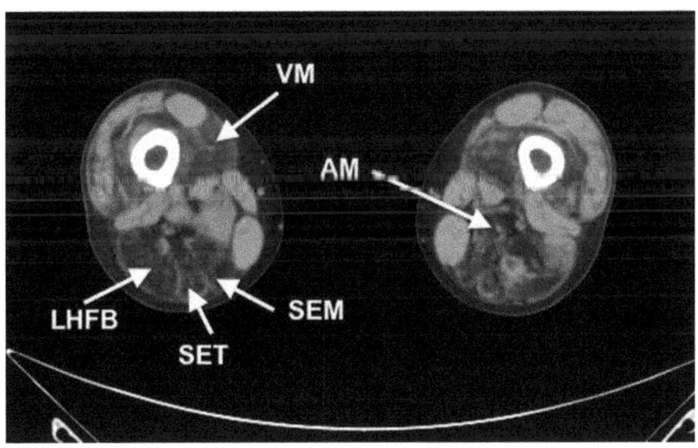

Fig. 18.8 Thigh muscles of a patient with the X-linked form of Emery–Dreifuss muscular dystrophy. Note the severe alterations in the semimembranosus muscle (*SEM*), vastii muscles (*VM*), adductor magnus (*AM*), and long head of the biceps femoris (*LHFB*)

one of the genes implicated in the synthesis of type IV collagen extracellular matrix proteins. Individuals with Bethlem myopathy show proximal muscle weakness associated with rigidity of the spine, contractures of the elbows, tendon Achilles, and long finger flexors. Imaging studies of the thigh in these subjects have revealed peculiar alterations at the periphery of vasti muscles and increased signal in the rectus femoris. Leg muscle imaging studies frequently reveal impairment at the periphery of both gastrocnemii muscles.

Another clinical condition that can mimic EDMD1 is RSMD1 related to *SEPN1* mutations (see Sect. 15.3). This disorder, usually slowly progressive, is characterized by hypotonia, proximal and axial weakness, and rigidity of the spine. In the later stages of RSMD1, patients frequently present with respiratory insufficiency and inconstant impairment of bulbar muscles. Imaging studies of the thigh show predominant compromise of the sartorius muscles. Legs muscle imaging shows no significant or only minimal alterations.

Individuals with LGMD2A (see Sect. 19.2) may have proximal muscle weakness and atrophy with an early scapular-humeral-pelvic distribution. Contractures of the elbows, paraspinal muscles, hamstrings, and Achilles tendons may also occur. Subjects with LGMD2A show predominant compromise of the adductor magnus and posterior thigh muscles. At calf level, alterations of the soleus muscle and the medial head of the gastrocnemius have been detected. LGMD2A is not usually associated with cardiac compromise, and respiratory failure in the later stages of the disease is limited to severe cases.

Emerinopathies and Laminopathies: X-Linked Emery–Dreifuss Muscular Dystrophy

Key Points

- EDMD1 is X-EDMD.
- EDMD1 is caused by a mutation of the *EMD/STA* gene, which encodes emerin, a protein of the inner nuclear membrane.
- Muscle biopsy may show variable changes, ranging from myopathic to overt dystrophic alterations.
- Immunohistochemistry shows absence of emerin labeling.
- The clinical phenotype includes a humeroperoneal pattern of muscular weakness, contractures, and cardiac compromise
- In EDMD1, imaging studies show marked involvement of calf muscles.
- EDMD1 patients may show variable compromise of thigh muscles including vastii, muscles, adductor magnus, and the long head of the biceps femoris.

Suggestions for Further Reading

Bonne G. Diseases associated with myonuclear abnormalities. In: George K, editor. Structural and Molecular Basis of Skeletal Muscle Disease, 1st ed. Basel: ISN Neuropath Press; 2002. p. 47–56.

Carboni N, Mura M, Mercuri E, et al. Cardiac and muscle imaging findings in a family with X-linked Emery–Dreifuss muscular dystrophy. Neuromuscul Disord. 2012;22:152–8.

Franke WW, Scheer U, Krohne G, et al. The nuclear envelope and the architecture of the nuclear periphery. J Cell Biol. 1981;91:39s–50s.

Mercuri E, Counsell S, Allsop J, et al. Selective muscle involvement on magnetic resonance imaging in autosomal dominant Emery–Dreifuss muscular dystrophy. Neuropaediatrics 2002;33:10–14.

Mercuri E, Clements E, Offiah A, et al. Muscle magnetic resonance imaging involvement in muscular dystrophies with rigidity of the spine. Ann Neurol. 2010;67:201–8.

Sakata K, Shimizu M, Ino H, et al. High incidence of sudden cardiac death with conduction disturbances and atrial cardiomyopathy caused by a nonsense mutation in the STA gene. Circulation 2005;111: 3352–58.

Toniolo D. Emery–Dreifuss muscular dystrophy. In: Emery AEH, editor. The Muscular Dystrophies, 1st ed. Oxford University Press, 2001. p. 95–108.

18.3 Autosomal Dominant Emery–Dreifuss Muscular Dystrophy

18.3.1 Synonyms, Abbreviations

Emery–Dreifuss muscular dystrophy (EDMD), (AD-EDMD, EDMD2)

18.3.2 Genetics and Pathophysiology

The autosomal dominant form of Emery–Dreifuss muscular dystrophy (OMIM#181350) is a disorder caused by mutations of the *LMNA* gene, which encodes lamins A and C, two proteins of the nuclear envelope.

Lamins of the A and C type are alternatively spliced products of the *LMNA* gene, located on chromosome 1q21.23. These proteins are essential scaffolding components of the nuclear lamina, forming a meshwork of intermediate filaments that is attached to the inner membrane of the nuclear envelope.

Lamins have a plethora of binding partners, including structural proteins, transcription fac-

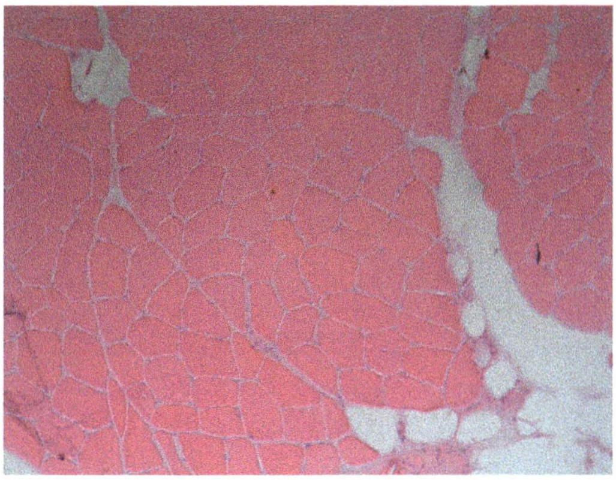

Fig. 18.9 Mild myopathic changes in a patient with an *LMNA* gene alteration. Note the variation in fiber size and shape and mild increase in connective tissue

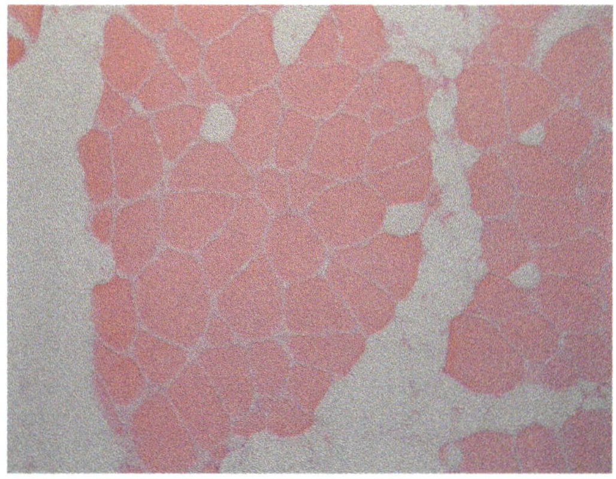

Fig. 18.10 Dystrophic alterations in a young patient with congenital-onset muscular dystrophy due to an *LMNA* gene mutation. Note the marked variability in fiber size and shape and the increased connective and adipose tissue

tors, chromatin components, signal transduction molecules, and several molecules with regulatory functions. Similar to emerin, lamins have several key functional roles: maintenance of nuclear integrity and mechanical stability, chromatin organization, regulation of the cell cycle, and metabolic, biochemical, and signal transduction pathways. Alterations of the *LMNA* gene associated with phenotypes of skeletal and/or cardiac muscle impairment are spread throughout the gene.

18.3.3 Histopathology

The histopathological findings of muscle biopsies from subjects with AD-EDMD are similar to those of patients with the X-EDMD. Histological findings mostly include mild to moderate changes in fiber size and shape, atrophic fibers, internal muscle nucleation, mild increase of adipose and connective tissue, and more rarely the presence of necrotizing and regenerating fibers. Other structural abnormalities may include decreased size of type 1 fibers and core formation (Fig. 18.9).

Muscle biopsies from patients with AD-EDMD may show markedly severe histological alterations (Fig. 18.10). In such cases, histopathology may reveal overt dystrophic changes including marked fiber size variability, increased connective tissue, and abundant necrotic/regenerating fibers; cellular infiltrates may also be present.

Immunohistochemistry studies clearly show normal labeling of emerin and lamins (Figs. 18.11 and 18.12). Also, all sarcolemmal membrane-associated proteins are present, with the exception of laminin β1, which may be reduced in adult patients with EDMD2.

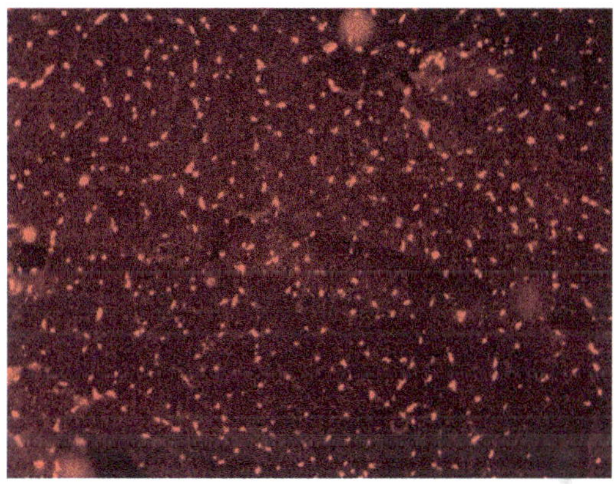

Fig. 18.11 Immunohistochemistry. Normal emerin labeling in a patient with EDMD2

18.3.4 Clinical Presentation

Skeletal muscle changes are prominent findings in AD-EDMD and are the same as those found in subjects with the X-linked form of EDMD (Fig. 18.13). Females carrying an *LMNA* gene mutation may have the same clinical phenotype as affected males. Patients almost invariably develop symptoms of cardiac impairment during the third decade of life.

Cardiac disease usually presents with conduction defects or other onset modalities, including supraventricular arrhythmias.

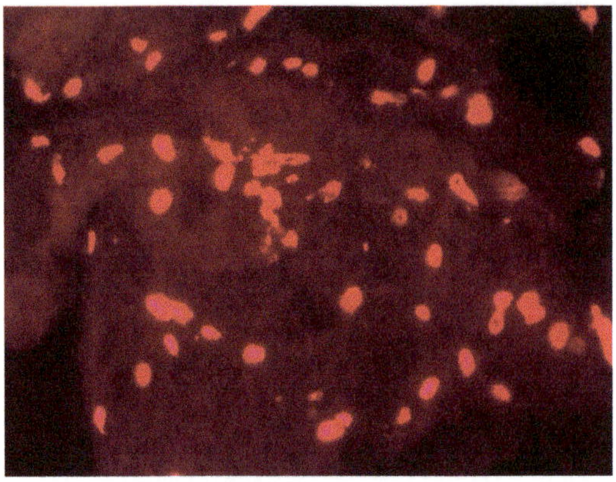

Fig. 18.12 Immunohistochemistry. Normal lamin A/C labeling in a patient with EDMD2

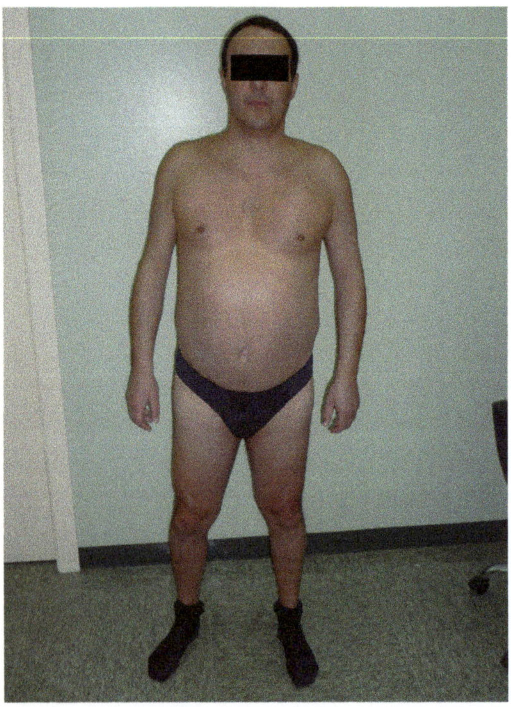

Fig. 18.13 Clinical features of a man with mild Emery–Dreifuss muscular dystrophy related to an *LMNA* gene mutation. Note the mild hypotrophy in the humeral-peroneal muscles, contractures of the elbows and Achilles tendons, and rigidity of the spine

With time, patients may develop dilatation of atria and ventricles—up to overt dilated cardiomyopathy. Individuals with *STA* gene mutations are at high risk of sudden cardiac death, generally due to severe bradyarrhythmias.

Also in EDMD2 patients, the risk of sudden death due to cardiac arrest can be dramatically reduced by pacemaker implantation.

18.3.5 Imaging Findings

See Sect. 18.7.

18.3.6 Differential Diagnosis

Differential diagnosis of AD-EDMD includes the forms of EDMD due to alterations of the *STA* (see Sect. 18.2), *FHL1*, *SYNE1*, and *SYNE2* genes.

Other disorders that have to be excluded are Bethlem myopathy (see Sect. 16.4), Rigid spine with muscular dystrophy 1 (see Sect. 15.3) and LGMD2A (see Sect. 19.2). Clinical and imaging findings of these clinical entities have been discussed in the section dealing with Emerinopathies (see Sect. 18.2).

Emerinopathies and Laminopathies: Autosomal Dominant Emery–Dreifuss Muscular Dystrophy

Key Points

- EDMD2 is the autosomal dominant form of Emery–Dreifuss muscular dystrophy.
- This clinical entity is due to alterations in the *LMNA* gene.
- Muscle biopsy may show variable histological alterations, ranging from mild, unspecific myopathic findings to severe dystrophic changes.
- The clinical phenotype is the same as that of EDMD1.
- In EDMD2, imaging studies show marked compromise of calf muscles.
- EDMD2 patients may have variable compromise of thigh muscles, including the vastii, adductor magnus, semimembranosus, and the long head of the biceps femoris.

Suggestions for Further Reading

Carboni N, Mura M, Marrosu G, et al. Muscle MRI findings in patients with an apparently exclusive cardiac phenotype due to a novel LMNA gene mutation. Neuromuscul Disord. 2008;18:291–8.

Dubowitz V, Sewry CA. Muscular dystrophies and allied disorders IV: Emery–Dreifuss muscular dystrophies and Bethlem myopathy. In: Dubowitz V, Sewry CA, editors. Muscle Biopsy A practical approach. 3rd ed. Saunders Edition. 2006. p. 377–94.

Mercuri E, Clements E, Offiah A, et al. Muscle magnetic resonance imaging involvement in muscular dystrophies with rigidity of the spine. Ann Neurol. 2010;67: 201–208.

Meune C, Van Berlo JH, Anselme F, et al. Primary prevention of sudden death in patients with lamin A/C gene mutations. N Engl J Med 2006;354:209–10.

Wu W, Muchir A, Shan J, et al. Mitogen-activated protein kinase inhibitors improve heart function and prevent fibrosis in cardiomyopathy caused by mutation in lamin A/C gene. Circulation 2011;123:53–61.

18.4 Limb Girdle Muscular Dystrophy Type 1B

18.4.1 Synonyms, Abbreviations

LGMD1B; autosomal dominant Emery–Dreifuss muscular dystrophy (EDMD2)

18.4.2 Genetics and Pathophysiology

The genetics and pathophysiology of LGMD1B are consistent with the autosomal form of Emery–Dreifuss muscular dystrophy due to *LMNA* gene mutations.

18.4.3 Histopathology

The histopathological findings of muscle biopsies from subjects with LGMD1B are not specific. They may include mild to moderate variability in fiber size and shape, internal nucleation, increased connective tissue, and fiber splitting consists in the division of a muscle fiber into different fibers. It is typically seen in most muscular dystrophies but it can also be detected in chronic neuropathies. In some cases, other structural abnormalities have been reported, including decreased size of type 1 fibers.

Immunohistochemistry shows normal labeling of lamins and all sarcolemmal membrane-associated proteins.

18.4.4 Clinical Presentation

Individuals with the autosomal dominant form of LGMD associated with *LMNA* gene mutations present with proximal muscle weakness and mild joint contractures. Cardiac compromise is the same as in EDMD2.

18.4.5 Therapy

The treatment approach is comparable to that of EDMD.

18.4.6 Imaging Findings

See Sect. 18.7.

18.4.7 Differential Diagnosis

Once the likely autosomal dominant inheritance has been established, the disorders that must be taken into account in the differential diagnosis of LGMD1B are all of the other currently known forms of autosomal dominant LGMD (see Chap. 19), Bethlem myopathy (see Sect. 16.4), and facioscapulohumeral muscular dystrophy (FSHD) (see Chap. 23).

LGMD1A (see Sect. 20.4) is a disorder due to alterations of the gene encoding the myotilin protein. The clinical phenotype is characterized by proximal weakness, mild contractures, and in some cases dysarthria. To date, there are no descriptions of cardiac compromise in these patients.

LGMD1C (see Sect. 19.5) in humans is associated with mutations in the *CAV-3* gene. This gene encodes caveolin-3, a protein that is expressed in cardiomyocytes and skeletal muscle fibers. Patients with LGMD due to *CAV-3* gene mutations generally experience early proximal weakness and calf hypertrophy. The disease course is variable, ranging from mild myopathy to moderate or severe compromise of muscle strength. As for LGMD1A, there are no reports of cardiac compromise in individuals with LGMD due to *CAV-3* mutations.

Another disorder to be considered in the differential diagnosis of LGMD1B is LGMD1D, a rare muscular dystrophy related to alteration of the genetic coding for the intermediate filament protein desmin. This form of muscular dystrophy is characterized by slow progression and mild proximal muscle weakness. Cardiac compromise is similar to that observed in patients with LGMD1B. The few studies of LGMD1D families report rhythm conduction defects in affected subjects and the possibility of developing dilated cardiomyopathy with advanced disease.

There are four other forms of LGMD with autosomal dominant inheritance. The causative genes for LGMD1E-H (recently linked to known loci) are yet to be identified. LGMD1E is linked to 7q36, LGMD1F to 7q32.1-q32.2, LGMD1G to 4q21, and LGMD1H to 3p25.1-p23. The clinical course of these forms is characterized by slow progression of proximal muscle weakness. There are no reports of cardiac compromise. Recent imaging studies performed on a group of subjects with the 7q36-linked disease revealed early compromise of the adductor magnus and semimembranosus as well as fibrous and fat replacement in all thigh muscles. Involvement of the sartorius and rectus femoris muscles was observed during the later stages of the disease. Imaging studies of leg muscle showed early compromise of the gastrocnemius and soleus and late compromise of deep toe flexors. There are no reports of skeletal muscle imaging findings in individuals with LGMD1F-H.

Bethlem myopathy (see Sect. 16.4) must also be included in the differential diagnosis of LGMD1B. The clinical and imaging features of this disorder have already been described in the section dealing with Emerinopathies.

Another disorder that can mimic LGMD1B is facioscapulohumeral dystrophy (FSHD) (see Chap. 23). This autosomal dominant disorder results from deletion of D4Z4 tandem repeats on chromosome 4q35. Facial weakness is often the earliest sign of the disease, but involvement of scapular, humeral, and hip girdle muscles may prompt the initial clinical evaluation. Several cases with a scapuloperoneal distribution of weakness have been described. Typically, many familial cases have been reported with marked phenotypic variability among relatives carrying the same genetic alteration. Several cases with proximal muscle involvement and only mild impairment of facial expression have been described. In such cases, it may be difficult to differentiate this form from the other autosomal dominant forms of LGMD. Muscle imaging studies in patients with the classic form of FSHD showed asymmetrical compromise of the adductor magnus, hamstrings, rectus femoris, and tibialis anterior.

Emerinopathies and Laminopathies: Limb Girdle Muscular Dystrophy Type 1B

Key Points

- Patients with LGMD1B present with proximal muscle weakness and mild contractures.
- LGMD1B is due to alterations of the gene coding for A-type lamins.
- Histopathology may show mild to moderate alterations of skeletal muscle fibers.
- Immunohistochemistry shows normal labeling of lamins and all sarcolemmal membrane-associated proteins.
- Imaging studies of LGMD1B patients show compromise of posterior leg muscles.
- LGMD1B patients may also show compromise of posterior thigh muscles.

Suggestions for Further Reading

Carboni N, Floris M, Valentini M, et al. A novel mutation in lamin A/C gene: phenotype and consequences on the protein structure and flexibility. SRX Biol. Volume 2010, Article ID 301679.

Carboni N, Mura M, Marrosu G, et al. Muscle imaging analogies in a cohort of patients with different clinical phenotypes caused by LMNA gene mutations. Muscle Nerve. 2010;41:458–63.

Hermans MC, Pinto YM, Merkies IS, et al. Hereditary muscular dystrophies and the heart. Neuromuscul Disord. 2010;20:479–92.
Muchir A, Bonne G, van der Kooi AJ, et al. Identification of mutations in the gene encoding lamins A/C in autosomal dominant limb girdle muscular dystrophy with atrioventricular conduction disturbances (LGMD1B). Hum Mol Genet. 2000;9:1453–9.
Satu S, Sanna H, Jaakko S, et al. The enigma of 7q36 linked autosomal dominant limb girdle muscular dystrophy. J Neurol Neurosurg Psychiatry 2010;81:834–9.
van der Kooi AJ, van Meegen M, Ledderhof TM, et al. Genetic localization of a newly recognized autosomal dominant limb-girdle muscular dystrophy with cardiac involvement (LGMD1B) to chromosome 1q11-21. Am J Hum Genet. 1997;60:891–5.
Volpi L, Ricci G, Passino C, et al. Prevalent cardiac phenotype resulting in heart transplantation in a novel LMNA gene duplication. Neuromuscul Disord. 2010;20:512–6.

18.5 Dilated Cardiomyopathy with Conduction Defects

18.5.1 Synonyms, Abbreviations

Dilated cardiomyopathy with conduction defects (CMD1A)

18.5.2 Genetics and Pathophysiology

The genetics and pathophysiology of CMD1A are consistent with the autosomal form of Emery–Dreifuss muscular dystrophy due to *LMNA* gene mutations.

18.5.3 Histopathology

Muscle biopsy from subjects with CMD1A typically shows no histological or immunohistochemical abnormalities.

18.5.4 Clinical Presentation

CMD1A, an allelic disorder to LGMD1B and EDMD2, is characterized by progressive dilated cardiomyopathy with conduction abnormalities, poor ejection fraction, and the absence of clinically detectable skeletal muscle weakness or contractures. Cardiac conduction defects are commonly the leading clinical manifestations, often followed by supraventricular/ventricular arrhythmias and left and/or right atrial enlargement. The prognosis is generally poor with a high risk of sudden cardiac death from recurrent ventricular tachyarrhythmias or, more rarely, heart failure.

Patients with this syndrome require scheduled routine clinical and instrumental investigations, including standard electrocardiography (ECG), Holter ECG, and echocardiograpy. ICD implantation should be considered.

18.5.5 Imaging Findings

See Sect. 18.7.

18.5.6 Therapy

There is currently no curative treatment for CMD1A patients. Therapeutic strategies focus primarily on the symptomatic manifestations of the disease. In particular, correct management of cardiac compromise can ameliorate the quality of life and life expectancy of these patients. Recent experimental studies have identified molecules that are potentially useful for treating cardiomyopathy caused by *LMNA* mutations. It has been shown how mitogen-activated protein kinase inhibitors improve cardiac function in hearts of Lmna H222P knock-in mice. These results are promising and give hope to CMD1A patients for more therapeutic benefits in the future.

18.5.7 Differential Diagnosis

Before pointing to a genetic cause for dilated cardiomyopathy, it is worth excluding common underlying causes such as arterial disease. Although less common, other causes of dilated cardiomyopathy include inflammatory processes (e.g., sarcoidosis, giant cell myocarditis) and infectious diseases (e.g., Chagas disease).

Familial dilated cardiomyopathies can be differentiated according to their inheritance. The most common forms have an autosomal dominant inheritance. So far, more than 30 genes responsible for dominant forms of dilated cardiomyopathies have been identified. *LMNA* is the gene most frequently responsible for these clinical entities. The majority of genetically identified familial dilated cardiomyopathy are due to alterations of the gene coding for A type lamins. Other genes associated with familial dilated cardiomyopathies are *MYH6*, *MYH7*, *MYBPC3*, *TNNT2*, and *SCN5A*.

More rarely, dilated cardiomyopathies have an X-linked (X-linked dilated cardiomyopathy due to mutations of the genes coding for the dystrophin or tafazzin proteins) or autosomal recessive inheritance. Alternatively, they may be due to mitochondrial DNA (mtDNA) alterations.

Emerinopathies and Laminopathies: Dilated Cardiomyopathy with Conduction Defects

Key Points

- Subjects with an *LMNA* gene mutation may show a phenotype with isolated dilated cardiomyopathy and cardiac conduction defects.
- The muscle biopsy is normal.
- Subjects with selective cardiac compromise due to *LMNA* gene mutations may have subclinical alterations of skeletal muscles detectable by imaging studies.
- There may be subclinical involvement of posterior leg muscles in subjects with selective cardiac compromise associated with *LMNA* gene mutations.

Suggestions for Further Reading

Carboni N, Mura M, Marrosu G, et al. Muscle MRI findings in patients with an apparently exclusive cardiac phenotype due to a novel LMNA gene mutation. Neuromuscul Disord. 2008;18:291–8.

Carboni N, Mura M, Marrosu G, et al. Muscle imaging analogies in a cohort of patients with different clinical phenotypes caused by LMNA gene mutations. Muscle Nerve. 2010;41:458–63.

Carboni N, Floris M, Mateddu A, et al. Aberrant splicing in the LMNA gene caused by a novel mutation on the polypyrimidine tract of intron 5. Muscle Nerve. 2011;43:688–93.

Fatkin D, Mac Rae C, Sasaki T, et al. Missense mutations in the rod domain of the lamin A/C gene as causes of dilated cardiomyopathy and conduction-system disease. N Engl J Med. 1999;341:1715–24.

Hersberger RE. Update 2011: clinical and genetic issues in familial dilated cardiomyopathy. J Am Coll Cardiol. 2011;57:1641–9.

Malhotra R, Mason PK. Lamin A/C deficiency as a cause of familial dilated cardiomyopathy. Curr Opin Cardiol. 2009;24:203–8.

Pasotti M, Klersy C, Pilotto A, et al. Long-term outcome and risk stratification in dilated cardiolaminopathies. J Am Coll Cardiol. 2008;52:1250–60.

18.6 Familial Partial Lipodystrophy of the Dunnigan Type

18.6.1 Synonyms, Abbreviations

Familial partial lipodystrophy of the Dunnigan type (FPLD)

18.6.2 Genetics and Pathophysiology

Familial partial lipodystrophy of the Dunnigan type (FPLD) is a rare autosomal dominant disorder resulting from mutations in the *LMNA* gene. Although a direct correlation between *LMNA* gene alterations and clinical manifestations has not been established, FPLD tends to be associated with mutations located in known regions. For example, several, but not all, subjects with FPLD have alterations at exon 8 of the *LMNA* gene.

The pathogenetic mechanism underlying this complex disease remains unclear. Several studies have associated FPLD with the accumulation of lamin A protein precursors (pre-lamin A) inside the nucleus. Pre-lamin A sequesters the adipocyte transcription factor sterol regulatory element-binding protein-1 (SREBP1) at the nuclear rim, thereby reducing the pool of SREBP1 that normally activates peroxisome proliferator-activated receptor (PPARγ), causing impaired adipocyte differentiation.

18.6.3 Histopathology

In the classic forms of FPLD, the muscle biopsy is histologically and immunohistochemically normal. However, the FPLD phenotype may be associated with muscular dystrophy, producing an overlapping syndrome. In these subjects, muscle biopsy may reveal myopathic/dystrophic changes similar to those found in LGMD1B and EDMD2.

18.6.4 Clinical Presentation

The condition is characterized by progressive loss of subcutaneous fat tissue from the upper and lower limbs, trunk, and buttocks, leading to a typical appearance of extreme muscularity. Conversely, fat accumulates on the neck, face, axillae, back, and genitalia. Intraabdominal fat deposits are also increased. Metabolic complications such as insulin resistance, diabetes mellitus, dyslipidemia, and atherosclerosis are generally associated. The onset is at puberty, and phenotypic expression is more pronounced in women.

18.6.5 Imaging Findings

See Sect. 18.7.

18.6.6 Therapy

Patients suffering from FPLD are at high risk for cardiovascular disease and diabetes.

Glitazone and oral antidiabetic agents are usually used to reduce hyperglycemia and plasma lipid levels. Several trials have recently tested the usefulness and safety of leptin in patients with severe metabolic problems related to FPLD.

18.6.7 Differential Diagnosis

Dunnigan-type familial partial lipodystrophy must be differentiated from the other forms of lipodystrophies that have so far been identified, including those due to alterations of genes other than *LMNA* or secondary to acquired disorders affecting fat tissue.

Genetically inherited lipodystrophies usually have an autosomal dominant or recessive trait and may be characterized by generalized, partial reduction or even absence of subcutaneous fat tissue. Generalized forms of lipodystrophy may be due to mutations of genes such as *AGPAT2*, *BSCL2*, *CAV-1*, and *PTRF*, whereas the currently known forms of partial lipodystrophies other than the Dunnigan type may be caused by alterations of *PPARG*, *PLIN1*, and *AKT2*. Rare cases of partial lipodystrophy associated with alterations of the *CIDEC* or *ZMPSTE24* genes have also been reported.

Subjects with congenital lipodystrophy due to *PTRF* gene mutations present with a complex phenotype characterized by an absence of body fat, skeletal muscle weakness, cardiac compromise, and pyloric stenosis.

Imaging studies in subjects with generalized forms of lipodystrophy reveal a marked reduction of fat in subcutaneous tissue, thorax, and abdomen. Different from subjects with *CAV1* and *PTRF* mutations, individuals with lipodystrophy due to *AGPAT2* or *BSCL2* alterations also show a loss of fat in bone marrow.

All currently known variants of partial lipodystrophy show reduced subcutaneous adipose tissue that affects all four limbs. In partial lipodystrophy due to *PPARG* mutations, fat loss in the calves and forearms is particularly striking. Like patients with FPLD, patients with PPARG and PLIN1 mutations may accumulate excess fat on the neck and face.

The rare reports of patients carrying *ZMPSTE24* mutations describe a progeroid phenotype with a partial or generalized reduction of subcutaneous body fat combined with skeletal alterations.

Imaging studies in a young woman carrying a homozygous mutation of the *CIDEC* gene showed prominent muscularity, hepatic steatosis, and marked reduction of fat tissue in the abdomen, forearms, and gluteal and femoral regions.

Lipodystrophy due to *LMNA* gene alterations also must be distinguished from acquired forms of lipodystrophy. It is particularly important to exclude lipodystrophy induced by antiretroviral therapy. Patients with acquired immunodeficiency syndrome (AIDS) often show a marked loss of subcutaneous fat tissue in the face and limbs with sparing of fat in the abdomen and neck. Some patients receiving antiretroviral treatment may even show overt accumulation of fat on the neck.

Emerinopathies and Laminopathies: Familial Partial Lipodystrophy of the Dunnigan Type

Key Points

- Alterations of the *LMNA* gene may be associated with FPLD.
- Familial partial lipodystrophy is characterized by reduction of subcutaneous adipose tissue in the extremities, trunk, and buttocks, with fat preservation or even accumulation in selected regions including the face, neck, back, and genitalia.
- Subjects with the isolated form of partial lipodystrophy related to *LMNA* gene mutations are histologically and immunohistochemically normal.
- Imaging studies may help reveal the abnormal distribution of subcutaneous fat tissue in FPLD.
- Patients with FPLD may also present with skeletal muscle compromise, indicating an overlapping syndrome.

18.7 Imaging Findings of Disorders Due to *LMNA* Gene Alterations

Several imaging studies of muscle involvement have been performed in EDMD2 patients. Leg muscle imaging shows selective compromise of calf muscles with varying degrees of alteration in the soleus, the medial head of the gastrocnemius, and to a lesser extent the lateral head of the gastrocnemius (Fig. 18.14).

At the level of the thigh, magnetic resonance imaging (MRI) and computed tomography (CT) scans have revealed changes predominantly in vastii muscles. They may be confined to the vastus intermedius or selectively compromise all vastii muscles. Other muscles that may be involved in the autosomal dominant form of EDMD are the adductor magnus, the semimembranosus, and the long head of the biceps femoris (Fig. 18.15). Patients with diffuse and unspecific alterations of all thigh muscles have also been described.

There are only a few reports of imaging findings in LGMD1B patients. Leg muscle imaging studies of seven individuals with LGMD1B showed alterations of the soleus and medial head of the gastrocnemius (Fig. 18.16). Mild impairment of the lateral head of the gastrocnemius can also be detected. At the thigh level, alterations in the adductor magnus, semimembranosus, and long head of the biceps femoris can be observed (Fig. 18.17). Some patients display diffuse unspecific alterations.

One study reported a patient with alterations in the posterior thigh muscles and relative sparing of gracile and sartorius muscles. Leg muscle imaging showed compromise of the medial and lateral head of the gastrocnemius.

So far, only a few imaging studies have been performed in CMDA1 patients with the aim of individuating the eventual presence of skeletal muscle alterations.

In one report, five members of a family with an *LMNA* gene mutation presenting with isolated cardiac involvement had subclinical alterations of leg and thigh muscles similar to those observed in EDMD2. At the thigh level, gluteal, adductor magnus and adductor longus, vastii, and semimembranosus muscles and the long head of the femoral biceps were variably involved (Fig. 18.17).

Leg muscle MRI scans have shown alterations of the soleus muscle, the medial head of the gastrocnemius, and to a lesser extent the lateral head of the gastrocnemius (Fig. 18.18).

A subsequent imaging study, performed on a larger cohort of individuals with different *LMNA* gene alterations confirmed the alterations of the posterior calf muscles but showed no involvement of the thigh muscles.

In another report, the authors discussed skeletal muscle imaging findings in a cohort of individuals with different phenotypes due to *LMNA*

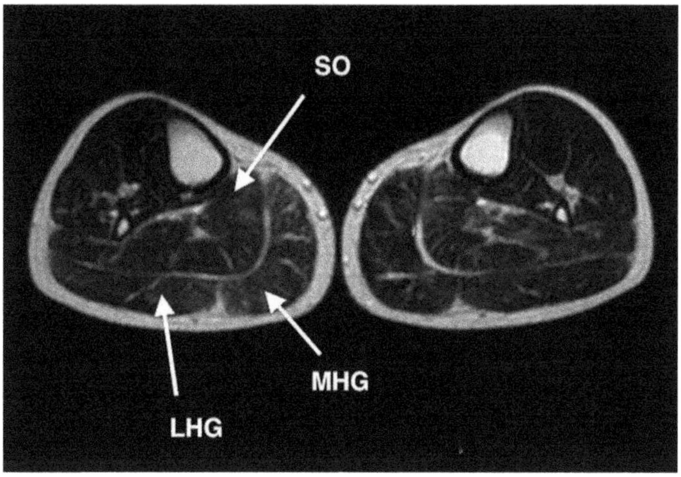

Fig. 18.14 T2-weighted magnetic resonance imaging (MRI) scans of leg muscles in a patient with Emery–Dreifuss muscular dystrophy due to an *LMNA* gene mutation. Note the moderate alterations of the soleus (*SO*), medial head of the gastrocnemius (*MHG*), and lateral head of the gastrocnemius (*LHG*). Adapted from Carboni N, Mura M, Marrosu G, et al (2010) Muscle imaging analogies in a cohort of patients with different clinical phenotypes caused by LMNA gene mutations. J Muscle Nerve. 41:458–63. With permission from Wiley Blackwell

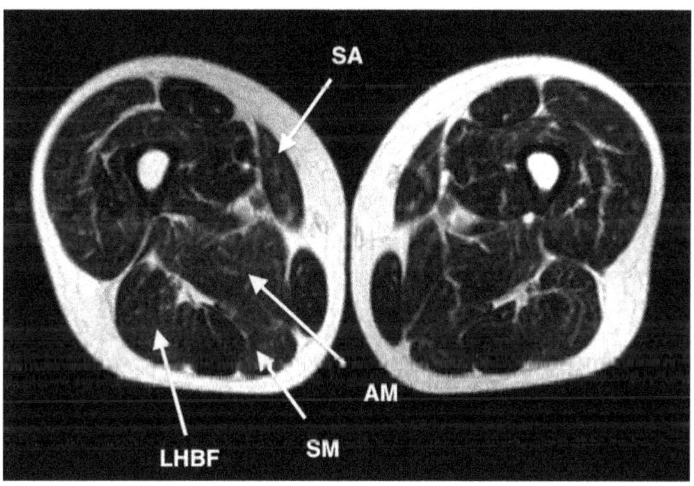

Fig. 18.15 MRI scan of thigh muscles in a patient with Emery–Dreifuss muscular dystrophy due to an *LMNA* gene mutation. Note alterations in the adductor magnus (*AM*), semimembranosus (*SM*), sartorius (*SA*), and the long head of the biceps femoris (*LHBF*)

mutations. The study cohort included the five patients of the previous report.

In this larger cohort, all patients presenting with selective cardiac abnormalities showed analogous patterns of leg muscle compromise. Conversely, thigh muscle alterations were observed only in the five subjects of the previous report and were not detected in the other subjects with an apparently exclusive cardiac phenotype.

These authors also report muscle alterations associated with *LMNA* gene mutations in another family group. Imaging studies of five mutated relatives showed two with the LGMD1B phenotype and three with clinically isolated cardiac

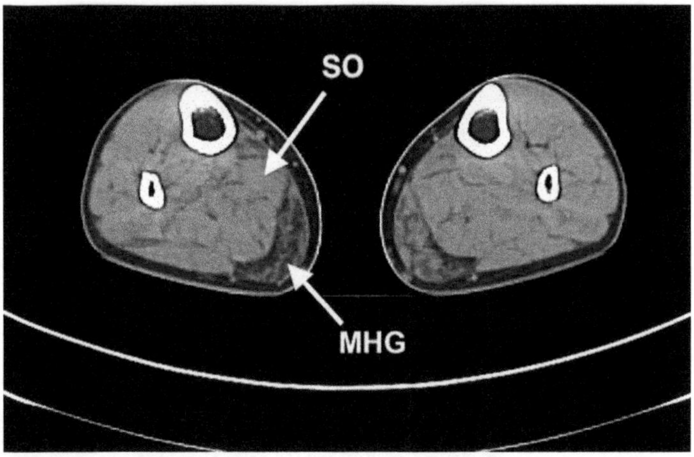

Fig. 18.16 CT scans of leg muscles in a patient with limb-girdle muscular dystrophy due to an *LMNA* gene mutation. Note the mild alterations in the soleus (*SO*) and severe alterations in the medial head of the gastrocnemius (*MHG*)

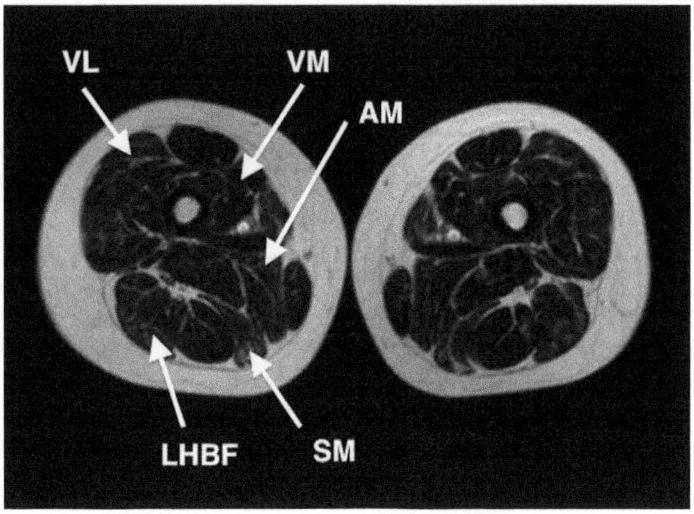

Fig. 18.17 T2-weighted MRI scans of thigh muscles in a patient with apparently selective cardiac compromise due to an *LMNA* gene mutation. Note the mild alterations in the adductor magnus (*AM*), the vastus lateralis (*VL*), vastus medialis (*VM*), semimembranosus (*SM*) muscles and the long head of the biceps femoris (*LHBF*)

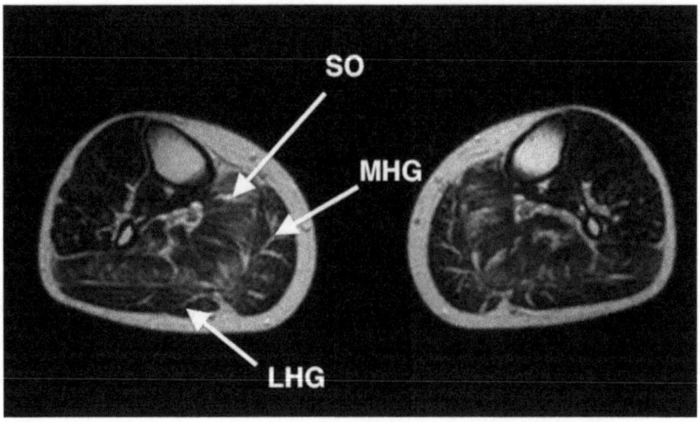

Fig. 18.18 T2-weighted MRI scans of leg muscles in a patient with selective cardiac compromise due to an *LMNA* gene mutation. Note the severe alterations in the soleus (*SO*), moderate alterations in the medial head of the gastrocnemius (MHG), and mild alterations in the lateral head of the gastrocnemius (*LHG*)

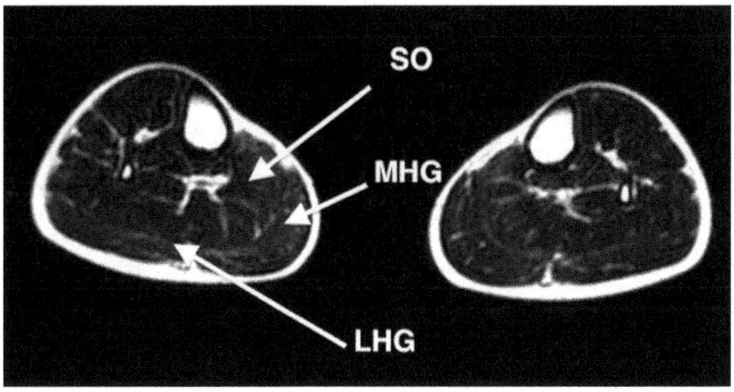

Fig. 18.19 T2-weighted MRI scans of leg muscles in a patient with cardiac compromise and early lipodystrophy due to an *LMNA* gene mutation. Note the mild alterations in the soleus (*SO*), medial head of the gastrocnemius (*MHG*), and lateral head of the gastrocnemius (*LHG*). Please note the marked reduction of subcutaneous fat tissue

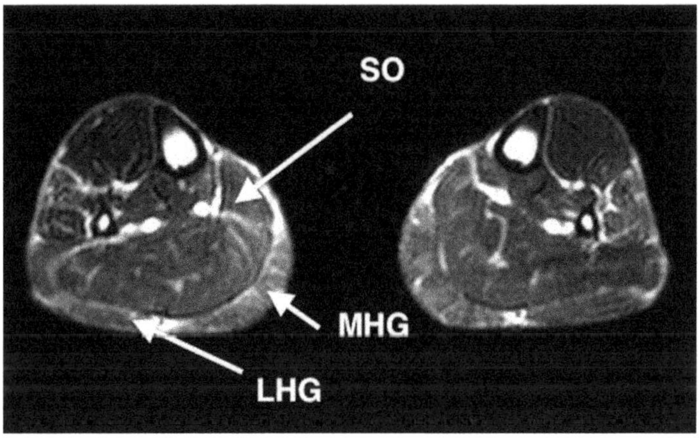

Fig. 18.20 T2-weighted MRI scans of leg muscles in a patient with cardiac compromise, lipodystrophy, and peripheral neuropathy due to an *LMNA* gene mutation. Note the moderate alterations in the medial head of the gastrocnemius (*MHG*) and mild alterations in the soleus (*SO*) and lateral head of the gastrocnemius (*LHG*)

compromise. Imaging patterns of muscle involvement were similar in all the subjects examined: diffuse and unspecific alterations in thigh muscles and compromise of leg muscles involving the soleus and the medial and lateral head of the gastrocnemius.

Imaging studies of individuals suffering from FPLD showed marked reduction (up to absence) of subcutaneous fat tissue in gluteal regions and limbs with preservation of intermuscular fat stores. Less extensive subcutaneous fat loss is observed in the trunk and breast regions. Reduction in subcutaneous fat tissue in the truncal area is more prominent anteriorly than posteriorly.

Fat is typically preserved within the intraabdominal and intrathoracic regions, perineum, buccal, temporal and periarticular regions, orbits, palms, soles, and scalp. Imaging studies also show accumulation of excess adipose tissue in selected sites, including the posterior cervical area, neck, face, labia majora, chin and axillae.

MRI studies have been performed in members of a family presenting with early CMD1A and late FPLD. In two cases, there was axonal peripheral neuropathy associated with the heterogeneous exon 1 c.178 C/G, p.Arg 60 Gly *LMNA* gene mutations. None of the family members with mutations of the *LMNA* gene had any clinically detectable signs of skeletal muscle compromise.

In the thighs and legs, we detected the typical loss of subcutaneous fat associated with normal preservation of intermuscular fat stores. Muscle MRI revealed mild to moderate compromise of posterior leg skeletal muscles primarily involving the soleus and medial head of the gastrocnemius and to a lesser extent the lateral head of the gastrocnemius (Figs. 18.19 and 18.20).

Acknowledgments We are grateful to the patients who agreed to participate in the imaging studies. We also thank the colleagues who made the writing of this chapter possible. In particular, we are deeply indebted to Professor Maria Giovanna Marrosu, MD, for her critical reading of the manuscript and continuous support and to all colleagues, clinicians, radiologists, biologists, and technical assistants for their kind help and cooperation.

Suggestions for Further Reading

Ahmad Z, Zackai E, Medne L, et al. Early onset mandibuloacral dysplasia due to compound heterozygous mutations in ZMPSTE24. Am J Med Genet A. 2010;152A(11):2703–10.

Capanni C, Mattioli E, Columbaro M, et al. Altered prelamin A processing is a common mechanism leading to lipodystrophy. Hum Mol Genet. 2005;14:1489–502.

Garg A, Peshock RM, Fleckenstein JL. Adipose tissue distribution pattern in patients with familial partial lipodystrophy (Dunnigan variety). J Clin Endocrinol Metab. 1999;84:170–4.

Garg A, Vinaitheerthan M, Weatherall PT, et al. Phenotypic heterogeneity in patients with familial partial lipodystrophy (Dunnigan variety) related to the site of missense mutations in lamin A/C gene. J Clin Endocrinol Metab. 2001;86:59–65.

Rubio-Cabezas O, Puri V, Murano I, et al. Partial lipodystrophy and insulin resistant diabetes in a patient with a homozygous nonsense mutation in CIDEC. Embo Mol Med. 2009;1:280–7.

Simha V, Garg A. Phenotypic heterogeneity in body fat distribution in patients with congenital generalized lipodystrophy caused by mutations in the AGPAT2 or seipin genes. J Clin Endocrinol Metab. 2003;88(11): 5433–7.

Speckman RA, Garg A, Du F, et al. Mutational and haplotype analyses of families with familial partial lipodystrophy (Dunnigan variety) reveal recurrent missense mutations in the globular C-terminal domain of lamin A/C. Am J Hum Genet. 2000;66:1192–8.

Vigouroux C, Magré J, Vantyghem MC, et al. Lamin A/C gene: sex-determined expression of mutations in Dunnigan-type familial partial lipodystrophy and absence of coding mutations in congenital and acquired generalized lipoatrophy. Diabetes. 2000;49:1958–62.

Limb Girdle Muscular Dystrophies 19

Maggie C. Walter and Dirk Fischer

19.1 Introduction

Autosomal dominant and recessive limb-girdle muscular dystrophies (LGMD) are a heterogeneous group of genetic diseases with a wide spectrum of clinical involvement and severity. In contrast to the more common X-linked dystrophinopathies, disease onset is often delayed into late childhood or adult age. LGMD patients usually show progressive weakness predominantly affecting proximal limb musculature. Onset, progression, and distribution of the weakness and wasting can vary between individual patients and genetic subtypes. Most LGMD patients have typical histopathological dystrophic changes consisting of degeneration and regeneration of muscle fibers which usually leads to elevated serum creatine kinase levels. Diagnosis can often be confirmed by protein immunostaining or-blotting. In addition, a specific pattern of muscular involvement on muscle magnetic resonance imaging (MRI) can be observed in many LGMD subtypes. There is considerable clinical and pathological overlap with other early onset congenital myopathies, distal myopathies, and myofibrillar myopathies. Not all of these entities are described in this chapter as some of these LGMD causing genes may also manifest with a different clinical (e.g., distal) or histopathological phenotype. Autosomal recessive forms are much more common and have been referred to as LGMD2, whereas autosomal dominant forms are referred to as LGMD1. For myotilinopathy (LGMD1A) see Sect. 20.4; for Laminopathies (LGMD1B), see Chap. 18; for dystroglycan-related myopathies (LGMD2I, LGMD2K, LGMD2M, LGMD2N) see Sect. 16.5; for titin-related limb-girdle myopathy (LGMD2J) see Sect. 21.2.1; and for Anoctamin (ANO5)-related myopathy (LGMD2L) see Sect. 21.3.2.

M.C. Walter (✉)
Friedrich-Baur-Institute, Department of Neurology, Ludwig-Maximilians-University of Munich, Ziemssenstr. 1, 80336 Munich, Germany
e-mail: maggie.walter@lrz.uni-muenchen.de

D. Fischer
Division of Neuropaediatrics, University Childrens Hospital Basel, 4056 Basel, Switzerland

Department of Neurology, University Hospital Basel, 4031 Basel, Switzerland
e-mail: Dirk.Fischer@ukbb.ch

19.2 Calpainopathy

19.2.1 Synonyms, Abbreviations

Limb girdle muscular dystrophy type 2A (LGMD2A).

19.2.2 Genetics and Pathophysiology

Limb-girdle muscular dystrophy type 2A (OMIM 114240, 253600) is associated with mutations in the human *CAPN3* gene located on chromosome 15q15.1-q21.1 that comprises 24 exons. Depending on the geographical region, LGMD2A

M.P. Wattjes and D. Fischer (eds.), *Neuromuscular Imaging*, DOI 10.1007/978-1-4614-6552-2_19,

is one of the most common forms of LGMD, accounting for around 20–30 % of LGMD patients. The frequency ranges from 20 % in the Netherlands, 25–30 % in Italy, to about 80 % in northern Spain. The *CAPN3* gene encodes a 94-kDa translated protein of 821 amino acids called calpain-3, but also other alternatively spliced variants. Calpain-3 is the muscle-specific member of Ca^{2+}-activated neutral proteases that is able to cut other proteins into shorter (poly)-peptides. It comprises several domains among them a regulatory, a proteolytic, and a Ca^{2+}-binding domain. The exact physiological role of calpain-3 is still unknown, but it has been suggested that it might process proteins involved in signalling pathways and in sarcomere remodeling.

Many hundreds disease-causing mutations are known, the majority of them are unique mutations. There are no identified mutation hotspots, the mutations are located within all regions of the gene. More than two thirds of known mutations are single nucleotide missense mutations. Other mutations such as small insertions or deletions causing a premature stop codon have been reported. Mutations in the *CAPN3* gene usually have a loss-of-function effect. Most calpainopathy patients have complete or partial calpain-3 protein deficiency. A normal amount of protein is observed in about 15–20 % of LGMD2A patients. In these cases it is supposed that calpain-3 has lost its autocatalytic activity leading to a functionally inactive enzyme.

19.2.3 Histopathology

Muscle biopsy histopathology in LGMD2A shows nonspecific dystrophic changes, including variation in fiber size, increased central nuclei, fiber degeneration and regeneration, and increased endomysial connective tissue. There is sometimes inflammation with perimysial and perivascular infiltrates without vacuoles. Other nonspecific myopathic features (fiber splitting, lobulated fibers) can be present. Later in the disease course, normal muscle tissue is commonly replaced by deposition of fat and connective tissue. Protein analyses in LGMD2A may show an absent immunohistochemical (IHC) reaction

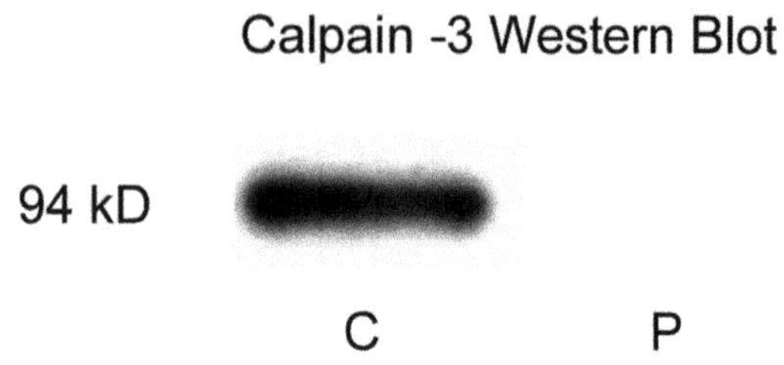

Fig. 19.1 Calpain-3 western blotting. Note the absent 94 kDa band in a LGMD2A patient (P) when comparing to a normal control (C)

against calpain-3, but IHC is not established as a diagnostic marker. In patients with partial protein deficiency, western blotting might not show any abnormalities. Therefore, calpain-3 western blot analysis of muscle biopsy protein extracts is the most useful diagnostic test for detecting a primary calpainopathy. About 80 % of patients with calpainopathy show pathologically absent or reduced levels of calpain-3 protein, and approximately 20 % show a normal protein expression on immunoblotting (with loss of protein function) (Fig. 19.1).

19.2.4 Clinical Presentation

Patients with calpainopathy frequently present with progressive symmetric proximal limb girdle weakness. Early motor milestones are usually normal, but asymptomatic HyperCKemia may be present before the onset of muscle symptoms. The age of symptom onset varies, but in most patients it occurs within the first two decades of life. Some affected LGMD2A patients complain of exercise related muscle pain before overt muscle weakness becomes evident. One of the first clinical findings is often tiptoe walking. Scapular winging, difficulties in running and walking, and a waddling gait are also commonly observed early in the disease. Achilles tendon contractures, hyperlordosis, a slight scoliosis, and laxity of the abdominal muscles are often present. Muscle hypertrophy is uncommon. In contrast marked calf or generalised atrophy is often present in patients with LGMD2A. On clinical examination the posterior compartment muscles of the pelvis (gluteus maximus), thigh (hamstrings and adductors), and lower legs

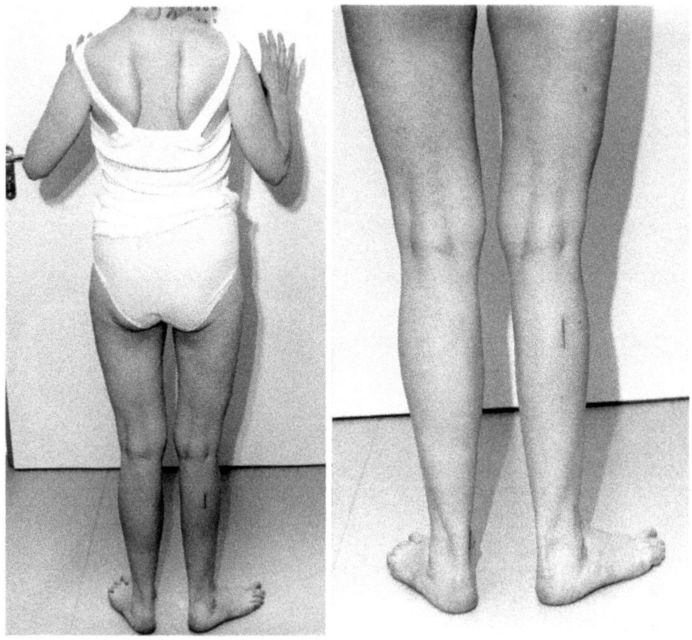

Fig. 19.2 Clinical phenotype of a LGMD2A patient. Note the marked shoulder winging and muscle atrophy in the posterior thigh compartment. The calf is rather slim instead of hypertrophic as observed in other muscular dystrophies

(soleus, gastrocnemius) as well as scapular fixator muscles (supraspinatus, infraspinatus) are the most affected muscles (Fig. 19.2). Prominent weakness of shoulder adduction and internal rotation, hip flexion and adduction, knee flexion and ankle dorsiflexion can be detected. Facial, neck, and tongue muscles are usually spared. In later, more advanced stages of calpainopathy, climbing stairs, rising from a chair, and getting up from the floor become increasingly difficult or impossible. The disease is invariably progressive and loss of ambulation occurs between 10 and 30 years after the onset of weakness. Joint contractures in the hips, knees, elbows, and fingers are often present. Respiratory muscles can be involved leading to respiratory insufficiency. Cardiac affection is uncommon, and there is no cognitive impairment in patients with LGMD2A.

19.2.5 Imaging Findings

Patients with calpainopathy show a consistent pattern of muscle involvement on MRI studies. At the pelvic level (Fig. 19.3a, d, g), the gluteus maximus muscle is usually more involved than the gluteus medius and minimus muscles. Often there is moderate to severe atrophy of the gluteus maximus muscle. At the thigh level (Fig. 19.3b, e, h) the medial (adductors) and posterior compartment (hamstring) muscles are usually the most severely affected, whereas the quadriceps muscle is much less affected. Involvement of the adductor magnus and semimembranosus muscles is the most common finding. Sartorius and gracilis are usually spared. Later in the course of the disease the adductor longus, biceps femoris and semitendinosus, vastus medialis, and vastus intermedius become involved. In the lower legs (Fig. 19.3c, f, i), the first muscles to be involved are the medial head of the gastrocnemius muscle and the soleus muscle with relative sparing of lateral head of the gastrocnemius muscle. There may be diffuse but less severe involvement of the anterior lower leg muscles.

19.2.6 Differential Diagnosis

Primary calpainopathies may be confounded with autosomal recessive (or sporadic) LGMDs with early onset and high CK levels [e.g., the sarcoglycanopathies (LGMD2C, LGMD2D, LGMD2E, LGMD2F, see Sect. 19.4], dysferlinopathy (LGMD2B, see Sect. 19.3); and dystrophinopathy type Becker (BMD, see Chap. 17).

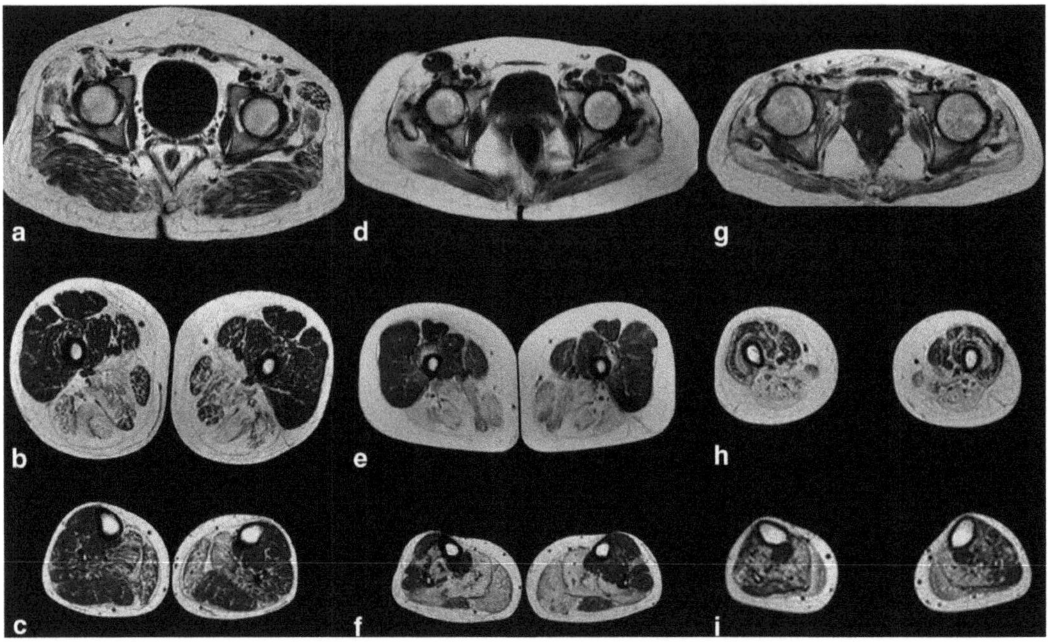

Fig. 19.3 Muscle MR images of three patients with genetically confirmed primary calpainopathy (LGMD2A) with a mild (**a–c**), moderate (**d–f**) and severe (**g–i**) clinical phenotype. It's noteworthy that, at the pelvic level there is progressive atrophy of the gluteaus maximus muscle (**a**, **d**, **g**), which is not seen in LGMD2I and LGMD2B. At the thigh level (**b**, **e**, **h**), similar to LGMD2I, the earliest and most severe changes are observed in the adductor and posterior compartment muscles, whereas in patients with a severe phenotype additional changes are seen in the quadriceps muscle (**g**). In the lower legs, there is a characteristic pattern of relatively homogeneus and selective involvement of the medial head of the gastrocnemius and the soleus muscle, which is not seen in other LGMD's. From Fischer D, et al. (2005) Diagnostic value of muscle MRI in differentiating LGMD2I from other LGMDs. J Neurol. 252;538–547. Reprinted with permission from Springer

Limb Girdle Muscular Dystrophies: Calpainopathy (LGMD2A)

Key Points

- Primary calpain-3 deficiency is one of the most common forms of LGMD, especially in Europe.
- Common clinical findings in calpainopathy include prominent scapular winging, marked calf or generalized atrophy, and weakness and atrophy of gluteus maximus, adductor posterior thigh (hamstrings), and lower leg (calf) muscles.
- About 15–20 % of patients exhibit normal protein expression on immunoblotting and may therefore be missed.
- There is a consistent pattern of muscular involvement on muscle imaging with affection of the gluteus maximus, adductor magnus, semimembranosus, medial gastrocnemius and soleus muscle. The vastus lateralis, gracilis, and sartorius muscles are often relatively spared.

Suggestions for Further Reading

Fardeau M, Hillaire D, Mignard C, et al. Juvenile limb-girdle muscular dystrophy. Clinical, histopathological and genetic data from a small community living in the Reunion Island. Brain. 1996;119:295–308.

Fischer D, Walter MC, Kesper K, et al. Diagnostic value of muscle MRI in differentiating LGMD2I from other LGMDs. J Neurol. 2005;252;538–47.

Gallardo E, Saenz A, Illa I. Limb-girdle muscular dystrophy 2A. Handb Clin Neurol. 2011;101:97–110.

Mercuri E, Bushby K, Ricci E, et al. Muscle MRI findings in patients with limb girdle muscular dystrophy with calpain 3 deficiency (LGMD2A) and early contractures. Neuromuscul Disord. 2002;15(2):164–71.

Pollitt C, Anderson LV, Pogue R, et al. The phenotype of calpainopathy: diagnosis based on a multidisciplinary approach. Neuromuscul Disord. 2001;11(3):287–96.

19.3 Dysferlinopathies

19.3.1 Synonyms, Abbreviations

Limb girdle muscular dystrophy type 2B (LGMD2B), Miyoshi muscular dystrophy (MMD1), Distal myopathy with anterior tibial onset (DMAT).

19.3.2 Genetics and Pathophysiology

The disease spectrum of dysferlinopathies includes Miyoshi muscular dystrophy (MMD1) and distal anterior compartment myopathy (DMAT), both of which are allelic distal muscle disorders that preferentially affect the gastrocnemius or tibial muscle, and Limb-girdle muscular dystrophy type 2B (LGMD2B, OMIM#253601) with characteristic proximal weakness at onset.

Dysferlin is a ubiquitously expressed 230 kDa molecule that is localized in the periphery of skeletal muscle fibers, linked to the sarcolemmal membrane. Given the homology of dysferlin to a nematode spermatogenesis factor that is required for successful membrane fusion, it has been suggested that the lack of dysferlin might cause faulty myotube fusion and impair muscle regeneration. Because of the large size of the dysferlin gene, and the absence of any apparent mutation hotspot region, no clear-cut genotype/phenotype correlations have been identified to date. However, identical mutations in patients with LGMD2B or MM suggest involvement of modifier genes.

The incidence of LGMD2B is comparable to LGMD2A and LGMD2I, 10 % of autosomal recessive LGMDs constitute LGMD2B. LGMD2B may be the most prevalent form (35–45 %) in some populations such as in the Cajun/Arcadian population of North America. It is the second most prevalent form of autosomal recessive LGMD in Brazil, accounting for 22 % of the classified forms.

19.3.3 Histopathology

Light microscopy shows a dystrophic muscle with necrosis and degeneration of muscle fibers, increased endomysial connective tissue, fiber size variation and sometimes inflammation with perimysial and perivascular infiltrates without vacuoles (Fig. 19.4a). Because vacuoles are a histological hallmark of several distal myopathies, lack of vacuoles suggest dysferlinopathy in patients with initial distal myopathy presentation. Protein analyses in LGMD2B have shown a total deficiency of dysferlin, in both IHC and immunoblotting (Fig. 19.4b–d). Although a partial deficiency has been reported in LGMD2B, dysferlin deficiency seems to be specific to LGMD2B. However, some patients IHC show a secondary reduction of caveolin-3.

19.3.4 Clinical Presentation

Symptoms of LGMD2B usually start during the late second decade of life with weakness pre-

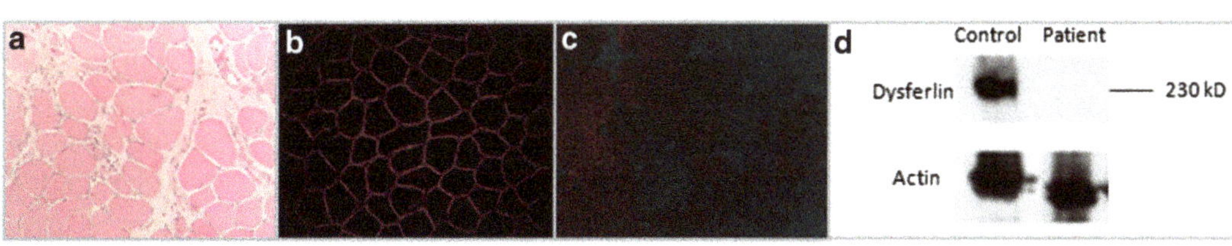

Fig. 19.4 Typical histological findings in dysferlinopathy. (**a**) H&E staining shows fiber size variation, rounded fibers, increased fatty and connective tissue along with inflammatory-like infiltration. Immunohistochemistry in dysferlinopathy (**c**) compared to normal muscle (**b**) shows negative dysferlin staining. Immunoblotting (**d**) shows absent dysferlin in skeletal muscle, while it is clearly detectable at the expected size in a normal control. Reprobing with an antibody to α-actin reveals equal loading

dominantly in proximal muscles, although the gastrocnemius muscle may show subclinical involvement on MRI. In MMD1 symptoms usually start in the posterior lower leg compartment, whereas in DMAT, it is the anterior lower leg compartment that is mainly affected. However, within the same pedigree, both LGMD2B and MMD1 phenotypes were identified that were caused by the identical dysferlin mutation. Although the initial presentation may be different, the distinction between patients with distal or proximal onset is difficult after many years of progression. Even in LGMD there is often characteristic early involvement of the gastrocnemius and soleus muscle, which might lead to wasting and difficulties in walking on the toes. This can also be seen on imaging. This form of LGMD arises from mutations in the dysferlin gene, which contains more than 55 exons and spans a region of 150 kb. The clinical picture is usually less severe than in the other autosomal recessive LGMD forms although there is wide intrafamilial and interfamilial variability. Calf hypertrophy is rare but is also observed in some cases. Interestingly, patients often lose their ability to walk on tiptoes before the ability to walk on their heels, a feature that might be helpful in the differential diagnosis. The mean age of onset is 19 years (range 12–39 years). However, a new clinical phenotype with congenital onset was recently described, widening the spectrum of the disease. Confinement to a wheelchair may occur, on average 10–20 years after onset of the disease but it is usually less frequent and occurs later than in patients with calpainopathy (LGMD2A, Sect. 19.2). Cardiac and respiratory muscles are not involved in either phenotype, and patients have normal intelligence. Serum CK is always elevated (10–72 fold) among these patients even during the preclinical stages. In some patients, hyperCKemia may be the only abnormality for years (Fig. 19.5).

19.3.5 Imaging Findings

Patients with mutations in the dysferlin gene can present with either more proximal (LGMD2B) or more distal muscle involvement (MMD1 or DMAT, respectively). Over the course of the disease these phenotypes often overlap and patients show both proximal and distal involvement, especially of the leg muscles. Almost every muscle can be affected in the dysferlinopathies (Fig. 19.6). The phenotypic presentations (LGMD2B, MMD1, DMAT) do not show differences in their rate of progression. In the thigh, muscle pathology generally seems to start in the adductor magnus muscle and then affects the semimembranosus and the vastus lateralis muscles (Fig. 19.7). There is no clear difference in the extent of thigh muscle pathology between MMD1 and LGMD2B patients. Similarly to many of the other LGMD and to Pompe disease (Sect. 14.2.1), the rectus, gracilis, and sartorius muscles are usually spared. In the calf, there is no relevant difference between LGMD2B and MMD1, the posterior compartment is predominantly affected, mainly the gastrocnemius medialis and lateralis and the soleus muscles (Fig. 19.8). Only in rare cases of DMAT the anterior lower leg compartment is more prominently involved. Overall, there is no clear correlation between disease onset, disease progression and muscle MRI findings. Interestingly, muscle pathology in dysferlinopathies can be asymmetrical.

The pattern of muscle involvement is quite variable in dysferlinopathy patients. The calf muscles seem to be the earliest and most severely affected in LGMD2B and MMD1. As in many other LGMDs, the tibialis anterior muscle is well preserved until later stages of the disease. The gluteus minimus muscle is almost always affected in patients with dysferlinopathy, whereas the gluteus maximus is sometimes spared.

19.3.6 Differential Diagnosis

Autosomal recessive LGMD with adult onset and high CK levels, especially Anoctaminopathy (LGMD2L, see Sect. 21.3.2), Calpainopathy (LGMD2A, see Sect. 19.2), Dystrophinopathy type Becker (BMD, see Chap. 17) can be easily mistaken for a Dysferlinopathy. Also because of the potential for inflammation in muscle biopsy specimens from Dysferlinopathy patients, a subset of patients is still misdiagnosed as having polymyositis.

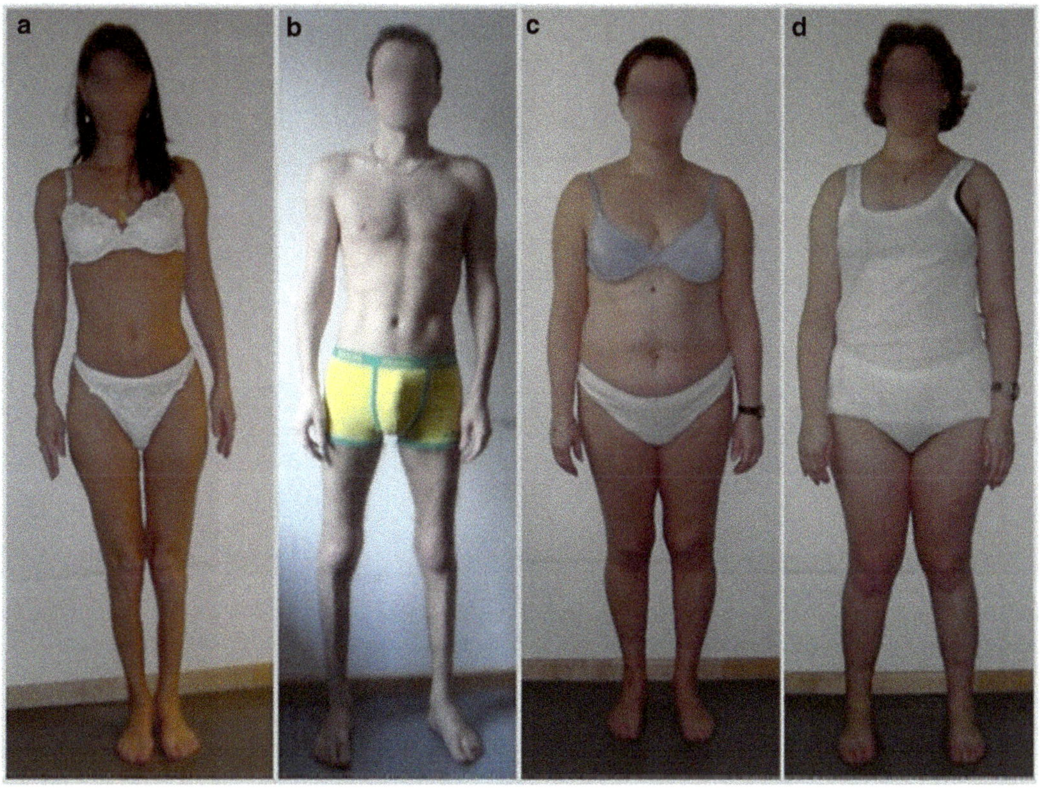

Fig. 19.5 Four German patients with dysferlinopathy. Patients **a** (c.638 C>T/c.5249delG, age 38) and **b** (homozygous deletion of exons 37–40, age 26) initially presented as MM D1, while, patients **c** (age 30) and **d** (age 33) as LGMD2B phenotype (c.1237insA/c.3570ins6). Patients **c** and **d** are siblings, patient **c** is 3 years older, but clinically much less affected than her younger sister

Limb Girdle Muscular Dystrophies: Dysferlinopathies (LGMD2B/MMD1/DMAT)

Key Points

- Muscle affection in Dysferlinopathy is more wide-spread early in the disease course than suggested by the clinical presentation. Myoedema can be seen long before the onset of clinical symptoms.
- The pattern of muscular involvement in dysferlinopathies is quite variable: The predominant muscle pathology can be in the anterior or posterior thigh compartment. Calf muscles are often the earliest and most severely affected muscles in LGMD2B and MMD1. Gracilis and sartorius muscles are relatively spared.
- There are no differences in the rate of progression or MRI pattern of muscle involvement in MMD1 and LGMD2B.
- The adductor magnus and gastrocnemius medialis are the first muscles to be impaired in both phenotypes. The biceps femoris and rectus femoris muscles are relatively spared, and the sartorius and gracilis muscles remain largely unaffected.

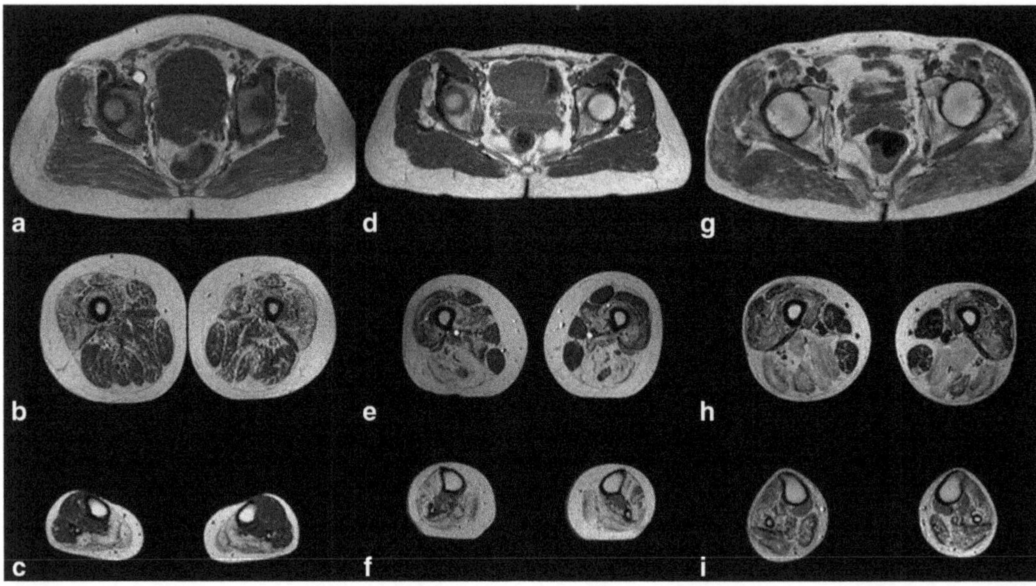

Fig. 19.6 Muscle MRI in dysferlinopathy in three patients with a mild (**a**–**c**), moderate (**d**–**f**) and severe (**g**–**i**) clinical phenotype. At the pelvic level, there are mild to moderate signal changes in the gluteus minimus muscle in all patients. At the thigh level, there is predominant anterior compartment involvement in some patients (**b**), whereas the posterior compartment muscle exceeds the anterior compartment muscle involvement in others (**e**, **h**). A similar heterogeneity is observed in the lower legs. Some patients show a relative selective involvement of the gastrocnemius and soleus muscle (**c**), whereas others show marked hyperintense signal abnormalities in the anterior lower leg compartment, too (**f**). In a patient with a severe clinical phenotype, all muscles in the lower leg show a similar pattern of involvement (**i**). From Fischer D, et al. (2005) Diagnostic value of muscle MRI in differentiating LGMD2I from other LGMDs. J Neurol. 252:538–47. Reprinted with permission from Springer

Suggestions for Further Reading

Amato AA, Brown RH Jr. Dysferlinopathies. Handb Clin Neurol. 2011;101:111–118.

Brummer B, Walter MC, Palmbach M, et al. Long-term MRI and clinical follow-up of symptomatic and presymptomatic carriers of dysferlin gene mutations. Acta Myol. 2005;24:6–16.

Kesper K, Kornblum C, Reimann J, et al. Pattern of skeletal muscle involvement in primary dysferlinopathies: a whole-body 3.0-T magnetic resonance imaging study. Acta Neurol Scand. 2009;120:111–8.

Krahn M, Illa I, Lévy N, et al. 172nd ENMC International Workshop: Dysferlinopathies 29–31 January 2010, Naarden, The Netherlands. Neuromuscul Disord. 2011;21:503–12.

Paradas C, Llauger J, Diaz-Manera I, et al. Redefining dysferlinopathy phenotypes based on clinical findings and muscle imaging studies. Neurology 2010;75: 316–23.

19.4 Sarcoglycanopathies

19.4.1 Synonyms, Abbreviations

Limb girdle muscular dystrophy type 2C (γ-sarcoglycanopathy, LGMD2C); type 2D (α-sarcoglycanopathy, Adhalinopathy, LGMD2D); type 2E (β-sarcoglycanopathy, LGMD2E); 2F (δ-sarcoglycanopathy, LGMD2F).

19.4.2 Genetics and Pathophysiology

The sarcoglycans [α-(SGCA), β-(SGCB), γ-(SGCG), δ-(SGCD)] are transmembrane glycoproteins that, together with sarcospan, dystrophin,

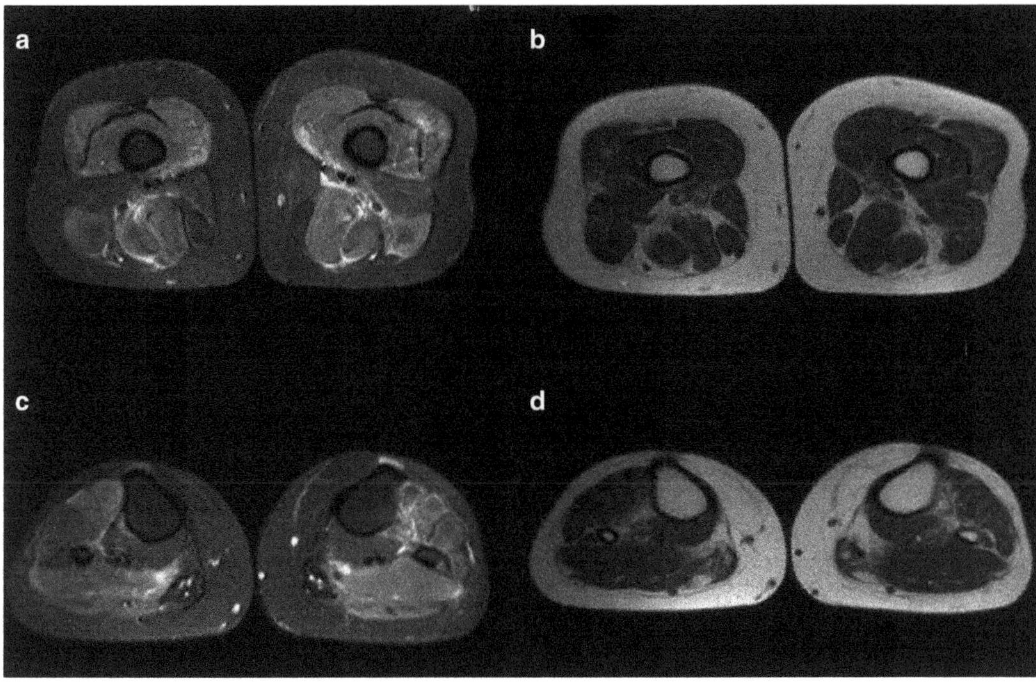

Fig. 19.7 Muscle MRI findings in a dysferlinopathy patient with initial symptomatology. STIR sequences visualize widespread edema in posterior and anterior compartments of distal (**c**) and proximal leg muscles (**a**). Initial fatty degeneration is present in the medial posterior compartment of the lower legs (**d**), but not in proximal leg muscles (**b**). From Brummer et al. Long-term MRI and clinical follow-up of symptomatic and presymptomatic carriers of dysferlin gene mutations. Acta Myol. 2005;XXIV:6–16. Reprinted with permission from the Mediterranean Society of Myology

dystroglycans, syntrophins and α-dystrobrevin, constitute the dystroglycancomplex (DGC). The DGC acts as a link between the cytoskeleton of the muscle cell and the extracellular matrix, providing mechanical support to the plasma membrane during myofiber contraction. In addition to this structural function, there is now increasing evidence that the DGC might play a role in cellular communication. Some frequent alterations (e.g., R77C in SGCA) have been associated with both severe and mild forms and with discordant phenotypes among affected siblings. Adult-onset forms with respiratory insufficiency as a presenting symptom have also been described.

The prevalence of sarcoglycanopathies is estimated at 0.56/100,000, population, and the incidence of sarcoglycanopathies is around 10 % within the LGMD group. The most frequent sarcoglycanopathy is LGMD2D, followed by LGMD2E and LGMD2C. LGMD2C is most frequent in Tunisia, North Africa and in Gypsies. LGMD2D is spread in Europe, the United States, and Brazil; LGMD2E is frequent in Brazilian sarcoglycanopathy patients, in Switzerland, and the Amish population in Indiana (USA). LGMD2F patients are rare worldwide and frequently share African-Brazilian ancestry

19.4.3 Histopathology

Light microscopy shows a dystrophic muscle with necrosis and degeneration of muscle fibers, increased endomysial connective tissue and fiber size variation without inflammation and without vacuoles (Fig. 19.9). Protein analyses (IHC and imunoblotting) show reduction or loss of all sarcoglycans (SCGA, SCGB, SCGC, SCGD) (Fig. 19.9b–g). In the majority of muscle biopsies from patients with a mutation in one of the sarcoglycan genes, the primary loss or deficiency of any one of the four sarcogylcan proteins leads to secondary deficiency of the whole subcomplex. However, exceptions may

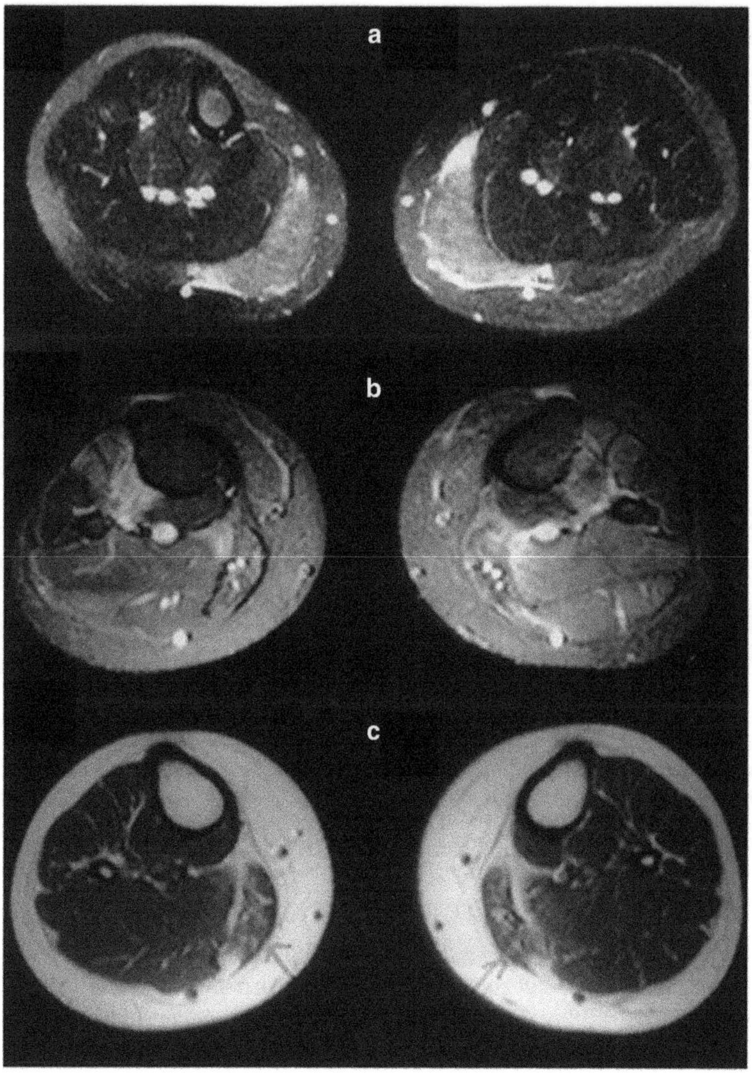

Fig. 19.8 MRI follow-up in presymptomatic and symptomatic periods of a dysferlinopathy patient. First MRI shows bilateral prominent edema in the medial gastrocnemius muscles (**a**). MRI at second follow-up discloses extensive edema spreading from the soleus and gastrocnemius muscles to the dorsiflexor group (**b**) and beginning fatty degeneration again to be seen in the medial gastrocnemius muscles (**c**). From Brummer et al. Long-term MRI and clinical follow-up of symptomatic and presymptomatic carriers of dysferlin gene mutations. Acta Myol. 2005;XXIV:6–16. Reprinted with permission from the Mediterranean Society of Myology

occur, such as minor deficiencies of SGCG with partial preservation of the other three sarcoglycan proteins in LGMD2C or a partial deficiency of only SCGA with the retention of the other three in LGMD2D. The observation of complete deficiency of one sarcoglycan protein with partial deficiency of the others may indicate which gene to evaluate first for mutations. Patients with sarcoglycan mutations may also have a secondary reduction in dystrophin.

19.4.4 Clinical Presentation

This group comprises defects of α-sarcoglycan (SGCA, LGMD2D), β-sarcoglycan (SGCB, LGMD2E), γ-sarcoglycan (SGCG, LGMD2C) and δ-sarcoglycan (SGDG, LGMD2F). Sarcoglycan defects frequently lead to severe LGMDs. The onset of symptoms is usually between toddler and school age. However, adult onset of LGMD2D has been reported. The clinical picture although

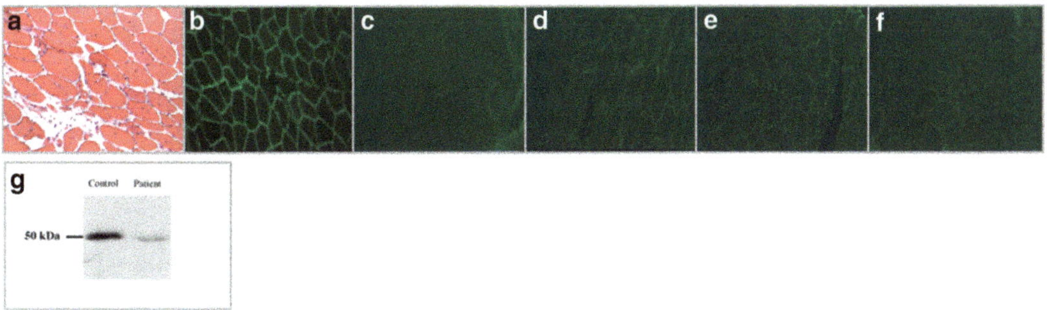

Fig. 19.9 Typical histological (**a**, H&E) and proteinchemical (**c–f**, α-, β-, γ-, δ-SG staining) findings in sarcoglyanopathy. H&E staining revealed a degenerative myopathy, compared to the normal control muscle (**b**), all sarcoglycans were reduced, most prominently α-SG staining (**c**). Immunoblotting (**g**) revealed severely reduced expression of α-SG protein as compared to normal muscle

more variable resembles in many aspects that of Duchenne muscular dystrophy (Fig. 19.10). The course is invariably progressive with loss of ambulation often occurring during the second decade of life. However, especially in cases with later onset ambulation may be preserved until adult life (mainly LGMD2D, Fig. 19.10). There is no cognitive involvement and overt cardiomyopathy is less common. However, in about 30 % of patients subclinical findings on electrocardiography or echocardiography indicate dilative cardiomyopathy. Patients with β- or δ-sarcoglycan mutations may be at higher risk for clinically relevant cardiac manifestations. CK levels are elevated 10–50 fold, respiratory involvement is usually seen during the course of the disease. Common clinical symptoms are scapular winging, lumbar hyperlordosis, and calf and tongue hypertrophy (Fig. 19.11). Interestingly, there is no clear-cut correlation between severity of disease and age of onset.

19.4.5 Imaging Findings

Although the four autosomal recessive sarcoglycanopathies (LGMD2C-2F) are among the best clinically characterized LGMDs, there are few muscle imaging data available. Similar to Duchenne and Becker muscular dystrophy, the most severe changes are seen in the anterior compartment of the thigh with little pathology in the lower legs. At early stages of the disease the calf muscles are normally not involved. The tibialis anterior muscles become affected during the course of the disease, whereas the gastrocnemius muscles remain relatively spared (Fig. 19.12).

19.4.6 Differential Diagnosis

Sarcoglycanopathy patients may exhibit IHC evidence of secondary reduction of dystrophin which should be taken into account for the differential diagnosis with X-linked Becker dystrophy (see Chap. 17) in patients with no identified mutation.

Limb Girdle Muscular Dystrophies: Sarcoglycanopathies (LGMD2C, LGMD2D, LGMD2E, LGMD2F)

Key Points

- In LGMD2D and BMD, there is more predominant involvement of the anterior thigh compartment.
- In the lower limbs in BMD, the most severe changes are observed in the soleus and gastrocnemius muscles, changes that are often not seen in LGMD2D.
- Whereas mutations in genes encoding proteins of the DGC (dystrophin, α-SG) predominantly affect the anterior thigh muscles, proteins with enzyme function (calpain-3, FKRP) predominantly involve the posterior thigh muscles.

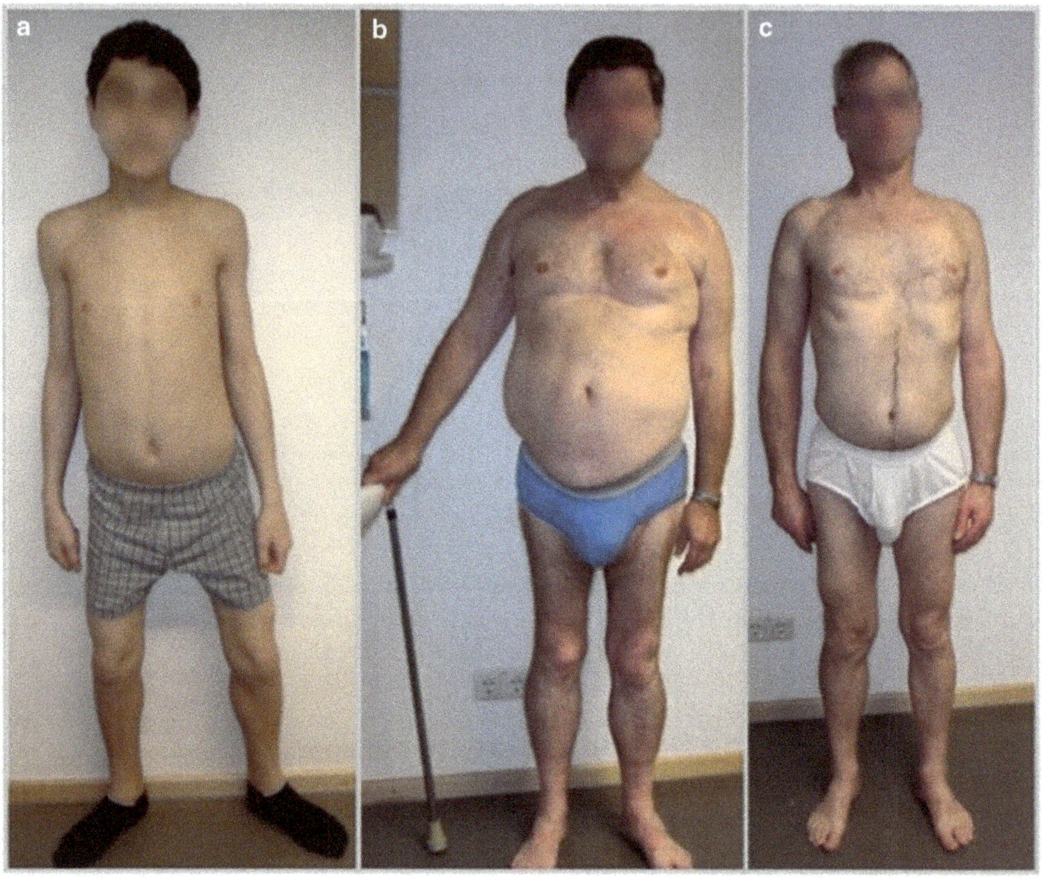

Fig. 19.10 Three patients with sarcoglycanopathies. Patient **a** (homozygous point mutation Met1Val) is 13 years old, of Arabic origin and suffers from LGMD2E (β-sarcoglycanopathy), while patients **b** (SGCA Tyr134STOP/Thr208Ala) and **c** (SGCA Arg77Cys/Val247Met) are both 60 years of age, of German descend, showed adult onset and are diagnosed with LGMD2D (α-sarcoglycanopathy). Note the muscle atrophy in proximal leg muscles along with calf hypertrophy in all patients. Interestingly, all patients are still able to walk independently

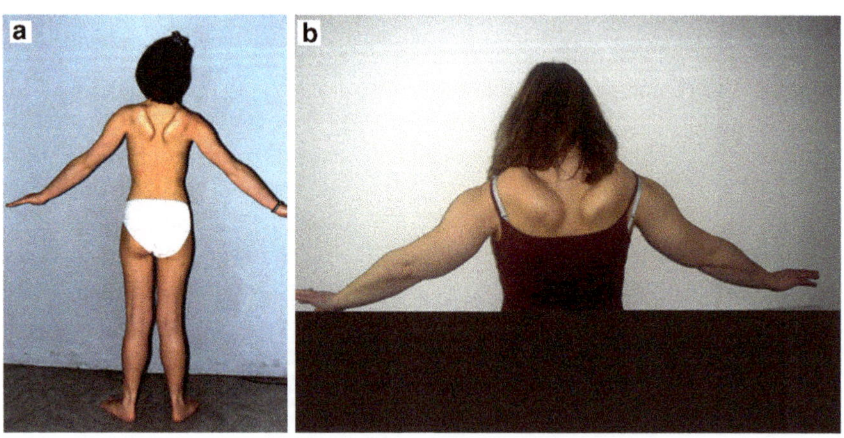

Fig. 19.11 Two patients with sarcoglyanopathies. Patient **a** is 12 years old and of Serbian origin. Genetically, LGMD2C (γ-sarcoglycanopathy) was identified [homozygous c.549_550InsT (p.Cys183fsX9)]. Patient **b** is German, 43 years of age, and showed adult onset of the disease, LGMD2D (α-sarcoglycanopathy) was genetically confirmed [c.229C>T (p.Arg 77Cys)/c.850C>T (p. Arg284Cys)]. Of notice calf hypertrophy, marked scapular winging and reduced arm elevation

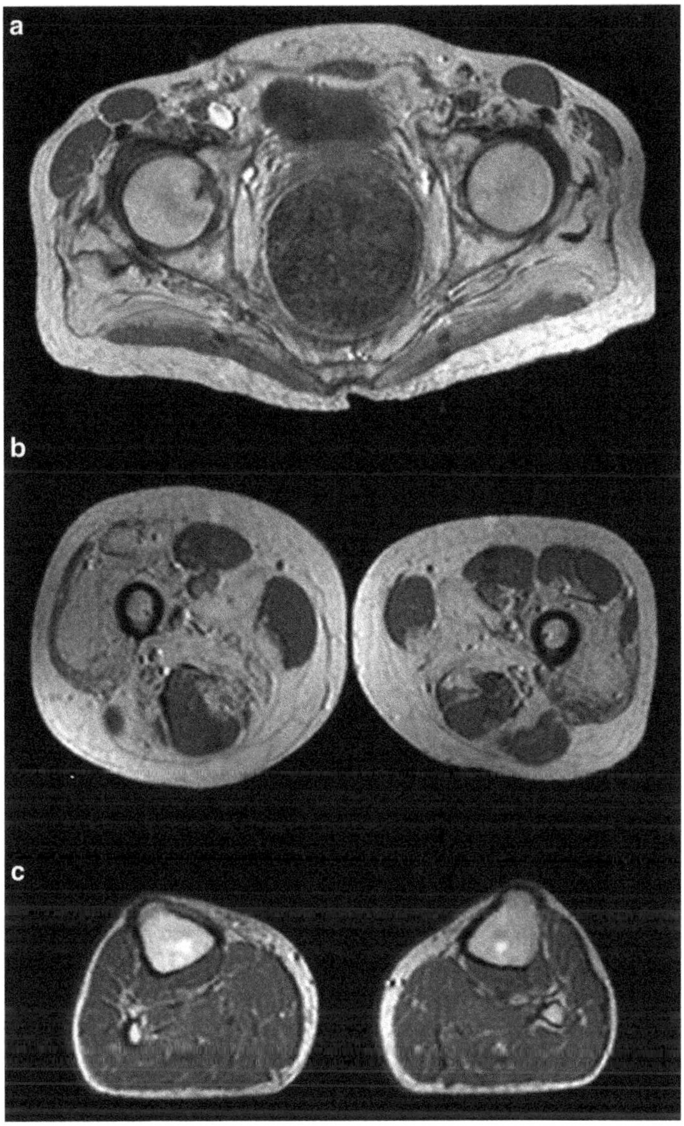

Fig. 19.12 Muscle MRI of a patient with α-sarcoglycanopathy (**a–c**). Involvement of the quadriceps muscle is more prominent than the affection of the posterior thigh compartment muscles (**b**). In the lower limbs, no severe changes are visible yet (**c**). From Fischer D, et al. (2005) Diagnostic value of muscle MRI in differentiating LGMD2I from other LGMDs. J Neurol. 252;538–47. Reprinted with permission from Springer

Suggestions for Further Reading

Fischer D, Walter MC, Kesper K et al. Diagnostic value of muscle MRI in differentiating LGMD2I from other LGMDs. J Neurol. 2005;252:538–47.

Kirschner J, Lochmüller H. Sarcoglycanopathies. Handb Clin Neurol. 2011;101:41–46.

Klinge L, Dekomien G, Aboumousa A, et al. Sarcoglycanopathies: can muscle immunoanalysis predict the genotype? Neuromuscul Disord. 2008;18:934–41.

Sandonà D, Betto R. Sarcoglycanopathies: molecular pathogenesis and therapeutic prospects. Expert Rev Mol Med. 2009;11:e28.

Trabelsi M, Kavian N, Daoud F, et al. Revised spectrum of mutations in sarcoglycanopathies. Eur J Hum Genet. 2008;16:793–803.

19.5 Caveolin-3 Related Myopathies

19.5.1 Synonyms, Abbreviations

Limb girdle muscular dystrophy type 1C (LGMD1C), rippling muscle disease (RMD).

19.5.2 Genetics and Pathophysiology

Mutations in the human caveolin-3 gene (*cav-3*) on chromosome 3p25 (OMIM *601253) have been described in limb girdle muscular dystrophy type 1C (LGMD1C), rippling muscle disease (RMD), asymptomatic hyperCKemia, distal myopathy, and various types of (hypertrophic and dilated) cardiomyopathy as well as the long QT syndrome. Caveolin-3 is the muscle specific caveolin isoform. Mutations may affect any region in the gene, but most mutations are located in the scaffolding domain of the protein. The mutations usually have a negative dominant effect. Cav-3 mutant/Cav-3 wild type proteins form unstable, high-molecular-weight protein aggregates that are retained within the Golgi complex where they undergo rapid degradation via the 26S-proteasome dependent pathway. As a result, there is marked reduction or an absence of normal sarcolemmal caveolin-3 expression. Rarely, autosomal recessive mutations have also been described.

Caveolin proteins (21–24 kDa) are the principal components of caveolae, which are flask-shaped invaginations of the plasma membrane that participate in signal transduction events and vesicular traffic processes. Caveolin proteins have been implicated in the formation of caveolae by acting as scaffolding proteins, that organize and concentrate specific-caveolin-interacting lipids and proteins. Caveolins are also associated with receptor tyrosine kinases and G-proteins implying an important role in signal transduction. The exact pathophysiology remains to be elucidated, but the loss of sarcolemmal caveolin-3 impairs caveolae formation, lipid functioning, and signal transduction.

19.5.3 Histopathology

Morphological analysis of a muscle biopsy usually reveals relatively mild myopathic changes consisting of slightly increased endomysial connective tissue, pathological fiber-size variability, and increased internalization of nuclei (Fig. 19.13). Some patients show more severe changes consisting of excessive fiber splitting and degeneration. IHC and Western blotting show that Caveolin-3 protein expression is markedly reduced or absent (Fig. 19.14).

19.5.4 Clinical Presentation

The clinical presentation in patients with a *cav-3* mutation is heterogeneous. Asymptomatic hyperCKemia, exercise-induced cramps, and myalgias are probably the most common clinical manifestations. The clinical hallmarks of RMD are percussion induced rapid muscle contractions (PIRCs), localized (painful) muscle moundings, and percussion or stretching induced rolling movements across a muscle group (rippling) (Fig. 19.15). Careful examination reveals signs of RMD in most *cav-3* mutation carriers even in patients with so-called asymptomatic hyperCKemia. Calf and generalized hypertrophy is common, but overt muscle weakness is often not as marked. Many patients walk preferentially on their toes during early childhood. Isolated distal foot and toe extensor weakness can be observed in patients with a mild distal myopathy phenotype (Fig. 19.16). LGMD1C with marked proximal weakness is probably the least common phenotype observed in patients with *cav-3* mutations (Fig. 19.17).

19.5.5 Imaging Findings

Data on muscle imaging in caveolinopathies is limited. There are few published data and anecdotal reports on a only few patients. These data suggest that in the thighs the most affected muscles are the rectus femoris, adductor magnus, adductor longus, and posterior thigh compartment muscles (Fig. 19.18). In the lower legs tibialis anterior and gastrocnemius muscles are most affected (Fig. 19.16d).

19.5.6 Differential Diagnosis

In patients with signs of RMD, the most important differential diagnosis includes myotonic dystrophies (see Chap. 22) and non-dystrophic myotonias (see Sect. 13.2). In patients with hyperCKemia the differential diagnosis is broad and includes all other LGMD. In particular dysferlinopathies (see Sect. 19.3) and Fukutin-related protein (FKRP)

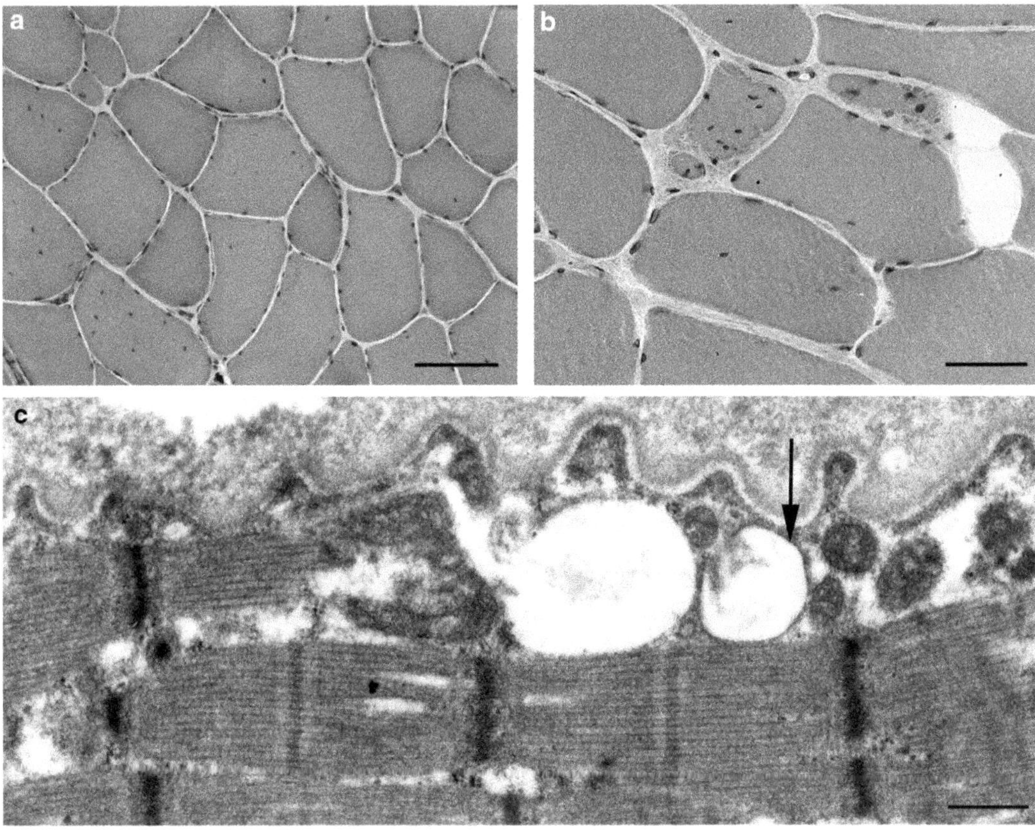

Fig. 19.13 Morphological analysis of cav-3 deficient muscle. (**a**) HE staining of skeletal muscle showed mild myopathic changes consisting of a slight increase of endomysial connective tissue, pathological fiber-size variability and increased internalisation of nuclei, bar = 100 μm. (**b**) HE staining of skeletal muscle from another patient with RMD and LGMD additionally showed an abnormal cytoplasmic configuration representing either fiber degeneration or excessive fiber splitting, bar = 50 μm. (**c**) Ultrastructural analysis of skeletal muscle from the index patient showed the presence of multiple vesicular structures in the subsarcolemmal region (*arrow*) and an abnormal folding of plasma membrane (bar = 0.3 μm). From Fischer D, et al. (2003) Consequences of a novel caveolin 3 mutation in a large German family. Ann Neurol. 53:233–41. With permission from John Wiley and Sons

related myopathies (see Sect. 16.5) need to be considered as in some of these patients IHC has revealed secondary caveolin-3 reduction.

Limb Girdle Muscular Dystrophies: Caveolinopathies

Key Points

- Caveolinopathy presents with (asymptomatic) hyperCKemia, a rippling muscle phenotype, distal myopathy, LGMD-1C), and various cardiac manifestations.
- Diagnosis is usually based on IHC and Western blotting on muscle biopsy tissue demonstrating an abnormal caveolin-3 expression.
- Muscle imaging studies are limited but suggest that the rectus femoris, adductor, and hamstrings in the thigh and the tibial anterior muscles in the lower leg are those most involved.

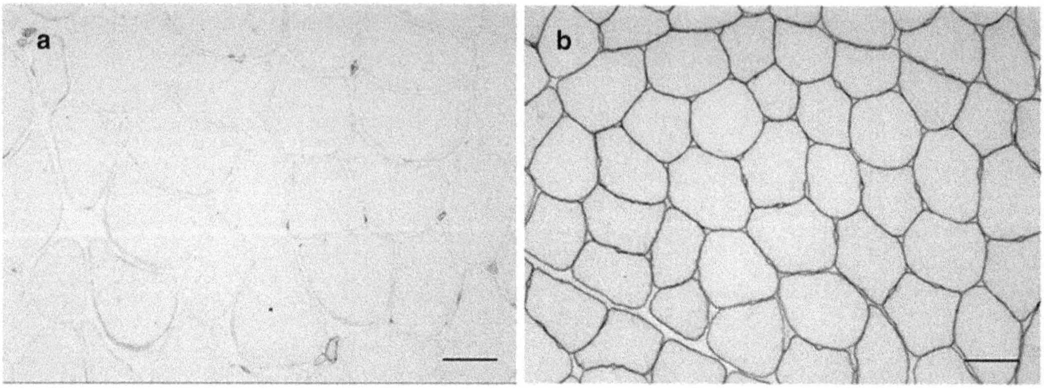

Fig. 19.14 Cav-3 immunostaining of diseased (**a**) and normal human skeletal muscle (**b**). Note the dramatic decrease of cav-3 expression when compared to normal controls, bar = 60 μm. From Fischer D, et al. (2003) Consequences of a novel caveolin-3 mutation in a large German family. Ann Neurol. 53:233–41. With permission from John Wiley and Sons

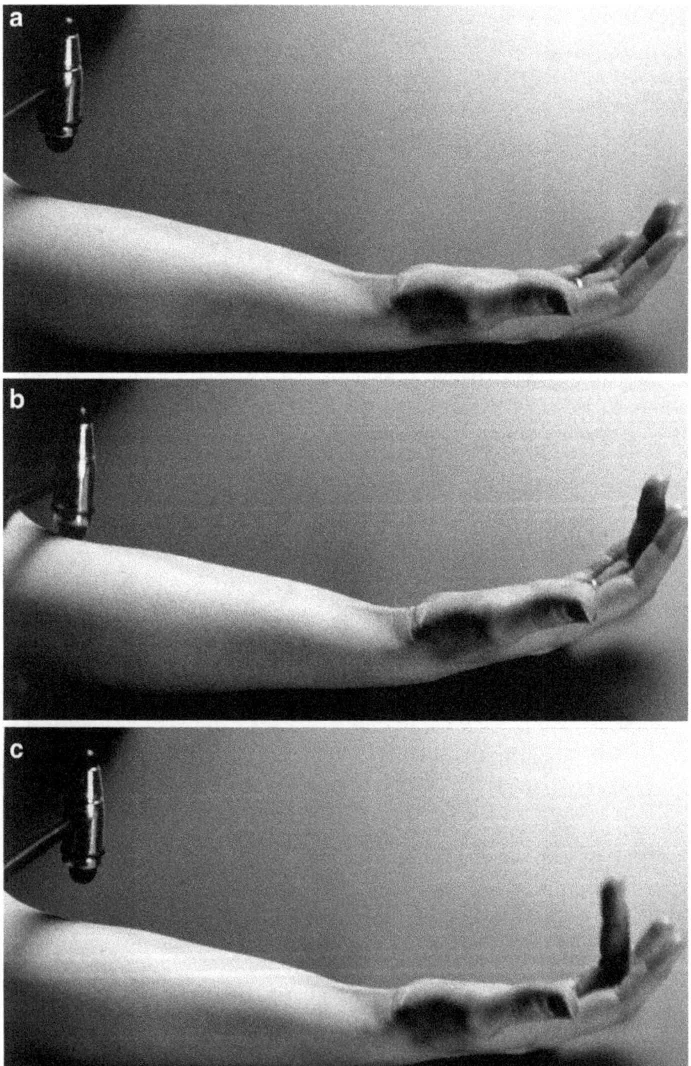

Fig. 19.15 Percussion-induced rapid muscle contractions: the clinical hallmark of rippling muscle disease. Note the the normal position at rest (**a**), flexion of the ring finger (**c**) in response to mild percussion (**b**) of the flexor digitorum muscle. From Fischer D, et al. (2003) Consequences of a novel caveolin-3 mutation in a large German family. Ann Neurol. 53:233–41. With permission from John Wiley and Sons

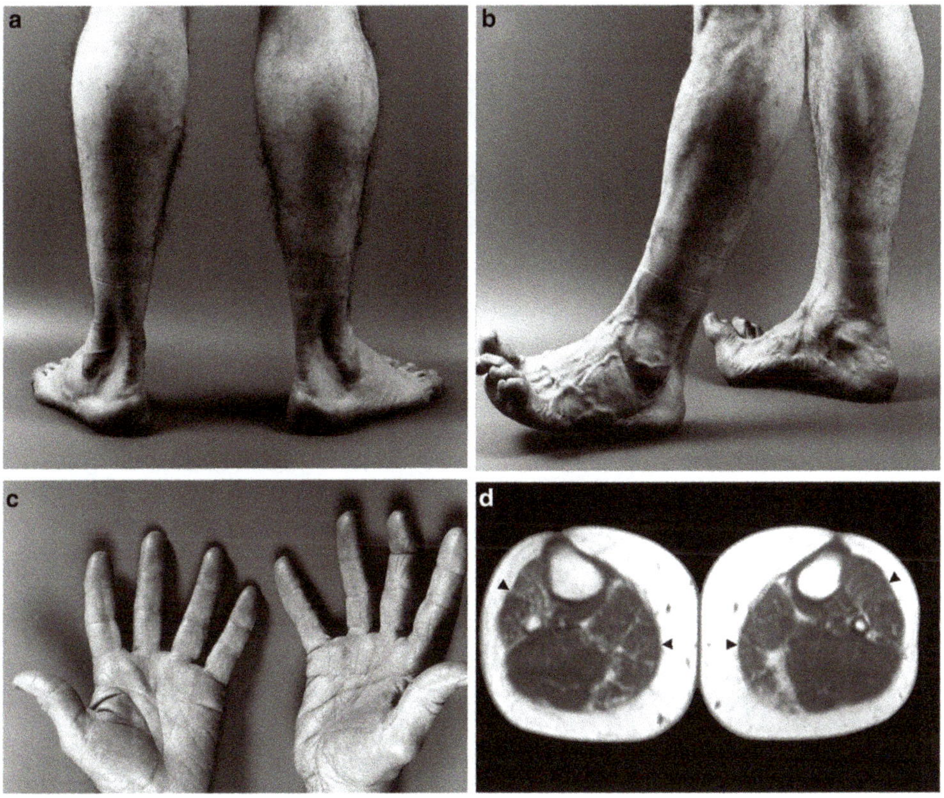

Fig. 19.16 Clinical and MRI features of a patient with caveolinopathy and distal myopathy: (**a**) calf hypertrophy, (**b**) weakness of foot dorsiflexion, (**c**) slight atrophy of intrinsic hand muscles, (**d**) MRI signal abnormalities (*arrowheads*) in the anterior leg compartment and medial gastrocnemius muscle on T2-weighted images. From Fischer D, et al. (2003) Consequences of a novel caveolin-3 mutation in a large German family. Ann Neurol. 53:233–41. With permission from John Wiley and Sons

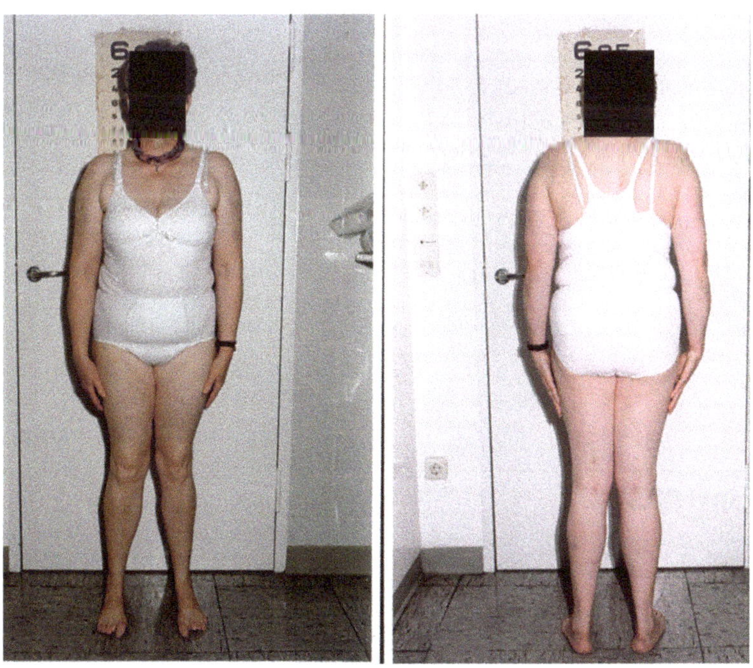

Fig. 19.17 Clinical phenotype of a LGMD1C patient. Note the rather hypertrophic phenotype compared to most other muscular dystrophies and the calf hypertrophy

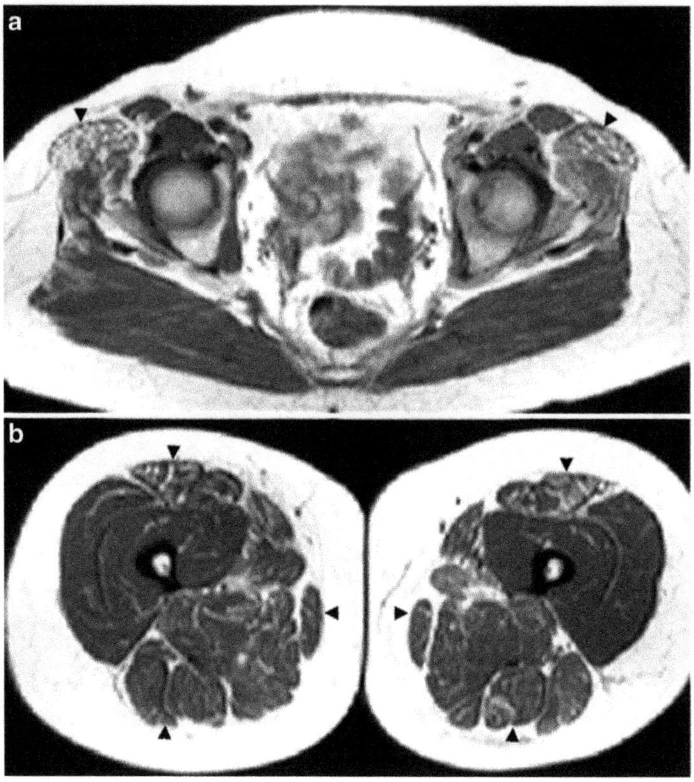

Fig. 19.18 MRI of a patient with caveolinopathy and LGMD1C phenotype: (**a**, **b**) MRI signal abnormalities (*arrowheads*) in hip and thigh muscles with predominant changes in hip abductor, hip adductor, rectus femoris and hamstring muscles on T2-weighted images. From Fischer D, et al. (2003) Consequences of a novel caveolin-3 mutation in a large German family. Ann Neurol. 53:233–41. With permission from John Wiley and Sons

Suggestions for Further Reading

Betz RC, Schoser BG, Kasper D, et al. Mutations in CAV3 cause mechanical hyperirritability of skeletal muscle in rippling muscle disease. Nat Genet. 2001;28:218–9.

Fischer D, Schroers A, Blümcke I, et al. Consequences of a novel caveolin-3 mutation in a large German family. Ann Neurol. 2003;53:233–41.

Papi L, Fischer D, Trajanoski S, et al. SNP-array based whole genome homozygosity mapping: a quick and powerful tool to achieve an accurate diagnosis in LGMD2 patients. Eur J Med Genet. 2011;54:214–9.

Walter MC, Braun C, Vorgerd M, et al. Variable reduction of caveolin-3 in patients with LGMD2B/MM. J Neurol. 2003;250:1431–8.

19.6 Therapy: All LGMD

To date, curative therapy is not available, although the development of promising new treatment modalities is underway. In the future, molecular therapy may be available to address the molecular defects that cause LGMD but this might still be years away to evaluate treatment modalities, we differentiate between symptomatic strategies (e.g., pharmacological therapies) and supportive treatment and causative treatment schedules (e.g., gene or cell therapy).

Nevertheless, life expectancy and life quality of LGMD patients has steadily improved. This has been achieved by improved symptomatic treatment and care, such as assisted ventilation, drug therapy for heart failure and surgical therapy to prevent complications. Despite these efforts, there are still few pharmacological options available specifically to prevent or delay the dystrophic process in muscle fibers. Currently, corticosteroids are the most effective drugs for patients with Duchenne muscular dystrophy (DMD). There are single reports on their efficacy in other LGMDs, but therapy is limited by the high frequency and severity of side effects. The exact mechanism of how steroids work in DMD remains unknown. Future studies should attempt to unravel this mechanism, hopefully leading to an equally potent but less toxic drug. Creatine monohydrate seems to be of some efficacy and has no remarkable side effects. Therefore, short-term administration may be helpful in individual cases.

New molecular therapeutic approaches such as exon skipping or stop-codon-read-through have been invented in recent years and are currently being investigated in clinical trials with DMD patients. Although molecular therapies promise causal intervention and curative treatment, a large number of technical and methodological problems still need to be solved. Molecular therapies should be applied to LGMD patients only if they are considered reasonably safe. Therefore, the majority of LGMD patients today must rely on standard symptomatic therapy, with molecular approaches continuing to hold promise for the future.

Suggestions for Further Reading

Amato AA, Griggs RC. Overview of the muscular dystrophies. Handb Clin Neurol. 2011;101:1–9.

Barthélémy F, Wein N, Krahn M, et al. Translational research and therapeutic perspectives in dysferlinopathies. Mol Med. 2011;17:875–82.

Bushby K. Diagnosis and management of the limb girdle muscular dystrophies. Pract Neurol. 2009;9:314–23.

Bushby K, Lochmüller H, Lynn S, et al. Interventions for muscular dystrophy: molecular medicines entering the clinic. Lancet 2009;374:1849–1856.

Manzur AY, Muntoni F. Diagnosis and new treatments in muscular dystrophies. J Neurol Neurosurg Psychiatr. 2009;80:706–714.

Schara U, Walter MC. Update on congenital and limb girdle muscular dystrophies. Neuropädiatrie 2006;6: 1–11.

Myofibrillar Myopathies

20

Montse Olivé and Rudolf Andre Kley

20.1 Introduction and Classification

The term myofibrillar myopathy (MFM) refers to a group of hereditary muscle disorders having in common myopathological features of focal disintegration of myofibrils and accumulation of degradation products into inclusions containing desmin and other myofibrillar and ectopic proteins. These highly clinical heterogeneous disorders are caused by mutations in the sarcomeric and Z-disc-supporting cytoskeletal proteins desmin (*DES*), αB-crystallin (*CRYAB*), myotilin (*MYOT*, *TTID*), Z-band alternatively spliced PDZ-containing protein (*ZASP*, *LDB3*), filamin C (*FLNC*), and Bcl-2-associated athanogene-3 (*BAG3*). The corresponding diseases are named accordingly: desminopathy, αB-crystallinopathy, myotilinopathy, ZASPopathy, filaminopathy, and BAG3-myopathy.

Mutations in LIM domain 2 of four and a half LIM domain 1 protein (FHL1) cause reducing body myopathy, a disease fulfilling the morphological criteria of MFM. Further genetic heterogeneity is suspected because the causative gene remains to be discovered in many patients suffering from MFM.

Clinical phenotypes associated with MFMs are widely heterogeneous. Individual MFM subtypes have distinct clinical, morphological and muscle imaging features depending on the disease-causative gene. MFMs with their causative genes and main phenotypes are summarized in Table 20.1. MFMs represent the paradigm of conformational protein diseases of skeletal muscles. The mechanisms leading to protein aggregation in MFM are not well known. However, disturbances of protein quality control mechanisms are important factors in the pathogenesis of these diseases. Several factors including mutant proteins, aggresome formation, generation of reactive oxygen species (ROS) as a result of mitochondrial dysfunction among others may compromise the ubiquitin–proteasome system and the autophagic–lysosomal pathway, promoting the accumulation of potentially toxic protein aggregates in muscle cells.

Muscle imaging particularly MRI is a powerful diagnostic tool that allows differentiation between gene-dependent subtypes of MFM. They allow differentiation of patients carrying mutations in the Z-disc supporting proteins desmin, and αB-crystallin from patients carrying mutations in the Z-disc proteins myotilin, ZASP and filamin C (Table 20.2). This chapter focuses on MFM caused by mutations in *DES*, *CRYAB*, *MYOT*, *ZASP* and *FLNC*.

M. Olivé
Institute of Neuropathology, Department of Neurology and Neuromuscular Unit, Department of Neurology, IDIBELL-Hospital de Bellvitge, Hospitalet de Llobregat, Barcelona, Spain
e-mail: 25169mop@comb.cat

R.A. Kley (✉)
Department of Neurology, Neuromuscular Center Ruhrgebiet, University Hospital Bergmannsheil, Ruhr-University Bochum, Buerkle-de-la-Camp-Platz 1, 44789 Bochum, Germany
e-mail: rudolf.kley@rub.de

M.P. Wattjes and D. Fischer (eds.), *Neuromuscular Imaging*, DOI 10.1007/978-1-4614-6552-2_20,

Table 20.1 Myofibrillar myopathies: clinical presentation

Gene	Disease	Inheritance	Onset	Main clinical phenotypes
DES	Desminopathy	AD AR De novo	Young adulthood	Distal or less frequently proximal myopathy preceded, accompanied or followed by cardiopathy frequently associated to respiratory insufficiency Scapuloperoneal syndrome Isolated cardiomyopathy
CRYAB	αB-crystallinopathy	AD AR	Young adulthood	Distal or less frequently proximal myopathy preceded, accompanied or followed by cardiopathy, with or without lens opacities, frequently associated with respiratory insufficiency
MYOT	Myotilinopathy	AD	Late adulthood	LGMD 1 A Distal > proximal weakness, less frequently initially mixed or proximal weakness Respiratory insufficiency in a minority of patients
LDB3	ZASPopathy	AD	Late adulthood	Distal > proximal weakness, sometimes associated with cardiopathy, associated peripheral neuropathy in some cases
FLNC	Filaminopathy	AD	Middle adulthood	Proximal > distal weakness similar to LGMD Regular involvement of respiratory muscles in advanced disease

Table 20.2 Myofibrillar myopathies: pattern of muscle involvement on muscle imaging

Desminopathy/αB-crystallinopathy		Myotilinopathy/ZASPopathy/filaminopathy	
Most affected muscles			
Thigh	Leg	Thigh	Leg
Semitendinosus Gracilis Sartorius	Peroneal group muscles Anterior tibialis Gastrocnemius	Semimembranosus Biceps femoris Adductor magnus	Soleus Gastrocnemius medial head Anterior tibialis
Least affected muscles			
Vastus intermedius Vastus lateralis Rectus femoris Vastus medialis	Soleus	Semitendinosus Gracilis Sartorius Rectus femoris	Gastrocnemius lateral head Peroneal group

20.2 Desminopathy

20.2.1 Synonyms

Desmin myopathy; desmin-related myopathy.

20.2.2 Genetics and Pathophysiology

Desmin is a type III intermediate filament protein that is highly expressed in skeletal, cardiac and smooth muscles. In mature skeletal muscle, desmin localizes at the Z-lines where it plays a major role in maintaining the structural integrity of myofibrils by connecting adjacent myofibrils laterally and linking peripheral myofibrils to the sarcolemma and nuclei. Desmin interacts with other intermediate filament proteins to form an intracytoplasmic network that maintains spatial relations between the contractile apparatus and other structural elements of the cell. In the heart, desmin is increased at intercalated discs and is the major component of Purkinje fibers. Human

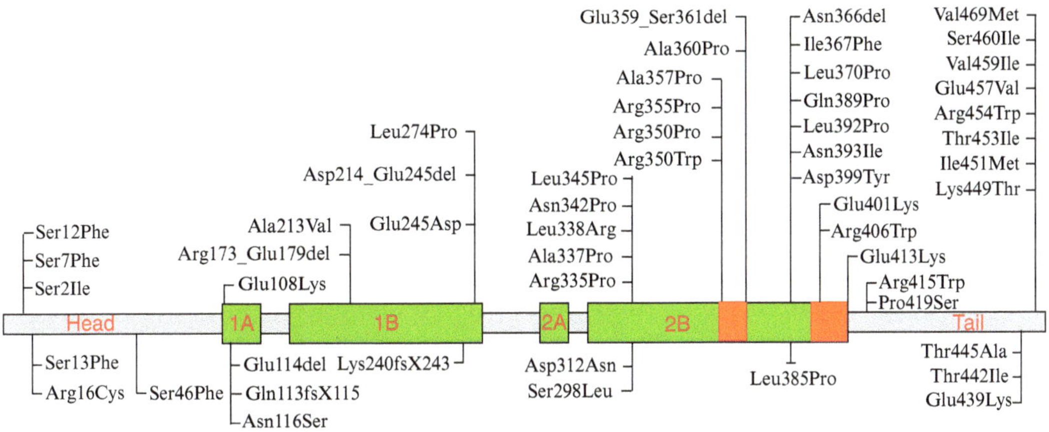

Fig. 20.1 Schematic representation of the desmin protein domains and positions of pathogenic mutations identified to date. Figure kindly provided by Lev G. Goldfarb (updated from J Clin Invest. 2009;119:1806–13)

desmin is encoded by a single copy gene (*DES*) located in chromosome 2q35 band; it encompasses nine exons and codes for 476 amino acids. The desmin molecule is organized into three domains: a highly conserved α-helical core flanked by globular N- and C-terminal ("head" and "tail") structures. The α-helical rod domain consists of four segments: 1A, 1B, 2A, 2B. The first desmin-associated mutations were described in 1998. So far, the number of disease-causing *DES* mutations has reached 45. Most of them are missense mutations that reside in the 2B α-helical rod domain (Fig. 20.1).

Transfection experiments and in vitro assembly studies indicate that the majority of mutant desmins are incapable of generating an intracellular filamentous network or disrupt pre-existing endogenous intermediate filament structures.

20.2.3 Histopathology

Muscle biopsies of affected muscles in desminopathy reveal the presence of amorphous eosinophilic regions that stain dark green or bluish with modified trichrome (Fig. 20.2a). These areas are typically devoid of oxidative enzymes giving rise to a rubbed-out appearance of muscle fibers (Fig. 20.2b). Other nonspecific myopathic features, such as variation in fiber size, scattered atrophic fibers, and an increased number of internal nuclei are also frequently observed. Abnormal fiber areas display strong immunoreactivity for desmin (Fig. 20.2c), α-B-crystallin, dystrophin, filamin C and many other proteins. Electron microscopy (EM) shows that the ultrastructural hallmark of desminopathies is the accumulation of granulofilamentous material underneath the sarcolemma and among the myofibrils (Fig. 20.2d). Areas in the vicinity of these aggregates show variable streaming of the Z-line. Mitochondria are sometimes located alongside the granulofilamentous deposits, forming sandwich-like structures. Autophagic vacuoles with polymorphous and myelin-like debris are additional findings.

20.2.4 Clinical Presentation

Myofibrillar myopathies (MFMs) resulting from mutations in desmin are probably the most frequent subtype. Age at onset usually varies between 15 and 40 years. The pattern of inheritance is autosomal dominant in the majority of cases, but not infrequently patients carry de novo mutations. Recessive mutations are rare. In patients carrying recessive mutations, the disease manifests in childhood and has a more devastating course.

Desminopathy usually manifests as a distal myopathy with later involvement of the proximal

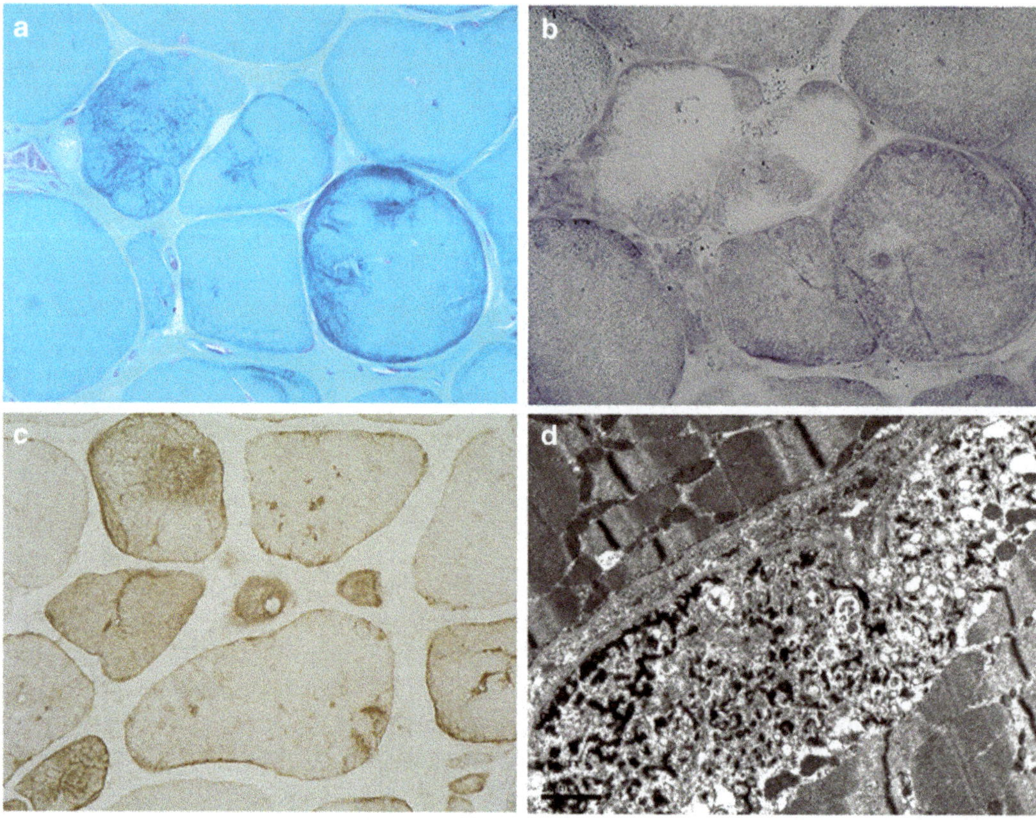

Fig. 20.2 Characteristic pathological features in desminopathy. Several fibers contain dark-bluish cytoplasmic inclusions (**a**: modified Gomori trichrome staining) which are devoid of oxidative activity (rubbed-out fibers) (**b**: SDH staining). Desmin-immunoreactive deposits (**c**). Under EM granulofilamentous material originating at the Z-line level accumulates under the sarcolemma and among the myofibrils (**d**)

muscles, although in some patients it presents as a limb-girdle myopathy with distal progression. In some families the disease presents as a scapuloperoneal syndrome. Involvement of bulbar and facial muscles is frequently observed, sometimes at disease onset. Respiratory insufficiency requiring nocturnal ventilatory support frequently occurs during the course of the illness. Up to 75 % of patients with desminopathy develop signs of cardiac involvement before, during, or following the skeletal myopathy. In the majority of cases cardiomyopathy manifests with atrioventricular conduction blocks with recurrent episodes of syncopes, and less frequently with arrhythmias. Many patients eventually require a pacemaker or a defibrillator implant. In advanced disease, many patients develop cardiac failure as a result of dilated, hypertrophic or restrictive cardiomyopathy. A patient suffering from desminopathy is shown in Fig. 20.3.

20.2.5 Imaging Findings

Patients with desminopathy show a recognizable pattern of muscle involvement on CT or MRI studies. As stated before, many patients with desminopathy eventually require a pacemaker or a defibrillator implant, thereby disallowing MRI studies. In these patients, muscle imaging can be performed with CT.

At the pelvic level (Fig. 20.4a–c), the gluteus maximus muscle is usually more involved than the gluteus medius and minimus muscles. At the mid thigh level (Fig. 20.4d–f) the sartorius, gracilis, and especially the semitendinosus muscles

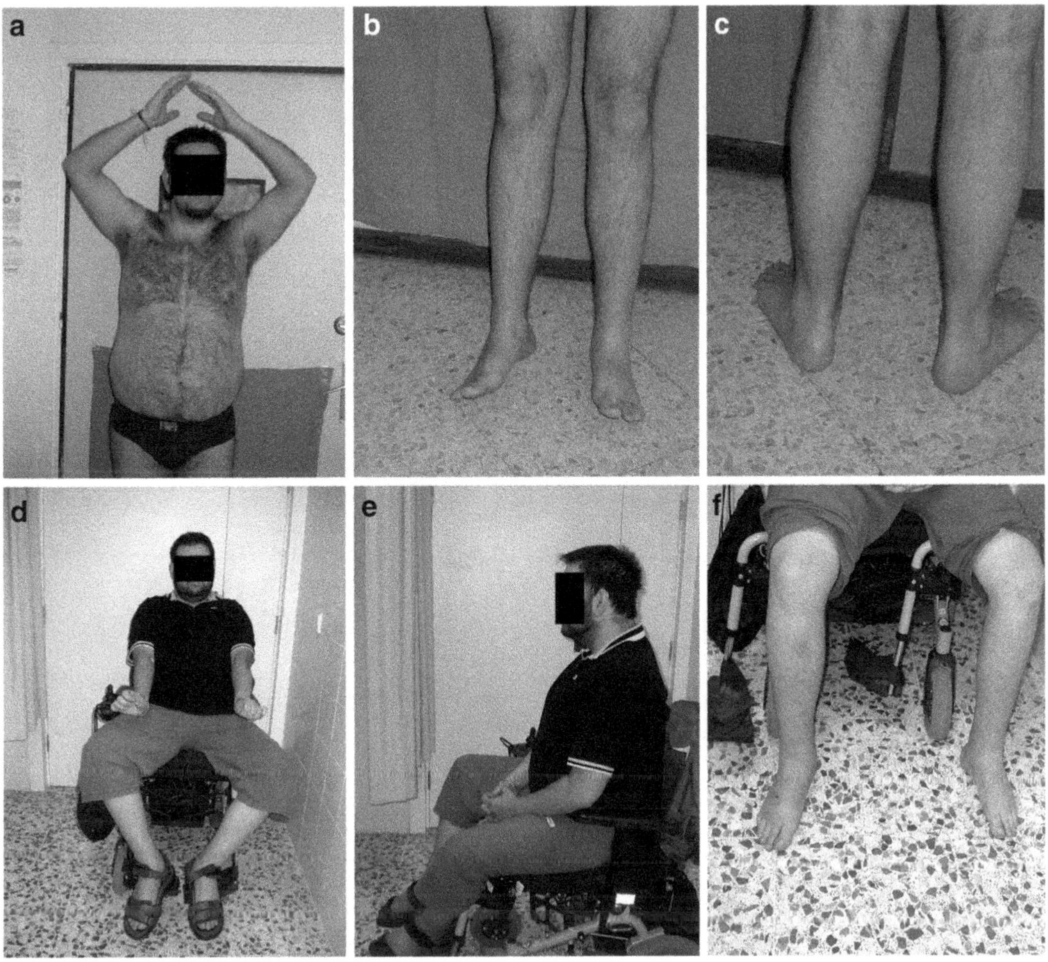

Fig. 20.3 Clinical phenotype of a patient carrying an Arg406Pro *DES* mutation at the age of 25 (**a–c**) and 29 years (**d–f**). This patient presented at the age of 14 with complete AV block, followed by progressive heart failure as a result of a dilated cardiomyopathy requiring heart transplantation. At the age of 25, weakness was restricted to the anterior compartment of legs. Four years later, he was severely disabled with prominent weakness in four limbs, neck extensors and respiratory muscles

are typically affected from very early stages of the illness. Later during the disease course the adductor magnus, biceps femoris and semimembranosus become involved. The anterior compartment muscles of the thigh (vastus lateralis, vastus intermedius, rectus femoris, vastus medialis) are less affected.

At the mid-leg level (Fig. 20.4g–i) the first muscles to be involved are the peroneal group, followed by the anterior tibialis muscle and muscles of the posterior compartment (soleus, medial gastrocnemius, lateral gastrocnemius).

20.3 αB-crystallinopathy

20.3.1 Synonyms

None.

20.3.2 Genetics and Pathophysiology

αB-crystallin is a chaperone that belongs to the "small heat shock protein" family. Although it

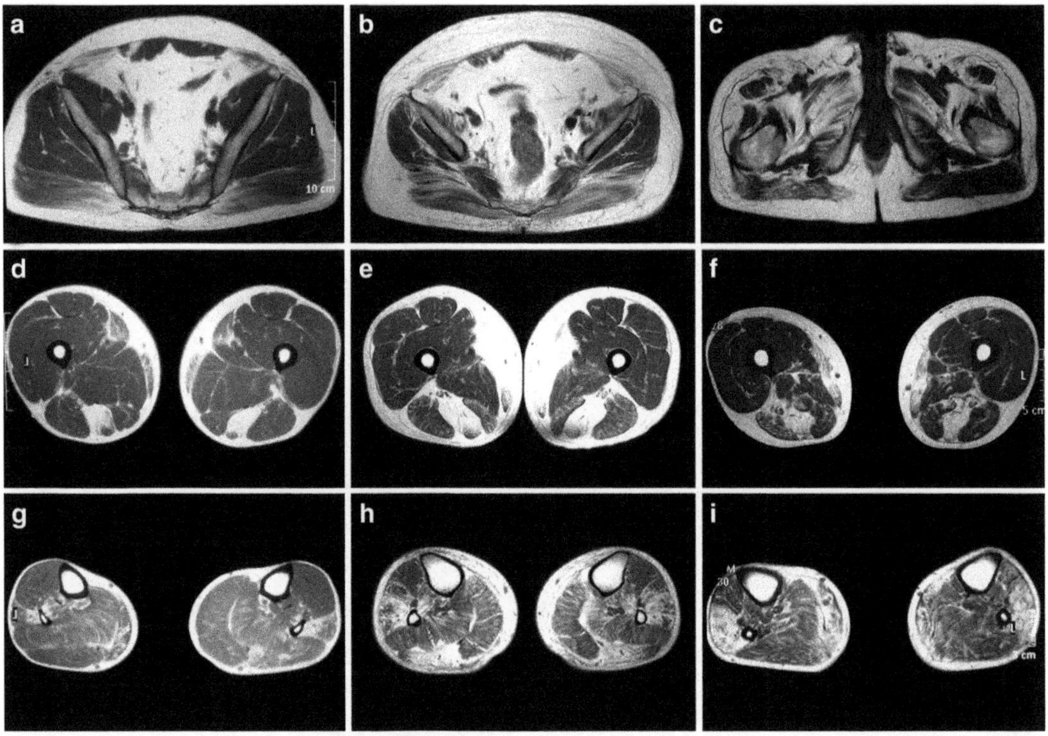

Fig. 20.4 Transverse T1-weighted MR images from three desminopathy patients at the pelvic (**a–c**), mid-thigh (**d–f**), and mid-leg level (**g–i**). In the pelvis, the gluteus maximus is the first muscle to be involved. At mid-thigh, the most severely affected muscle is always the semitendinosus followed by the sartorius and gracilis. At mid-leg changes are first observed in the peroneal group muscles (**i**), medial gastrocnemius and anterior tibialis

was originally discovered as a lens protein, αB-crystallin is found in nonlenticular tissues and is highly expressed in cardiac and skeletal muscle. Under stress conditions αB-crystallin binds to unfolded proteins to prevent their denaturation and aggregation. αB-crystallin is encoded by the gene *CRYAB* mapped to chromosome 11q22.3–q23.1; it encompasses three exons and codes for 175 amino acids.

Cell cultures transfected with mutant αB-crystallin show abnormal cytoplasmic aggregates containing desmin and αB-crystallin, suggesting similar disease mechanisms in desminopathy and αB-crystallinopathy.

20.3.3 Histopathology

Myopathological features in patients with αB-crystallinopathy are indistinguishable from those observed in desminopathy. They consist of patches of desmin and αB-crystallin-immunoreactive inclusions, characteristic rubbed-out areas on oxidative stains and typical granulofilamentous material accumulation when viewed by electron microscopy.

20.3.4 Clinical Presentation

αB-crystallinopathy is an infrequent subtype of MFM. A heterozygous *CRYAB* p.Arg120Gly mutation was identified in 1998 in a large multigenerational French family with a clinical and myopathological phenotype indistinguishable from desminopathy. Affected members presented around the age of 30 years with proximal upper limb and distal lower limb weakness, involvement of the velopharyngeal muscles, respiratory failure and cardiomyopathy. A distinctive feature in this family was the presence of lens opacities. The pattern of inheritance was autosomal dominant.

Only a few additional cases have been reported since then; they presented in adulthood with cervical and limb-girdle weakness and respiratory failure, or with proximal and distal limb weakness and peripheral neuropathy. There was no cardiac involvement or lens opacities. Recently, recessive mutations in *CRYAB* have been identified as the cause of a severe infantile myopathy causing limb and axial muscle stiffness and severe respiratory insufficiency leading to early death.

20.3.5 Imaging Findings

Only limited data regarding the pattern of muscle involvement on imaging studies in patients with αB-crystallinopathy have been reported. Muscle CT scans performed in four individuals carrying the p.Arg120Gly *CRYAB* mutation revealed a pattern of muscle involvement similar to that observed in desminopathy patients. It was characterized by early involvement of the semitendinosus, sartorius and gracilis muscles at the thigh level (Fig. 20.5a) later spreading to hip adductors and quadriceps femoris. At the mid-calf level (Fig. 20.5b), the first changes were seen in the peroneal group, followed by involvement of the anterior tibialis and the posterior group.

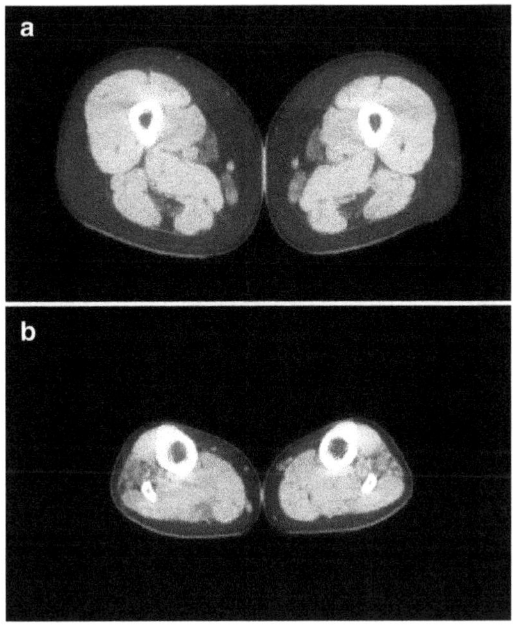

Fig. 20.5 Transverse muscle CT images from a patient carrying a R120G *CRYAB* mutation early in the course of the disease. At mid-thigh (**a**), there is a selective involvement of the semitendinosus, sartorius and gracilis. At mid leg (**b**), changes are observed in the peroneal group muscles. This pattern of involvement is identical to that observed in patients carrying mutations in *DES* (see Fig. 20.4 for comparison)

Myofibrillar Myopathies: Desminopathy and alphaB-Crystallinopathy

Key Points

- Desminopathy and αB-crystallinopathy are hereditary disorders caused by mutations in the *DES* and *CRYAB* genes respectively.
- Desminopathy and αB-crystallinopathy usually manifests in young adults with distal or less often proximal weakness. A large proportion of patients develop signs of cardiac involvement before, during or following skeletal myopathy. Respiratory failure is a frequent complication in desminopathy and αB-crystallinopathy. The presence of lens opacities is a distinctive feature in αB-crystallinopathy.
- Muscle biopsies from desminopathy and αB-crystallinopathy patients show patches of desmin-immunoreactive inclusions, rubbed-out areas on oxidative stains, and granulofilamentous material accumulation under electron microscopy.
- Muscle imaging of lower limbs shows a characteristic pattern of muscle involvement. At the mid-thigh level, the semitendinosus, gracilis and sartorius are the first muscles to be involved. At the mid-leg level, the peroneal group are the first affected muscles.
- Currently there is no curative therapy for desminopathy or αB-crystallinopathy, although some of the complications and premature death can be prevented.

Suggestions for Further Reading

Clemen CS, Herrmann H, Strelkov SV, Schröder R. Desminopathies: pathology and mechanisms. Acta Neuropathol. 2013;125:47–75.

Fardeau M, Vicart P, Caron A, et al. Familial myopathy with desmin storage seen as a granulo-filamentar, electron-dense material with mutation of the alphaB-crystallin gene. Rev Neurol. (Paris) 2000;156:497–504.

Ferrer I, Olivé M. Molecular pathology of myofibrillar myopathies. Expert Rev Mol Med. 2008;10:e25.

Fischer D, Kley RA, Strach K, et al. Distinct muscle imaging patterns in myofibrillar myopathies. Neurology 2008;71:758–65.

Forrest KM, Al-Sarraj S, Sewry C, et al. Infantile onset myofibrillar myopathy due to recessive CRYAB mutation. Neuromuscul Disord. 2011;21:37–40.

Goldfarb LG, Dalakas MC. Tragedy in a heartbeat: malfunctioning desmin causes skeletal and cardiac muscle disease. J Clin Invest. 2009;119:1806–13.

Goldfarb LG, Olivé M, Vicart P, Goebel HH. Intermediate filament diseases: desminopathy. Adv Exp Med Biol. 2008;642:131–64.

Goldfarb LG, Vicart P, Goebel HH, Dalakas MC. Desmin myopathy. Brain 2004;127:723–34.

Olivé M, Odgerel Z, Martínez A, et al. Clinical and myopathological evaluation of early- and late-onset subtypes of myofibrillar myopathy. Neuromuscul Disord. 2011;21:533–42.

Schröder R, Schoser B. Myofibrillar myopathies: a clinical and myopathological guide. Brain Pathol. 2009;19: 483–92.

Schröder R, Vrabie A, Goebel HH. Primary desminopathies. J Cell Mol Med. 2007;11:416–26.

Selcen D. Myofibrillar myopathies. Neuromuscul Disord. 2011;21:161–71.

Vicart P, Caron A, Guicheney P, et al. A missense mutation in the alphaB-crystallin chaperone gene causes a desmin-related myopathy. Nat Genet. 1998;20:92–95.

Wattjes MP, Kley RA, Fischer D. Neuromuscular imaging in inherited muscle diseases. Eur Radiol. 2010;20:2447–60.

20.4 Myotilinopathies

20.4.1 Synonyms

Myotilin myopathy, Limb girdle muscular dystrophy type 1A (LGMD1A).

20.4.2 Genetics and Pathophysiology

Myotilin is a sarcomeric Z-disc protein expressed strongly in skeletal muscle and weakly in cardiac muscle. Myotilin plays a significant role in sarcomere assembly, acting together with α-actinin and filamin C to cross-link actin into tightly packed bundles. Myotilin is encoded by a single copy gene (*MYOT*, *TTID*) located on chromosome 5q31. It encompasses 10 exons and codes for 498 amino acids. Myotilin molecule contains a serine-rich amino-terminal region, two immunoglobulin-like domains and a carboxy terminal tail. To date, eight missense mutations in *MYOT* have been identified. Except for one, all mutations are located in the serine-rich amino-terminal domain. The pattern of inheritance is autosomal dominant, but many patients do not have a family history of the disease.

20.4.3 Histopathology

Muscle biopsies in myotilinopathies show variable myopathic changes including variation in fiber size, fiber splitting, and internal nuclei, as well as variable degrees of fatty and fibrous tissue replacement. Typically, muscle fibers contain nonhyaline and dense hyaline deposits, visualised with modified trichrome stain as dark blue or blue–red inclusions. Small cytoplasmic bodies and nemaline-like bodies often clustered in groups are frequently observed. The hyaline inclusions display strong congophilia. Spheroid bodies are frequently observed. Rimmed and nonrimmed vacuoles are found in the majority of cases. Oxidative enzyme activity is absent in the fiber areas containing the inclusions, but is frequently enhanced at their periphery. Immunohistochemical studies reveal dense protein aggregates containing myotilin, desmin, dystrophin and many other proteins. Under electron microscopy, streaming of the Z-line is a prominent feature of early lesions in myotilinopathy. In more damaged fibers disrupted sarcomeres are replaced by remnants of myofibrils, filamentous bundles and filamentous debris that often coalesce to form dense globoid inclusions. Collections of 15–20 nm tubulofilaments are frequently found in myotilinopathies. Mitochondrial abnormalities are usually observed at the periphery of disrupted sarcomeres. Autophagic vacuoles filled with polymorphous and dense osmiophilic material,

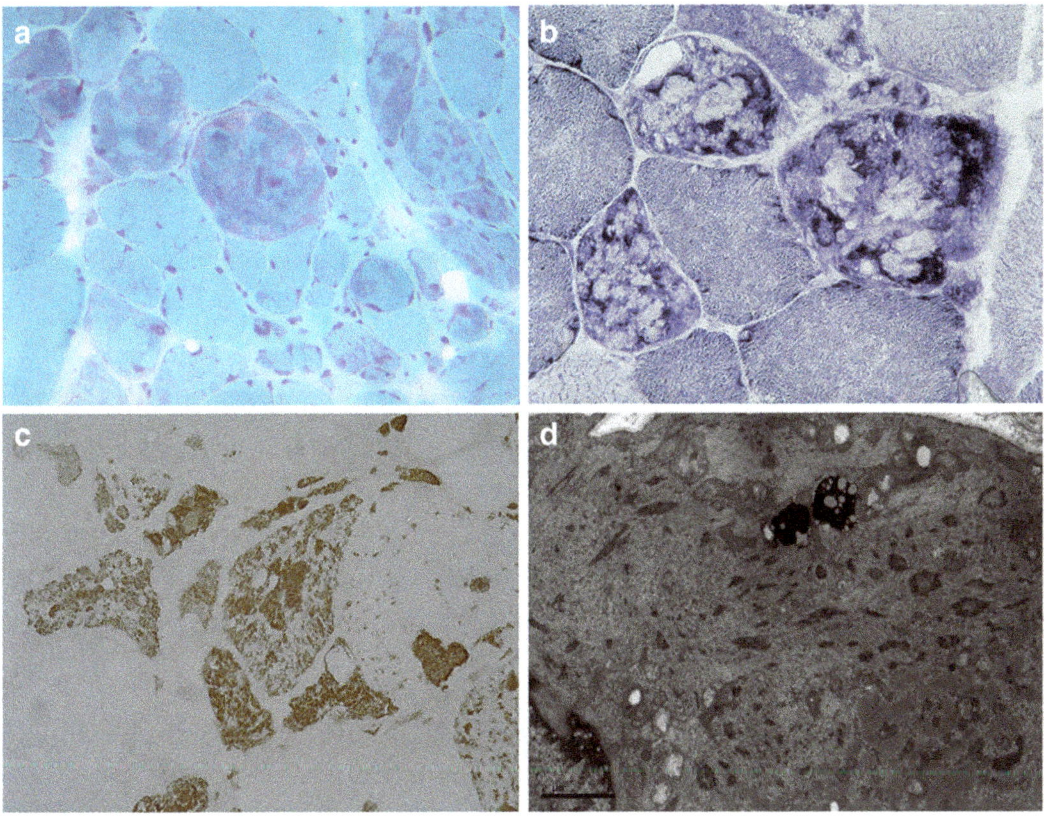

Fig. 20.6 Muscle biopsy findings in a patient with myotilinopathy showing polymorphous inclusions in several fibers (**a**: modified Gomori trichrome staining). Abnormal fiber areas are devoid of oxidative enzyme activity (**b**: NADH staining). Prominent myotilin accumulation in abnormal fibers (**c**). Under EM, areas of sarcomeric disorganisation are replaced by remnants of fine filaments, filamentous bundles, fine electron-dense granular material, small vacuoles and some lipofucsin granules (**d**)

myelin-like inclusions and membranous structures are additional features. Characteristic myopathology in myotilinopathies is shown in Fig. 20.6.

20.4.4 Clinical Presentation

MYOT mutations were originally discovered in two families suffering from limb-girdle muscle dystrophy type 1A (LGMD1A). They were also later identified in a subset of patients with MFM and in a family originally described as having spheroid body myopathy. To date, 50 patients from 40 families with *MYOT* mutations have been identified. Most myotilinopathy patients present between the ages of 42 and 77 years with distal weakness of lower limbs manifested by bilateral foot drop and later spreading to proximal muscles (Fig. 20.7). In other cases, however, the disease manifests as a limb girdle syndrome, with later involvement of distal muscles. Nasal speech which was a prominent symptom in the first reported families is rarely seen. Peripheral neuropathy, respiratory failure and cardiomyopathy are rare associated findings.

20.4.5 Imaging Findings

The pattern of muscle involvement in patients with myotilinopathy is sharply different from that observed in desminopathy or αB-crystallinopathy, but is almost identical to that seen in ZASPopathy. At the pelvic level (Fig. 20.8a–c), the gluteus medius and minimus muscles are usually more affected than the gluteus maximus.

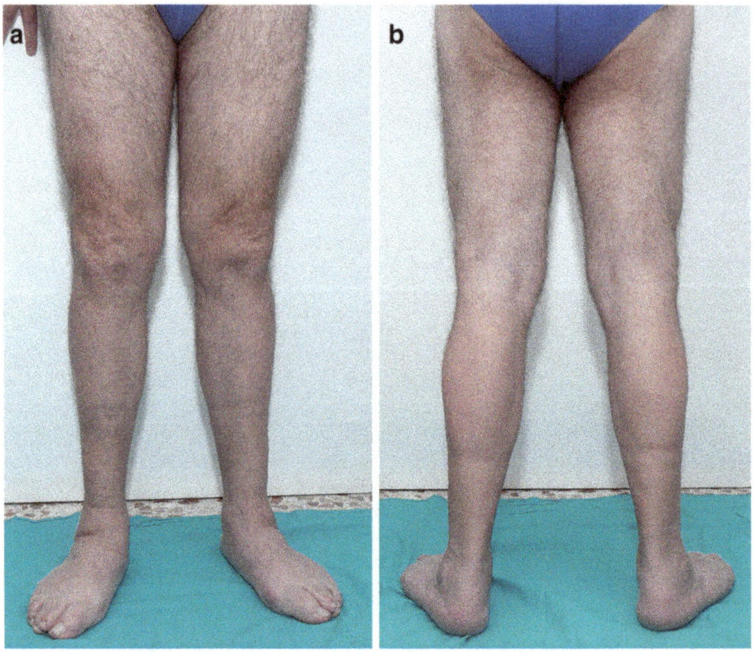

Fig. 20.7 Clinical picture of a 69-year-old man (**a**, **b**) carrying a Ser55Phe MYOT mutation, showing weakness and atrophy in the anterior compartment of legs

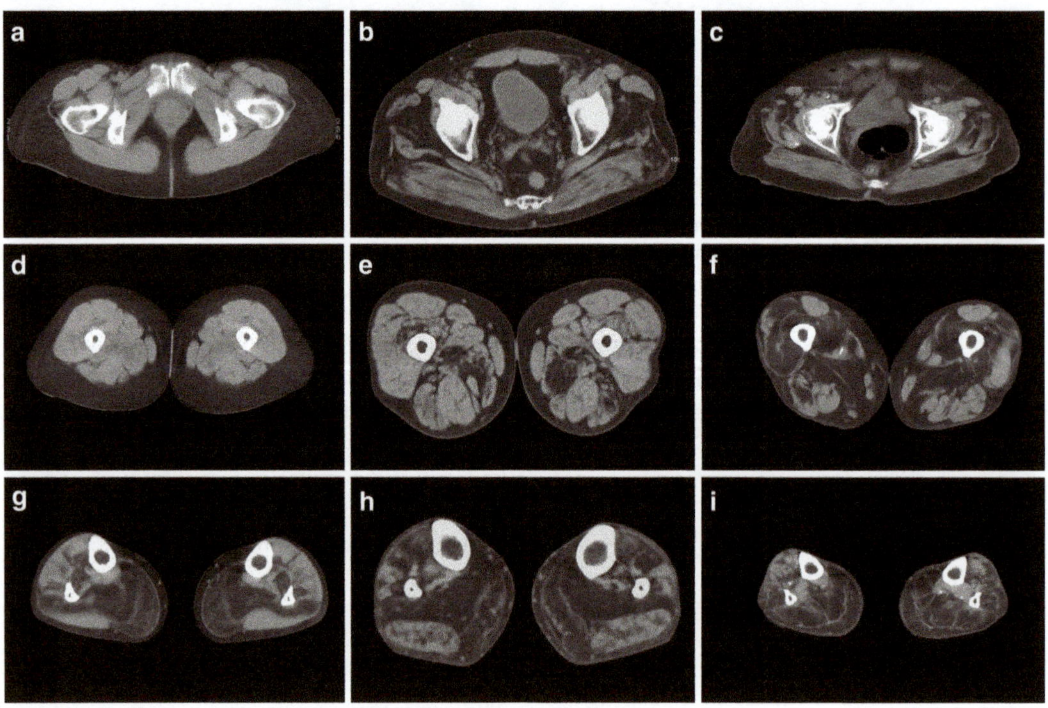

Fig. 20.8 Transverse muscle CT at the pelvis (**a–c**), mid-thigh (**d–f**), and mid-leg level (**g–i**) in three myotilinopathy patients 2, 4 and 6 years after the disease onset. No abnormalities are observed at the pelvis and mid-thigh level in the very early course of the illness (**a, d**). At more advanced disease, the gluteus medius and gluteus minimus are more affected than the gluteus maximus (**b, c**). At mid-thigh the semimbranosus, adductor magnus and biceps femoris are the first to be involved (**e**), followed by the vastus intermedius and vastus medialis muscles (**f**). Note that the semitendinosus, rectus femoris, sartorius and gracilis are well preserved (**f**). In the lower legs, the soleus and medial gastrocnemius (**g**) are the first to be affected, followed by the anterior tibialis (**h**). At more advanced disease, the peroneal and lateral gastrocnemius also become affected (**i**)

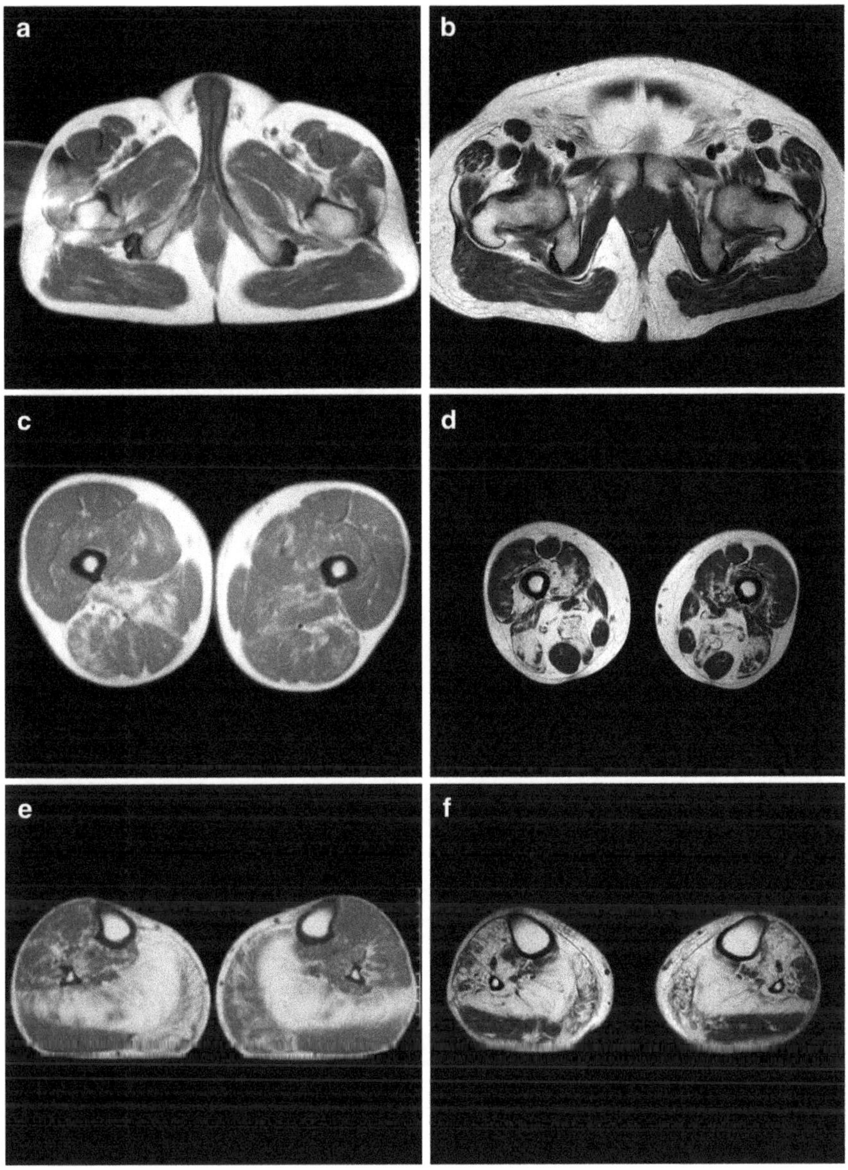

Fig. 20.9 Transverse T1-weighted MR images of the pelvis (**a**, **b**), mid-thigh (**c**, **d**), and mid-leg level (**e**, **f**) in two myotilinopathy patients 1 and 6 years after the first symptoms. Initial changes are observed in the semimembranosus and adductor magnus (**c**). Later on, there is involvement of the biceps femoris, vastus intermedius and vastus medialis muscles (**d**). In the lower legs, the soleus is the first and more severely affected muscle, followed by the medial gastrocnemius (**g**). At more advanced disease the anterior tibialis and peroneal group are involved (**f**)

In contrast to desminopathy and αB-crystallinopathy, at mid-thigh (Figs. 20.8d–f and 20.9c, d) the semimembranosus, biceps femoris and adductor magnus are the first muscles to be involved followed by the vastus medialis and vastus intermedius. The vastus lateralis, rectus femoris and especially the sartorius, gracilis and semitendinosus are much less severely affected and remain well preserved even in patients at very advanced stages of illness. At the mid-leg level (Figs. 20.8g–i and 20.9e, f), the soleus muscle is the first to be involved followed by the medial gastrocnemius. Later, the lateral gastrocnemius, peroneal group and anterior tibial muscle are affected.

Myofibrillar Myopathies: Myotilinopathies

Key Points

- Myotilinopathy is an autosomal dominant disease caused by mutations in MYOT.
- Late-onset distal myopathy is the most frequent clinical phenotype associated with myotilinopathy.
- Cardiopathy and respiratory failure rarely occur in patients with myotilinopathy.
- Muscle biopsies from myotilinopathy patients show prominent polymorphous inclusions that react with antibodies against desmin, myotilin and many other proteins that correspond at the ultrastructural level to fragmented and compacted filaments.
- In the myotilinopathies, imaging of lower limbs shows a characteristic pattern of muscle involvement. At the mid-thigh level, the semimembranosus, adductor magnus, and biceps femoris are the first affected. At the mid-leg level, the soleus muscle is the first affected. At mid-thigh level, the semitendinosus, gracilis, and satorius are the first muscles involved. At mid-leg level, the muscles of the peroneal group are those first affected.

Suggestions for Further Reading

Berciano J, Gallardo E, Domínguez-Perles R, et al. Autosomal-dominant distal myopathy with a myotilin S55F mutation: sorting out the phenotype. J Neurol Neurosurg Psychiatr. 2008;79:205–8.

Olivé M, Goldfarb L, Shatunov A, Fischer D, Ferrer I. Myotilinopathy: refining the clinical and myopathological phenotype. Brain 2005;128:2315–26.

Olivé M, Odgerel Z, Martínez A, et al. Clinical and myopathological evaluation of early- and late-onset subtypes of myofibrillar myopathy. Neuromuscul Disord. 2011;21:533–42.

Penisson-Besnier I, Talvinen K, Dumez C, et al. Myotilinopathy in a family with late onset myopathy. Neuromuscul Disord. 2006;16:427–31.

Schramm N, Born C, Weckbach S, Reilich P, Walter MC, Reiser MF. Involvement patterns in myotilinopathy and desminopathy detected by a novel neuromuscular whole-body MRI protocol. Eur Radiol. 2008;18:2922–36.

Selcen D, Engel AG. Mutations in myotilin cause myofibrillar myopathy. Neurology 2004;62:1363–71.

20.5 Filaminopathy

20.5.1 Synonyms

Filamin myopathy, C-filaminopathy.

20.5.2 Genetics and Pathophysiology

Filamins are a family of large cytoskeletal proteins that crosslink F-actin filaments into parallel bundles or dynamic three-dimensional meshwork and act as a scaffold for transmembrane receptors, signaling and adapter proteins. Filamin C, the muscle-specific filamin isoform cross-links actin at the Z-disc level. It interacts with myotilin, mopodin and FATZ and seems to play an important role during myofibrillogenesis and in maintaining muscle structural integrity. At the sarcolemma, filamin C interacts with γ- and δ-sarcoglycan in costameres and with Xin in myotendinous junctions.

The filamin C gene (*FLNC*) is located in the chromosomal band 7q32–q35 and contains 48 exons that code for 2,725 amino acids. The filamin molecule is composed of an amino-terminal actin-binding domain (ABD) followed by a semiflexible rod comprising 24 highly homologous immunoglobulin (Ig)-like modules. The most carboxy-terminally situated Ig-like domain 24 is required and sufficient for dimerization, which enables filamin C to cross-link and bundle actin filaments.

Filaminopathy leading to MFM is caused by mutations in the rod domain of *FLNC*. The pattern of inheritance is autosomal dominant. Mutations in the ABD domain of *FLNC* are associated with a distal myopathy that is described

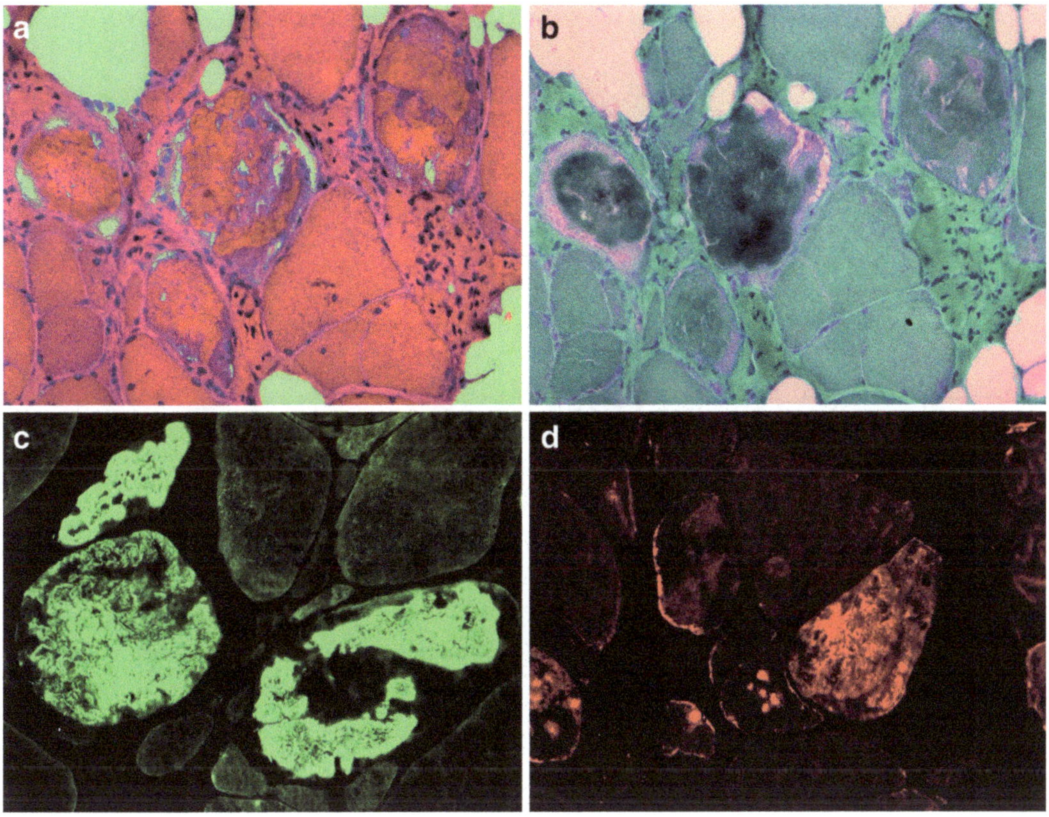

Fig. 20.10 Histological findings in filaminopathy. (**a**, **b**) Abnormal fibres harbouring polymorphous inclusions and vacuoles, increased fibre size variability, fibre splitting, internal nuclei, endomysial fibrosis and fatty replacement (**a**: H&E staining, **b**: modified Gomori trichrome staining). (**c**, **d**) Immunofluorescence stainings show strong immunoreactivities for filamin C (**c**) and myotilin (**d**) in abnormal fibre areas

in a separate chapter (see Sect. 21.2.4). The most frequent and best characterized mutation is located in the dimerization domain of filamin C (p.W2710X). This mutation causes a deletion of the carboxy-terminal 16 amino acids. In vitro studies revealed a less stable secondary structure of Ig-like domain 24 and a reduced structural stability of the mutant protein. As a consequence, the mutant protein does not dimerize properly and has a strong tendency for uncontrolled aggregation. A variety of proteins including filamin C binding partners are subsequently recruited into these aggregates, thereby destabilizing tissue homeostasis in decaying muscle fibers. Impairment of the ubiquitin–proteasome system seems to play an important role in the pathogenesis of filaminopathy.

20.5.3 Histopathology

Early signs of filaminopathy are cytochrome oxidase (COX)-negative fibers and core-like lesions along with unspecific changes including increased fiber size variability. In advanced stages, dystrophic changes occur, including fiber necrosis and regeneration, endomysial fibrosis, fiber splitting and fatty replacement (Fig. 20.10a). Another common feature is type 1 fiber predominance.

The most impressive findings are abnormal fibers harboring polymorphous inclusions characterized as single or multiple plaque-like formations in the cytoplasm, convoluted serpentine inclusions of varying thickness, granular deposits and/or spheroid bodies. The aggregates appear

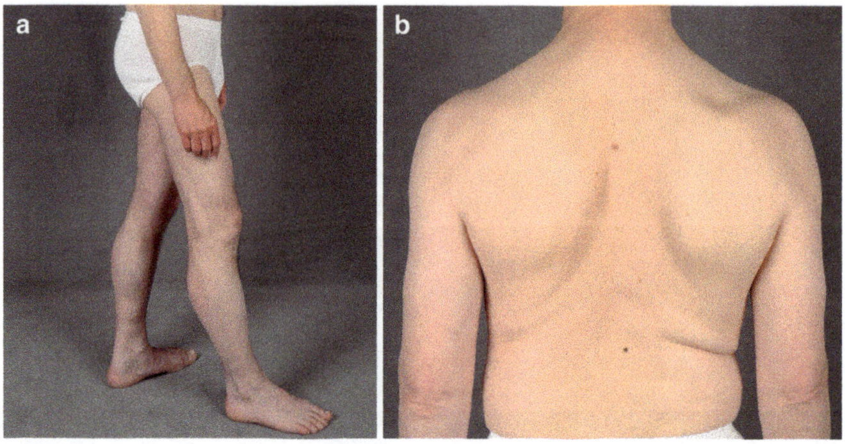

Fig. 20.11 Clinical pictures of a 50-year-old man with filaminopathy (p.W2710X mutation). (**a**) Predominantly proximal muscle atrophy in lower extremities. (**b**) Atrophy of proximal upper limb muscles with winged scapula

eosinophilic on H&E stain (Fig. 20.10a) and dark-blue to purple on modified trichrome staining (Fig. 20.10b). They mostly display strong congophilia. Abnormal fibers typically occur in uneven distribution across the fascicles and often show increased acid phosphatase levels. Some fibers harbor vacuoles of variable size and location that are partly rimmed or filled with basophilic membranous material. Non-rimmed vacuoles frequently show strong periodic acid-Schiff (PAS) positivity. Activities of oxidative enzymes and ATPase are decreased or lacking in abnormal fibre regions. Immunofluorescence analyses show strong immunoreactivities for filamin C (Fig. 20.10c), myotilin (Fig. 20.10d), desmin, αB-crystallin, BAG3, Xin and multiple other proteins in areas corresponding to protein aggregates.

Ultrastructural analyses show widespread myofibrillar pathology including rod formation, Z-disc remnants, Z-disc streaming and myofibrillar lysis. Many fibers display subsarcolemmal and intermyofibrillar pathological protein aggregates consisting of filamentous or desmin-positive granulofilamentous material. Additional findings may include sarcoplasmic paired helical filaments, tubulofilaments, and large autophagic vacuoles containing myelin-like figures and cellular debris.

20.5.4 Clinical Presentation

Usually between the fourth and sixth decades of life, muscle weakness appears in the proximal lower limbs (Fig. 20.11a) manifesting as difficulty rising from a chair and climbing stairs. Weakness slowly progresses to inability to walk and of the need for support. Other muscle groups also become involved with disease progression, primarily muscles of the proximal upper limbs (Fig. 20.11b), distal lower and distal upper limbs and axial muscles, but rarely facial muscles. Respiratory weakness occurs regularly in disease progression and seems to be the main reason for shortened life expectancy. About 40 % of patients have cardiac abnormalities including left ventricular hypertrophy, diastolic dysfunction and in particular conduction blocks. Creatine kinase (CK) levels are mostly elevated up to tenfold the upper limit of normal. Chronic gastroenteritis occurs in a small number of patients and may be caused by smooth muscle involvement.

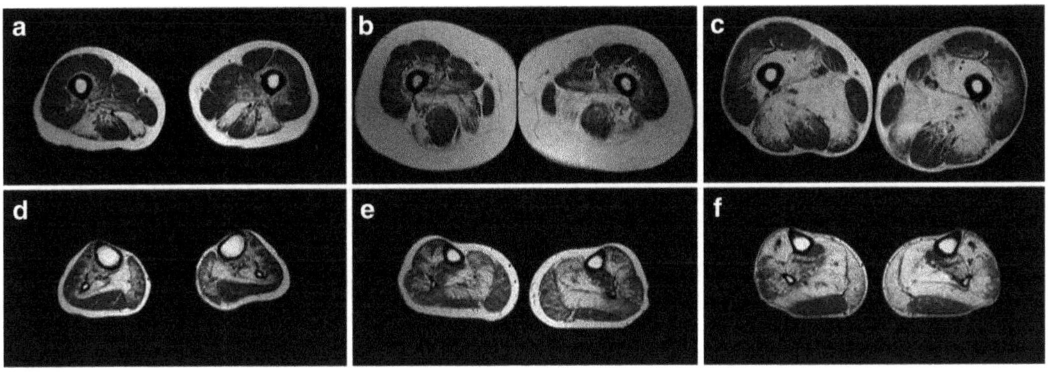

Fig. 20.12 Transverse T1-weighted muscle MR images of filaminopathy patients (p.W2710X mutation) of the mid-thigh (**a–c**) and mid-lower leg level (**d–f**). **a**, **d** (Sixty-year-old man, disease duration 3 years): on the thigh level (**a**), semimembranosus and biceps femoris are most affected. The semitendinosus, adductor magnus vastus intermedius and vastus medialis show less pronounced lipomatous changes. In lower legs, the soleus is most affected, followed by medial head of gastrocnemius. **b**, **e** (Fifty-four-year-old woman, disease duration 5 years): the pattern of muscle involvement is similar to the first patient but lipomatous alterations are more pronounced. In lower legs, the tibialis anterior, extensor hallucis longus and extensor digitorum longus are a little more affected than peroneal group muscles. **c**, **f** (Fifty-eight-year-old man, disease duration 13 years): the superficial parts of the quadriceps femoris, sartorius, gracilis and the lateral head of gastrocnemius are almost spared even in more advanced disease

20.5.5 Imaging Findings

The MRI scans of lower limbs show a rather homogeneous pattern of muscle involvement across filaminopathy patients with different mutations. T1-weighted images show a reticular pattern of hyperintensity in less affected patients, whereas homogeneous areas of T1-weighted hyperintensity are visible in individuals with progressive disease. At the level of the thigh, semimembranosus, adductor magnus and longus, biceps femoris, vastus intermedius and vastus medialis are most affected. The superficial parts of the quadriceps femoris, sartorius and gracilis muscles appear almost normal even in patients with a more advanced clinical course (Fig. 20.12a–c). In the lower legs, the soleus, medial head of the gastrocnemius, tibialis anterior, extensor hallucis longus, and extensor digitorum longus are more involved than the lateral gastrocnemius and peroneal muscles (Fig. 20.12d–f). Muscular signal intensities on T2-weighted fat suppressed MRI scans are only mildly elevated indicating an absence of distinct intramuscular edema.

Myofibrillar Myopathies: Filaminopathy

Key Points

- Filaminopathy is caused by mutations in the rod or dimerization domain of *FLNC* and inherited in an autosomal dominant manner.
- Histological features are typical of MFM, including polymorphous cytoplasmic inclusions and in advanced disease dystrophic changes.
- Muscle weakness usually starts between the fourth and sixth decade of life in proximal lower limbs.
- The clinical phenotype is similar to LGMD.
- About half of the patients show cardiac abnormalities.
- Muscle imaging of lower limbs shows a characteristic pattern of muscle involvement.

Suggestions for Further Reading

Fischer D, Kley RA, Strach K, et al. Distinct muscle imaging patterns in myofibrillar myopathies. Neurology 2008;71:758–65.

Fürst DO, Goldfarb LG, Kley RA, et al. Filamin C-related myopathies: pathology and mechanisms. Acta Neuropathol. 2013;125:33–46.

Kley RA, Hellenbroich Y, van der Ven PFM, et al. Clinical and morphological phenotype of the filamin myopathy: a study of 31 German patients. Brain 2007;130: 3250–64.

Kley RA, Serdaroglu-Oflazer P, Leber Y, et al. Pathophysiology of protein aggregation and extended phenotyping in filaminopathy. Brain 2012;135: 2642–60.

Lowe T, Kley RA, van der Ven PFM, et al. The pathomechanism of filaminopathy: altered biochemical properties explain the cellular phenotype of a protein aggregation myopathy. Hum Mol Genet. 2007;16: 1351–58.

Luan X, Hong D, Zhang W, Wang Z, Yuan Y. A novel heterozygous deletion-insertion mutation (2695–2712 del/GTTTGT ins) in exon 18 of the filamin C gene causes filaminopathy in a large Chinese family. Neuromuscul Disord. 2010;20:390–6.

Odgerel Z, van der Ven PF, Fürst DO, Goldfarb LG. DNA sequencing errors in molecular diagnostics of filamin myopathy. Clin Chem Lab Med. 2010;48:1409–14.

Shatunov A, Olivé M, Odgerel Z, et al. In-frame deletion in the seventh immunoglobulin-like repeat of filamin C in a family with myofibrillar myopathy. Eur J Hum Genet. 2009;17:656–63.

van der Ven PFM, Wiesner S, Salmikangas P, et al. Indications for a novel muscular dystrophy pathway. Gamma-filamin, the muscle-specific filamin isoform, interacts with myotilin. J Cell Biol. 2000;151: 235–48.

Vorgerd M, van der Ven PFM, Bruchertseifer V, et al. A mutation in the dimerization domain of filamin c causes a novel type of autosomal dominant myofibrillar myopathy. Am J Hum Genet. 2005;77:297–304.

20.6 ZASPopathy

20.6.1 Synonyms

Markesbery-Griggs disease.

20.6.2 Genetics and Pathophysiology

Z-band alternatively spliced PDZ-motif containing protein [ZASP, also known as LIM-domain-binding-3 (*LDB3*)] is a Z-disc-associated protein expressed in human cardiac and skeletal muscle. The ZASP gene (*ZASP*) is located at chromosome 10q22.3–q23.2 and consists of 16 exons. Three differentially spliced isoforms are expressed in skeletal muscle. All ZASP isoforms have an N-terminal PDZ domain important for protein–protein interactions and a ZASP-like motif (ZM motif) that is required and sufficient for interaction with α-actinin, which cross-links thin filaments in adjacent sarcomeres. ZASP also interacts with calsarcin and protein kinase C subtypes.

Three mutations in exon 6 and exon 9 of the ZASP gene are associated with MFM. The most frequent p.A165V mutation is in the ZM motif which is needed for the interaction with α-actinin. The pathomechanism of ZASPopathy has not yet been clarified. *ZASP* mutations also may cause dilated cardiomyopathy.

20.6.3 Histopathology

Histopathological findings include nonspecific myopathic alterations such as variation of fiber size, central nuclei, fiber splitting, regenerating and necrotic fibers, endomysial fibrosis and fatty replacement (Fig. 20.13a). In addition, rimmed and non-rimmed vacuoles are regularly present (Fig. 20.13b). Cytoplasmic bodies, spheroid inclusion bodies and nemaline-like bodies are also frequent findings. Core-like lesions surrounded by increased oxidative enzyme activity are regularly found whereas rubbed-out fibers are rare. Characteristic polymorphous hyaline deposits (Fig. 20.13b) often show a strong congophilia. Immunofluorescence analyses indicate a strong accumulation of desmin (Fig. 20.13c), myotilin (Fig. 20.13d), αB-crystallin and various other proteins in abnormal fibers.

Ultrastructural analyses reveal streaming and disintegration of Z-discs as early pathological alteration. More affected fiber areas show an accumulation of filamentous bundles of Z-disc origin and filamentous debris in the cytoplasm and subsarcolemmal regions. Autophagic vacuoles contain granulofilamentous material and dislocated membranous organelles.

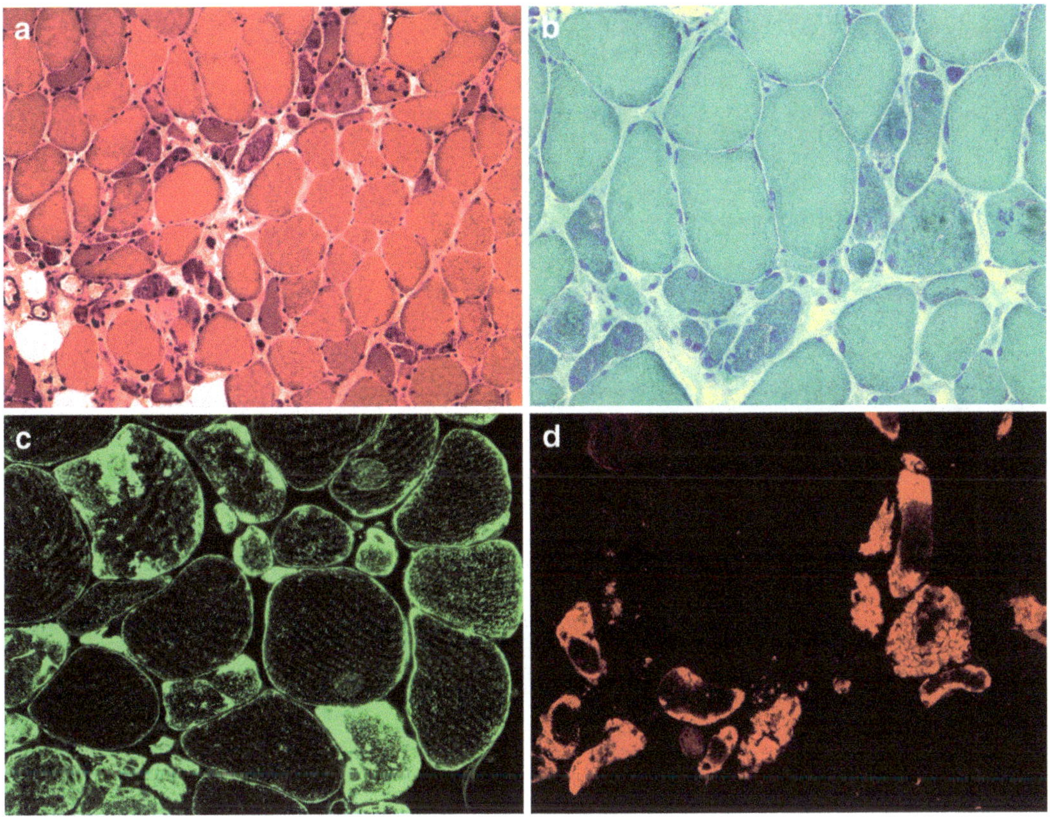

Fig. 20.13 Histological findings in ZASPopathy. (**a**) Dystrophic pattern with variation of fibre size, internal nuclei, muscle fibre necrosis and regeneration, endomysial fibrosis and fatty replacement (H&E staining). (**b**) Hyaline deposits and vacuoles in abnormal fibres (modified Gomori trichrome staining). (**c**, **d**) Immunofluorescence stainings reveal accumulations of desmin (**c**) and myotilin (**d**) in abnormal deposits

20.6.4 Clinical Presentation

First clinical symptoms of ZASPopathy usually occur during the sixth decade (range 31–73 years). Muscle weakness regularly starts in the distal lower limbs followed by an involvement of intrinsic hand muscles combined with wrist extensors. In later disease stages, mild to moderate proximal weakness occurs. Disease progression is very slow and patients remain ambulatory until a late age. Respiratory weakness has not been reported. CK levels are normal or slightly elevated. Peripheral neuropathy and/or cardiac involvement may be associated features in a small number of cases.

20.6.5 Imaging Findings

The involvement pattern in ZASPopathy as revealed by muscle MRI or CT is similar to that observed for myotilinopathy. At the pelvic level, the gluteus maximus and minimus muscles are most affected (Fig. 20.14a). At the thigh level, the semimembranosus and adductor magnus muscles are involved early followed by the biceps femoris, vastus medialis, vastus intermedius and vastus lateralis. The semitendinosus, sartorius and gracilis are relatively spared (Fig. 20.14b).

In the lower legs, imaging indicates early involvement of the soleus and medial gastrocnemius muscle whereas the lateral gastrocnemius is

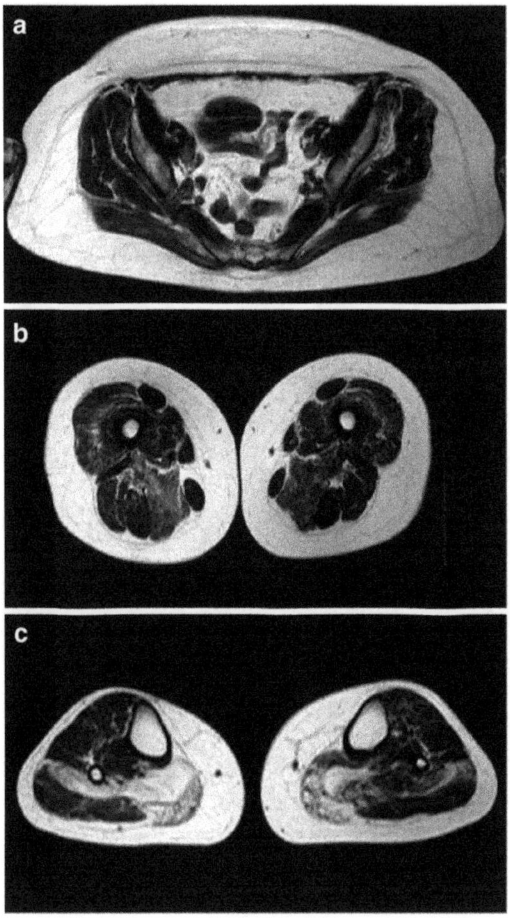

Fig. 20.14 Transverse T1-weighted muscle MR images of a 60-year-old woman with ZASPopathy (p.A147T mutation). At the pelvic level (**a**), gluteus maximus and minimus show slight to moderate lipomatous alterations. At the mid-thigh level (**b**), semimembranosus and adductor magnus are most involved. In the lower legs (**c**), the soleus is most affected, followed by the medial gastrocnemius

initially preserved (Fig. 20.14c). Later in the disease course, all lower leg muscles show distinct changes.

Myofibrillar Myopathies: ZASPopathy

Key Points

- ZASPopathy is caused by mutations in the ZASP gene.
- Histological changes are characteristic of MFM.
- Slowly progressive muscle weakness usually starts during the sixth decade in the distal lower limbs.
- Cardiomyopathy and/or peripheral neuropathy are associated features in a small number of cases.
- Muscle imaging of the lower legs shows early involvement of the soleus and medial gastrocnemius. It also reveals distinct lipomatous changes in all lower leg muscles when the disease becomes advanced.
- Muscle imaging of thigh show an early involvement of semimembranosus and adductor magnus.

Suggestions for Further Reading

Au Y, Atkinson RA, Guerrini R, et al. Solution structure of ZASP PDZ domain; implications for sarcomere ultrastructure and enigma family redundancy. Structure 2004;12:611–22.

Faulkner G, Pallavicini A, Formentin E et al. ZASP: a new Z-band alternatively spliced PDZ-motif protein. J Cell Biol. 1999;146:465–75.

Griggs R, Vihola A, Hackman P, et al. Zaspopathy in a large classic late-onset distal myopathy family. Brain 2007;130:1477–84.

Klaavuniemi T, Ylanne J. Zasp/Cypher internal ZMmotif containing fragments are sufficient to co-localize with alpha-actinin-analysis of patient mutations. Exp Cell Res. 2006;312:1299–311.

Olivé M, Odgerel Z, Martínez A, et al. Clinical and myopathological evaluation of early- and late-onset subtypes of myofibrillar myopathy. Neuromuscul Disord. 2011;21:533–42.

Selcen D, Engel AG. Mutations in ZASP define a novel form of muscular dystrophy in humans. Ann Neurol. 2005;57:269–76.

Vatta M, Mohapatra B, Jimenez S, et al. Mutations in Cypher/ZASP in patients with dilated cardiomyopathy and left ventricular non-compaction. J Am Coll Cardiol. 2003;42:2014–27.

20.7 Therapy of Myofibrillar Myopathies

There is no specific treatment for MFMs, but some of the complications can be prevented. Early detection and treatment of cardiac arrhythmias and conduction defects, frequently occurring in desminopathy, αB-crystallinopathy and filaminopathy, can be lifesaving. Pacemaker and implantable cardioverter defibrillator devices should be considered in individuals with arrhythmia and/or cardiac conduction defects. Patients with progressive or life-threatening cardiomyopathy may be candidates for cardiac transplantation. Respiratory support with continuous or bilevel positive airway pressure is indicated in patients with hypercapnia and other signs of ventilatory failure. Physical therapy including aerobic exercise training may help to maintain functional performances, but extreme exercise should be avoided. Assistive devices should be used in individuals with advanced muscle weakness. There have been reports of some filaminopathy patients benefiting from creatine supplementation, but it has not yet been confirmed in randomized controlled trials.

20.8 Differential Diagnoses of Myofibrillar Myopathies

The clinical phenotype of MFM is extremely heterogeneous. Desminopathy, for example, may present with limb-girdle (LGMD; see Chap. 19), scapuloperoneal (FSHD; see Chap. 23) or distal myopathy phenotype, even in patients harboring the same mutation. This results in a broad spectrum of differential diagnoses including not only various myopathies but also peripheral neuropathies. As MFM is characterized and defined by histological features, a muscle biopsy is usually necessary for diagnostic purposes. However, in the early stages of the disease or in unaffected or minimally affected muscles, the histopathological results may be false negative. Muscle imaging is a powerful tool to help select a suitable skeletal muscle for biopsy and to avoid misdiagnosis.

Histological hallmarks of MFM are focal destruction of myofibrils and protein aggregation in skeletal muscle fibers. Intracytoplasmic inclusions are also observed in some hereditary and acquired myopathies, e.g., sporadic and hereditary inclusion body myopathy (see Chap. 26), nemaline myopathies (Sects. 15.6, 15.7 and 21.3.3), cytoplasmic body myopathies. Intracytoplasmic accumulation of proteins seen in MFM should be distinguished from the non-specific accumulation of proteins that occurs whenever the structural integrity of the sarcomere is compromised, including core lesions seen in core myopathies and target formations observed during muscle fiber denervation and reinnervation. Clinical characteristics, additional histological findings and ultrastructural analyses normally allow differentiation of these diseases from MFM.

Acknowledgements We would like to thank the clinicians who provided some of the figures included in the present chapter especially Drs. M Fardcau, R Zabalza, and JJ Poza.

21 Distal Myopathies

Bjarne Udd

21.1 Introduction and Classification

The term distal myopathies refers to a group of primary genetic muscle diseases that share the clinical feature of causing predominantly distal weakness in the hands and/or feet early in the disease evolution. However, the range of phenotypic variability is large including both early childhood-onset forms and very late-onset forms. Both autosomal dominant and recessive transmission is present. The pathology is highly variable even though many of the diseases share the finding of rimmed vacuolation without major or prominent protein aggregations (as seen with desmin immunostaining). The number of distinct genetic disorders is expanding, and muscle imaging has become a well accepted diagnostic tool to aid and restrict the number of molecular genetic procedures.

The distal myopathies and causative genes are summarized in Table 21.1. Distal myopathies are in fact muscular dystrophies that are hereditary and cause progressive loss of muscle tissue. The molecular mechanisms leading to preferential involvement of distal muscles are not well understood. Interestingly, all the five genes causing myogenic distal arthrogryposis are all coded for well-known sarcomeric proteins. This group would thus qualify for a category of congenital distal myopathies.

Muscle imaging studies performed with computed tomography (CT) or magnetic resonance imaging (MRI) are powerful diagnostic tools that allow important differentiation between genetic subtypes of the distal myopathies. Particularly, they allow differentiation of patients with mutations in genes causing anterior compartment leg muscle involvement from those with distinct posterior calf muscle involvement or with equal affection of both anterior and posterior compartments.

The following diseases are covered in this chapter: titinopathy (tibial muscular dystrophy, Udd); Welander distal myopathy; MYH7 distal myopathy (Laing); distal ABD-filaminopathy; distal VCP myopathy; KHLH9 distal myopathy; distal anoctaminopathy; distal nebulin myopathy; GNE distal myopathy (Nonaka). Distal dysferlinopathy (Miyoshi) is covered in Chap. 19.

There is no specific treatment for any of the distal myopathies. Fortunately, complications such as progressive or life-threatening cardiomyopathy are not present in these diseases. Mild cardiomyopathy may occur with Laing distal MYH7 myopathy but this is rare. Respiratory failure and dysphagia are exceptions. Rehabilitation measures and various aids and orthoses are needed to compensate for foot drop and finger weakness. If foot drop, foot deformities, or contractures are severe, early surgical corrective measures, including tendon transpositions, can be an option.

B. Udd (✉)
Neuromuscular Research Center, Tampere University Hospital, 33520 Tampere, Finland
e-mail: bjarne.udd@pshp.fi

M.P. Wattjes and D. Fischer (eds.), *Neuromuscular Imaging*, DOI 10.1007/978-1-4614-6552-2_21,

Table 21.1 List of genetically confirmed distal myoopathies

	Gene	Protein
1. *Late adult-onset autosomal dominant forms*		
(a) Welander distal myopathy	TIA1	TIA1
(b) Tibial muscular dystrophy (TMD, Udd myopathy)	*TTN*	Titin
(c) Distal myotilinopathy	*TTID*	Myotilin
(d) ZASPopathy (Markesbery–Griggs)	*LDB3*	ZASP
(e) Matrin3 distal myopathy (VCPDM, MPD2)	*MATR3*	Matrin3
(f) VCP-mutated distal myopathy	*VCP*	VCP
(g) αB-Crystallin mutated distal myopathy	*CRYAB*	αB-Crystallin
2. *Adult-onset autosomal dominant forms*		
(a) Desminopathy	*DESM*	Desmin
(b) Distal ABD filaminopathy	*FLNC*	Filamin-C
(c) Finnish MPD3	nd	nd
(d) Oculopharyngeal distal myopathy, OPDM	nd	nd
3. *Early-onset autosomal dominant forms*		
(a) Laing distal myopathy (MPD1)	*MYH7*	β-MyHC
(b) *KLHL9*-mutated distal myopathy	*KLHL9*	KLHL9
4. *Early-onset autosomal recessive forms*		
(a) Distal nebulin myopathy	*NEB*	Nebulin
5. *Early adult-onset autosomal recessive forms*		
(a) Miyoshi myopathy (MM)	*DYSF*	Dysferlin
(b) Distal anoctaminopathy	*ANO5*	Anoctamin-5
(c) Distal myopathy with rimmed vacuoles (DMRV)	*GNE*	GNE
(d) Oculopharyngeal distal myopathy, OPDM	nd	nd

21.2 Autosomal Dominant Distal Myopathies

21.2.1 Titinopathy

21.2.1.1 Synonyms, Abbreviations

Tibial muscular dystrophy (TMD); Udd myopathy; OMIM #600334.

21.2.1.2 Genetics and Pathophysiology

Titin protein is the biggest single polypeptide in nature, consisting of up to 38,000 amino acids expressed in a number of isoforms in skeletal and heart muscle. Titin proteins form the third filament system of the sarcomeric myofilaments (the other two are the thick and thin filaments). This system integrates a huge number of interacting protein ligands as a backbone of the sarcomere. The titin molecule starts at the Z-disc and stretches over 1 μm to the M-band. Human titin is encoded by a single copy gene (*TTN*) located in chromosome 2q31. It contains 363 exons with a cDNA of 100 kb—almost 10 times the size of dystrophin. Titin is organized into a large number of domains, many of which are repeats of immunoglobulin and fibronectin domains. Many others, however, have unique sequences and a distinct vital kinase domain in the C-terminus. The first titin mutations to cause skeletal muscle disease (i.e., autosomal dominant TMD and recessive LGMD2J) were described in 2002 as being located in the last exon of the gene. The number of disease-causing *TTN* mutations is continuously increasing. Most of them are missense mutations causing cardiomyopathy, but one dominant mutation in the kinase domain is associated with hereditary myopathy with early respiratory failure (HMERF). Other recessive mutations in the C-terminus may cause lethal cardiac and skeletal myopathies. Consequently, there are different molecular pathomechanisms depending on the underlying mutation.

21.2.1.3 Histopathology

Muscle biopsies of affected muscles in TMD show dystrophic changes, including rimmed vacuolated fibers. Fiber necrosis is rare. Other nonspecific myopathic features, such as variation in fiber size, scattered atrophic fibers, and an increased number of internal nuclei, are usually present (Fig. 21.1). The corresponding ultrastructural hallmark consists of autophagic vacuoles with polymorphous debris and myeloid bodies without consistent filamentous bodies.

21.2.1.4 Clinical Presentation

Age at onset varies between 25 and 60 years. The disease presents with ankle dorsiflexion weakness progressing to foot drop (Fig. 21.2a). Proximal muscles remain less affected even at older age, thus preserving walking capacity. Upper limb muscles, bulbar and facial muscles, respiratory muscles, and myocardium are usually not involved, in keeping with the normal life expectancy of the patients. The prevalence of TMD is high (20/100,000) in Finland because of the founder mutation effect. In addition, a few Rare families have been described in other populations.

21.2.1.5 Imaging Findings

Tibial muscular dystrophy exhibits a distinctive pattern of muscle involvement in terms of fatty degenerative change on CT scans and/or MRI studies. At the pelvic level, the gluteus minimus

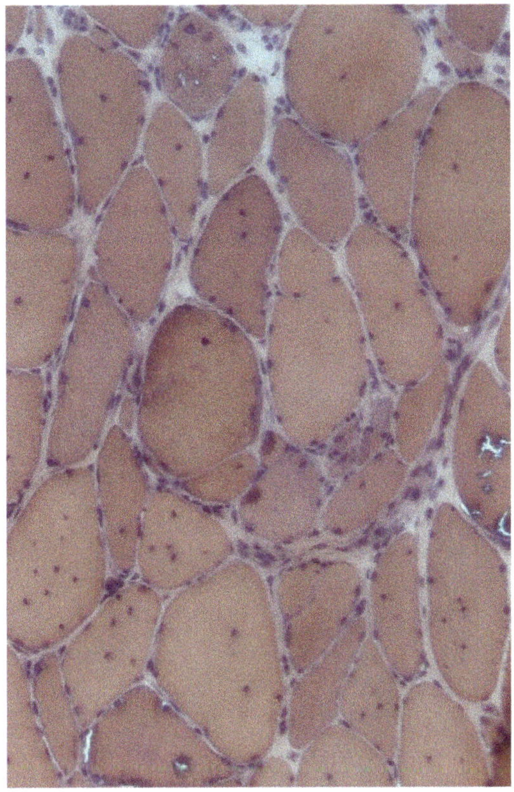

Fig. 21.1 Tibialis anterior muscle biopsy specimen from a 45-year-old man with tibial muscular dystrophy (TMD) prior to the severe dystrophic stage. Note the rimmed vacuolated fibers, variation in fiber size, atrophic fibers, and increased number of internal nuclei

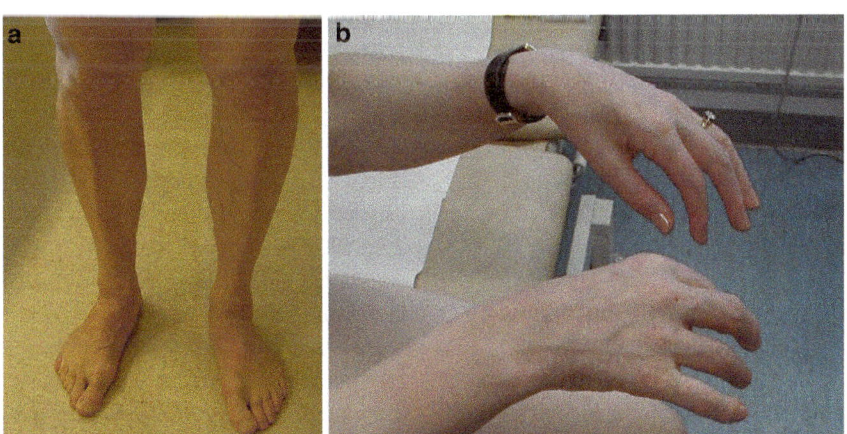

Fig. 21.2 (**a**) A 54-year-old man with TMD. Note the atrophy of the anterior tibialis muscles with preserved extensor digitorum brevis muscle bulk. (**b**) A 52-year-old woman with Welander distal myopathy. Note the impaired finger extension (most prominently in the index finger) and mild atrophy of small hand muscles

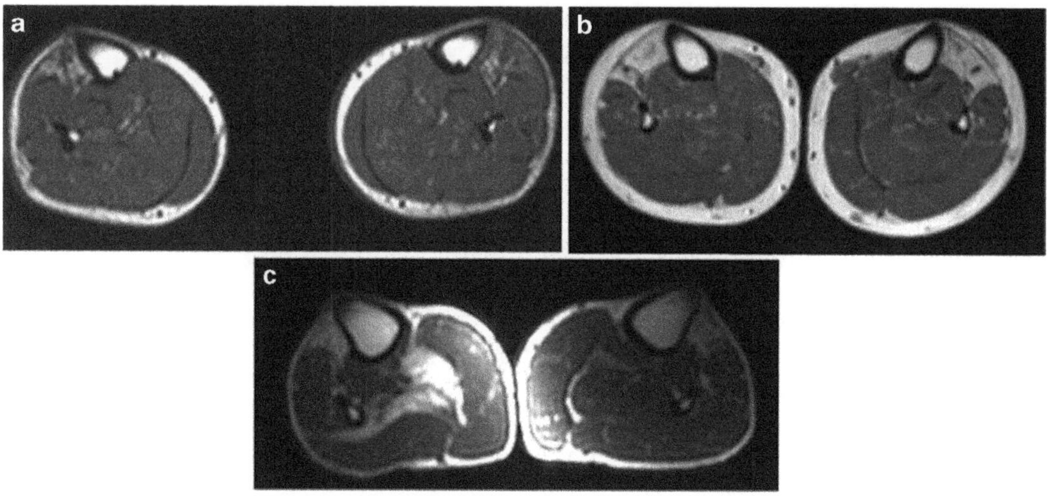

Fig. 21.3 Axial T1-weighted magnetic resonance imaging (MRI) demonstrates the fatty degenerative changes of Titinopathy (TMD) at the mid-leg level. First muscles to be involved are the anterior tibialis (**a**) followed by the extensor hallucis and digitorum longus muscles (**b**). Occasionally, anterior compartment lesions are combined with asymmetrical soleus involvement (**c**)

muscle is selectively involved. At the mid-thigh level, the hamstrings with the semimembranosus, semitendinosus, and biceps femoris muscles are typically affected at later stages of the disease. At the mid-leg level, the first muscle to be involved is the anterior tibialis (Fig. 21.3a), followed by the extensor hallucis and digitorum longus muscles (Fig. 21.3b). Infrequently, the soleus and the medial gastrocnemius asymmetrically show changes in addition to the typical replacement of anterior compartment muscles (Fig. 21.3c).

21.2.2 Welander Distal Myopathy

21.2.2.1 Synonyms, Abbreviations

Welander distal myopathy (WDM); OMIM# 604454.

21.2.2.2 Genetics and Pathophysiology

The autosomal dominant disease was linked to a locus on chromosome 2p13 more than a decade ago, and the genetic defect responsible for WDM, TIA1, was recently identified. So far only Swedish and Finnish families have been conclusively linked to this locus. They all share one identical haplotype and the founder mutation.

21.2.2.3 Histopathology

Muscle biopsies of affected muscles in WDM show dystrophic changes with rimmed vacuolated fibers. Fiber necrosis is rare, but internal nuclei are frequent. Variation in fiber size and scattered atrophic angulated fibers are usually present. Morphological changes cannot be differentiated from those in other distal myopathies with rimmed vacuoles.

21.2.2.4 Clinical Presentation

Age at onset varies between 30 and 70 years. Two-thirds of patients first present with index finger extension weakness later progressing to weakness and atrophy of all hand muscles (Fig. 21.2b). In a small number of patients the disease appears first in the lower legs with mild foot drop. Proximal muscles are rarely affected, even at older age. Upper limb muscles, bulbar and facial muscles, respiratory muscles, and myocardium are not involved. The prevalence has been estimated at 8/100,000 in Sweden and at 3/100,000 in Finland. It is rarely reported elsewhere.

21.2.2.5 Imaging Findings

The WDM pattern of muscle involvement in terms of fatty degenerative changes on CT or

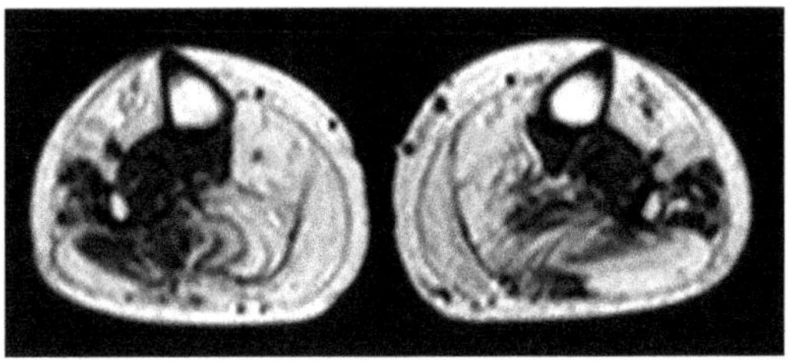

Fig. 21.4 Axial T1-weighted muscle MRI scan of a patient presenting with Welander distal myopathy. Anterior and posterior calf muscles are severely involved in both lower legs at late stages of the disease

MRI scans is more variable than in TMD. In the lower legs (Fig. 21.4) usually both anterior and posterior calf muscles show changes if weakness is present in the legs. At the early stages when finger extension weakness is the exclusive clinical presentation, imaging of the lower legs may be normal. In patients presenting with symptoms in the legs, the anterior compartment is more degenerated than the posterior compartment. Patients with more prominent hand than leg weakness show more severe involvement of the posterior compartment than the anterior compartment. The involvement of the lateral peroneal muscles is less prominent.

21.2.3 MYH7 Distal Myopathy

21.2.3.1 Synonyms, Abbreviations

Laing myopathy, MPD1; OMIM#160500.

21.2.3.2 Genetics and Pathophysiology

Laing myopathy is caused by dominant mutations in the *MYH7* gene, which is localized on chromosome 14q. Mutations affect the coiled coil tail of the β-myosin heavy-chain dimer. Most mutations are located within the amino acid positions 1500–1750, whereas mutations in the N-terminal usually cause cardiomyopathy and those in the finding C-terminus cause hyaline body myopathy. Mutations causing Laing myopathy rarely cause cardiomyopathy and are supposed to disrupt the sterical heptad structure of the coil. The mutations frequently arise de novo and have been identified in many populations.

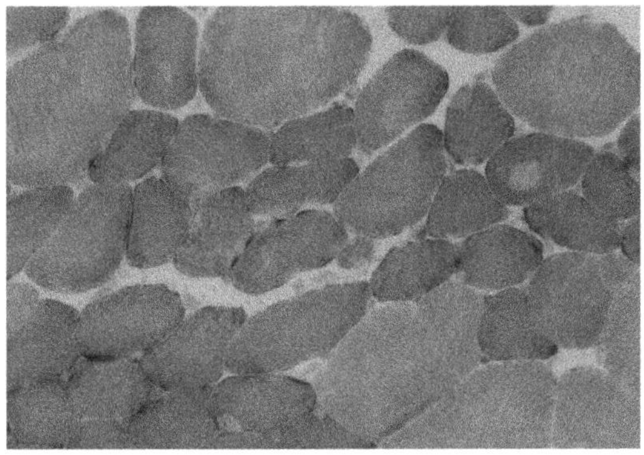

Fig. 21.5 Muscle biopsy specimen from a 35-year-old woman with an *MYH7* mutation. Note the smaller, type 1 fibers, the fiber type disproportion, and a few fibers with core changes (NADH stain)

According to recent data, should occur with a frequency of more than 1/1,000,000.

21.2.3.3 Histopathology

Tissues from muscle biopsies present a range of myopathic findings. Fiber type disproportion is the most consistent. Fiber necrosis and rimmed vacuoles are rare, whereas core-like findings are common (Fig. 21.5).

21.2.3.4 Clinical Presentation

Patients may present with drop foot symptoms from early childhood. Because the disease develops slowly, its onset is often not clearly defined. There is later progression of weakness to proximal muscles, which may cause loss of free ambulation at the age of 60–70 years in the more severe forms. Neck flexor weakness is a consistent clinical finding on examination. In its severe form, patients also have scoliosis and loss of finger extension in addition to proximal weakness.

21.2.3.5 Imaging Findings

The pattern of muscle involvement in terms of fatty degenerative changes in the lower legs (Fig. 21.6) always includes the tibialis anterior muscle. Depending on the severity and duration of the disease, the soleus muscles are infrequently affected. The medial gastrocnemius may also show mild hypertrophy at early stages and more degeneration later in the disease course. Proximal

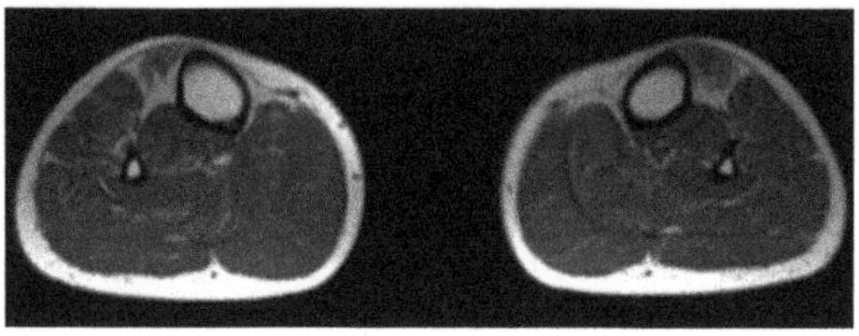

Fig. 21.6 Axial T1-weighted muscle MRI scan of a patient carrying an *MYH7* mutation. At mid-leg, fatty degenerative changes are selectively found in the tibialis anterior, whereas the medial gastrocnemius is mildly hypertrophic

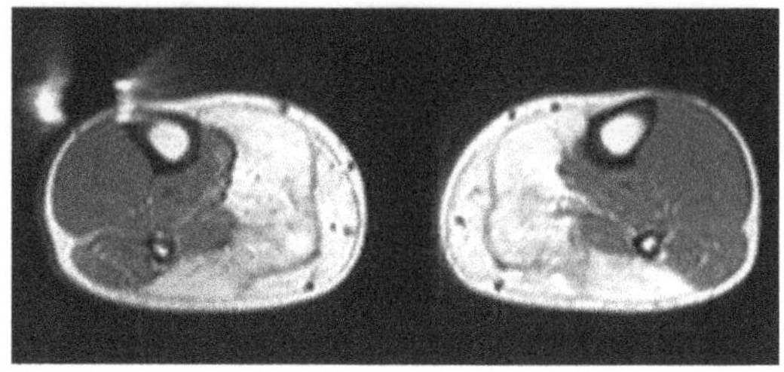

Fig. 21.7 Axial T1-weighted muscle MRI scan of the lower legs of a patient with distal ABD filaminopathy. Note the extensive and total fatty replacement in the calf muscles, medial and lateral gastrocnemii, and soleus, whereas all other muscles are more or less normal

thigh muscles are involved very late in parallel with clinical weakness. More changes are observed in the vastii than in the rectus femoris or the medial and posterior thigh muscles.

21.2.4 Distal Actin-Binding Domain Filaminopathy

21.2.4.1 Synonyms, Abbreviations

Distal ABD filaminopathy, OMIM#614065.

21.2.4.2 Genetics and Pathophysiology

Dominant mutations in the rod domain of the large muscle-specific filamin-C are known to cause myofibrillar myopathy (see Chap. 20). A different disease caused by dominant mutations in the N-terminal actin-binding domain (ABD) of the gene was recently identified. Whether these two different pathologies and clinical outcomes of these mutations are mediated through actin dynamics or other interactions has not been determined. The disease has so far been recognized in only a few families.

21.2.4.3 Histopathology

Muscle biopsies show nonspecific alterations. There are scattered atrophic fibers, no rimmed vacuoles, and no protein aggregations—similar to myofibrillar pathology. At the final stage, the muscle fibers diseappear and are replaced by fat and connective tissue.

21.2.4.4 Clinical Presentation

In patients who are physically active, the first symptom may be weakness of the hand grip during early adulthood. This develops into atrophy of thenar muscles and, later, other hand muscles. After 30 years of age, calf muscle weakness causes changes in walking, but free ambulation is usually preserved into late senescence despite mild proximal weakness. No respiratory, symptoms dysphagia, or cardiomyopathy have been recorded.

21.2.4.5 Imaging Findings

The pattern of muscle involvement was essential to identify the second reported family. It showed extensive fatty degenerative changes in all calf muscles (Fig. 21.7), sparing the anterior and to a lesser extent the lateral compartment muscles of the lower legs. Proximal thigh muscles are involved later in the disease course. Changes in the hamstrings exceed those in the quadriceps, while relative sparing of adductors and short head of the biceps femoris is common.

21.2.5 Valosin-Containing Protein Distal Myopathy

21.2.5.1 Synonyms, Abbreviations

Distal IBMPFD, VCP, OMIM#167320.

21.2.5.2 Genetics and Pathophysiology

Valosin-containing protein (VCP) is a ubiquitous multifunctional molecule involved in many of the processes that regulate the turnover and degradation of proteins. It is thus not surprising that mutations usually cause multi-organ disease first identified as autosomal dominant inclusion body myopathy with Paget and frontotemporal dementia (IBMPFD). However, in some circumstances mutations manifest as a much more restricted disorder, such as the pure distal myopathy recently described in one family.

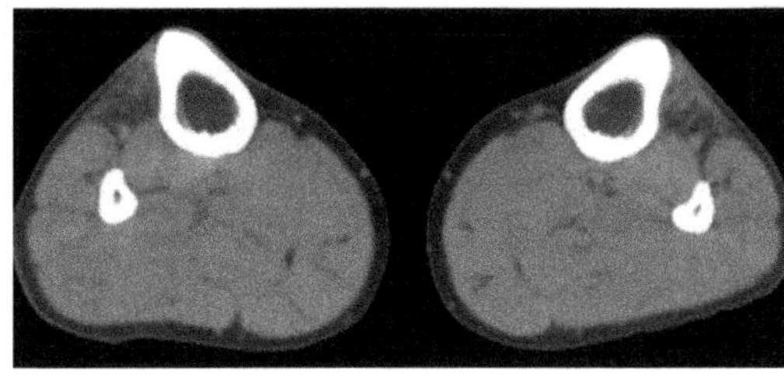

Fig. 21.8 Axial muscle computed tomography (CT) scan of a VCP distal myopathy patient. In the lower legs, the anterior tibialis, extensor hallucis longus, and extensor digitorum longus show fatty degenerative change. At the very early stage, the first muscle to show changes is the extensor hallucis longus

21.2.5.3 Histopathology

Muscle biopsies show a range of unspecific myopathic findings and rimmed vacuoles but no overt protein aggregations as is seen with the myofibrillar myopathies (MFMs). Instead, there may be peculiar lobulated ring fibers.

21.2.5.4 Clinical Presentation

Patients present with ankle dorsiflexion weakness after the age of 30 years. Clinically, the phenotype is indistinguishable from that of TMD or leg-onset WDM disease. In some patients, there is mild hands and feet interosseus muscle atrophy later in the disease course, but the typical finding of scapular winging common with IBMPFD is lacking even in the long run. In the reported family, rapidly progressive frontotemporal dementia developed more than two decades after clinical onset of the distal myopathy. No cardiac complications were observed.

21.2.5.5 Imaging Findings

The pattern of muscle involvement in terms of fatty degenerative change in the lower legs is somewhat different from that of TMD. During the early stages, the first changes are observed in the extensor hallucis longus and extensor digitorum longus muscles, followed by tibialis anterior involvement (Fig. 21.8). Proximal thigh muscles and calf muscles remain intact during the first two decades of disease progression.

21.2.6 KLHL9 Distal Myopathy

21.2.6.1 Synonyms, Abbreviations

Kelch-like homologue 9 protein distal myopathy.

21.2.6.2 Genetics and Pathophysiology

Kelch-like homologue 9 protein distal myopathy is an autosomal dominant disease based on a mutation in *KLHL9* on chromosome 3p22. It has been described in one family. The mechanisms that links the mutation defect in the Kelch-like homologue 9 protein to pathways currently known to be involved in distal myopathies are not well understood.

21.2.6.3 Histopathology

Muscle biopsy findings show nonspecific myopathic changes.

21.2.6.4 Clinical Presentation

Patients may present with droped foot that starts at the early childhood. The disease develops slowly with some later progression to weakness of proximal muscles but with preserved walking.

21.2.6.5 Imaging Findings

The few reported images of the muscle involvement in terms of fatty degenerative changes in the lower legs documented a less selective pattern when compared to those in previously described in distal myopathies. Diffuse changes occur in the posterior and anterior muscle groups. During adulthood there are also changes in the proximal thigh muscles.

Distal Myopathies: Autosomal Dominant Distal Myopathies

Key Points

- Distal myopathies are hereditary disorders caused by dominant mutations in *TTN, TIA1, MYH7, MATR3, VCP,* N-terminal *FLNC, KLHL9,* or recessive mutations in *DYSF, GNE, ANO5,* or *NEB* genes. Moreover, most of the myofibrillar myopathies present with distal weakness.
- In patients with *MYH7, KLHL9,* and *NEB* mutations, the disease usually manifests during childhood and with *DYSF, GNE, ANO5,* and N-terminal *FLNC* mutations during early or middle adulthood. *TTN, MATR3, VCP,* and Welander distal myopathies are late-onset disorders.
- Cardiomyopathy is rarely present with *MYH7* mutations, and respiratory failure has not been reported with these distal myopathies.
- Muscle imaging of the lower limbs shows a characteristic pattern of muscle involvement in most of the distal myopathies. At the mid-thigh level, the hamstrings are the first muscles to be involved in titinopathy and GNE myopathy, whereas the semimbranosus, adductor magnus, and biceps femoris are the first affected in anoctaminopathy and the quadriceps in dysferlinopathy. At the mid-leg level, the anterior compartments are the first affected muscles in titinopathy, myosinopathy, and VCP and GNE myopathy, whereas the calf muscles are the first clearly involved in dysferlinopathy, anoctaminopathy and ABD filaminopathy.
- Currently there is no curative therapy for distal myopathies. Active management to prevent complications is recommended.

Suggestions for Further Reading

Ahlberg G, Jakobsson F, Fransson A, et al. Distribution of muscle degeneration in Welander distal myopathy: a magnetic resonance imaging and muscle biopsy study. Neuromuscul Disord. 1994;4:55–62.

Cirak S, Deimling F, Sahdev S, et al. Kelch-like homologue 9 mutation is associated with an early onset autosomal dominant distal myopathy. Brain 2010;133: 2123–35.

Duff R, Tay V, Hackman P, et al. Mutations in the N-terminal actin-binding domain of filamin C (FLNC) cause a distinct distal myopathy. Am J Hum Genet. 2011;88:729–40.

Durmus H, Laval S, Deymeer F, et al. Oculopharyngeal distal myopathy is a distinct entity. Neurology 2011;76: 227–35.

Feit H, Silbergleit A, Schneider L, et al. Vocal cord and pharyngeal weakness with autosomal distal myopathy: clinical description and gene localization to chromosome 5q31. Am J Hum Genet. 1998;63: 1732–44.

Griggs R, Vihola A, Hackman P, et al. Zaspopathy in a large classic late onset distal myopathy family. Brain 2007;130:1477–84.

Mahjneh I, Haravuori H, Paetau A, et al. A distinct phenotype of distal myopathy in a large Finnish family. Neurology 2003;61:87–92.

Muelas N, Hackman P, Luque H, et al. MYH7 gene tail mutation causing myopathic profiles beyond Laing distal myopathy. Neurology 2010;75:732–41.

Palmio J, Sandell S, Suominen T, et al. Distinct distal myopathy phenotype caused by VCP gene mutation in a Finnish family. Neuromusc Disord. 2011;21(8): 551–5.

Penisson-Besnier I, Talvinen K, Dumez C, et al. Myotilinopathy in a family with late onset myopathy. Neuromuscul Disord. 2006;16:427–31.

Reilich P, Schoser B, Schramm N, et al. The p.G154S mutation of the alpha-B crystallin gene (CRYAB) causes late-onset distal myopathy. Neuromuscul Disord. 2010;20(4):255–9.

Senderek J, Garvey SM, Krieger M, et al. Autosomal-dominant distal myopathy associated with a recurrent missense mutation in the gene encoding the nuclear matrix protein, matrin 3. Am J Hum Genet. 2009;84: 511–8.

Udd B, Partanen J, Halonen P, et al. Tibial muscular dystrophy: late adult-onset distal myopathy in 66 Finnish patients. Arch Neurol. 1993;50:604–8.

Udd B. 165th ENMC international workshop: distal myopathics III. Neuromusc Disord. 2009;19:429–438.

Welander L. Myopathia distalis tarda hereditaria. Acta Med Scand. 1951;141:1–124.

21.3 Autosomal Recessive Distal Myopathies

21.3.1 GNE Myopathy

21.3.1.1 Synonyms, Abbreviations

Distal myopathy with rimmed vacuoles (DMRV); Nonaka myopathy; OMIM #605820; quadriceps sparing myopathy (QSM), hereditary inclusion body myopathy (HIBM).

21.3.1.2 Genetics and Pathophysiology

GNE myopathy is caused by recessive mutations in the UDP-*N*-acetylglucosamine 2-epimerase/*N*-acetylmannosamine kinase (*GNE*) gene on chromosome 9, which is the rate-limiting enzyme in the production of sialic acid. Hyposialylation of muscle proteins occurs and is a proposed pathomechanistic explanation for the disease. However, reported results of gene expression profiling of patient muscle samples, reported interactions of GNE with α-actinin, and the reported sarcomeric location of GNE together suggest that other molecular pathways may also be involved. Mutations have been identified in many populations with one common founder mutation in the Middle East producing a quadriceps-sparing myopathy phenotype (HIBM). In populations outside the founder regions, the disease occurs with a frequency of ~1/1,000,000.

21.3.1.3 Histopathology

Muscle biopsies show prominent rimmed vacuolar pathology also in proximal muscles, which is less common with the dominant rimmed vacuolar distal myopathies.

21.3.1.4 Clinical Presentation

Patients develop ankle dorsiflexion weakness during early adulthood, but the disease markedly progresses during the following years to weakness of proximal muscles and loss of ambulant capability 10–20 years after onset. Milder forms have been described. Respiratory and bulbar muscles are relatively spared. Cardiomyopathy has not been reported.

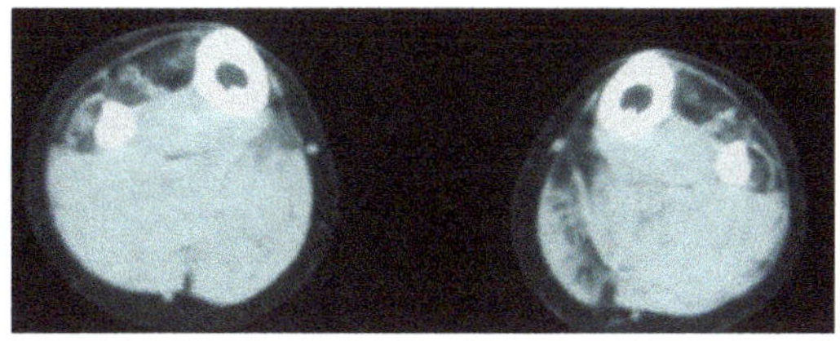

Fig. 21.9 Axial muscle CT scan of a patient with GNE distal myopathy (Nonaka). In the lower legs, the tibial anterior, extensor hallucis longus, extensor digitorum longus, lateral peroneal, and medial gastrocnemius muscles show fatty degenerative change

21.3.1.5 Imaging Findings

Muscle changes with fatty degeneration occur in parallel to clinical weakness, starting in the anterior compartment of the lower legs (Fig. 21.9). Proximal posterior thigh muscles are involved early. The quadriceps is usually spared. Depending on the severity and duration of the disease, involvement of other muscles is more generalized later in the disease course.

21.3.2 ANO5 Distal Myopathy

21.3.2.1 Synonyms, Abbreviations

Distal anoctaminopathy, OMIM#608662.

21.3.2.2 Genetics and Pathophysiology

ANO5 distal myopathy is caused by recessive mutations in any part of the anoctamin-5 protein encoded by the *ANO5* (*TMEM16E*) gene on chromosome 11p. These mutations cause a wide range of clinical phenotypes, from asymptomatic hyperCKemia over decades to severe LGMD during late adulthood. One clinical phenotype is distal myopathy. In one report a common European mutation was thought to cause the limb-girdle muscular dystrophy (LGMD) phenotype, whereas another was associated with the distal phenotype. Later studies have discarded this phenotype–genotype correlation. The molecular functions of the protein are not well understood. The overall frequency of the disease is not yet determined, but mutated *ANO5* is a common cause of muscular dystrophy.

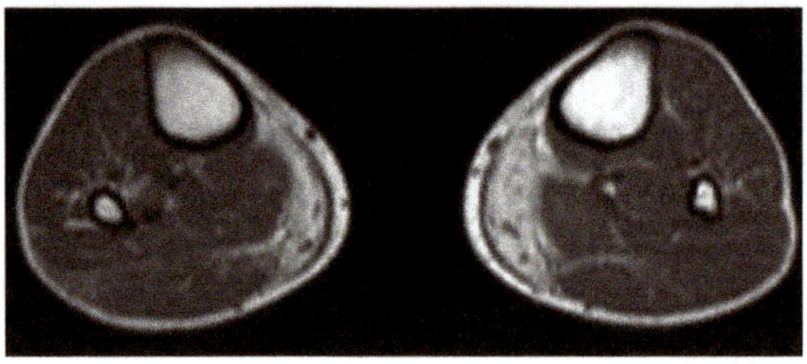

Fig. 21.10 Axial T1-weighted muscle MRI scan of a patient with *ANO5* distal myopathy. In the lower legs, the medial gastrocneumius muscles show fatty degeneration on both sides. Frequently, the change is more asymmetrical than in this patient

21.3.2.3 Histopathology

Muscle biopsy findings are nonspecific, showing scattered fiber necrosis that in many cases has been interpreted as immune-mediated polymyositis.

21.3.2.4 Clinical Presentation

Patients with the distal phenotype present with calf pain, infrequently with early hypertrophy, and high CK levels (100–500 times the normal values). It presents asymmetrically during the early adulthood and with clear male predominance. Within a few years, the calf muscles are atrophic. Progression during the following decades is slow involving also proximal muscles in later disease stages. The upper limbs, respiratory, and masticatory muscles are spared. Cardiomyopathy has not been reported.

21.3.2.5 Imaging Findings

The MRI findings are highly variable. The medial gastrocnemius muscle is the first target of the disease, with more reduced volume in some patients and in others regular dystrophic fatty replacement (Fig. 21.10). The soleus and lateral gastrocnemius are the next muscles to be involved. Asymmetrical tibial anterior replacement has been observed. Proximal thigh muscles are involved in advanced disease stages in parallel with clinical weakness. Changes are observed in the adductor magnus, semitendinosus, and biceps femoris muscles, with relative sparing of the quadriceps.

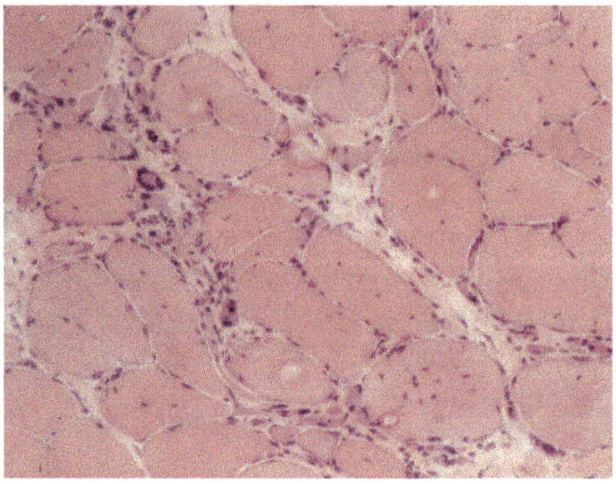

Fig. 21.11 Extensor digitorum superficialis muscle biopsy specimen from an 18-year-old patient with distal nebulin myopathy. Note the extensive pathology with group atrophy resembling neurogenic atrophy but without any nemaline rods (H&E, light microscopy)

21.3.3 Distal Nebulin Myopathy

21.3.3.1 Synonyms, Abbreviations

Nemaline (NEB-related) myopathy, OMIM# 161650.

21.3.3.2 Genetics and Pathophysiology

Recessive truncating mutations in nebulin (gene on chromosome 2q) are well known causes of congenital nemaline myopathy. The milder distal nebulin myopathy phenotype is caused by recessive missense mutations. So far, the disease has been identified in only a few families in Finland, but missense mutations in nebulin are presumed to occur in any population.

21.3.3.3 Histopathology

Missense mutations in nebulin are apparently less disruptive for the thin filament structure because nemaline rods, the hallmark of nemaline myopathy, are missing in biopsy specimens examined by light microscopy. On electron microscopy, a few small rods were identified in some biopsies and were completely absent in others, showing only disintegration of the myofibrillar structure (Fig. 21.11).

21.3.3.4 Clinical Presentation

Patients may have drop foot symptoms from early childhood or during adolescence. Slow

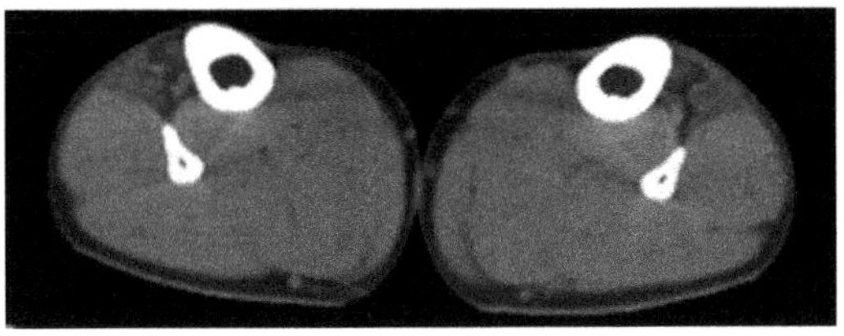

Fig. 21.12 Axial muscle CT scan of a 48-year-old man with distal nebulin myopathy. In the lower legs, the tibial anterior, extensor hallucis longus, and extensor digitorum longus show fatty degenerative changes. The other muscles are normal

progression includes weakness of neck flexors and, in some, of finger extensors with atrophy of hand muscles. Proximal muscles remain relatively spared without loss of ambulant capability despite late joint deformities.

21.3.3.5 Imaging Findings

The pattern of muscle involvement in terms of fatty degenerative changes in the lower legs (Fig. 21.12) always includes the tibialis anterior. Later, the extensor hallucis longus, extensor digitorum longus, gastrocnemius medialis, and more diffusely the proximal thigh muscles are involved.

Distal Myopathies: Autosomal Recessive Distal Myopathies

Key Points

- Distal recessive myopathies are caused by mutations in *DYSF, GNE, ANO5*, or *NEB* genes.
- In patients with *NEB* mutations the disease usually manifests during childhood and with *DYSF, GNE*, or *ANO5* mutations during early or middle adulthood.
- Cardiomyopathy has not been reported with these distal myopathies.
- Muscle imaging of the lower limbs shows a characteristic pattern of muscle involvement in most of the distal myopathies. At the mid-thigh level, the hamstrings are the first muscles to be involved in GNE myopathy, whereas the semimembranosus, adductor magnus, and biceps femoris are the first affected in anoctaminopathy. The quadriceps is first affected in dysferlinopathy. At the mid-leg level, the anterior compartments are the first affected muscles in GNE myopathy, whereas the calf muscles are the first clearly involved in dysferlinopathy and anoctaminopathy.
- Currently there is no curative therapy for distal myopathies. Active management to prevent complications is recommended.

Suggestions for Further Reading

Bolduc V, Marlow G, Boycott KM, et al. Recessive mutations in the putative calcium-activated chloride channel anoctamin 5 cause proximal LGMD2L and distal MMD3 muscular dystrophies. Am J Hum Genet. 2010;86:213–21.

Durmus H, Laval S, Deymeer F, et al. Oculopharyngeal distal myopathy is a distinct entity. Neurology. 2011;76: 227–35.

Illa I, Serrano-Munuera C, Gallardo E, et al. Distal anterior compartment myopathy: a dysferlin mutation causing a new muscular dystrophy phenotype. Annal Neurol. 2001;49:130–4.

Miyoshi K, Kawai H, Iwasa M, Kusaka K, Nishino H. Autosomal recessive distal muscular dystrophy as a new type of progressive muscular dystrophy. Brain 1986;109:31–54.

Nonaka I, Sunohara N, Ishiura S, Satoyoshi E. Familial distal myopathy with rimmed vacuole and lamellar (myeloid) body formation. J Neurol Sci. 1981;51: 141–55.

Paradas C, Llauger J, Diaz-Manera J, et al. Redefining dysferlinopathy phenotypes based on clinical findings and muscle imaging studies. Neurology 2010;75:316–23.

Penttilä S, Palmio J, Suominen T, et al. Eight new mutations and the expanding phenotype variability in muscular dystrophy caused by ANO5. Neurology 2012;78:897–903.

Udd B. 165th ENMC international workshop: distal myopathies III. Neuromusc Disord. 2009;19: 429–438.

Wallgren-Pettersson C, Lehtokari V-L, Kalimo H, et al. Distal myopathy caused by homozygous missense mutations in the nebulin gene. Brain 2007;130: 1465–76.

Myotonic Dystrophies

22

Cornelia Kornblum

22.1 Introduction

22.1.1 Synonyms, Abbreviations

Myotonic dystrophy type 1 (DM1), Steinert's disease, Curschmann–Steinert-disease, Myotonic dystrophy type 2 (DM2), Proximal Myotonic Myopathy (PROMM).

22.1.2 Introduction and Classification

Myotonic dystrophy type 1 (DM1) and type 2 (DM2) are complex and multi-systemic inherited disorders with several clinical and genetic features in common. These disorders are characterized by progressive skeletal muscle weakness, wasting and myotonia. DM1 and DM2 typically involve a wide range of tissues including cardiac and smooth muscles as well as skeletal muscle tissue, which is the most frequently affected tissue in both disease entities.

Myotonic dystrophy type 1 is the most common form of muscular dystrophy in adults, affecting approximately one person in 8000 worldwide. Estimates of the prevalence of DM1 are 3–15:100,000 in Europe to 1:500 in Quebec, Canada, where founder effects may have increased the prevalence. In Europe, DM2 may be as common as DM1, but reliable epidemiological data are still lacking. Worldwide, DM2 seems to be rarer than DM1, and most DM2 families are of European, especially German/Polish origin.

22.1.3 Genetics and Pathophysiology

DM1 and DM2 are dominantly inherited disorders caused by pathogenic expansions of polynucleotide microsatellite repeat units within non-coding regions at two distinct genetic loci. DM1 results from a trinucleotide CTG-repeat expansion in the 3´UTR of the dystrophia myotonica-protein kinase gene (*DMPK* gene, OMIM #160900) on chromosome 19q. DM2 results from a tetranucleotide CCTG-repeat expansion in the intron 1 of the zinc finger protein 9 gene (*ZNF9* gene, OMIM#602668) on chromosome 3q. The overall disease range of CTG-repeat numbers in DM1 is 50–4000. Repeat sizes of 38–49 are usually clinically asymptomatic ("pre-mutation phenotype"). Repeat sizes of 50–80 may be associated with mild or late-onset clinical phenotypes, and repeat sizes of 50–1,000 are usually associated with the classic juvenile- or adult-onset phenotypes and occasionally with childhood-onset disease subtypes. Large repeat expansions up to 4,000 are often found in severe, mostly congenital forms of DM1. In DM1, CTG-repeat expansions of more than 37 repeats in length are unstable and may expand in length during gametogenesis,

C. Kornblum (✉)
Universitätsklinikum Bonn, Klinik und Poliklinik für Neurologie, Sigmund-Freud-Str. 25, 53105 Bonn, Germany
e-mail: cornelia.kornblum@ukb.uni-bonn.de

M.P. Wattjes and D. Fischer (eds.), *Neuromuscular Imaging*, DOI 10.1007/978-1-4614-6552-2_22,

meiosis and mitosis. The presence of larger repeat sizes usually results in earlier ages of onset and more severe disease phenotypes, occasionally leading to the severe "congenital" phenotype of DM1. Children with congenital disease phenotypes almost always inherit the expanded mutant *DMPK* allele from their mothers through the maternal lineage. The phenomenon of intergenerational repeat instability with expanding CTG-repeat sizes causes "anticipation," which means the occurrence of increasing disease severity and earlier ages of onset in successive generations. Repeat numbers usually increase most with maternal transmission, however, changes from the mild or late-onset clinical phenotypes harbouring small repeat expansions to the classic clinical phenotypes most frequently occur with paternal transmission. Because of marked somatic mosaicism of the CTG-repeat lengths, there are considerable tissue variations in repeat sizes with often rather small expansions in blood and much larger expansions in heart or skeletal muscle tissue. Moreover, repeat sizes may increase throughout life even in post-mitotic tissues which suggests that repeat lengths in blood that are routinely determined in DM1 might not correlate with repeat lengths in other tissues.

The repeat expansions in DM2 are generally much larger than in DM1, ranging from 75 to over 11,000 repeats (mean of ~5,000 repeats). Somatic instability with different repeat sizes in different tissues has also been described in DM2. Unlike DM1, the repeat size in DM2 does not correlate with the age of onset or disease severity, and repeat expansions sizes are usually not determined in molecular genetic routine analyses. Anticipation in DM2 is, if present at all, mild and less evident clinically. In contrast to DM1, a congenital form of DM2 has not been reported.

In myotonic dystrophies, the pathogenic mechanism of microsatellite repeat expansions results from the aberrant RNA transcripts, long sequence tracts of $(CUG)_n$ or $(CCUG)_n$ in the DM1 and DM2 transcripts, respectively. The expanded mutant RNA transcripts are retained in the nucleus and accumulate to form ribonuclear inclusions called foci, however inclusions are also present in cytoplasm. The nuclear retention of mutated transcripts of *DMPK* might be responsible for DMPK haploinsufficiency in DM1. More important, the expanded messenger RNA (mRNA) causes a toxic-gain-of-function RNA effect in DM1 and DM2 that is mediated by a variety of pathogenic structural interactions, which include the binding and altered function of at least two RNA-binding proteins that regulate splicing and translation: the sequestration within foci and loss-of-function of the splicing factor muscleblind-like protein 1 (MBNL1) as well as upregulation and gain-of-function of CUG triplet repeat RNA-binding protein 1 (CUGBP1, synonyms CELF1 or ETR3-like factor 1) through a mechanism of hyperphosphorylation via aberrant activation of protein kinase C. Downstream effects of sequestration and/or upregulation of RNA-binding proteins result in altered RNA stability and RNA processing with aberrant pre-mRNA splicing of several transcripts and global dysregulation of alternative splicing. Consequently, the molecular defects result in a global "spliceopathy" which is responsible for the multi-systemic nature of the diseases. Moreover, increased CUGBP1 and decreased MBNL1 in DM1 possibly cause a reversion to more fetal mRNA species, and the loss of several adult mRNA species results in specific defects in diverse tissues. Molecular effects of altered splicing factors have been shown to result in misregulated alternative splicing of several pre-mRNAs and finally altered production of various proteins including the insulin receptor, muscular chloride channel CLCN1 and CaV1.1 calcium channel, cardiac troponin T, ryanodine receptor 1 (RYR-1), myotubularin MTM1, muscular bridging integrator-1 (BIN1), N-methyl-D-aspartate (NMDA) receptor 1, amyloid precursor protein APP, and microtubule-associated protein tau in DM1 and DM2, respectively. Recently, new advances have added complexity to the basic aberrant splicing model. In DM1, elevation of CUGBP1 has been reported to increase translation and splicing of CUGBP1 targets, CUG repeats seem to cause oxidative and endoplasmatic reticulum stress in DM1 cells thus inhibiting mRNA translation, and soluble mutant CUG repeats outside of foci have been shown to sequester transcription factors from active chromatine. In DM2, recent data postulated that CCUG repeats reduce translation of mRNA coding for proteins of the translational apparatus leading to a reduction of the global protein synthesis rate. In myotonic dystrophies in general, mutant transcripts cause additional cellular dysfunction by altering the processing and metabolism of several microRNAs. Recent findings indicate that RNA transcripts with expanded CAG repeats can be translated in the complete absence of a starting ATG, and this Repeat Associated Non-ATG translation (RAN-translation) occurs across expanded CAG repeats in all reading frames to produce long polyglutamine, polyserine, and polyalanine tracts. Expanded CUG transcripts also show RAN-translation occurring in all three reading frames to produce homopolymeric proteins. These RAN-translation products can be toxic, which gives evidence of an additional toxic-gain-of-protein function in myotonic dystrophies.

22.1.4 Clinical Presentation

DM1 and DM2 present with distinct, although overlapping, clinical phenotypes. The pattern of clinical skeletal muscle affection in DM1 usually differs from that of DM2. However, profound general weakness may emerge during the late stages of both disorders. DM1 and DM2 primarily affect skeletal muscle with myotonia, muscle weakness and wasting as the leading symptoms. Major extra-muscular clinical manifestations in both disorders involve cardiac defects, endocrinological problems, cataracts, gastrointestinal complaints, daytime sleepiness and/or fatigue, and neuropsychological and cognitive deficits. Myalgia is characteristic for DM2 but may also occur in DM1.

The DM1 patients can be divided into four main clinical phenotypes that are partly associated with CTG-repeat expansion sizes:

1. Patients with mild or late-onset disease.
2. Classic juvenile- or adult-onset phenotype with ages of onset approximately 10–30 years.
3. Childhood-onset phenotype showing first symptoms at 1–10 years of age.
4. Severe congenital phenotype with prenatal onset or latest age of onset at birth.

Age of onset best correlates with CTG-repeat size lengths when sizes are < 400 repeats. The classical adult-onset DM1 phenotype is characterised by distal muscle weakness. Weakness and wasting of forearm and lower leg muscles with pareses of ankle dorsiflexors, foot drop and steppage gait are early and frequent signs. Neck flexors and forearm muscles with early finger/wrist flexor involvement are also common. Temporal muscle atrophy, frontal balding, mild upper eyelid ptosis, facial and masticatory muscle weakness with lack of facial expression and problems with mouth closure lead to a typical appearance ("myotonic facies"). Weakness of tongue, palatal and pharyngeal muscles often result in indistinct speech and dysarthria, and pharyngeal or esophageal dysphagia sometimes develops. Pelvic girdle and ankle plantar flexor muscles are often clinically less affected. Muscle weakness usually progresses slowly over time and proximal muscles are involved later in the disease course. Clinical muscular impairment in DM1 patients is often categorized using the five-point Muscular Impairment Rating Scale (MIRS) for DM1: 1, no muscular impairment; 2, minimal signs (myotonia, facial weakness, ptosis, nasal speech, jaw and temporal wasting, neck flexor weakness, no distal weakness except isolated digit flexor weakness); 3, distal weakness (no proximal weakness except isolated elbow extensor weakness); 4, mild to moderate proximal weakness (Medical Research Council muscle strength scale MRC between 3 and +4); 5, severe proximal weakness (MRC < 3). Myotonia is evoked by muscle percussion and contraction, and a "warm up phenomenon" is frequently seen. Myotonia rarely causes disability and sometimes is alleviated during the course of the disease when dystrophic muscle changes become more evident.

Posterior subcapsular cataracts develop in most patients during early adulthood. Cardiac conduction disturbances, tachyarrhythmias, atrial fibrillation, ventricular arrhythmias, and cardiomyopathy with left ventricular dysfunction usually developing later in life are common in DM1. Malignant arrhythmia and sudden cardiac death may be the most fatal complications of the disorder, and cardiac involvement contributes significantly to the morbidity and mortality of the disease. Respiratory insufficiency due to diaphragm and respiratory muscle weakness as well as aspiration pneumonia from swallowing problems constitute common complications particularly in the advanced stages.

Endocrine abnormalities may include disturbances of the thyroid, hypothalamus, gonads and pancreas, the latter resulting in insulin resistance. Testicular atrophy may cause infertility in men, and habitual abortion and menstrual irregularities are common in women. Gastrointestinal complaints are frequent and may be due to smooth muscle involvement with hypokinesis, megacolon, constipation and pseudo-obstruction. Cholelithiasis is a frequent finding.

Apathy, daytime sleepiness, and fatigue are extremely common and often seriously disabling symptoms. Obstructive and primary central apnea and an abnormal ventilatory response to hypercapnia and hypoxia have been documented in DM1. The hypersomnia, however, may be related to central nervous system dysfunction (e.g., at the brain stem level). Depression may be prominent and seems to be more pronounced during the early disease stages. There is ample evidence of cerebral involvement in DM1. Mental impairment and neuropsychological deficits especially of executive and visuospatial functions have been frequently described. Avoidant personality traits, apathy, and "lack of self-awareness"—eventually deteriorating with age—are common findings in DM1 patients.

In congenital and childhood-onset forms of DM1, mental impairment, low intelligence, learning difficulties, and psychosocial and behavioral abnormalities often constitute the most prominent and disabling symptoms of the disorder. Congenital DM1 is a distinct clinical phenotype. After delivery, diseased children present with a typical appearance including severe facial weakness with a characteristic "tented" upper lip, feeding difficulties, generalized muscle weakness, hypotonia ("floppy infant"), and respiratory problems.

In comparison with DM1, clinical symptoms of DM2 are usually milder and manifest later in life, most frequently during the third decade but sometimes at ages up to ≥ 60 years. Skeletal muscle affection is characterized by myotonia, stiffness, proximal and axial muscle weakness with early affection of hip girdle and paraspinal muscles and muscle pain predominantly present in the thighs. Calf hypertrophy, mild facial weakness, hearing loss, hyperhidrosis, tremor, diabetes mellitus type 2, further endocrinological problems, posterior subcapsular cataracts, testicular failure, cardiac conduction defects and -less frequently-cardiomyopathy may present in DM2. Similar to DM1, fatigue and depression are common in DM2. Brain affection has equally been demonstrated in DM2, and impaired frontal lobe function is a predominant finding in both forms of DM. Mental impairment in DM2 may be milder than that in DM1. Neuropsychological deficits particularly affect executive, attentional, and visuospatial functions.

Electromyographic (EMG) investigations may show myotonia in affected skeletal muscles. In contrast to DM1, myotonic discharges are more frequent in proximal limb muscles in DM2 (e.g., iliopsoas muscles). Laboratory examinations usually show elevated serum creatine kinase (CK) levels in both disorders, although the increase can be rather mild. Normal levels do not exclude the diagnosis. In DM2, high serum cholesterol levels are common. In DM1, elevated serum GGT activities are characteristic and can be mistaken as indicating liver involvement. Serum IgG levels may be reduced in both disease entities. Testosterone and insulin-like growth factor-1 (IGF-1) levels can also be reduced, in contrast to follicle-stimulating hormone levels, which are frequently increased in DM1 and DM2 patients.

22.2 Myotonic Dystrophy Type I (DM1)

22.2.1 Genetics, Pathophysiology, and Clinical Presentation

See Sect. 22.1

22.2.2 Histopathology

Light microscopic changes in skeletal muscle tissue in patients with DM1 range from mild to grossly abnormal in clinically affected individuals. Pathological histological findings in DM1 may include myopathic changes with fiber size variation; numerous internal nuclei that are occasionally located in longitudinal chains; a disordered internal architecture of muscle fibers with

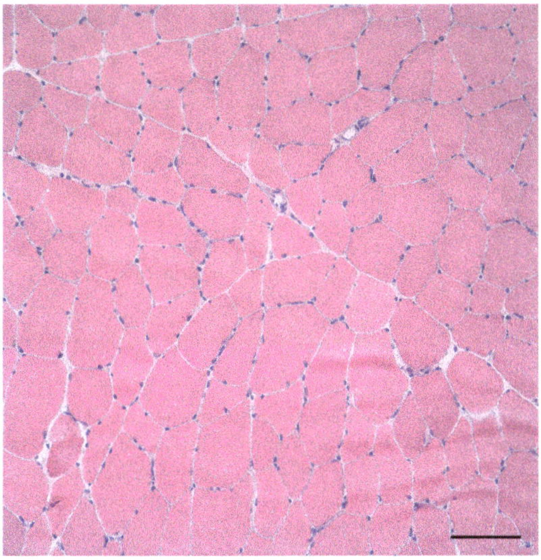

Fig. 22.1 DM1 in a 50-year-old woman with advanced disease, 150–250 CTG repeats, Muscular Impairment Rating Scale (MIRS) grade 4, moderate myotonia, mildly elevated serum creatine kinase (mild hyperCKemia). Open skeletal muscle biopsy of vastus lateralis muscle at age 46 years showed mild variation in fiber size without other relevant changes. Scale bar = 100 μm. Corresponding 3T T1-weighted magnetic resonance imaging (MRI) scans of the thighs at age 50 years showed a moderately moth-eaten appearance with numerous scattered T1-weighted hyperintense areas of vastus medialis muscles indicating moderate fatty degeneration. In contrast, the vastus lateralis muscles did not have fatty degeneration (data not shown)

the presence of ring fibers, sarcoplasmic masses, and acid phosphatase-positive sarcoplasmic granules; early type-1 fiber atrophy and type-2 fiber hypertrophy; pyknotic nuclear clumps; increased numbers of intrafusal muscle fibers; dystrophic tissue changes with slight necrosis and degeneration of muscle fibers with absence of regenerative activity; mildly increased endomysial connective tissue; fibroadipose tissue replacement (usually present only in severely affected muscles and more advanced disease stages). Type-1 fiber predominance may be seen in severely affected muscles. In the congenital form of DM1, small muscle fibers with increased numbers of internal nuclei may be present, and fiber type differentiation is generally poor (Fig. 22.1).

In general, the histological findings in skeletal muscle tissue of DM1 and DM2 patients are not specific and may be rather mild. Further immunohistochemistry and immunoblotting techniques do not contribute to the diagnostic process. Based on clinical experience, numerous internal nuclei and pyknotic nuclear clumps are nonspecific, but particularly frequent findings in both disease entities. For diagnostic purposes, DNA testing is the method of choice in individuals who are clinically suspected to have DM1 or DM2.

Neuropathological findings in brain tissue of DM1 patients include abnormalities such as intracytoplasmic inclusions in the thalamus, striatum, cerebral cortex, and brainstem. Other studies in DM1 and DM2 brains found evidence of neurofibrillary degeneration with intracellular aggregation of microtubule-associated tau protein. Most changes are located in neurons, although white matter abnormalities including disordered arrangement of myelin sheaths and axons have been described.

22.2.3 Neuromuscular Imaging

Muscular imaging has proven useful for the phenotypical characterization of DM1 during the past two decades. Early imaging techniques applied included ultrasonography, computed tomography (CT), and low field musculoskeletal magnetic resonance imaging (MRI). Musculoskeletal MRI studies in DM1 are mostly restricted to lower limbs, although a few data on upper limb involvement are available. In comparison with DM1, there are fewer musculoskeletal imaging data available for DM2. Recently, 3T whole body MRI systems were applied to characterize skeletal muscle involvement in myotonic dystrophies. In a recent study on muscle affection in DM1 and DM2 using a 3T whole-body MRI system, clinical muscular impairment in DM1 patients was categorised using the MIRS, and muscular strength in DM2 patients was evaluated according to the MRC Scale.

Analyzing the current data on DM1, shows that there is selective involvement of specific muscle groups, suggesting a characteristic pattern of skeletal muscle deterioration. With regard to the lower limbs, the anterior compartment is more predominantly affected than the posterior compartment of the thighs, and the calf muscles are more preferentially affected than the anterior compartment. These are consistent findings in MRI studies of DM1. In DM1, the anterior thighs and the calf muscles are most frequently and severely degenerated and demonstrate a distinct pattern of MRI signal abnormalities including fatty degeneration and edema-like changes. The rectus femoris and gracilis muscles are relatively spared, whereas the vastus muscles typically show a semilunar anterolateral perifemoral area of fatty degeneration. This characteristic perifemoral muscle degeneration has been repeatedly reported in DM1 patients, with the vastus intermedius muscles most seriously affected, followed by deep parts of the vastus medialis and lateralis muscles. In contrast to the long and short heads of the biceps femoris, hamstring internal muscles (semimembranosus, semitendinosus) frequently show moderate fatty degeneration as well (Fig. 22.2). In the lower legs of DM1 patients, the gastrocnemius muscles show early and frequent involvement. Frequent and early degeneration of the medial heads of the gastrocnemius and soleus muscles is a consistent, characteristic finding. The medial heads of the gastrocnemius muscles are usually more vulnerable to degeneration than the lateral heads (Fig. 22.3). Some DM1 patients show fatty changes of the medial heads and isolated edema-like changes of the lateral heads, and occasionally the medial heads are more severely (or solely) fatty degenerated in comparison with the lateral heads. Correlation with data on disease duration as well as rare longitudinal observations might indicate a sequential involvement of gastrocnemius muscles with an early affection of medial heads and fatty degeneration of lateral heads in advanced disease stages. In a variety of neuromuscular disorders, it has been postulated that fatty deterioration proceeds only after development of edema-like changes seen on MRI. In DM1 as well, edema-like abnormalities have been described as early MRI markers of the disease characterizing an early stage of muscle degeneration (see Chap. 4). However, this has not been finally proven, and intraindividual longitudinal data are still limited. The significance and histological correlates of edema-like changes in skeletal muscles of DM1 patients are not well known. Strikingly, increased water content, inflammatory changes, edema, and serious necrosis are not typical for DM1 skeletal muscle biopsies. Previously, edema-like abnormalities have been associated with changes in muscle fiber type distribution, such as type-2 fiber hypertrophy which is a common histological finding in DM1. Also tibialis anterior muscles are frequently involved in DM1, although they are usually less severely affected than the posterior lower leg muscles. These MRI data are partly in contrast to abundant clinical data describing ankle dorsiflexor weakness as an early and common clinical sign in DM1. Tibialis posterior muscles of the lower legs are generally best preserved and relatively spared with regard to MRI signal changes.

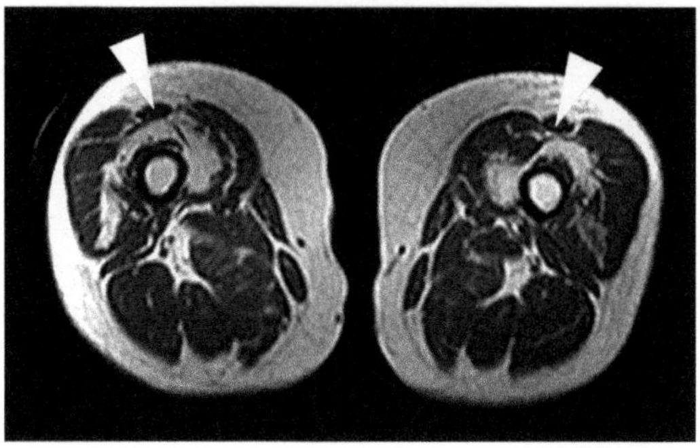

Fig. 22.2 A 48-year-old woman with advanced DMI, MIRS grade 3, moderate myotonia (also see Fig. 22.3) showing a semilunar perifemoral area of fatty degeneration of the vastus intermedius, medialis and lateralis sparing the rectus femoris (*white arrow heads*) and gracilis muscles (3T T1-weighted MRI). From Kornblum C, et al. Distinct neuromuscular phenotypes in myotonic dystrophy types 1 and 2: a whole body highfield MRI study. J Neurol. 2006 Jun;253(6):753–61. Reprinted with permission from Springer

Data on upper limb involvement in DM1 are limited primarily for technical reasons. Atrophy and fatty degeneration of triceps muscles and edema-like changes and mild to moderate fatty degeneration of forearm muscles (flexor and extensor carpi, flexor and extensor digitorum muscles) have been reported. Moderate to severe fatty changes of trunk muscles have been described in DM1 patients with more advanced disease affecting the neck flexors, erector spinae muscles, rectus abdominis, and obliquus externus and internus muscles.

In DM1, the scapular and pelvic girdle, posterior thighs, rectus femoris, gracilis, and tibialis posterior muscles are usually the best preserved.

Dysphagia is a common clinical symptom in DM1. Whole-body MRI protocols have revealed substantial dilatation of the esophagus in the proximal segment with prominent air-fluid

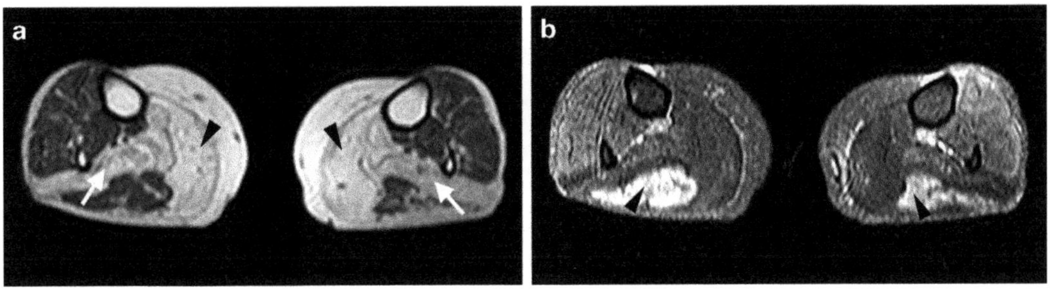

Fig. 22.3 A 48-year-old woman with DM1 (see Fig. 22.2). (**a**) The 3T T1-weighted images of the lower legs show severe fatty degeneration of the medial heads of the gastrocnemius muscles (*black arrow heads*) and soleus muscles (*white arrows*). (**b**) Corresponding fat-suppressed 3T MRI T2-weighted images (SPAIR sequences) show focal edema-like changes of the lateral heads of the gastrocnemius muscles (*black arrowheads*). From Kornblum C, et al. Distinct neuromuscular phenotypes in myotonic dystrophy types 1 and 2: a whole body highfield MRI study. J Neurol. 2006 Jun;253(6):753–61. Reprinted with permission from Springer

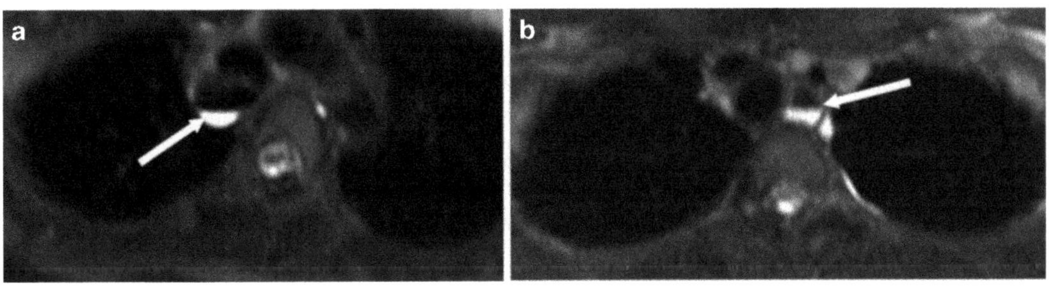

Fig. 22.4 DM1, transverse spectral fat-suppressed T2-weighted images obtained during 3T whole body muscle MRI. Both patients showed dysphagia. MRI demonstrated dilatation of the proximal esophageus with prominent air-fluid levels indicative of gastroesophageal reflux disease. (**a**) 37 year old woman. (**b**) 16 year old boy

levels indicative of gastroesophageal reflux disease (Fig. 22.4).

22.2.4 Brain Imaging

See Sect. 22.4

Myotonic Dystrophies: Myotonic Dystrophy Type I (DM1)

Key Points

- Anterior thigh compartments are predominantly involved in DM1, and vastus muscles typically show a semilunar anterolateral perifemoral area of fatty degeneration.
- Frequent and early degeneration of the medial heads of gastrocnemius and soleus muscles is a characteristic finding in the lower legs of DM1 patients.
- The posterior compartments of the thighs and the anterior compartments of the lower legs are usually better preserved than the anterior thigh compartments and the calves.
- Rectus femoris and gracilis as well as tibialis posterior muscles are relatively spared in DM1.
- Neuromuscular MRI data are usually in line with the clinical presentation in DM1.
- Brain involvement is frequent in DM1. Current neuroimaging techniques provide evidence of prominent white matter involvement with pronounced callosal body and limbic system involvement.

22.3 Myotonic Dystrophy Type II (DM2)

22.3.1 Genetics, Pathophysiology, and Clinical Presentation

See Sect. 22.1

22.3.2 Histopathology

In DM2, light microscopy of skeletal muscle tissue usually show multiple internal nuclei predominantly in type-2 muscle fibers, fiber size variation with predominantly type-2 fiber atrophy without fiber type grouping, numerous pyknotic nuclear clumps, acid phosphatase positive sarcoplasmic granules, and a disordered internal architecture of the muscle fibers. Histological changes and dystrophic skeletal muscle alterations may be less than in DM1 (Figs. 22.5 and 22.6).

22.3.3 Neuromuscular Imaging

In comparison with DM1, systematic muscular imaging data on DM2 are limited. In general, DM2 patients are less affected based on skeletal muscle MRI findings. A more proximal focus of fatty muscle degeneration is present in DM2 in contrast to DM1, and the number of affected muscles and the severity of fatty degeneration seems to be less pronounced. In a whole-body 3T MRI study most DM2 patients with early or less advanced disease stages as indicated by mild proximal pareses or the absence of muscle weakness showed normal MRI results. Even mild to moderate muscle weakness and DM2-characteristic myalgias were usually not reflected by MRI signal alterations. Edema-like changes have been shown in anterior thigh and posterior lower leg muscles and in the fibularis longus in a few DM2 patients. Interestingly, there are no systematic data concerning muscular MRI signal changes in patients with muscle pain. Inflammatory reactions or ischemic changes, both well-known causes of muscle pain, would be expected to result in muscle edema on MRI. However, edema-like signal changes, a common feature in DM1, have been less frequently reported in DM2. Correspondingly, DM2 patients do not show distinct histological correlates of muscle pain such as inflammation or serious fiber necroses in their skeletal muscle biopsies. These findings might be indicative of a particular pathophysiological mechanism of musculoskeletal pain in DM2. Skeletal muscle signal changes on MRI and subclinical skeletal muscle involvement have been predominantly reported in DM2 patients with clinically advanced disease stages showing moderate to severe proximal pareses. In these patients, no highly specific pattern of muscle affection was present in contrast to DM1. However, most DM2 patients with MRI signal changes show fatty degeneration of trunk muscles, particularly of erector spinae muscles which seem to be the most frequently affected muscles in DM2, and—less frequently—of rectus abdominis and obliquus externus muscles (Fig. 22.7). Hip girdle and thigh muscles are often affected in addition to trunk muscles with gluteus maximus being the second most frequently altered muscles. In general, muscles of the anterior and posterior thigh compartments, particularly the quadriceps muscles and semimembranosus and semitendinosus muscles, are affected in DM2. In line with DM1, the posterior compartments of the thighs and anterior compartments of the lower legs are relatively better preserved than the anterior thigh compartments and the calves, the latter occasionally showing fatty degeneration and edema-like changes. As in DM1, rectus femoris and gracilis muscles are often spared in DM2 (Fig. 22.8). Data on upper limb involvement in DM2 are limited. Shoulder girdle muscles such as the latissimus dorsi might be affected as are the triceps brachii muscles and less frequently the deltoid and biceps brachii muscles. In contrast to DM1, a 3T whole-body MRI study found that pathological MRI findings were restricted to women with DM2 and emerged with increasing age. The latter finding may reflect the exclusive adult-onset phenotype and the chronic progressive disease course of DM2.

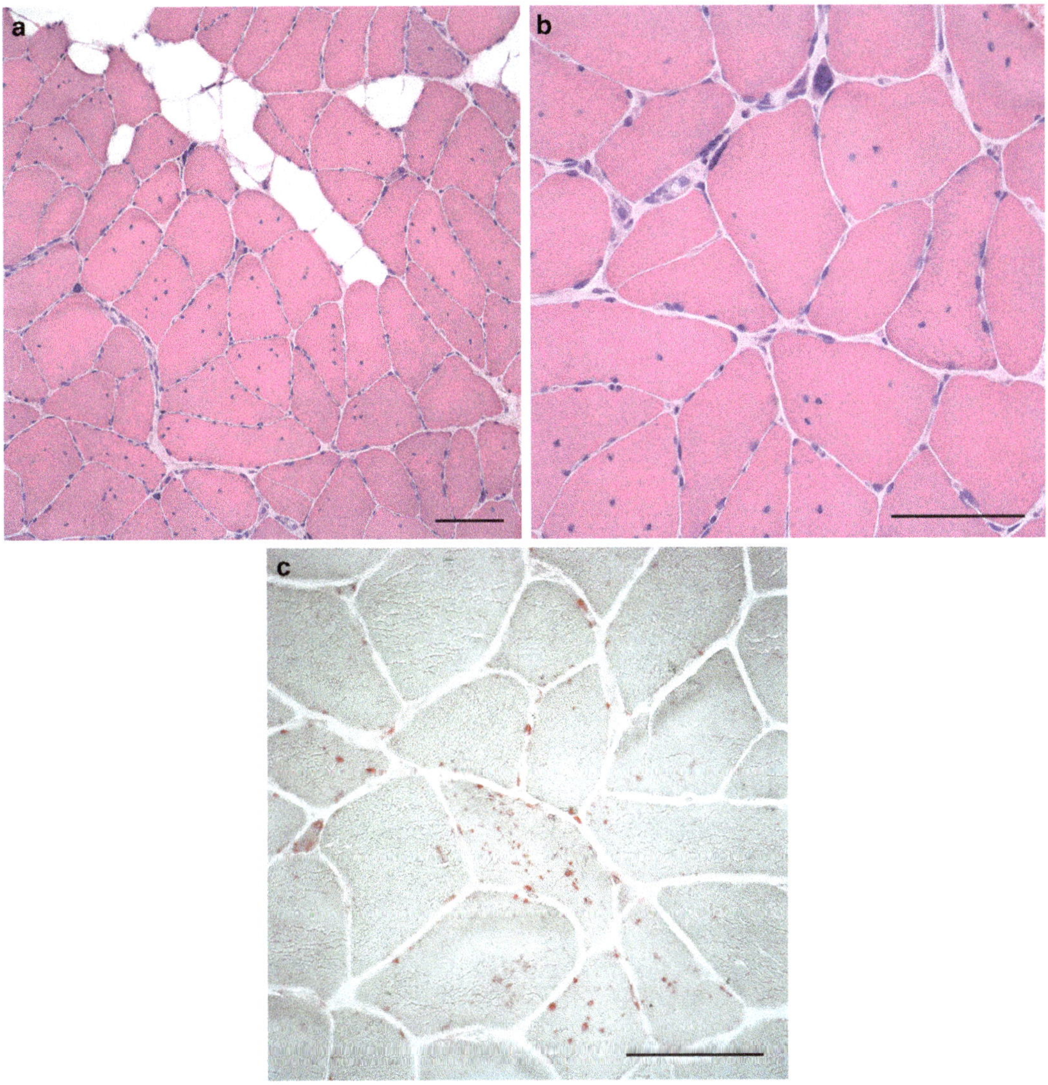

Fig. 22.5 DM2, 70 year old woman with advanced disease, severe proximal weakness of the shoulder girdle, hip girdle, and trunk muscles as well as moderate hyperCKemia. (**a**) Open skeletal muscle biopsy of vastus lateralis muscle at the age of 57 years showed increased fiber size variation with a number of atrophic fibres, marked increase of internalised myonuclei, pyknotic nuclear clumps, occasional fiber splitting, few fibers with degenerative sarcoplasmic changes, and areas of fatty replacement. H&E staining (×20 magnification). Scale bar = 100 μm. (**b**) gives a higher powered image of the same slide. H&E staining (×40 magnification). Scale bar = 100 μm. (**c**) shows fine acid phosphatase positive sarcoplasmic foci ("granules"). Acid phosphatase staining (×40 magnification). Scale bar = 100 μm. Corresponding 3T T1-weighted MR images of the thighs at the age of 70 years (see for Fig. 22.8) showed a moderate moth-eaten appearance with numerous scattered T1-hyperintense areas of vastus intermedius and lateralis muscles

Neuromuscular MRI data are usually in line with the clinical impression of DM1, in contrast to DM2 patients, who frequently show discrepancies between their clinical evaluation and MRI results. MRI proved to be a sensitive technique for detecting subclinical skeletal muscle involvement in subgroups of DM1 and DM2 patients, but in DM2 it was restricted to advanced disease stages. The differences in skeletal muscle involvement patterns on MRI may reflect

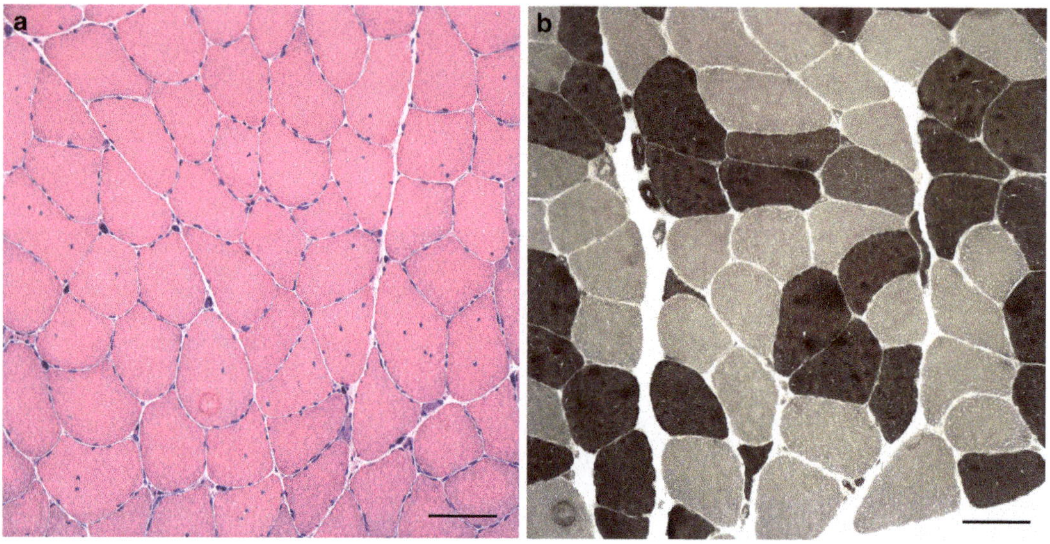

Fig. 22.6 DM2, 38 year old man with early disease stage. There were no fixed pareses, and the clinical phenotype was dominated by mild myotonia, severe myalgia predominantly of the thighs, and moderate hyperCKemia. (**a**) Open skeletal muscle biopsy of vastus lateralis muscle at the age of 35 years showed numerous atrophic fibres, pyknotic nuclear clumps, and increased internalised myonuclei. Scale bar = 100 μm. (**b**) demonstrates atrophic type II fibers in the ATPase reaction following pretreatment at pH 9.4. Dark staining of type II fibers, light staining of type I fibers. Scale bar = 100 μm. Corresponding 3T T1-weighted MR images of the thighs at the age of 38 years showed normal results (data not shown)

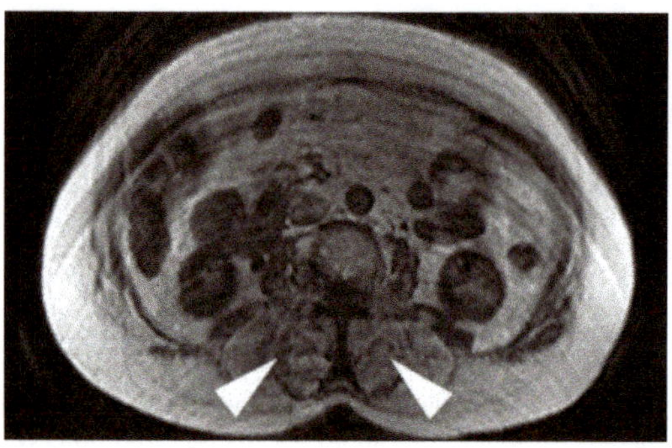

Fig. 22.7 DM2, 70 year old woman with advanced disease (see for Figs. 22.5 and 22.8) showing symmetric severe fatty degeneration of the lumbar erector spinae muscles (white arrow heads, 3T T1-weighted MR images). From Kornblum C, et al. Distinct neuromuscular phenotypes in myotonic dystrophy types 1 and 2: a whole body highfield MRI study. J Neurol. 2006 Jun;253(6):753–61. Reprinted with permission from Springer

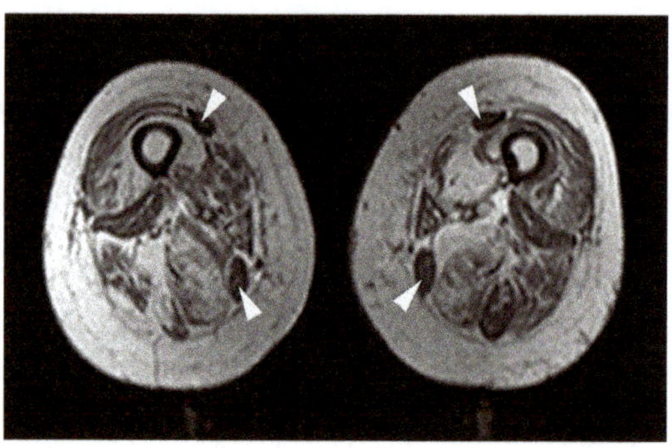

Fig. 22.8 DM2, 70 year old woman with advanced disease (see for Figs. 22.5 and 22.7) showing a moderate moth-eaten appearance with numerous scattered T1-hyperintense areas of vastus intermedius and lateralis muscles. Vastus medialis as well as the long heads of biceps femoris, semimembranosus and adductor muscles demonstrated a moth-eaten appearance with partly scattered and partly confluent areas of T1-hyperintensity, some areas showed complete replacement of muscle by connective tissue and fat. Rectus femoris and gracilis muscles were spared (white arrow heads, 3T T1-weighted MR images). From Kornblum C, et al. Distinct neuromuscular phenotypes in myotonic dystrophy types 1 and 2: a whole body highfield MRI study. J Neurol. 2006 Jun;253(6):753–61. Reprinted with permission from Springer

fundamental discrepancies in the pathophysiology of muscle degeneration between DM1 and DM2. Previous imaging results for myotonia congenita showed that chloride channel myotonia and/or myalgia alone does not result in MRI skeletal muscle signal changes. Fatty skeletal muscle alterations and edema-like changes seen in DM1 and DM2 are not the result of chloride channel dysfunction but clear consequences of myopathic and dystrophic disease processes.

22.3.4 Brain Imaging

See Sect. 22.4

> **Myotonic Dystrophies: Myotonic Dystrophy Type II (DM2)**
>
> **Key Points**
>
> - DM2 patients are often less affected than DM1 patients based on skeletal muscle MRI findings. DM2 patients with less advanced disease stages and/or myalgia may show normal MRI results.
> - Most DM2 patients with advanced disease show fatty degeneration of trunk muscles, particularly of the erector spinae. Hip girdle and thigh muscles are often affected, especially the gluteus maximus muscles.
> - As in DM1, the posterior compartments of the thighs and the anterior compartments of the lower legs are usually better preserved than the anterior thigh compartments and the calves.
> - Rectus femoris and gracilis muscles are relatively spared in DM2.
> - Brain involvement is frequent in DM2, although it may be less pronounced than that seen in DM1.

22.4 Brain Imaging in Myotonic Dystrophies

A variety of neuroimaging techniques have been applied to DM1 and DM2 patients to further analyze cerebral involvement, which is a prominent clinical finding. Morphological and functional brain involvement has been demonstrated in both disorders in vivo. Cerebral CT and MRI studies were first performed decades ago in DM1 patients. To date, numerous brain MRI studies have shown focal white matter lesions (WMLs) and diffuse brain atrophy in DM1 and—usually less pronounced—DM2 patients. WMLs located in anterior temporal lobes (ATWML) are a common, characteristic feature of DM1. Cellular and neuronal markers were determined by MR spectroscopy techniques in both DM1 and DM2 patients. They proved to be reduced in occipital and temporoparietal cortical regions and in frontal white matter. Single photon emission computed tomography and positron emission tomography studies showed more hypoperfusion and glucose hypometabolism of frontal and temporal lobes in DM1 than in DM2. In DM1, gray matter reductions have been described in several cortical regions, hippocampi, and thalami using voxel-based morphometry (VBM). T2 relaxometry, magnetization transfer imaging, and diffusion MRI studies applying diffusion tensor imaging (DTI) demonstrated white matter changes in DM1 using region of interest-based approaches. Atrophy or hypoplasia of the corpus callosum had first been reported mainly in the congenital form of DM1. Later, callosal body atrophy was also demonstrated in a small group of adult patients. White matter affection with prominent callosal body involvement was proven in adult DM1 patients in a diffusion MRI study using DTI techniques. Recent DTI analyses showed widespread white matter changes in congenital- and juvenile-onset DM1. In DM2 patients, callosal body affection was first demonstrated with VBM, and gray matter reduction was shown in thalamic, hypothalamic and brainstem regions as well as various cortical areas including hippocampi. Recently, a 3T MRI cerebral study applied VBM and DTI with a voxel-wise analysis approach to evaluate gray and white matter affection in DM1 and DM2. WMLs were more prevalent and severe in DM1 compared to controls, the frontal white matter was most seriously affected in both disorders, and temporal WMLs were restricted to DM1 patients. VBM analyses demonstrated white matter involvement in all cerebral lobes, brain stem, and the callosal body in DM1 and DM2. Gray matter was decreased in various cortical areas, the thalamus, and the putamen, a finding that was restricted to DM1. There was more prominent white matter affection in DM1 than in DM2, as demonstrated by DTI. Association fibers throughout the brain, limbic system fiber tracts, corpus callosum, and projection fibers were affected in both diseases (Fig. 22.9). Central motor pathways were exclusively impaired in the series of DM1 patients. White matter changes dominated by far the extent of gray matter affection in both diseases. These data suggest that myotonic dystrophies are predominantly white matter diseases with callosal body and limbic system affection. They link the myotonic dystrophies to the growing group of brain disconnection disorders.

22.5 Therapy

Curative therapy of myotonic dystrophies is not available to date. However, there has recently been substantial progress in the search for novel and innovative treatments targeting RNA and modulating pre-mRNA splicing to inhibit the toxic effects of pathogenic RNA expansions.

Symptomatic management strategies include monitoring and treating the expected complications of the diseases. As cardiorespiratory complications are the most common causes of serious morbidity and death, close cardiac monitoring and regular assessment of respiratory functions are indispensable. Early insertion of permanent cardiac pacemakers and/or implantable cardioverter defibrillators is recommended depending on the risk stratification of malignant or symptomatic cardiac arrhythmias and/or sudden cardiac death. Overnight sleep studies should be performed at least in patients with excessive daytime sleepiness or fatigue, and non-invasive ventilation should be offered if sleep disordered breathing is significant. Central nervous system stimulating drugs such as modafinil have proven to be useful in myotonic dystrophy patients with fatigue and excessive somnolence, although recently prescription of the drug was generally restricted because of potentially serious cardiac side effects. Dysphagia and gastrointestinal complaints may be treated by dietary modifications, antiflatulence and motility-modifying drugs and swallowing therapy. Impaired glucose tolerance, diabetes mellitus and other endocrinological problems are treated according to internal medicine practice guidelines. Patients with cataracts are usually referred for potential cataract surgery. Myotonia may be managed by sodium channel blockers such as tocainide, phenytoin, and a variety of other agents. As these drugs are potentially arrhythmogenic, however, alternative drugs have to be tested in individuals with disabling myotonic symptoms. In general, myotonia is not a major complaint of patients with myotonic dystrophies and medical treatment is mostly not needed. Physiotherapy, occupational therapy, and speech and language therapy are important for managing major neuromuscular symptoms and preventing secondary complications such as aspiration pneumonia and orthopedic deformities. Moderate intensity strength and aerobic exercise training should be encouraged provided that there are no cardiac contraindications. Creatine monohydrate has not proven to be successful in myotonic dystrophies yet, however there may be mild positive effects in DM2 patients with myalgia.

Insights into the dominant RNA toxic-gain-of-function pathogenic mechanism resulted in the development of various molecular genetic approaches to target the toxic RNA directly. These strategies intend to inhibit the effects of toxic expanded RNA or directly degrade the pathogenic RNA expansions. Inhibitors of pathogenic RNAs include small-molecule inhibitors (e.g., pentamidine) that inhibit binding and sequestration of MBNL1, and—most promising—innovative steric block antisense oligonucleotides (AON) (e.g., CAG25) that bind to the CUG microsatellite

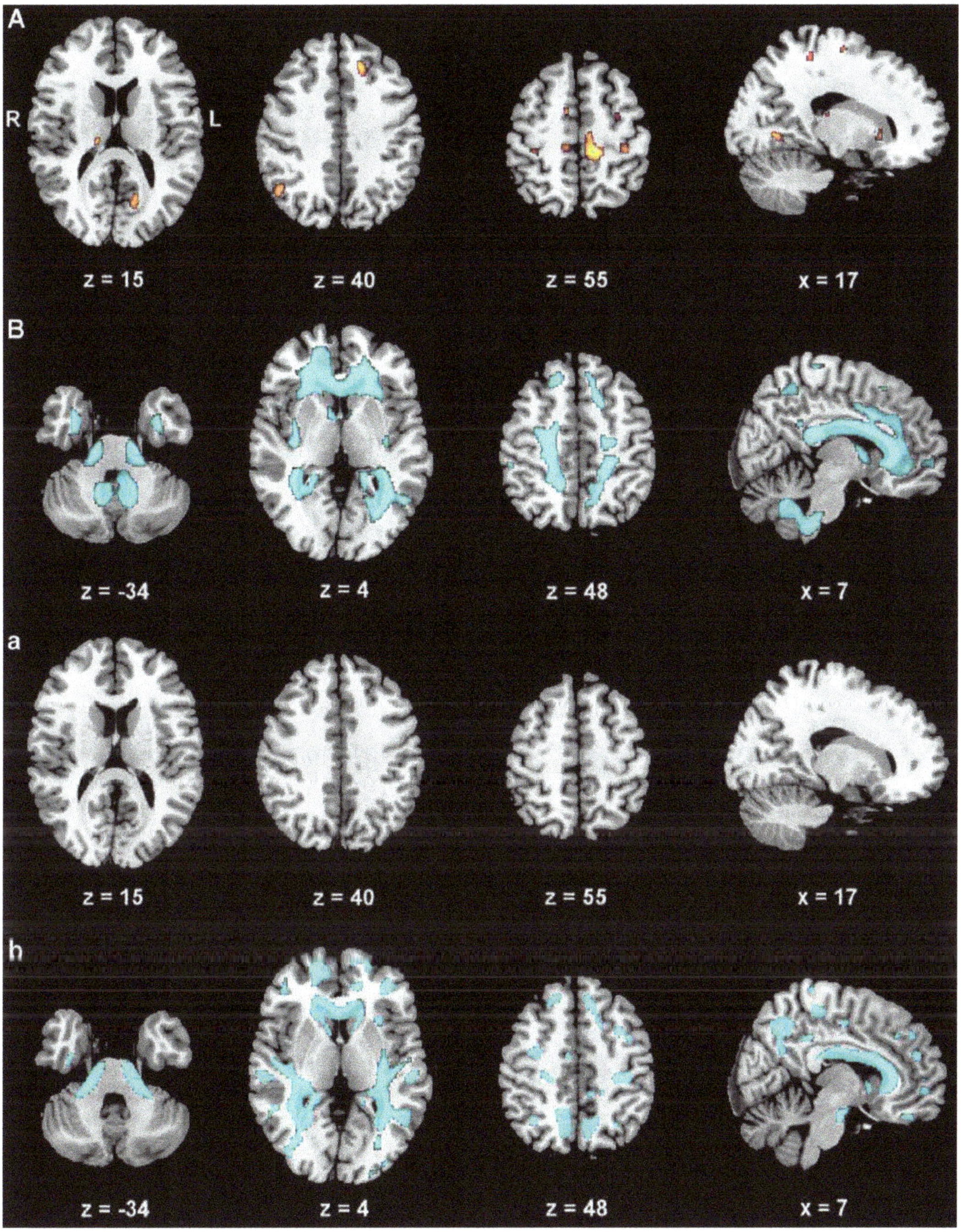

Fig. 22.9 Brain imaging results in DM1 and DM2 (Voxel-based morphometry/VBM, group comparisons). The displayed results are based on a threshold of $p_{FDR} < 0.05$ at voxel-level with an extended cluster threshold of 10 voxel. (**A**) Grey matter decrease in DM1 patients compared to controls. (**B**) White matter decrease in DM1 patients compared to controls. (**a**) Grey matter decrease in DM2 patients compared to controls (no clusters detected). (**b**) White matter decrease in DM2 patients compared to controls. From Minnerop M. et al. The brain in myotonic dystrophy 1 and 2: evidence for a predominant white matter disease. Brain 2011;134:3527–3543. Reprinted with permission from Oxford University Press

repeat expansions of the toxic mutated RNA. These AONs are designed to bind toxic RNAs with high affinity, inhibit the sequestration and binding of splicing factors to the mutated RNAs, redistribute splicing factors from nuclear foci, and probably result in final degradation of mutated RNAs. A reversal of global pathogenic effects thus might be achieved with the use of a single AON. Alternative degradation strategies of pathogenic RNAs include conventional AON-mediated RNA degradation and RNA interference (RNAi) or RNA silencing techniques. Finally, splice-correcting AONs have been developed to correct aberrantly spliced transcripts such as CLCN1. The development of targeted molecular treatments, especially antisense therapies, has already achieved great success in cell culture and animal models of the myotonic dystrophies. The translation of gene therapy strategies to human trials in DM1 is expected within the next few years.

22.6 Differential Diagnosis

Although DM1 patients usually show a characteristic clinical phenotype, the diagnosis might be missed in clinically atypical or mildly affected patients. Oculopharyngeal muscular dystrophy (OPMD) (Chap. 24) and early disease stages of chronic progressive external ophthalmoplegia (CPEO) (Sect. 14.3) with isolated upper eyelid ptosis can be mistaken for DM1 or DM2, although rarely.

At times, DM2 is misdiagnosed as LGMD (see Chap. 19), and a variety of other myopathies with predominant proximal and/or axial muscle affection might be suspected, especially when myotonia is mild or even absent. It is most helpful and important to search for the characteristic multisystemic features of myotonic dystrophies in clinically unclear cases as they usually help guide the examiner to appropriate genetic testing.

Neuromuscular imaging may be helpful regarding differential diagnosis. Similar to DM1, the anterior thigh compartment is preferentially degenerated in dystrophinopathies and LGMD-2D. In line with DM1 and DM2, the rectus femoris and gracilis muscles are usually spared in a variety of LGMD such as LGMD 2B (Sect. 19.3) and Pompe disease (Sect. 14.2.1). The posterior compartments of lower legs, particularly the medial heads of gastrocnemius muscles and soleus muscles, are predominantly affected in LGMD 2A (Sect. 19.2), 2B (Sect. 19.3), 2L and Filaminopathies (Sect. 20.5) similar to DM1.

Suggestions for Further Reading

Bachmann G, Damian MS, Koch M, et al. The clinical and genetic correlates of MRI findings in myotonic dystrophy. Neuroradiology. 1996;38:629–35.

Castillo J, Pumar JM, Rodriguez JR, et al. Magnetic-Resonance-Imaging of Muscles in Myotonic Dystrophy. Eur J Radiol. 1993;17:141–44.

Damian MS, Bachmann G, Herrmann D, et al. Magnetic resonance imaging of muscle and brain in myotonic dystrophy. J Neurol. 1993;240:8–12.

George A, Schneider-Gold C, Zierz S, et al. Musculoskeletal pain in patients with myotonic dystrophy type 2. Arch Neurol. 2004;61:1938–42.

Hamano T, Kawamura Y, Mutoh T, et al. Muscle MRI in myotonic dystrophy type 1 with foot drop. Eur Neurol. 2010;63:144–48.

Huichalaf C, Sakai K, Jin B, et al. Expansion of CUG RNA repeats causes stress and inhibition of translation in myotonic dystrophy 1 (DM1) cells. FASEB J. 2010;24:3706–19.

Hund E, Jansen O, Koch MC, et al. Proximal myotonic myopathy with MRI white matter abnormalities of the brain. Neurology. 1997;48:33–37.

Kley RA, Tarnopolsky MA, Vorgerd M. Creatine for treating muscle disorders. Cochrane Database Syst Rev. 2011;2:CD004760.

Kornblum C, Reul J, Kress W, et al. Cranial magnetic resonance imaging in genetically proven myotonic dystrophy type 1 and 2. J Neurol. 2004;251:710–14.

Kornblum C, Lutterbey G, Bogdanow M, et al. Distinct neuromuscular phenotypes in myotonic dystrophy types 1 and 2: a whole body highfield MRI study. J Neurol. 2006;253:753–61.

Kornblum C, Lutterbey G, Czermin B, et al. Whole-body high-field MRI shows no skeletal muscle degeneration in young patients with recessive myotonia congenita. Acta Neurol Scand. 2010;121:131–35.

MacDonald JR, Hill JD, Tarnopolsky MA. Modafinil reduces excessive somnolence and enhances mood in patients with myotonic dystrophy. Neurology. 2002; 59:1876–80.

Mathieu J, Boivin H, Meunier D, et al. Assessment of a disease-specific muscular impairment rating scale in myotonic dystrophy. Neurology. 2001;56:336–40.

Meola G, Sansone V. Cerebral involvement in myotonic dystrophies. Muscle Nerve. 2007;36:294–306.
Mercuri E, Talim B, Moghadaszadeh B, et al. Clinical and imaging findings in six cases of congenital muscular dystrophy with rigid spine syndrome linked to chromosome 1p (RSMD1). Neuromuscul Disord. 2002;12:631–38.
Minnerop M, Luders E, Specht K, et al. Grey and white matter loss along cerebral midline structures in myotonic dystrophy type 2. J Neurol. 2008;255:1904–9.
Minnerop M, Weber B, Schoene-Bake JC, et al. The brain in myotonic dystrophy 1 and 2: evidence for a predominant white matter disease. Brain. 2011; 134:3527–43.
Muntoni F, Wood MJ. Targeting RNA to treat neuromuscular disease. Nat Rev Drug Discov. 2011; 10:621–37.
Ogata A, Terae S, Fujita M, et al. Anterior temporal white matter lesions in myotonic dystrophy with intellectual impairment: an MRI and neuropathological study. Neuroradiology. 1998;40:411–15.
Romeo V, Pegoraro E, Ferrati C, et al. Brain involvement in myotonic dystrophies: neuroimaging and neuropsychological comparative study in DM1 and DM2. J Neurol. 2010;257:1246–55.
Schedel H, Reimers CD, Nagele M, et al. Imaging techniques in myotonic dystrophy. A comparative study of ultrasound, computed tomography and magnetic resonance imaging of skeletal muscles. Eur J Radiol. 1992;15:230–38.
Schneider-Gold C, Timchenko LT. CCUG repeats reduce the rate of global protein synthesis in myotonic dystrophy type 2. Rev Neurosci. 2010;21:19–28.
Stramare R, Beltrame V, Dal Borgo R, et al. MRI in the assessment of muscular pathology: a comparison between limb-girdle muscular dystrophies, hyaline body myopathies and myotonic dystrophies. Radiol Med. 2010;115:585–99.
Trip J, Drost GG, van Engelen BGM, et al. Drug treatment for myotonia. Cochrane Database Syst Rev. 2007;4:CD004762.
Turner C, Hilton-Jones D. The myotonic dystrophies: diagnosis and management. J Neurol Neurosurg Psychiatry. 2010;81:358–67.
Vielhaber S, Jakubiczka S, Gaul C, et al. Brain (1)H magnetic resonance spectroscopic differences in myotonic dystrophy type 2 and type 1. Muscle Nerve. 2006;34: 145–52.
Weber YG, Roebling R, Kassubek J, et al. Comparative analysis of brain structure, metabolism, and cognition in myotonic dystrophy 1 and 2. Neurology. 2010;74: 1108–17.
Wozniak JR, Mueller BA, Ward EE, et al. White matter abnormalities and neurocognitive correlates in children and adolescents with myotonic dystrophy type 1: a diffusion tensor imaging study. Neuromuscul Disord. 2011;21:89–96.
Zu T, Gibbens B, Doty NS, et al. Non-ATG initiated translation directed by microsatellite expansions. Proc Natl Acad Sci USA. 2011;108:260–65.

Facioscapulohumeral Dystrophy 23

Hermien E. Kan, Barbara H. Janssen,
and Nicoline Berendina Maria Voet

23.1 Introduction and Classification

Facioscapulohumeral dystrophy (FSHD) is an autosomal dominant muscular dystrophy with an estimated incidence of approximately 1/20,000 worldwide. It is the third most common hereditary muscular dystrophy, after Duchenne muscular dystrophy and myotonic dystrophy. The disease was first described by Landouzy and Dejerine in 1885 and was originally known as Landouzy–Dejerine disease.

The onset of FSHD is usually during the second decade of life, even though age of onset and rate of progression vary greatly among patients. The disease is characterized by asymmetrical loss of force and atrophy of muscular tissue starting in the face and shoulder region. The muscle weakness is slowly progressive, and over time the lower leg muscles and pelvis muscles can become affected.

H.E. Kan (✉)
C.J. Gorter Center for High Field MRI, Department of Radiology - C3Q, Leiden University Medical Center, Albinusdreef 2, 2333 ZA Leiden, The Netherlands
e-mail: h.e.kan@lumc.nl

B.H. Janssen
Department of Radiology, Radboud University Nijmegen Medical Center, Nijmegen, The Netherlands

N.B.M. Voet
Department of Rehabilitation/Nijmegen Center for Evidence Based Practice, Radboud University Nijmegen Medical Center, Nijmegen, The Netherlands

23.1.1 Synonyms and Abbreviations

FSHD; infantile FSHD (IFSHD); Landouzy–Dejerine disease; OMIM#158900.

23.2 Genetics and Pathophysiology

In the majority of patients, FSHD is caused by contraction of a large repeat structure called D4Z4 on chromosome 4 (*FSHD1*) (Fig. 23.1). Although normally this repeat varies from 11 to 100 units, patients with *FSHD1* have one chromosome with 1–10 units. D4Z4 repeat contraction is associated with local chromatin relaxation and transcriptional derepression of the *DUX4* gene encoded in each D4Z4 unit. The *DUX4* gene encodes for a double homeobox transcription factor that, when ectopically expressed, is toxic to many cell types, including skeletal muscle. Only contractions on highly specific genetic backgrounds are associated with FSHD. Contractions of the repeat on other backgrounds of chromosome 4 and chromosome 10q, where a highly homologous repeat structure exists, seem to be nonpathogenic. The genetic basis for this difference in pathogenicity is the presence of a DUX4 polyadenylation site in pathogenic backgrounds that allows stabilization of the DUX4 transcript. Nonpathogenic backgrounds have polymorphisms in this polyadenylation site and therefore fail to generate stable DUX4 transcripts upon repeat contraction. A small subset of patients—FSHD2 patients—show the same chromatin relaxation and transcriptional

M.P. Wattjes and D. Fischer (eds.), *Neuromuscular Imaging*, DOI 10.1007/978-1-4614-6552-2_23,

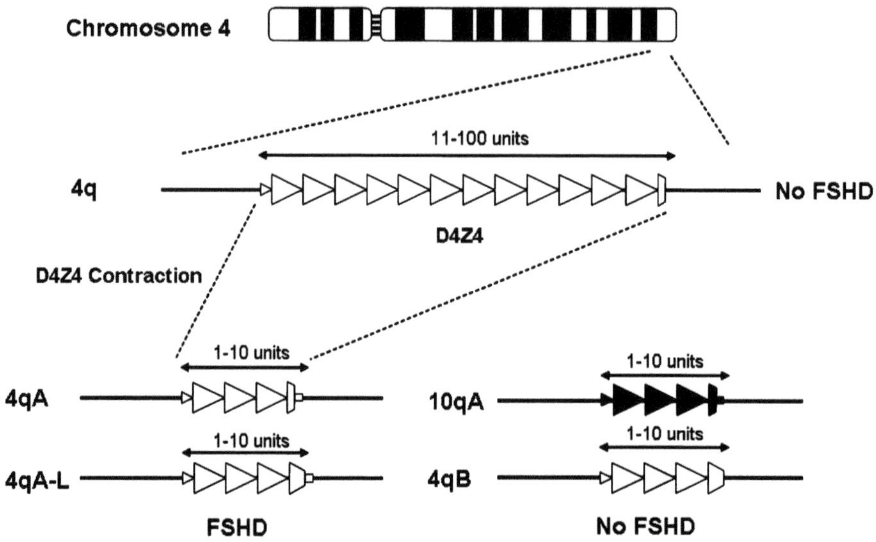

Fig. 23.1 Overview of the basic genetic background of facioscapulohumeral dystrophy type 1 (FSHD1). Note the D4Z4 repeat on chromosome 4q35 (*open triangles*) and its homologue on chromosome 10q26 (*closed triangles*). Only D4Z4 repeat array contractions on specific genetic backgrounds are associated with FSHD. Patients with FSHD1 carry a D4Z4 repeat array size of 1–10 units on chromosomes 4qA or 4qA-L. Short D4Z4 repeat arrays can also occur on 4qB or 10q chromosomes, but they do not cause FSHD. Modified from Lemmers RJ, et al (2010) A unifying genetic model for facioscapulohumeral muscular dystrophy. Science 329:1650–1653. With permission from The American Association for the Advancement of Science

derepression of DUX4 in the absence of repeat contraction. These patients also have at least one chromosome 4 with a disease-permissive genetic background.

Recently, the following categories for the disease have been suggested.

1. Severe disease: infantile form with onset usually before age 10 years; with one to three residual D4Z4 repeats (~4 % of patients).
2. Moderate disease: classic phenotype, with four to seven residual repeats; a widely variable course. It encompasses also a large percentage of asymptomatic carriers > 50 years of age. Approximately 60 % of patients have involvement of the lower limb, and 20 % are wheelchair-dependent.
3. Mild disease: with 8–10 residual D4Z4 repeats, probably with frequent nonpenetrant carriers; muscle involvement limited to the upper limbs. This category has not been explored in sufficient detail.

The pathogenesis of FSHD is largely unclear. So far as is known, instead of a single structural mutation causing the disease, it likely that a complex cascade of epigenetic events is involved. Overall, it is likely that muscle development pathways play a major role along with probable involvement of vascular development pathways.

The pathophysiology in FSHD also remains to be elucidated, and the affected muscles display general dystrophic features, such as atrophy, fatty infiltration, and transient edema. Interestingly, the disease appears to progress in a truly muscle-specific pattern, where muscles that are unaffected early in the disease process do not appear to show any abnormality. Muscle cell cultures derived from the vastus lateralis muscle of FSHD patients are morphologically and behaviorally indistinguishable from cell cultures derived from healthy muscle. Also, on a metabolic level, apparently unaffected muscles seem to be similar to healthy muscle, as shown by in vivo phosphorus-31 magnetic resonance spectroscopy (^{31}P-MRS).

23.3 Histopathology

Histopathological analyses of muscle biopsies in FSHD patients show changes similar to those of other muscular dystrophies. Hence, there is no specific marker for FSHD. Findings include increased variation in fiber size and type, fiber necrosis and fibrosis, and an increased number of internal nuclei. Fatty replacement of muscle tissue and mononuclear inflammatory cell infiltrates are common, and small angular fibers may also be present, which could be an indication of regeneration (Fig. 23.2). As the disease progression differs among muscles and significant differences are also present in muscles, findings can vary depending on the site of the biopsy and disease progression.

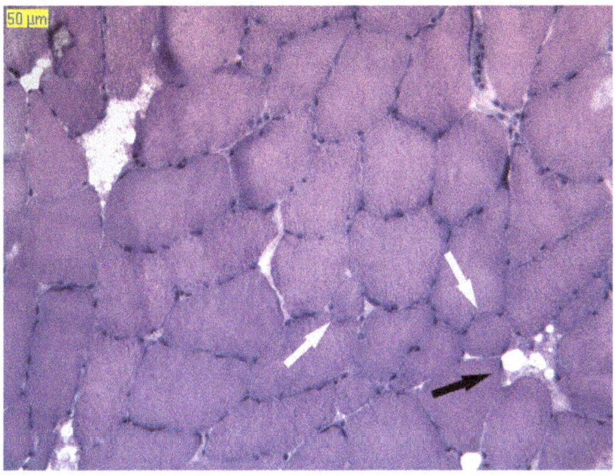

Fig. 23.2 FSHD histopathology. Muscle biopsy from the quadriceps muscle of a 47-year-old woman with FSHD who had relatively mild abnormalities. There is some variation in fiber size, with most fibers measuring 90–100 µm but also some small and round fibers of only 30–40 µm (*white arrows*). Small areas with interstitial fat are visible (*black arrow*) (hematoxyline-phloxine stain). Courtesy of M. Lammens, Nijmegen, The Netherlands

23.4 Clinical Presentation

FSHD derives its name from the muscle groups that are mainly affected first: facial and shoulder girdle muscles. In more than 90 % of cases, on first clinical examination the orbicularis oculi and orbicularis oris muscles are affected, leading to incomplete eye closure, asymmetrical lips, inability to whistle, and sometimes swallowing problems (Fig. 23.3). Shoulder girdle muscles, especially the scapular and pectoral muscles, are involved early. An initially fairly normal deltoid muscle contributes to winging of the scapula on elevation of the arms (Fig. 23.4). Tasks such as combing hair, brushing teeth, and reaching up become difficult if not impossible.

During disease progression, humeral, abdominal, and lower extremity muscles and the pelvic girdle can become involved as well. Lower abdominal muscles are weaker than the upper abdominal muscles, causing "Beevor's sign," a

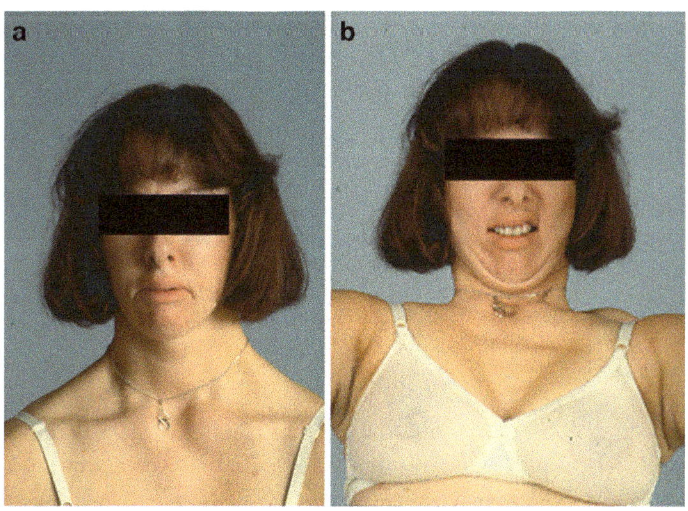

Fig. 23.3 Weakness of facial muscles. Typical myopathic facies in FSHD with decreased facial expression. (**a**) The lips are pouted, and dimples appear at the corners of the mouth. (**b**) There are no wrinkles in the forehead or around the eyes, and the patient is unable to close the eyes properly (some patients sleep with eyes partially open). Many patients cannot whistle or purse their lips and may have a transverse smile as the disease progresses

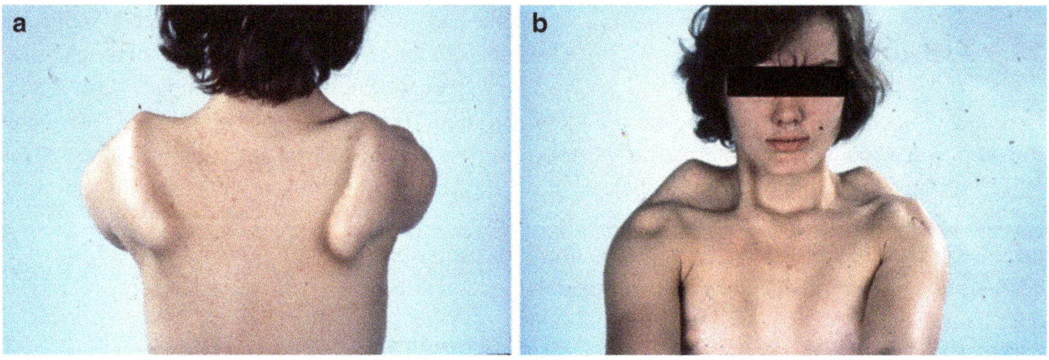

Fig. 23.4 Winging of the scapulae. Note the winging of the scapulae, back view (**a**) and frontal view (**b**); forward sloping of the shoulders, horizontal position of the clavicles due to the weight of the upper extremity and weakness of the trapezius muscle; prominence of sterno-clavicular joints. Preferential weakness of the lower trapezius muscle results in characteristic upward movement of the scapula when attempting to flex or abduct the arms

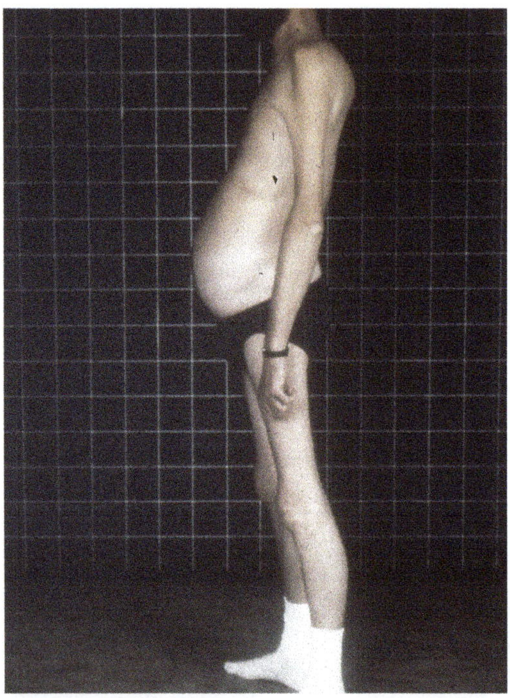

Fig. 23.5 Beevor's sign. Many FSHD patients have a protruding abdomen because the lower abdominal muscles are more severely affected than the upper abdominal muscles. This asymmetrical weakness leads to Beevor's sign: upward displacement of the navel while flexing the neck. It is a typical finding for FSHD during the clinical examination

movement of the navel toward the head on flexing the neck (Fig. 23.5). This physical finding is specific to FSHD. In the arm, only the upper arm muscles, the biceps and triceps, are selectively involved, resulting in atrophy of the upper arm and sparing of the forearm muscles, which results in the appearance of "Popeye arms" (Fig. 23.6). The onset of lower-extremity weakness is often but not always distal. It typically appears in the anterior leg compartment, presenting with foot drop. Asymmetrical muscle weakness is characteristic of FSHD (Fig. 23.7), but the underlying reason for it is unknown. Despite the asymmetrical weakness, the incidence of contractures or scoliosis is low. About 10 % of patients with FSHD have ankle contractures, and 30 % of FSHD patients develop scoliosis.

The most commonly described extramuscular manifestation in patients with FSHD is retinal telangiectasia, occurring in 60 % of affected individuals. Rarely and only in severely affected individuals, the retinal vascular abnormalities can cause potentially relevant retinal exudation, leading to retinal detachment (Coat's syndrome). Hearing loss and retinopathy were formerly considered part of the disease, but later studies disprove it.

Unlike many other muscular dystrophies, cardiac complications in FSHD are rare. Occasionally, cardiac conduction defects have been observed, although most authors claim no cardiac involvement. Symptomatic respiratory weakness occurs in about 1 % of affected individuals. Risk factors include severe involvement with wheelchair

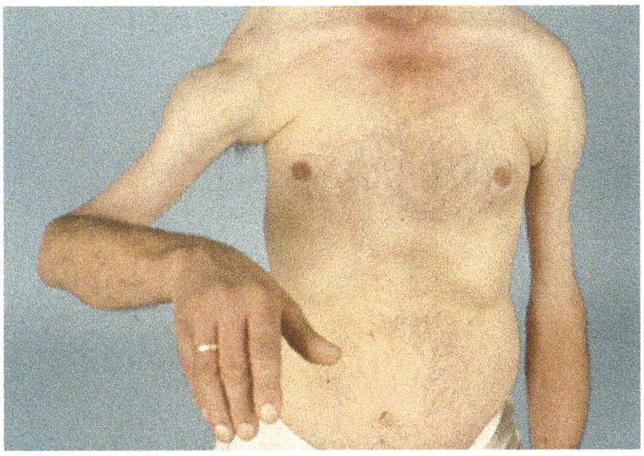

Fig. 23.6 "Popeye arm." The Popeye arm has selective atrophy of the upper arm muscles and relative preservation of the lower arm muscles. An axillary crease is often evident because of atrophy of the pectoralis muscles. Wrist extensors can also be involved

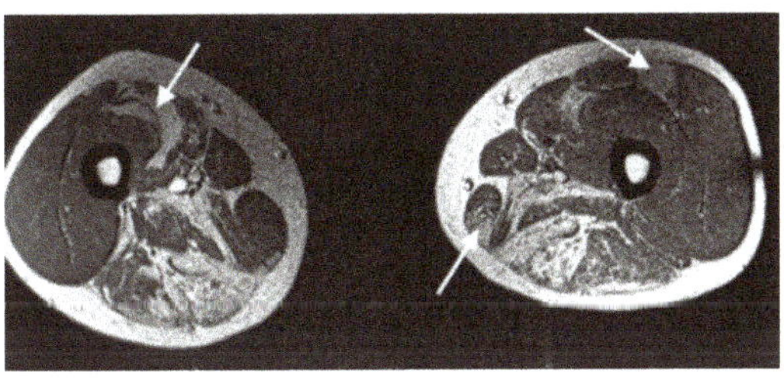

Fig. 23.7 Asymmetrical muscle involvement. Axial T1-weighted magnetic resonance imaging (MRI) scan of the upper legs of an FSHD patient shows asymmetry in muscle involvement in the two legs. (*Left*) The vastus medialis muscle in the right leg shows more fatty replacement compared to the same muscle of the contralateral leg. (*Right*) In contrast, in the left leg, the gracilis and vastus lateralis muscles are more affected (*white arrows*)

confinement, moderate to severe kyphoscoliosis, and the presence of pectus excavatum.

Pain is often reported by patients (although not commonly mentioned in the literature). More than 70 % of patients with FSHD experience pain more than 4 days per month and almost 60 % of patients for at least 4 days per week. Likewise, fatigue is a frequent and relevant problem: 60 % of patients with FSHD report severe fatigue associated with decreased quality of life.

The prevalence of FSHD is equal worldwide and has no particular racial, geographical, or ethnic distribution. The median age of FSHD onset is ~17 years—usually determined in retrospect—but can vary from infancy to the seventh decade. Men and women are affected equally, although women are more often asymptomatic or clinical less affected. The degree of involvement among patients is extremely variable, even within families, ranging from mild muscle weakness (patients are unaware that they are affected) to severe generalized weakness (Fig. 23.8). Eventually, approximately 20 % of patients require use of a wheelchair.

The course of FSHD is usually slowly progressive, and life expectancy is normal. Many patients report a relapsing course with long periods of quiescence interrupted by periods of rapid deterioration involving a particular muscle group. The latter is often heralded by pain in the affected limb. Regrettably, no prognostic tools are currently available to predict the course of the

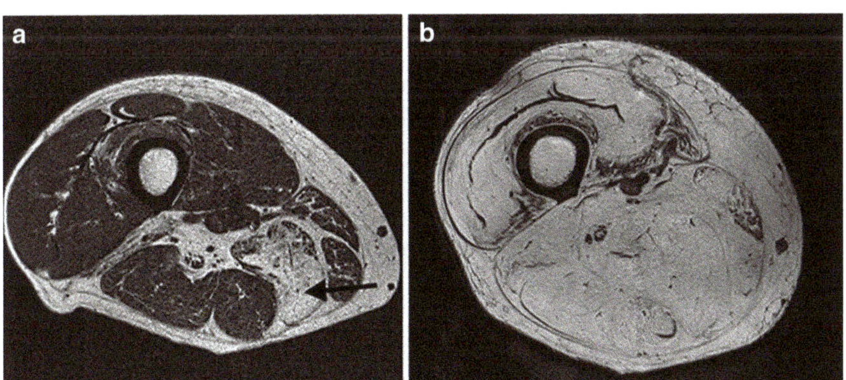

Fig. 23.8 Mild and severe changes in fatty replacement of muscle tissue. (**a**) Axial T1-weighted MRI of the middle of the right upper leg of a mildly affected FSHD patient. All thigh muscles appear normal except for the semimembranosus muscles, which display severe fatty replacement of the muscle tissue (*black arrow*). (**b**) Axial T1-weighted MRI of the same location in a severely affected FSHD patient. All muscles show almost complete fatty replacement of muscle tissue. The muscle boundaries are only barely visible

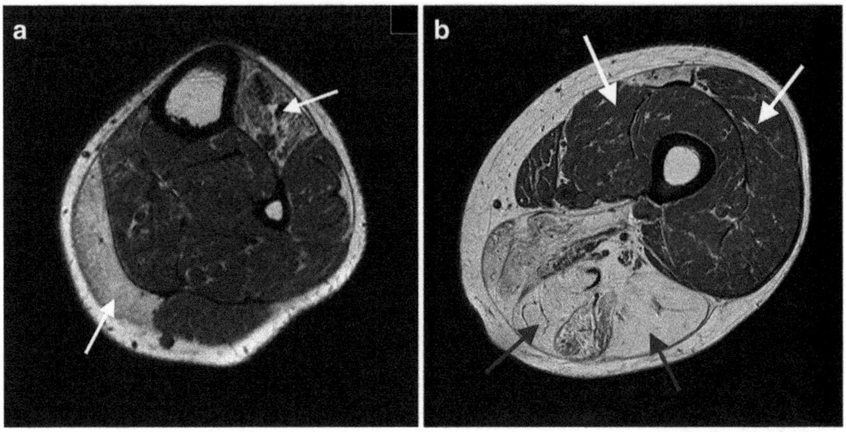

Fig. 23.9 Fatty replacement of muscle tissue in specific muscles. (**a**) Axial T1-weighted MRI of the calf muscles at the level of the mid-calf in the left leg of a FSHD patient with a typical pattern of involvement. Fatty infiltration is clearly seen in the gastrocnemius medialis and tibialis anterior muscles (*white arrows*). (**b**) Axial T1-weighted MRI of the thigh muscles at the level of the mid-thigh in the right upper leg of a typical FSHD patient. Fatty replacement of muscle tissue is apparent in the hamstring muscles (*grey arrows*), whereas the quadriceps muscles appear normal (*white arrows*)

disease in more detail. Despite all the advances in understanding the genetics of the disease, the exact mechanisms responsible for the clinical features are still not known.

Some 4 % of patients with FSHD have an infantile form called infantile FSHD (IFSHD). IFSHD is a more severe and progressive phenotype of FHSD. There are signs or symptoms of facial weakness before the age of 5 years with progressive shoulder-girdle weakness and the need of a wheelchair before the age of 10 years. Sensorineural hearing loss, retinal vasculopathy, and seizures have been documented in IFSHD. Cardiac and respiratory complications are rare.

Table 23.1 Muscles of the lower extremities in the order of their temporal involvement as found by US, CT, and MRI

Lower leg	Upper leg
1. Tibialis anterior	1. Semimembranosus
2. Gastrocnemius medialis	2. Biceps femoris
3. Extensor digitorum longus	3. Semitendinosus
4. Soleus	4. Adductor group
5. Peroneal (brevis and longus)	5. Vastus lateralis, intermedius, and femoris
6. Gastrocnemius lateralis	
7. Tibialis posterior	

23.5 Imaging Findings

Several imaging techniques such as ultrasonography (US), computed tomography (CT), and magnetic resonance imaging (MRI) have been used to study muscle involvement in FSHD. Muscle imaging in these patients has mainly focused on the lower extremities and has revealed a distinct pattern of muscle involvement in the upper and lower legs. In the lower leg, the tibialis anterior and gastrocnemius medialis show early signs of fatty infiltration. In the upper leg, the hamstring muscles usually show fatty infiltration (Fig. 23.9). Mixed results have been reported regarding involvement of the vasti muscles. Table 23.1 lists the muscles of the lower and upper leg in the order of their involvement in FSHD, as was found by the various imaging techniques.

23.5.1 Ultrasonography

Calf hypertrophy can be observed in FSHD patients using quantitative US. Absolute calf hypertrophy and relative calf hypertrophy—defined as an increased ratio of the calf muscles over the rectus femoris and vastus intermedius muscles—can be present. In the latter case, there is atrophy of the quadriceps muscles.

23.5.2 Computed Tomography

Fat replacement and/or atrophic lesions of the anterior muscles of the lower legs (mainly the tibialis anterior) and the posterior muscles from the upper legs (hamstrings) is common. Muscle damage in the leg muscles is observed even during early stages of the disease, which is one of the most interesting CT findings for FSHD. The asymmetry of the lesions, which is considered one of the main characteristics of the disease, is also apparent on CT, as is damage to the paraspinal muscles. In general, CT findings in FSHD patients are consistent, except regarding involvement of the upper arm muscles. In most patients, anomalies are found in the brachial biceps and triceps and the scapular girdle. In contrast, a patient with no involvement of the shoulder, midarm, or pelvic muscles has been reported.

23.5.3 Magnetic Resonance Imaging

The first MRI study in a FSHD patient was described in 1996. Since then, several MRI studies have been performed. In general, MRI findings in FSHD patients show that the tibialis anterior muscle presents with the most severe fatty replacement of muscle tissue, followed by the gastrocnemius muscle, especially the gastrocnemius medialis. The peroneal muscles are mostly unaffected (Fig. 23.9). In the upper legs, the hamstring and adductor muscles are most affected (semimembraneous, biceps femoris, semitendineous, adductor longus, adductor magnus), and the vastus muscles are least affected (vastus lateralis, vastus intermedius, vastus medialis) (Figs. 23.7 and 23.8). Usually, the psoas muscle shows no evidence of involvement. Remarkably, the asymmetrical involvement—considered a main characteristic of FSHD—is sometimes evident in only 15 % of the investigated leg muscle pairs.

The level of fatty replacement of muscle tissue can also be correlated with muscle strength. A four-point semi-quantitative visual scale is used to evaluate fatty replacement of muscle tissue based on T1-weighted images, and muscle strength is tested using the scale of the Medical Research Council (MRC scale). The level of fatty replacement usually correlates well with muscle strength for hip extension, hip abduction, hip adduction, knee flexion, knee extension, and ankle dorsal flexion. However, grading scores of the involved muscles of hip flexion and ankle plantar flexion do not correlate as well with the corresponding MRC scores. This could be due to the action of unaffected synergistic muscles, which may compensate for loss of force in affected muscles tested during the same maneuver. In the case of ankle plantar flexion strength, the weakness of the medial gastrocnemius muscle is often compensated for by other, relatively spared, flexor muscles in the calf. For hip flexion, the discrepancy between the MRC score and the MRI grading is probably due to the variable affection of muscles involved in flexion of the hip.

Energy metabolism in muscles of patients with FSHD is also affected. Spatially resolved ^{31}P-MRS of muscles with a high level of fat replacement shows higher tissue pH and a lower phosphocreatine/adenosine triphosphate (ATP) ratio than that of healthy controls. Muscles that appear normal on T1-weighted images—and therefore do not have extensive fatty replacement—do not show changes compared to control subjects. This likely indicates that disturbed energy metabolism and secondary mitochondrial dysfunction in FSHD is limited to muscles that have a high level of fatty replacement, and that the disease progresses in a truly muscle-specific fashion. Fat-suppressed T2-weighted images [turbo inversion recovery magnitude (TIRM)] sometimes show hyperintense areas in some of the muscles, indicating the presence of edema as a sign of inflammation (Fig. 23.10). These results correspond well with the biopsy findings, where mononuclear inflammatory cells are occasionally observed.

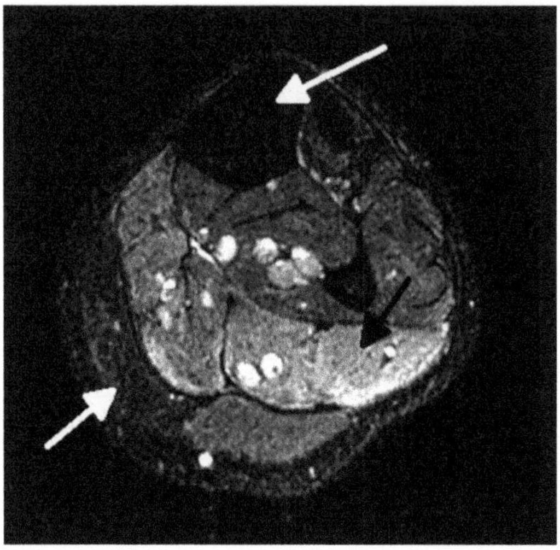

Fig. 23.10 Edema indicating inflammation. An axial turbo inversion recovery magnitude (TIRM) image of the calf muscles at the mid-level of the calf. The TIRM image has a nulled fat signal, as can clearly be seen by the absence of signal in the bone marrow and the muscles with high levels of fat replacement (*white arrows*). Inflammation or edema is illuminated. On this image, the soleus medialis shows muscle edema as a sign of inflammation (*black arrow*)

The MRI scans of limb and paraspinal muscles in FSHD patients with the camptocornmia phenotype (bent spine phenotype) show similar results of the lower extremities. That is, the tibialis anterior and gastrocnemius are the most affected muscles, whereas the peroneal muscles in the lower leg show less involvement. In the upper leg, the semimembranosus is the most affected muscle. In the shoulder and arm muscles, the latissimus dorsi muscle is most affected. Severe, asymmetrical involvement of the thoracic and lumbar spinal tract may be shown, but this result may be specific to the bent-spine phenotype.

23.6 Therapy

Currently, there is no curative therapy for FSHD. Unfortunately, the FSHD clinical trials that have been performed have not had great success. Positive effects generally do not persist or fail to significantly improve the quality of life for the patients. However, there are several therapeutic strategies that can alleviate symptoms and provide functional improvement, thereby improving the quality of life. Known complications of the disease can sometimes be prevented with these approaches as well.

Ankle-foot orthoses are helpful in the management of foot drop in patients with FSHD. Floor reaction ankle-foot orthoses can be used for patients with a foot drop combined with knee extensor weakness due to quadriceps atrophy. Surgical scapular fixation has been shown, in retrospective case series, to significantly enhance arm mobility. Symptomatic respiratory insufficiency can be managed with nighttime non-invasive pressure support. The role of exercise in many muscular dystrophies including FSHD remains largely untested, mostly because of the fear of worsening muscle weakness in dystrophies where the sarcolemmal membrane is structurally compromised. As this is not the case in FSHD, there may be a short-term beneficial effect of aerobic exercise in FSHD.

Pharmacological strategies such as corticosteroids fail to improve strength or muscle mass, even though inflammation is a common finding in FSHD muscle. Albuterol treatment shows a consistent anabolic effect in FSHD, but the magnitude of the increased muscle mass does not translate into significantly increased strength. Myostatin is a protein that inhibits muscle differentiation and growth. Myostatin inhibitors, however, do not produce any effect in FSHD patients. There is evidence that phosphocreatine stores are depleted in some dystrophic muscle and that creatine may have cell-protective characteristics. However, it is currently unclear if creatine supplementation has a positive effect on FSHD. Considering the complexity of the disease mechanism of FSHD, further refinement of the pathogenic mechanism will assist future research strategies, likely based on candidate gene approaches.

23.7 Differential Diagnosis

Despite the characteristic clinical presentation of FSHD, the combination of prominent winging of the scapula and facial weakness are also seen in other myopathies. Moreover, the wide clinical variability in the severity of the disease and atypical phenotypes makes recognition difficult in some patients, especially if the family history is negative.

Onset in the pelvic girdle muscles suggests alternative diagnoses, including limb-girdle muscular dystrophy (see Chapt. 19) or spinal muscular atrophy (see Sect. 29.2), especially in the absence of facial muscle weakness. However, regression of symptoms and signs as well as severe and diffuse contractures does not occur in FSHD and would exclude the diagnosis of FSHD. Cardiomyopathy is not part of the disease and when present suggests an alternative diagnosis.

In the more severe infantile-onset cases, facial weakness is the earliest, most prominent sign. The infant may be initially misdiagnosed as having Möbius syndrome, which is a static disorder in which facial diplegia occurs in association with abducens nerve dysfunction and skeletal defects.

The pattern of weakness in scapuloperoneal muscular dystrophy (SPMD) and scapuloperoneal muscular atrophy (SPMA) sometimes overlaps with that of FSHD. Although prominent ankle dorsiflexor weakness and scapular winging is seen in both conditions, disease onset is usually in the legs in SPMD and in the face and shoulders in FSHD. Moreover, facial weakness is not a prominent feature of SPMD.

Facioscapulohumeral Dystrophy

Key Points

- FSHD is characterized by asymmetrical loss of force as well as atrophy and fatty replacement of muscular tissue starting in the face and shoulder region. The disease is muscle-specific.
- In the majority of patients, FSHD is caused by contraction of a large repeat structure called D4Z4 on chromosome 4. However, the pathogenesis is largely unclear.
- In the lower limbs, fatty replacement of muscle tissue mostly occurs in the tibialis anterior, gastrocnemius medialis, and hamstring muscles, as shown by MRI, US, and CT.
- FSHD appears to progress in a truly muscle-specific fashion, where muscles with no fatty replacement of muscle tissue also show no metabolic abnormalities.
- Fatty replacement observed on T1-weighted MRI scans correlates with most muscle strength tests, which indicates that MRI can be helpful as a marker of disease progression.
- Currently, there is no curative therapy for FSHD, although therapeutic strategies exist that can alleviate the patient's symptoms and provide functional improvement.

Acknowledgments The authors thank the FSH Society, Sam E. and Mary F. Roberts Nutrition Research Fellowship Grant FSHS-SMRF-003, the FSHD Global Research Foundation, the Dutch Prinses Beatrixfonds WAR06-0217 and WAR 08-15, and ZonMW Grant 89000003 for financial support.

Suggestions for Further Reading

Friedman SD, Poliachik SL, Carter GT, et al. The magnetic resonance imaging spectrum of fascioscapulohumeral muscular dystrophy. Muscle Nerve. 2012;45:500–6.

Jiddane M, Gastaut JL, Pellissier JF, et al. CT of primary muscle diseases. AJNR Am J Neuroradiol. 1983;4:773–76.

Jordan B, Eger K, Koesling S, et al. Camptocormia phenotype of FSHD: a clinical and MRI study on six patients. J Neurol. 2010;58:866–73.

Kan HE, Klomp DW, Wohlgemuth M, et al. Only fat infiltrated muscles in resting lower leg of FSHD patients show disturbed energy metabolism. NMR Biomed. 2010;23:563–68.

Lemmers RJ, van der Vliet PJ, Klooster R, et al. A unifying genetic model for facioscapulohumeral muscular dystrophy. Science. 2010;329(5999):1650–53.

Olsen DB, Gideon P, Jeppesen TD, et al. Leg muscle involvement in facioscapulohumeral muscular dystrophy assessed by MRI. J Neurol. 2006;253:1437–41.

Padberg GW, van Engelen BG. Facioscapulohumeral muscular dystrophy. Curr Opin Neurol. 2009;22:539–42.

Phoenix J, Betal D, Roberts N, et al. Objective quantification of muscle and fat in human dystrophic muscle by magnetic resonance image analysis. Muscle Nerve. 1996;19:302–10.

Reimers CD, Schlotter B, Eicke BM, et al. Calf enlargement in neuromuscular diseases: a quantitative ultrasound study in 350 patients and review of the literature. J Neurol Sci. 1996;143:46–56.

Rose MR, Tawil R. Drug treatment for facioscapulohumeral muscular dystrophy. Cochrane Database Syst Rev. 2004;2:CD002276.

Tawil R. Facioscapulohumeral muscular dystrophy. Neurotherapeutics. 2008;5:601–6.

24 Oculopharyngeal Muscular Dystrophy

Arne Fischmann

24.1 Synonyms, Abbreviations

OPMD; OMIM#164300; variant: oculopharyngeodistal muscular dystrophy (OPDM).

24.2 Genetics and Pathophysiology

Oculopharyngeal muscular dystrophy (OPMD) is generally a rare, slowly progressive, autosomal dominant inherited muscular dystrophy, although rare cases of autosomal recessive inheritance have been reported. Both dominant and recessive forms have been found to be allelic and are caused by short GCN_{11-17} expansions in the first exon of the polyadenylate-binding protein nuclear 1 gene (PABPN1, previously called PABP2) localized on chromosome 14q11.2. The mutations cause lengthening of an N terminal polyalanine domain. The triplet repeat in PABPN1 is stable, and triplet repeat expansion is uncommon. The normal repeat length is GCN_{10} or GCG_6 (Fig. 24.1). Although large clusters of OPMD cases with defined founder mutations have been identified in various populations, the diversity of mutations suggests the existence of a large number of independent original mutation events. In addition, novel mutations (e.g., point mutations in the PABPN1 gene) have been identified.

Multiple lines of evidence suggest that gene dosage has an influence on age of onset and severity of the disease. Homozygous carriers of the dominant allele are most affected, with disease onset on average 18 years earlier than in heterozygote carriers. In addition, patients who are heterozygotes for the dominant mutation and have a GCN_{11} polymorphism in the other copy of the *PABPN1* gene develop more severe symptoms than the general population. The GCN_{11} polymorphism has a prevalence of 1–2 % in North America, Europe, and Japan. Homozygosis of the GCN_{11} allele is responsible for the autosomal recessive form of OPMD.

PABPN1 is an ubiquitous polyadenylation factor essential for the formation of poly(A) tails of eukaryotic mRNA. PABPN1 is important for muscle development and regeneration. Muscles expressing pathological PAPBN1 have atrophic changes and fatty degeneration. Preserved muscle cells show reduced cellular structures. Overexpression of PABPN1 readily produces the formation of intranuclear inclusions (INIs) associated with cell death. However, the exact pathophysiological mechanism remains unclear. Most hypotheses suggest that the expanded polyalanine stretch leads to a gain of function of the protein and causes increased aggregation and toxicity. On the other hand, increased expression of PABPN-1 with normal (GCN_{10}) polyalanine stretches also leads to nuclear aggregates, suggesting that INIs may not be a causative step in

A. Fischmann (✉)
Department of Radiology, University of Basel Hospital, 4031 Basel, Switzerland
e-mail: arne.fischmann@unibas.ch

M.P. Wattjes and D. Fischer (eds.), *Neuromuscular Imaging*, DOI 10.1007/978-1-4614-6552-2_24,

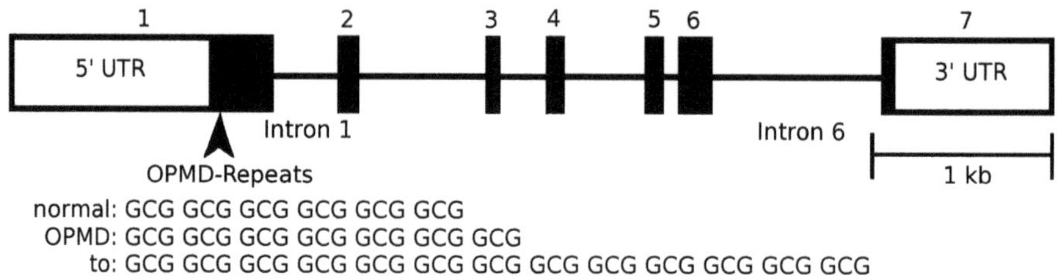

Fig. 24.1 Genetic structure of the *PABPN1* gene. Exons are numbered 1–7. Introns 1 and 6 are present in variable degrees. The GNC expansion in oculopharyngeal muscular dystrophy (OPMD) is located in exon 1. Modified from Brais et al (1998) Nat Genet. 164–7

disease progression but are, rather, a protective measure by the cells against PABPN-1 toxicity.

Although OPMD is primarily a myopathic disorder, electrophysiological nerve conduction studies showed signs of symmetrical polyneuropathy in several affected families, indicating involvement of peripheral nerves. Other pedigrees showed no signs of neuropathy. It is therefore probable that nerve involvement is dependent on certain genetic factors.

Oculopharyngeodistal myopathy (OPDM), a variation of OPMD, has a slightly different clinical presentation, with predominantly distal involvement. It has a mainly autosomal dominant hereditary pattern, although at least one family with an autosomal recessive pattern has been described. The underlying genetic defect has not been identified.

24.3 Histopathology

Although the histological diagnostic workup of OPMD has been largely replaced by direct genetic testing, it is still valuable in the evaluation of atypical manifestations of OPMD.

Nonspecific dystrophic changes can be detected using standard histological staining techniques. They include loss of muscle fiber, abnormal variation in fiber size, and increased interstitial fibrous and fatty connective tissue. Small angulated fibers can be detected in many cases, suggesting an additional underlying denervation process. Whether these changes represent denervation itself or secondary changes due to advanced aging processes is still under discussion. Autophagic rimmed vacuoles are another finding in OPMD. Usually, there are no necrotic or inflammatory changes. Immunohistochemical analysis can detect increased levels of a wide array of growth factors, many of which are also involved in hepatic fibrosis.

Ultrastructural studies with electron microscopy reveal tubulofilamentous INIs, which are unique for OPMD and are only found in muscle fibers. The INIs contain unbranched, sometimes striated filaments of up to 250 nm in length. One integral component of the INIs is PABPN-1. Other components are poly(T)RNA, transcription factors, part of the ubiquitin proteasome pathway, and other mRNA binding proteins. Inclusion body myositis (IBM)-type filaments have also been described in OPMD.

For a long time, INIs were considered to be the causative agent in disease progression. More recent data suggest that a soluble form of PABPN1 is responsible for the disease and that INIs are a protective mechanism in the cells to contain damage from PABPN1 overexpression.

Although PABPN1 is ubiquitously expressed, the clinical phenotype in OPMD is restricted to skeletal muscles. Fast glycolytic fibers are predominantly involved. Muscles containing mainly oxidative fibers (e.g., soleus) are relatively spared.

24.4 Clinical Presentation

Contrary to many other hereditary muscle dystrophies, OPMD is a late-onset muscle disease with manifestation during the fifth or sixth decade. It shows rather slow clinical progression. The average age at onset in autosomal dominant OPMD is around 50 years. Initial presentation beyond the age of 70 years is a rarity.

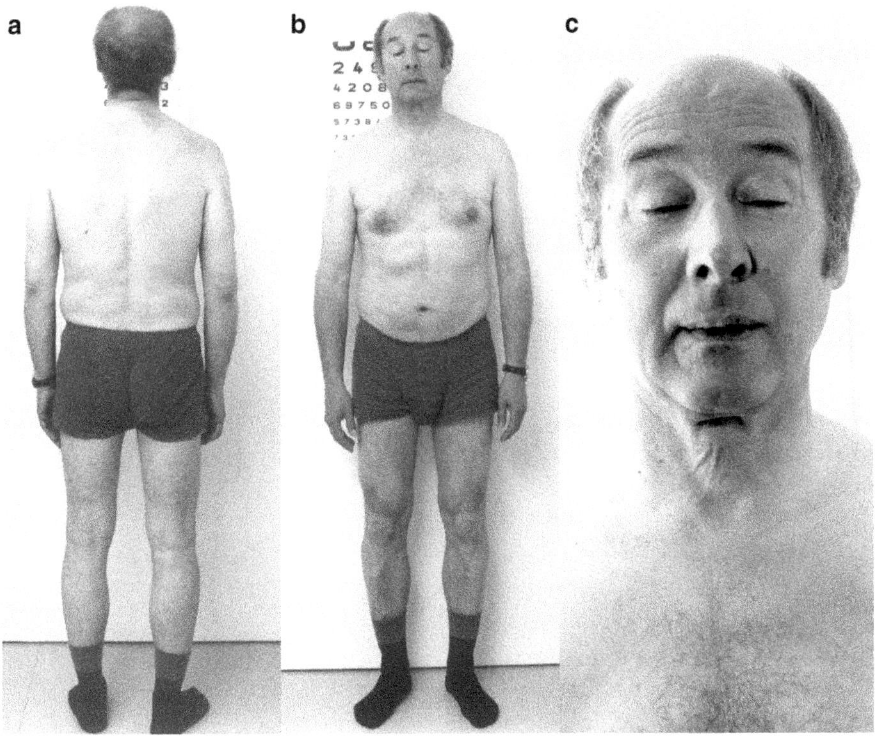

Fig. 24.2 Clinical presentation of OPMD in a male patient. He had limb-girdle weakness especially of the thighs (**a**, **b**) and prominent ptosis (**c**). Courtesy of Dr. Dirk Fischer, Basel, Switzerland

OPMD has an estimated prevalence of 1/100,000 worldwide, but it is much more common (1:1,000 to 1:600) in certain ethnic communities, such as French Canadians and Bukhara Jews. The late onset and slow progression of nonspecific symptoms cause diagnostic delay in most patients, with reported delays of up to 20 years before a correct diagnosis.

OPMD is usually diagnosed clinically. The patient must fulfill three diagnostic criteria for a diagnosis of autosomal dominant OPMD.

- Positive family history with at least two generations involved
- Presence of ptosis (defined as vertical separation or at least one palpebral fissure that measures <8 mm at rest) (Fig. 24.2)
- Presence of dysphagia (swallowing time more than 7 s when drinking 80 ml of ice-cold water)

Ptosis is initially restricted to the levator palpebrae with later involvement of all extraocular muscles, occasionally causing diplopia. Complete ophthalmoplegia is rather rare and differentiates OPMD from chronic progressive external ophthalmoplegia (CPEO). The clinical picture includes an elevated head to compensate for the ptosis with a downward gaze, also known as "the astrologers pose."

Dysphagia is initially noticed in regard to solid foods. In advanced disease stages, dysphagia can lead to malnutrition and aspiration pneumonia. Dysphagia is often worsened by the adaptive head position to compensate for the ptosis.

Involvement of peripheral muscles is common, usually in a limb-girdle distribution pattern. It presents with proximal weakness, especially of the proximal lower extremity muscles (Fig. 24.2). Although this weakness usually appears later in the disease course compared to ptosis and dysphagia, it represents the first complaint in many patients. Facial weakness causing an expressionless face and a nasal voice due to palatal weakness are manifestations in more-advanced stages.

Heterozygous patients with OPMD have a normal life-span, but patients who are homozygous for the CGN13 allele have a decreased life expectancy. Homozygotes also display signs of central nervous system involvement (e.g., reduced selective attention) more prominently than heterozygous patients. Patients with recessive OPMD, on the other hand, tend to be less affected, although more severe cases have been reported.

Clinical diagnosis of OPMD is usually possible if the disease is considered in the differential diagnosis. Definitive diagnosis, however, can be achieved only by testing for the polyalanin-repeat in the PABPN-1 gene by a polymerase gene reaction, which has sensitivity close to 100 % and is available through many laboratories worldwide.

OPDM is characterized by a generally younger age at onset of about 22 years and early death at an average age of 45. Ptosis and ophthalmoplegia are early symptoms of OPDM. Disease onset in extremity muscles, which is predominantly distal with involvement of the fingers and toes, and proximal muscle affection occurs only during later stages of the disease. Myotonic discharges are also reported without clinical signs of myotonia. OPDM is usually an exclusion diagnosis in patients negative for the *PABPN-1* gene mutation.

24.5 Imaging Findings

Probably because of the rare nature of the disease, there is only limited information about the pattern of muscle involvement in OPMD. The reports mainly described imaging of the legs.

Patients presenting clinically with weakness of certain muscle groups showed symmetrical fatty replacement and moderate atrophy in the clinically affected muscle groups. Involvement is more prominent in the thigh than in the calf, representing limb-girdle involvement. These changes correlate with clinical functional measures of movement and stance.

The pattern of involvement in the thigh is shown in Fig. 24.3, and involvement of the calves can be seen in Fig. 24.4.

In the neck, there is prominent involvement of the splenius capitis, with less prominent involvement of the sternocleidomastoid, the posterior neck, and the trapezius muscles as well as the shoulder girdle. No data on involvement of the arms are available. Some studies demonstrated fatty atrophy of the psoas muscle, the erector spinae (iliocostalis lumborum, longissimus dorsi), and the gluteus (gluteus maximus and medius) muscles.

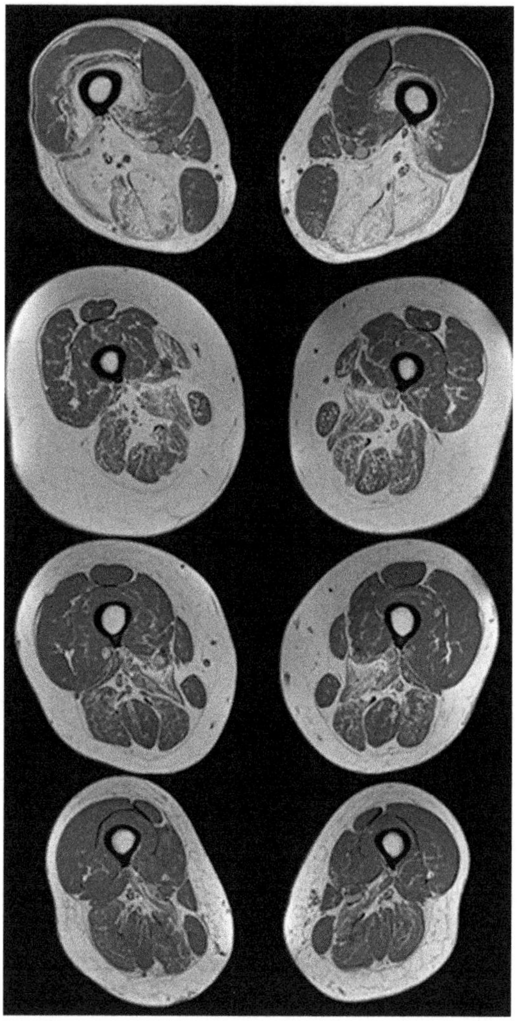

Fig. 24.3 Magnetic resonance imaging, T1-weighted sequence, show involvement of the thigh in four typical patients. From *bottom* to *top*: increasing stages of disease progression. The first muscle involved is the adductor magnus, followed by the hamstrings, especially the semimembranosus and long head of the biceps femoris. Involvement of the semitendinosus follows in later stages. The short head of the biceps, the sartorius, and the gracilis are relatively spared—a finding also present in several other myopathies (e.g., inclusion body myositis). The quadriceps muscles show a specific pattern of involvement, with prominent fatty replacement of the deeper layers of the vastus intermedius

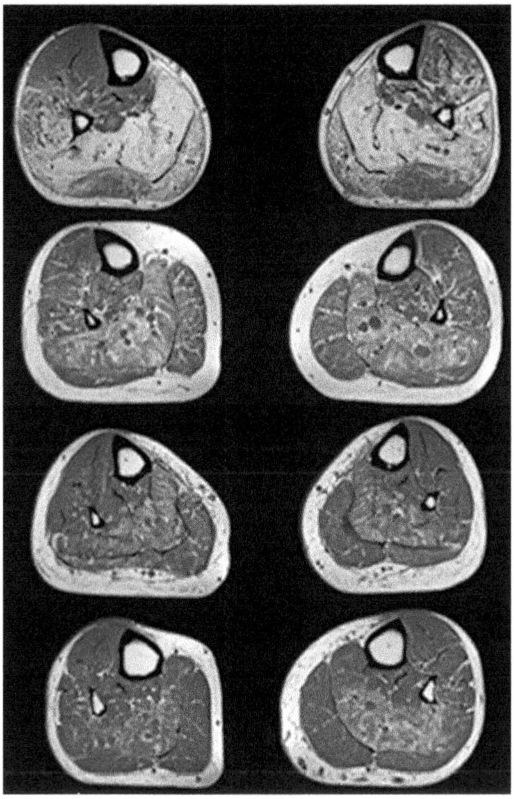

Fig. 24.4 Magnetic resonance imaging, T1-weighted sequences, of the calves in the patients from Fig. 24.3. Involvement of the posterior compartments is prominent in the calves. The first muscle involved (from *bottom* to *top*) is the soleus followed by the medial gastrocnemius. The peroneal muscles and the lateral gastrocnemius are involved only during later stages of the disease. The tibialis anterior and posterior groups are relatively spared even in more advanced stages of the disease

The facial muscles show fatty atrophy of the temporalis and pterygoid muscles. There is also evidence of extensive fatty atrophy of the tongue in patients with OPMD. The floor of the mouth is spared.

The muscular changes can be quantified with standard techniques such as two- or three-point Dixon fat separation or measurement of T2 relaxation times, as described in Chap. 5. These quantitative techniques can detect disease progression at an earlier stage and at shorter time intervals than clinical and functional measurement scales.

No pattern of involvement has been described in OPDM patients.

In addition to anatomical descriptions of muscle involvement, functional examination of dysphagia includes swallowing radiographic and manometric studies. These tests reveal prolonged and weak esophageal motility with normal contraction of the upper esophageal sphincter. Relaxation of the sphincter is delayed.

24.6 Therapy

Currently, there is no medical treatment for OPMD, although several promising compounds are under development: Antiprion drugs such as 6-aminophenanthridine (6AP) or guanabenzacetate, which prevent formation of amyloid fibers by prion proteins, have been shown to alleviate symptoms of OPMD in animal models. Cystamine can protect against PABPN1 toxicity in mouse models and human cell lines by reducing transaminase activity. Trehalose and doxycycline also have shown promising effects in mouse models of OPMD. None of these compounds has reached trial stage in humans.

As no causative treatment is available, interventions are currently limited to symptom relief. Treatment of pharyngeal dysfunction and better nutrition has greatly improved the quality of life. A high-protein diet is recommended in advanced cases, which tend to shy away from meat to avoid choking despite the extremely small risk. Overall muscle function should be maintained with light exercise, but strenuous exercise should be avoided.

Dysphagia can be treated with speech therapy to improve swallowing or by constrictor myotomy. Cricopharyngeal myotomy alleviates symptoms in most cases, although the dysphagia will slowly reappear over some years. Aspiration pneumonia is a common complication of OPMD. As it is a frequent cause of death, patients should be advised to seek medical attention whenever they have a productive cough and/or fever.

Ptosis can be treated surgically with resection of the levator palpebrae aponeurosis or frontal suspension of the eyelids. Both operations lead to overall good results.

The lack of preventive or causative treatment means that care should be taken before requesting genetic testing of an asymptomatic individual.

It should be performed only in a context where genetic counseling and psychological support can be offered, especially when considering the late onset and relatively mild course of the disease.

24.7 Differential Diagnosis

In more advanced stages of the disease, the differential diagnosis of OPMD is usually straightforward. The main reasons for delayed diagnosis are its slow progression and the low prevalence of the disease.

Considering the clinical presentation of OPMD patients, the differential diagnosis should include a limited number of other neuromuscular diseases. Ptosis and impaired ocular movements can occur in other muscle disorders such as myotonic dystrophy (see Chap. 22) and centronuclear myopathy (see Sects. 15.4 and 15.5), but ptosis is rarely the predominant finding in these disorders. CPEO (see Sect. 14.3) can be distinguished from OPMD by the patient's "astrologer's pose" that is apparent in OPMD patients. This compensatory mechanism is not possible in CPEO patients because of the limited downward movement of the eyes.

Myasthenia gravis is the most important disease to exclude in the workup of patients with OPMD. The fatigability and fluctuating course of the ptosis in myasthenia already hints at this diagnosis. The diagnosis can be verified by repetitive nerve stimulation, single-fiber electromyography, testing for acetylcholine receptor antibodies, and successful treatment with anticholinesterase drugs.

The differential diagnosis for dysphagia should include pharyngeal malignancies and paresis of the pharyngeal nerves. Inclusion body myositis (IBM) (see Chap. 26) can also present with dysphagia and limb muscle weakness. As neither of these diseases presents with ptosis, clinical differentiation usually poses no problem.

When considering the differential diagnosis of imaging findings, the pattern of involvement resembles the limb-girdle myopathies LGMD2A, LGMD2B, and LGMD2I (see Chap. 19), as well as Z-disc-related myofibrillar myopathies (see Chap. 20). However, clinical differentiation of these diseases is easy because of the prominent ocular involvement in OPMD.

A definitive diagnosis can be easily achieved by conducting a simple, standardized genetic test for the polyalanine repeat expansion in the *PABPN1* gene.

Newer studies indicate that special emphasis should be put on the age at symptom onset and the pattern of peripheral weakness, as OPDM has a slightly different clinical presentation despite similar symptoms. As patients with OPDM do not test positive for the polyalanine repeat, diagnosis of this rare subgroup depends on clinical findings.

Oculopharyngeal-Muscular Dystrophy

Key Points

- OPMD is a rare autosomal dominant disorder caused by a GCG-repeat expansion in the *PABPN-1* gene on chromosome 14q11.2.
- Disease onset is during later adult life (on average at 45–50 years) with ptosis and dysphagia as the initial symptoms and later development of weakness in a limb-girdle distribution.
- MRI of the legs shows predominant involvement of the posterior thigh and calf with a characteristic pattern.
- No curative therapy is available. Cricopharyngeal myotomy and surgical treatment of ptosis can provide symptom relief.

Suggestions for Further Reading

Brais B. Oculopharyngeal muscular dystrophy: a polyalanine myopathy. Curr Neurol Neurosci Rep. 2009;9:76–82.

Brais B, Rouleau GA. Oculopharyngeal muscular dystrophy. In: Pagon RA, Bird TD, Dolan CR, Stephens K, editors. GeneReviews [Internet]. Seattle: University of Washington, Seattle; 1993. 8 March 2001. Update 22 June 2006. Accessed 02 August 2011.

Dubbioso R, Moretta P, Manganelli F, et al. Executive functions are impaired in heterozygote patients with oculopharyngeal muscular dystrophy. J Neurol 2012; 259:833–837.

Durmus H, Laval SH, Deymeer F, et al. Oculopharyngodistal myopathy is a distinct entity: clinical and genetic features of 47 patients. Neurology 2011;76:227–35.

Fischmann A, Gloor M, Fasler S, et al. Muscular involvement assessed by MRI correlates to motor function measurement values in oculopharyngeal muscular dystrophy. J Neurol. 2011;258:1333–40.

Trollet C, Anvar SY, Venema A, Hargreaves IP, et al. Molecular and phenotypic characterization of a mouse model of oculopharyngeal muscular dystrophy reveals severe muscular atrophy restricted to fast glycolytic fibres. Hum Mol Genet. 2010;19:2191–207.

Diagnostic Algorithms and Differential Diagnosis

25

Rudolf Andre Kley and Dirk Fischer

25.1 Introduction

The aim of this chapter is to provide algorithms based on muscle imaging findings that might be of help for scheduling appropriate genetic testing in patients presenting with clinical and histopathological features consistent with a congenital myopathy, limb-girdle myopathy, or myofibrillar myopathy. As whole-body muscle imaging data are not yet available for most hereditary myopathies, we have used data dealing with imaging findings in the thighs and lower legs. With increasing use of whole body MRI protocols, we can expect extended involvement patterns to be described in the near future. In addition to imaging findings we include valuable clinical data that can be used to distinguish these genetic disorders.

R.A. Kley
Department of Neurology, Neuromuscular Center Ruhrgebiet, University Hospital Bergmannsheil, Ruhr-University Bochum, Bürkle-de-la-Camp-Platz 1, 44789 Bochum, Germany
e-mail: RudiKley@t-online.de

D. Fischer (✉)
Division of Neuropaediatrics, University Childrens Hospital Basel, 4056 Basel, Switzerland

Department of Neurology, University Hospital Basel, 4031 Basel, Switzerland
e-mail: Dirk.Fischer@ukbb.ch

25.2 Congenital Myopathies

Congenital myopathies (CMs) have been described in detail in Chap. 16. Figure 25.1 outlines an approach to distinguish the various CMs using muscle imaging findings of the lower limbs. The systematic analysis of muscle imaging findings starts with the distinction between patients with involvement predominantly of proximal thigh muscles and those with alterations predominantly in the (distal) lower legs. In the first group, the pattern observed in ryanodine receptor type 1 (RYR1) related patients is highly characteristic. These patients show more predominant involvement of the anterior than the posterior thigh compartment muscles, predominantly affecting the gluteus maximus, vasti, adductor magnus, and sartorius. In the lower legs, RYR1 patients show predominant involvement of soleus and the peroneal muscles. Sparing of the rectus femoris, adductor longus, and gracilis muscles is common. Selenoprotein 1 (SEPN1) related patients may present with similar changes. But evaluation of the lower legs usually allows a distinction: in contrast to the RYR1-patients, SEPN1-patients show more involvement of the medial and lateral gastrocnemius muscles and less of the soleus muscle. In dynamin 2 (DNM2) related-patients, there are some important imaging findings that are different from those of the RYR1- and SEPN1-patients: predominant involvement of the gluteus minimus muscle, relative sparing of the vasti and sartorius muscles, more involvement

M.P. Wattjes and D. Fischer (eds.), *Neuromuscular Imaging*, DOI 10.1007/978-1-4614-6552-2_25,

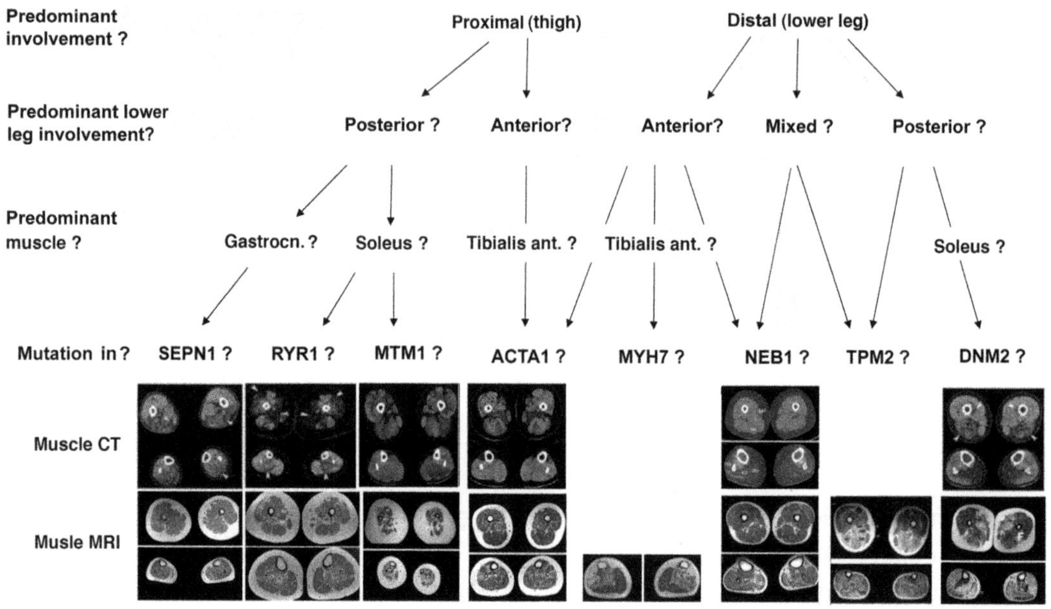

Fig. 25.1 Algorithm for the differential diagnosis of congenital myopathies (CM) based on muscle imaging data of lower extremities. Modified with permission from Springer, Wattjes MP, et al., Neuromuscular imaging in inherited muscle diseases. Eur Radiol. 2010;20:2447–60, and from Bevilacqua et al. "Necklace" fibers, a new histological marker of late-onset MTM1-related centronuclear myopathy. Acta Neuropathol. 2009 Mar;117(3):283–91. Reprinted with permission from Springer

of the adductor longus than the adductor magnus muscles, and predominant involvement of the medial gastrocnemius and soleus muscles in the lower legs. The overall pattern in patients with the myotubularin 1 (*MTM1*) gene is similar to the pattern observed in RYR1-patients. However, the vastus lateralis is more affected than the vastus medialis in RYR1-patients, whereas the opposite seems to be the case in MTM1-patients. The biceps femoris is involved early in MTM1-patients, whereas it is often spared in RYR1-patients. In addition, tibialis anterior involvement can be seen in MTM1- patients but not in RYR1-patients. A reliable distinction cannot be made, though, before further data are available. In contrast to SEPN1-, RYR1-, and MTM1-patients, which have predominant proximal weakness, ACTA1-patients present with anterior rather than posterior lower leg involvement. Also Nebuline (NEB) related patients, that sometimes present with predominant proximal weakness, show involvement of the tibialis anterior muscle, which should help to distinguish these patients from RYR1- and SEPN1-patients, in whom the tibialis anterior muscle is spared.

By contrast, there is another group of congenital myopathy patients who present with predominantly distal lower leg weakness. Most DNM2-patients have isolated distal involvement on muscle imaging. In the lower legs, the medial gastrocnemius and soleus muscles are often severely involved, and the posterior tibialis and anterior lower leg compartment muscles are spared. TPM2 patients show a similar pattern as DNM2 patients but have less affection of the soleus muscle. Other congenital myopathies with distal affection related to mutations in the NEB, ACTA1, and MYH7 genes, by contrast, show predominantly anterior lower leg involvement. Congenital (nemaline) myopathies related to ACTA1 gene mutations show predominantly distal anterior lower leg and mild diffuse thigh compartment involvement. In contrast, MYH7 gene associated myopathies (Chap. 21) spare the thigh muscles and have selective distal involvement of the tibialis anterior, tibialis posterior, and soleus muscles. In cases of thigh muscle involvement, there is more posterior compartment affection than involvement of the vasti muscle in patients with ACTA1 and NEB mutations, whereas the opposite has been observed in patients with MYH7 mutations. Thus, a reliable distinction between NEB, ACTA1 and MYH7 patients is currently almost impossible. As these myopathies are rare, and sometimes only case reports have been described, evolutions of the algorithm will be possible when more published data are available in the future.

25.3 Dystrophinopathies and Limb-Girdle Muscular Dystrophies

Dystrophinopathies and limb girdle muscular dystrophies (LGMDs) have been described in detail in Chaps. 17 and 19. Figure 25.2 shows a flowchart demonstrating an approach to distinguish the various LGMDs using muscle imaging and clinical findings for the differential diagnosis. We suggest analyzing systematically muscle imaging findings in LGMDs first according to the degree of anterior compared to posterior thigh involvement. Most LGMD patients show more-pronounced muscle alterations in the posterior than in the anterior thigh compartment. In contrast, patients presenting with a limb girdle pattern of muscle weakness (see also Chap. 12, Fig. 12.1) caused by dystrophin mutations (e.g., such as female carriers, patients with late onset Becker-type dystrophinopathy) or sarcoglycanopathy often have important involvement of the quadriceps muscle. These two disease groups can normally be distinguished in a second step based on the lower leg involvement. Dystrophinopathy often presents with early, marked changes in the gastrocnemii or soleus muscles. These muscles are not affected in sarcoglycanopathy patients.

Patients with dysferlinopathy most often display posterior thigh and posterior lower leg involvement with sparing of the sartorius, gracilis and biceps femoris although the pattern of muscle involvement can be variable. However, calf atrophy and the absence of scapular winging are common clinical findings. Calpain-3 related and Fukutin-related protein (FKRP) related patients present with predominantly posterior thigh and posterior lower leg involvement. Calpain-3 patients usually show marked involvement of the

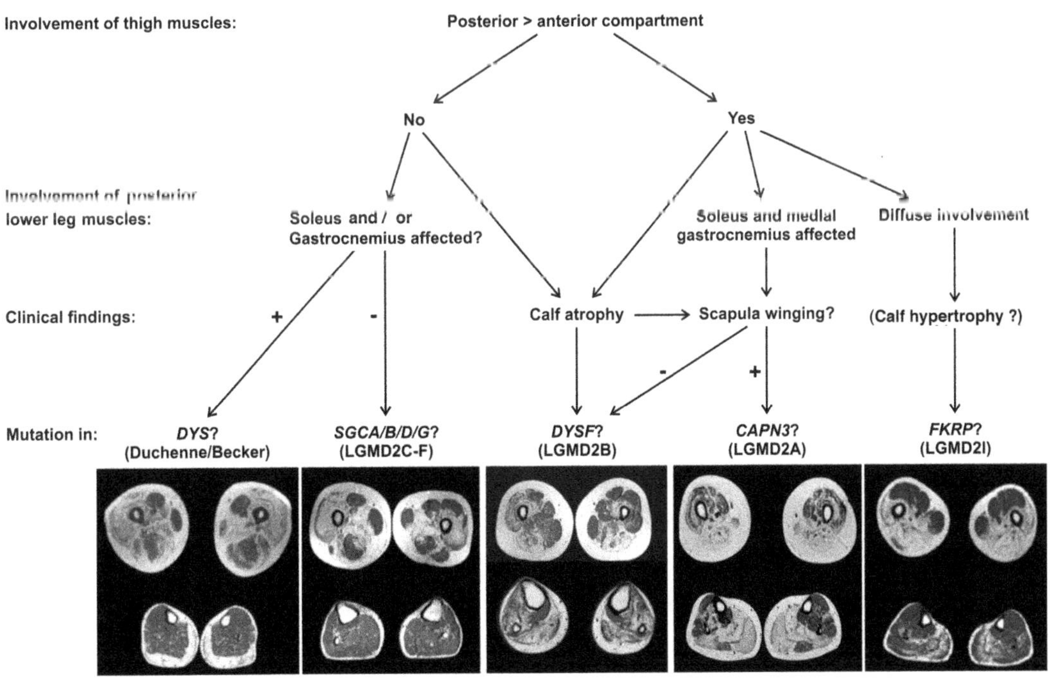

Fig. 25.2 Algorithm for the differential diagnosis of dystrophinopathies and limb girdle muscular dystrophies (LGMD) based on muscle imaging data of lower limbs. From Wattjes MP, et al., Neuromuscular imaging in inherited muscle diseases. Eur Radiol. 2010;20:2447–60. Reprinted with permission from Springer

soleus and medial gastrocnemius muscles. Calf atrophy and scapular winging are also usually observed. In contrast, FKRP patients have a more diffuse involvement of the posterior lower leg muscles, and the tibialis anterior muscle is often spared or even hypertrophied.

25.4 Myofibrillar Myopathies

Myofibrillar myopathies (MFMs) are described in detail in Chap. 20. Figure 25.3 provides an algorithm to distinguish MFM subtypes based on muscle imaging findings in the lower limbs. Only limited data are available regarding α(alpha)B-crystallinopathy, but the pattern of muscle involvement seems to be quite similar to that observed in desminopathy. A specific finding in both diseases that helps to distinguish them from myotilinopathy, filaminopathy, and ZASPopathy is equal or more involvement of the semitendinosus than of the biceps femoris and at least equal involvement of the peroneal group muscles in relation to the tibialis anterior. In addition, the gracilis and sartorius muscles are more involved in desminopathy and α-B-crystallinopathy than in the other mentioned MFM subtypes. A characteristic feature of myotilinopathy is at least equal involvement of the sartorius compared to the semitendinosus and more involvement of the adductor magnus than the gracilis muscle. The pattern of muscle alterations in the lower legs is helpful for distinguishing filaminopathy from ZASPopathy patients as the medial head of the gastrocnemius is regularly more affected than the lateral head in filaminopathy but not in ZASPopathy.

In addition to the muscle imaging findings, other clinical features may be helpful in the differential diagnosis of MFMs. Cataract, for instance, has been described in αB-crystallinopathy. An LGMD-like distribution of muscle weakness is a characteristic feature of filaminopathy but may also be observed in other MFMs. The age

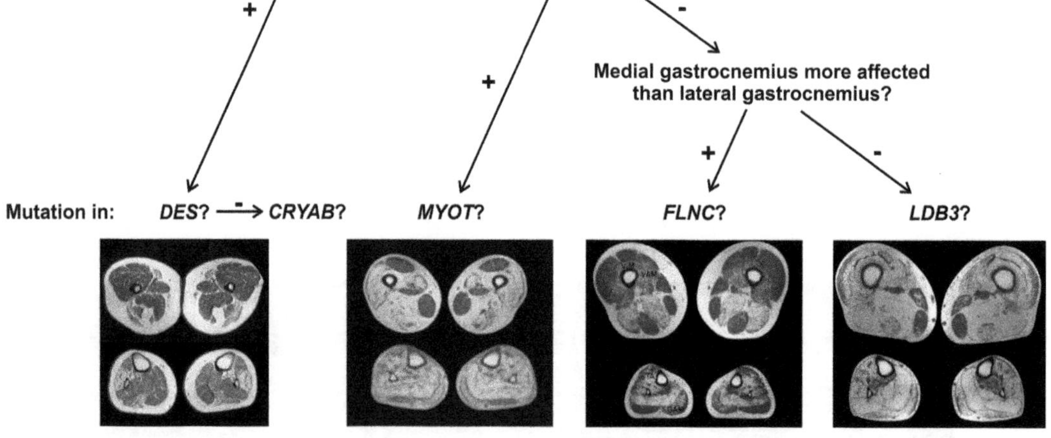

Fig. 25.3 Algorithm for the differential diagnosis of myofibrillar myopathies (MFM) based on muscle imaging findings in lower limbs. From Wattjes MP, et al., Neuromuscular imaging in inherited muscle diseases. Eur Radiol. 2010;20:2447–60. Reprinted with permission from Springer

of onset is variable in all MFM subtypes but on average, desminopathy and αB-crystallinopathy manifest during the fourth decade, filaminopathy and ZASPopathy during the fifth decade, and myotilinopathy during the sixth decade of life. More details on the clinical findings of the MFM subtypes are provided in Chap. 20.

25.5 Other Muscular Dystrophies

The diagnosis of common muscular dystrophies such as myotonic dystrophy type 1, facioscapulohumeral muscular dystrophy, and oculopharyngeal muscular dystrophy is usually not difficult due to because of their classic clinical presentation. Therefore, the role of muscle imaging has yet to be defined for these muscular dystrophies. Recent studies performed on these myopathies suggested that some characteristic findings are present (Fig. 25.4), even if there is less diagnostic value than for CMs, LGMDs and MFMs. Myotonic dystrophy type I (Fig. 25.4A) is typically characterized by distal more than proximal muscle involvement, with predominant affection of the soleus, medial gastrocnemius, and proximally the anterior thigh compartment with relative sparing of the rectus femoris. Myotonic dystrophy type II

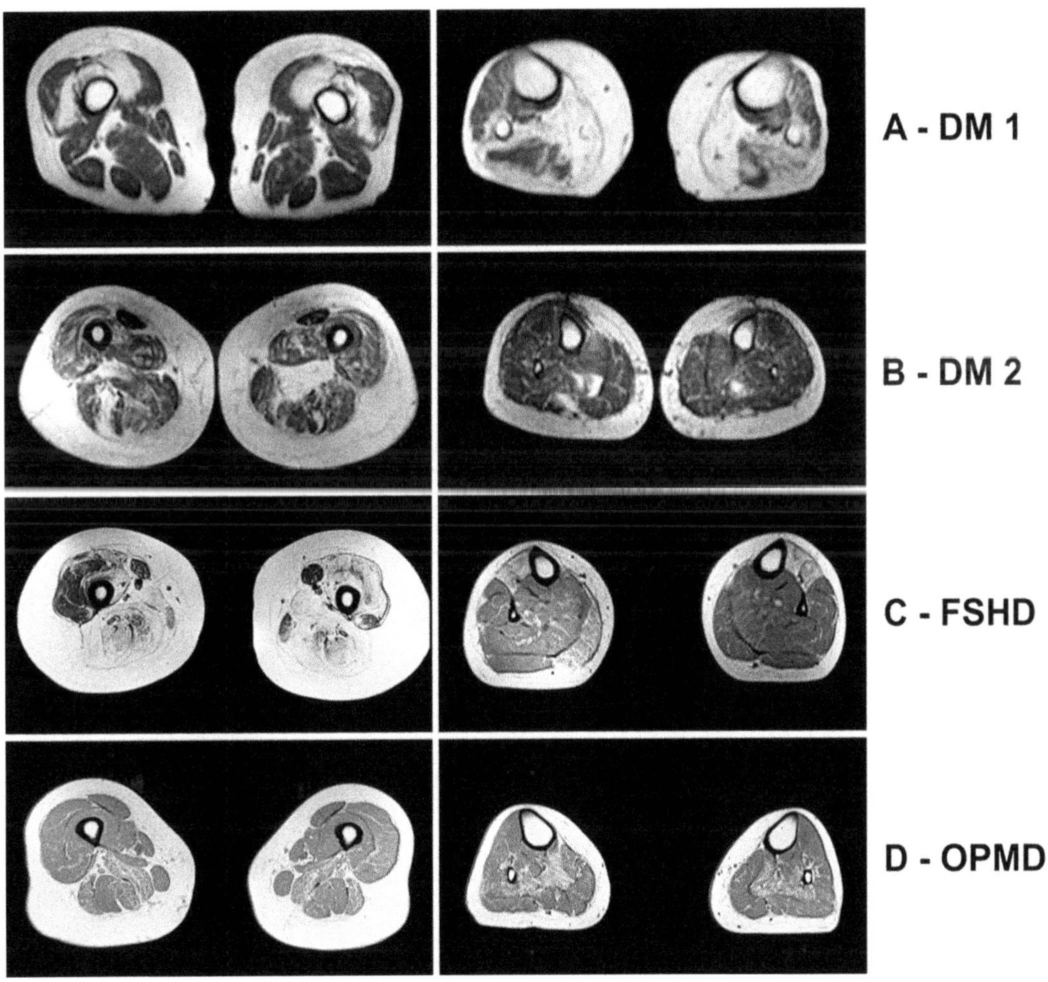

Fig. 25.4 Muscle MRI of lower extremities in other muscular dystrophies. From Wattjes MP, et al., Neuromuscular imaging in inherited muscle diseases. Eur Radiol. 2010;20:2447–60. Reprinted with permission from Springer

(proximal myotonic myopathy) often has less involvement and shows no fatty degeneration. Affected patients show more involvement of the proximal muscles with affection of the quadriceps and sparing of the rectus femoris and gracilis muscles (Fig. 25.4B). FSHDs are often characterized by marked asymmetry with the adductor magnus, hamstrings, rectus femoris, and tibial anterior muscles being those most often involved (Fig. 25.4C). OPMD patients show predominantly posterior thigh (adductor magnus, semimembranosus biceps femoris muscles) and posterior lower leg (soleus) muscle involvement (Fig. 25.4D).

Suggestions for Further Reading

Fischer D, Walter MC, Kesper K, et al. Diagnostic value of muscle MRI in differentiating LGMD2I from other LGMDs. J Neurol. 2005;252:538–47.

Fischer D, Kley RA, Strach K, et al. Distinct muscle imaging patterns in myofibrillar myopathies. Neurology 2008;71:758–65.

Quijano-Roy S, Carlier RY, Fischer D. Muscle imaging in congenital myopathies. Semin Pediatr Neurol. 2011; 18:221–9.

Wattjes MP, Kley RA, Fischer D. Neuromuscular imaging in inherited muscle diseases. Eur Radiol. 2010;20: 2447–60.

Part IV

Clinical Applications in Acquired Myopathies

Inflammatory Myopathies

26

Jan Verschuuren, Fieke M. Cox, Baziel van Engelen, Marianne de Visser, and Umesh A. Badrising

26.1 Introduction and Classification

Idiopathic inflammatory myopathies (IIMs) represent a heterogeneous group of muscular disorders characterized by acquired muscle weakness and inflammatory infiltrates in skeletal muscle tissue. The three main disease entities in this group are sporadic inclusion body myositis (IBM), polymyositis (PM), and dermatomyositis (DM). These diseases differ strongly from each other in terms of clinical and pathological features. Since 1975, the Bohan and Peter criteria have been applied, allowing only a distinction between dermatomyositis and polymyositis based on the presence or absence of skin abnormalities. Histopathologically, there was no difference between PM and DM. At that time, IBM was not generally recognized as a separate disease entity and usually was not differentiated from PM. It was considered a "treatment-resistant" polymyositis. In 1984, IIMs were looked at from a histopathological point of view, which allowed PM, DM, and IBM to be discriminated particularly on histopathological criteria. A cytotoxic CD8-positive T-cell reaction is the main feature of PM and IBM, whereas in DM a B-cell-mediated microangiopathy is most prominent. Recently, this classification has been challenged as numerous cases of histopathologically defined PM have been described that were nonresponsive to immunosuppressants and immunomodulating therapies, eventually mimicking the clinical picture of IBM. However, differentiation between PM and IBM is crucial because of the different therapeutic approaches required. This chapter focuses on the three most relevant IIMs: IBM, PM, and DM.

26.2 Sporadic Inclusion Body Myositis

26.2.1 Synonyms, Abbreviations

IBM

26.2.2 Genetics and Pathophysiology

Sporadic inclusion body myositis is, as the name implies, not hereditary. There are rare descriptions of a familial form of IBM that is probably no more frequent than in other autoimmune diseases. There is a strong association with the auto-

J. Verschuuren (✉) • F.M. Cox • U.A. Badrising
Department of Neurology, Leiden University Medical Center, Postbox 9600, 2300 RC Leiden, The Netherlands
e-mail: j.j.g.m.verschuuren@lumc.nl; m.devisser@amc.uva.nl

B. van Engelen
Department of Neurology, Radboud University Nijmegen Medical Center, Nijmegen, The Netherlands
e-mail: b.vanengelen@neuro.umcn.nl

M. de Visser
Department of Neurology, Academic Medical Center, Amsterdam, The Netherlands
e-mail: m.devisser@amc.uva.nl

M.P. Wattjes and D. Fischer (eds.), *Neuromuscular Imaging*, DOI 10.1007/978-1-4614-6552-2_26,

immune prone ancestral HLA 8.1 haplotype and with other autoimmune disorders, such as Sjögren's disease, thyroid disorders, celiac disease, rheumatoid arthritis, and type I diabetes mellitus. Hereditary IBMs are a group of rare myopathies with a genetic origin that share some histopathological characteristics such as inclusions and tubulofilamentous structures with sporadic IBM but lack cellular infiltrates on muscle biopsies. They include IBM1 (desmin-related myopathy), a form of myofibrillar myopathy caused by mutations in the *Desmin* gene on chromosome 2q35; Japanese distal myopathy with rimmed vacuoles or Nonaka myopathy, allelic to IBM2, with a similar clinical and pathological picture with quadriceps sparing and mutations in the UDP-*N*-acetylglucosamine-2-epimerase/*N*-acetylmannosamine kinase (*GNE*) gene mapped on chromosome 9p13-p12; IBM3 characterized by joint contractures, external opthalmoplegia, and proximal weakness resulting from mutations in the gene encoding myosin heavy chain IIa (MYHC2A or MYH2) on chromosome 17p13.1; and inclusion body myopathy with Paget disease and frontotemporal dementia, caused by missense mutations in the valosin-containing protein (*VCP*) gene on chromosome 9p13.3-p12. ZASPopathy, another subtype of myofibrillar myopathy, is a late-onset distal myopathy with its responsible gene located on chromosome 10q22.2-q23.3 and coding for Z-band alternatively spliced PDZ-motif containing protein (*ZASP*). It is a hereditary myopathy with overlap. These hereditary myopathies are not considered inflammatory muscle disorders or myositis. Most are discussed in Chap. 20 (myofibrillar myopathies) and Chap. 21 (distal myopathies).

The pathophysiology in IBM is still unknown. Histopathological features based on muscle biopsy findings suggest the presence of inflammation and degeneration. Which of these processes is the primary etiological factor is a matter of debate.

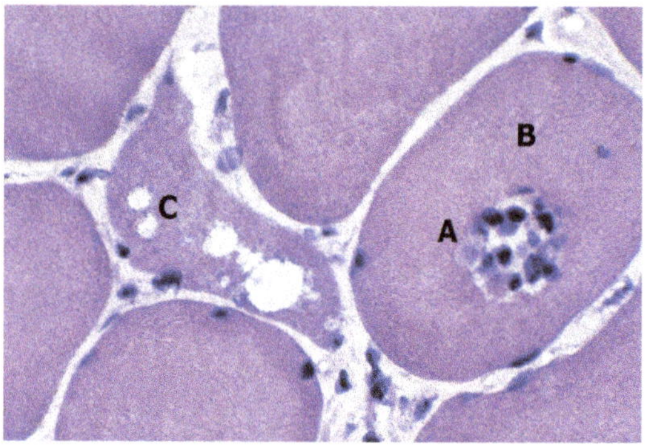

Fig. 26.1 Muscle biopsy of a patient with sporadic inclusion body myositis. This biopsy shows mononuclear cell invasion (*A*) of a non-necrotic muscle fiber (*B*) and rimmed vacuoles. (H&E)

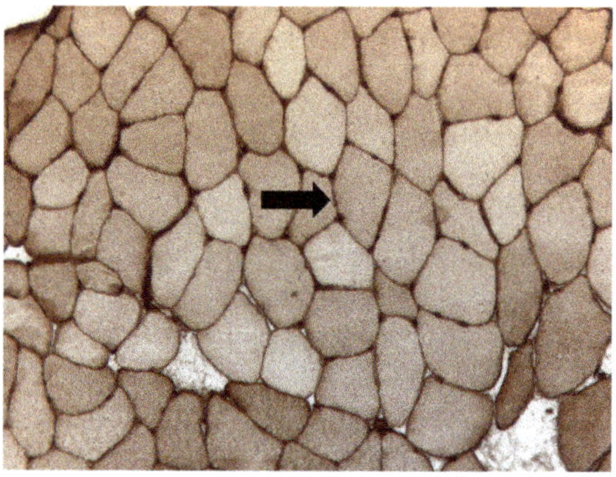

Fig. 26.2 Pathological sarcolemmal major histocompatibility complex type I (MHC-I) expression (*arrow*) in a muscle biopsy of a patient with sporadic inclusion body myositis. The muscle fiber membrane is darkly colored, as are capillaries. Normally, capillaries stain darker than the membrane (see Fig. 26.3)

26.2.3 Histopathology

Muscle biopsy shows atrophic fibers and inflammatory and degenerative changes. Inflammation is mainly located endomysially and consists of mononuclear cells, including T lymphocytes and to a lesser extent B cells and macrophages. CD8-positive cytotoxic T cells invade non-necrotic muscle fibers (Fig. 26.1). Similar to PM, pathological expression of major histocompatibility complex type I (MHC-I) on the sarcolemma can be observed in sporadic IBM (Figs. 26.2 and 26.3). Degenerative changes include the "rimmed vacuoles," which are seen with hematoxylin-eosin (H&E) or Gomori trichrome staining of fresh frozen muscle biopsy specimens. The vacuoles are filled with

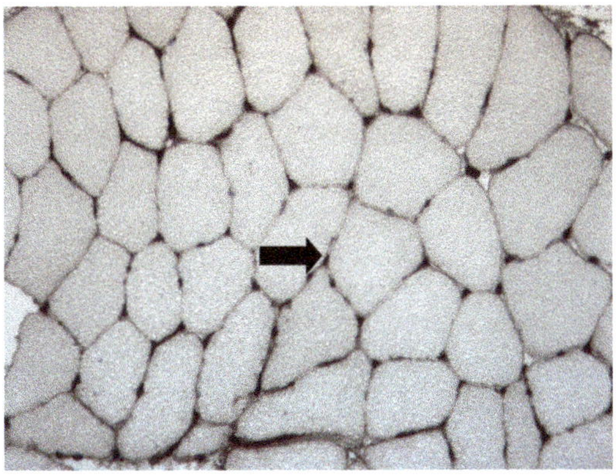

Fig. 26.3 Negative MHC-I stain to compare with Fig. 26.2. It was obtained using the same microscope and similar light exposure. Capillaries (*arrow*) normally take up more stain than does the muscle fiber membrane, as can be seen here

amorphous material. Eosinophilic inclusions are rarely seen in the nucleus or cytoplasm, and their presence is not mandatory for the diagnosis of IBM. On electron microscopy, tubulofilamentous structures can be visualized in the cytoplasm of 15- to 21-nm diameter, as well as in the nucleus or near the rimmed vacuoles. Degenerative proteins such as β-amyloid and hyperphosphorylated tau accumulate near these tubulofilamentous structures.

26.2.4 Clinical Presentation

Inclusion body myositis is the most frequent acquired myopathy after 50 years of age. The first symptoms of weakness usually start after age 40 years (average 60 years). The male to female ratio is 2:1. The most frequent first clinical manifestation is weakness of the quadriceps muscles, leading to falls onto the knees and difficulty rising from a chair. Other muscle groups that are frequently affected at clinical onset are the finger flexors and pharyngeal muscles, the latter leading to dysphagia with obstructive symptoms such as inability to swallow and aspiration. Weakness of the finger flexors results in the inability to make a tight fist in which the fingernails are no longer visible (Fig. 26.4). The clinical involvement pattern is often asymmetrical. As the disease progresses over time, preferential muscle involvement

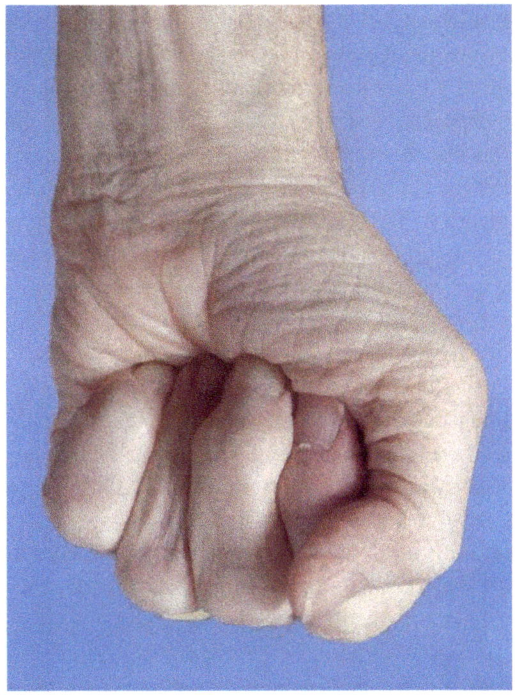

Fig. 26.4 Finger flexor weakness in inclusion body myositis. The patient is unable to conceal the fingernails when making a fist

continues, with ventral muscles of the legs and arms being most weakened. At the end stage, all muscles of the lower leg are experiencing weakness. Pain and malaise are usually not associated with IBM. IBM is slowly progressive and leads to major disabilities at the end-stage of the disease.

The serum creatine kinase (CK) activity is usually normal to mildly elevated (two to five times the upper limit). About half of IBM patients show reactivity toward a not yet specified 43-kDa muscle protein autoantigen.

26.2.5 Imaging Findings

26.2.5.1 Magnetic Resonance Imaging and Computed Tomography

The main findings visualized on magnetic resonance imaging (MRI) are fatty infiltration, inflammation, and atrophy of muscles. Fatty infiltration is the most common abnormality, and computed tomography (CT) can also be used to demonstrate it. The asymmetrical clinical manifestations are reflected in an asymmetrical involvement pattern on CT and MRI. The degree of fatty infiltration correlates with the duration of symptoms, the severity of weakness, and the functional disabilities. The extent of fatty infiltration is much greater than that seen in polymyositis. Changes suggestive of muscle edema on fat-suppressed T2-weighted MRI sequences—which are considered to indicate inflammation—are seen less frequently and do not correlate with disease duration or with severity of the disease.

The deep finger flexor is the first muscle in the forearm that shows signs of fatty degeneration. In the case that the deep finger flexor muscle is unaffected, the other forearm muscles are not likely to show abnormalities. Signs of discrete fatty infiltration of the deep finger flexors on MRI or CT may be clinically silent and can precede clinical symptoms of weakness (Fig. 26.5).

Fatty infiltration in the upper arm has no distinct involvement pattern. The shoulder girdle is less frequently affected by fatty degeneration than the upper arm. The subscapular muscle is most frequently affected in the shoulder girdle.

The legs are more commonly and more severely affected than the upper extremities or the pelvis. Overall, the lower legs usually have relatively less preserved muscle bulk than the upper legs. Anterior thigh compartment muscles are more affected than the posterior compartment muscles. The quadriceps femoris muscle frequently exhibits severe fatty degeneration, with a relative sparing of the rectus femoris muscle. Complete sparing of the entire quadriceps muscle is rather rare (Fig. 26.6). In general, all muscles of the lower legs can be involved, in particular the medial head of the gastrocnemius muscle, although it may not appear to be the clinically most involved lower leg muscle. The anterior compartment muscles are usually those most involved clinically. The lateral head is often relatively spared (Fig. 26.7). Atrophy is a common finding and shows a pattern similar to that of fatty infiltration. A combination of severe fatty infiltration of the deep finger flexors and the medial head of the gastrocnemius muscle, with sparing of the rectus femoris muscle, in an elderly

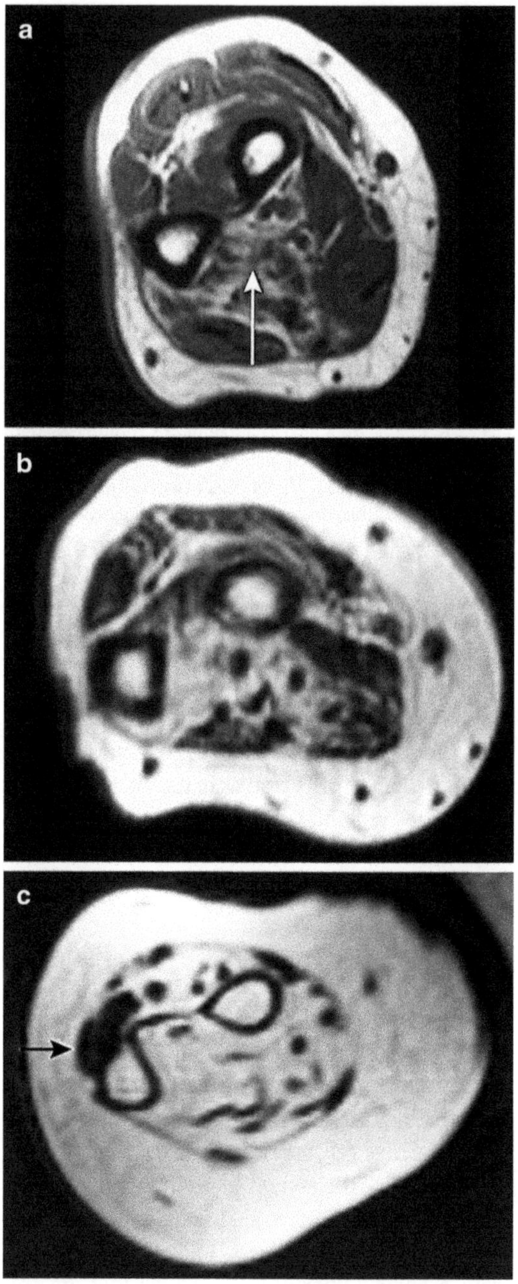

Fig. 26.5 Axial T1-weighted magnetic resonance imaging (MRI) scans of the right forearms of patients with inclusion body myositis. (**a**) Mild and isolated fatty infiltration of the deep finger flexor (*white arrow*). (**b**) Moderate fatty infiltration of the flexors (especially the deep finger flexors), in contrast to the less severely infiltrated extensor compartment. (**c**) Severely fatty infiltrated muscles, with relative sparing of the extensor carpi ulnaris (*black arrow*) muscle

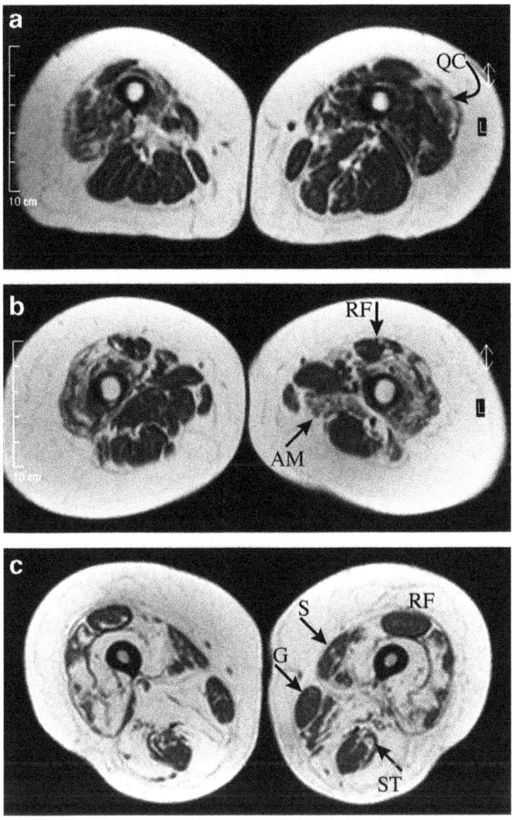

Fig. 26.6 Axial T1-weighted MRI scans of the thighs of patients with inclusion body myositis. (**a**) Mild, asymmetrical fatty infiltration of the quadriceps muscles (*QC*), with relative sparing of the rectus femoris muscle. (**b**) Moderate fatty infiltration of the quadriceps muscles with relative sparing of the rectus femoris muscle (*RF*). The left adductor magnus muscle (*AM*) is more severely affected than the right adductor magnus. (**c**) Severe fatty infiltration of almost all muscle groups with relative sparing of the rectus femoris (*RF*), semitendinosus (*ST*), sartorius (*S*), and gracilis (*G*) muscles

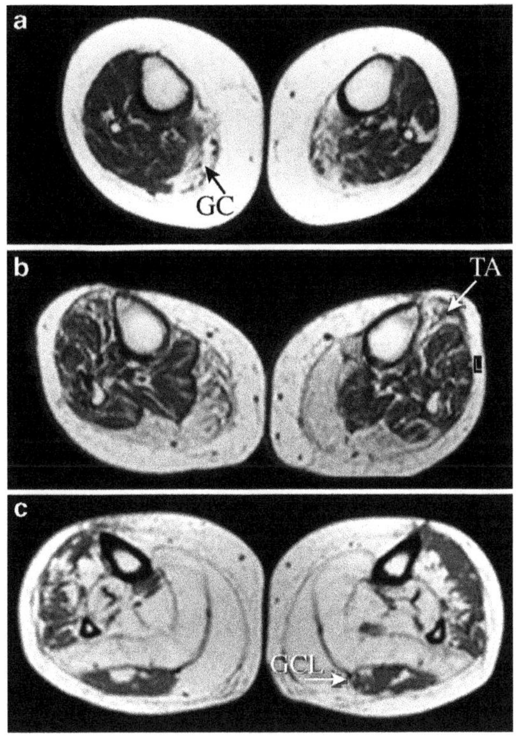

Fig. 26.7 Axial T1-weighted MRI scans of the lower legs of patients with inclusion body myositis. (**a**) Isolated fatty infiltration of the gastrocnemius muscles (*GC*). (**b**) More pronounced fatty infiltration of the gastrocnemius muscles and anterior tibial muscles (*TA*). (**c**) Severe, relatively symmetrical fatty infiltration of almost all posterior compartment muscles, with relative sparing of the lateral head of the gastrocnemius muscle (*GCL*). The anterolateral compartment is affected to a lesser degree

patient with no family history should prompt for a search for IBM. Hyperintensity on fat-suppressed T2-weighted images indicating edema suggestive of inflammation is randomly present. It is most frequently found in the extensor carpi ulnaris muscle in the forearms and the dorsal muscles of the lower leg (Fig. 26.8). In a series of 32 patients, inflammation was absent in the gluteal, obturatorius, and pectineus muscles and therefore should be regarded as highly uncommon in sporadic IBM.

26.2.5.2 Swallowing Video-fluoroscopy

Dysphagia, as described above, is common in IBM and can be visualized by video-fluoroscopy of the patient swallowing. Typically, repetitive swallowing, residues in the vallecular and piriform sinuses, and cricopharyngeal dysfunction (Fig. 26.9) can be observed. Diverticula and frank aspiration are seen less frequently.

26.2.6 Therapy

There is no effective treatment to slow progression of the disease. Immunosuppressive and immunomodulating therapy, including corticosteroids,

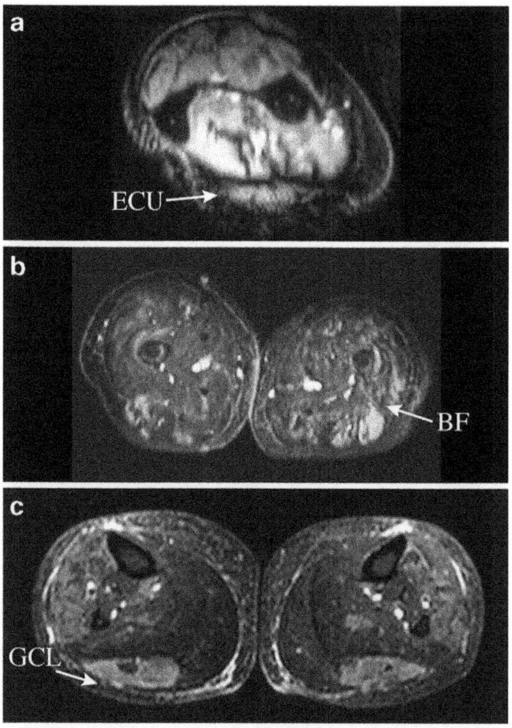

Fig. 26.8 Axial fat-suppressed T2-weighted MRI (short tau inversion recovery, STIR) scans of patients with inclusion body myositis. (**a**) Edema in the right extensor carpi ulnaris muscle (*ECU*). (**b**) Edema in the biceps femoris muscle (*BF*). (**c**) Edema in the lateral head of the gastrocnemius muscle (*GCL*). Corresponding T1-weighted images are shown in Fig. 26.7c

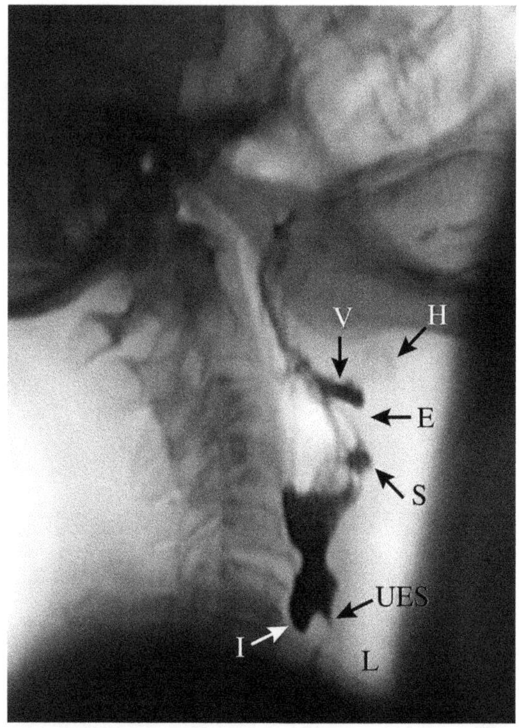

Fig. 26.9 Video-fluoroscopy of swallowing radiopaque fluid in upright position. Note the indentation (*I*) of the cricopharyngeal muscle near the upper esophageal sphincter (*UES*) and residues in the vallecular (*V*) and piriform (*S*) sinuses. Also shown are the hyoid bone (*H*), epiglottis (*E*), and larynx (*L*)

azathioprine, methotrexate, intravenous immunoglobulins, and β-interferon have not been shown to be effective. Obstructive dysphagia can sometimes be treated by cricopharyngeal myotomy or botulinum toxin injections. A percutaneous endoscopic gastrostomy tube is sometimes necessary in others to maintain nutrition and to prevent aspiration of oral intake.

26.2.7 Differential Diagnosis

Differentiation from polymyositis (PM) (see Sect. 26.3) is based on clinical information—presence or absence of pain and malaise, symmetrical versus asymmetrical weakness, waddling gait versus nonwaddling gait, high versus low serum CK activity—and histopathological criteria. However, the histopathological findings in IBM, particularly early in the disease course, are not always conclusive according to current diagnostic criteria. Muscle MRI can be helpful in the distinction as it shows more fatty infiltration in sporadic IBM than in PM. Furthermore, the combination of fatty infiltration of the flexor digitorum profundus and medial gastrocnemius muscles, with relative sparing of the rectus femoris muscle, may be highly indicative of sporadic IBM.

Compared to sporadic IBM, motor neuron disease (see Sect. 29.3) is a rapidly progressive disorder often presenting also with muscle cramps and fasciculations. The distribution of weakness is different, finger extensors are usually more affected than finger flexors—in contrast to the usual pattern in sporadic IBM. Welander myopathy (see Sect. 21.2.2), an autosomal dominantly inherited late-onset myopathy, presents with similar predominantly finger extensor weakness. Miyoshi myopathy (see Sect. 19.3) has early adult onset in the distal lower leg. It is caused by mutations in the dysferlin gene. Inflammation in muscle tissue may also be evident both histopathologically and on MRI. Markedly elevated serum CK activity, often 10–100 times normal, is usually present. Multifocal motor neuropathy presents with asymmetrical selective muscle weakness, often initially affecting the finger extensors. In contrast to sporadic IBM, electromyography often shows conduction blocks.

Inflammatory Myopathies: Sporadic Inclusion Body Myositis

Key Points

- IBM is the most frequent acquired myopathy of the elderly.
- Fatty infiltration is far more extensive than inflammation on muscle MRI.
- Fatty infiltration is present proximally as well as distally, and asymmetry is common.
- Signs of fatty degeneration are seen more frequently in anterior thigh muscles (with relative sparing of the rectus femoris) than in posterior thigh compartment (hamstring) muscles.
- Deep finger flexors are the first muscles in the forearm to be involved.
- A combination of severe fatty infiltration of the medial head of the gastrocnemius muscle, with relative sparing of the rectus femoris, and affliction of the deep finger flexors are indicative of IBM.

Suggestions for Further Reading

Cox FM, Verschuuren JJ, Verbist BM, et al. Detecting dysphagia in inclusion body myositis. J Neurol. 2009;256:2009–13.

Cox FM, Reijnierse M, van Rijswijk CS, et al. Magnetic resonance imaging of skeletal muscles in sporadic inclusion body myositis. Rheumatology (Oxford). 2011;50:1153–61.

Degardin A, Morillon D, Lacour A, et al. Morphologic imaging in muscular dystrophies and inflammatory myopathies. Skeletal Radiol. 2010;7:1219–27.

Dion E, Cherin P, Payan C, et al. Magnetic resonance imaging criteria for distinguishing between inclusion body myositis and polymyositis. J Rheumatol. 2002;29: 1897–1906.

Needham M, Mastaglia FL. Inclusion body myositis: current pathogenetic concepts and diagnostic and therapeutic approaches. Lancet Neurol. 2007; 6:620–31.

Phillips BA, Cala LA, Thickbroom GW, et al. Patterns of muscle involvement in inclusion body myositis: clinical and magnetic resonance imaging study. Muscle Nerve. 2001;24:1526–34.

Sekul EA, Chow C, Dalakas MC. Magnetic resonance imaging of the forearm as a diagnostic aid in patients with sporadic inclusion body myositis. Neurology. 1997;48:863–66.

26.3 Polymyositis

26.3.1 Synonyms, Abbreviations

PM

26.3.2 Genetics and Pathophysiology

Polymyositis (PM) is an inflammatory myopathy with presumed autoimmune pathogenesis. The current pathophysiological concept is based on CD8-positive cytotoxic T cells that attack nonnecrotic muscle fibers. The presence of proinflammatory cytokines and chemokines and overexpression of MHC-I on the surface of muscle fibers seem to play a key role in the formation of infiltrates of CD8-positive T cells, which persist over time. The antigenic target of the autoimmune attack is still unknown. Viruses are a potential trigger of the immune response, but auto-antigens expressed on the sarcolemma of the muscle fiber itself may be involved. Myositis-specific antibodies (MSAs) (e.g., anti-Jo antibodies) directed against histidyl-tRNA synthetase and antibodies against anti-aminoacyl-tRNA synthetases (ARS) have been found. The latter are rare and include anti-PL-7, anti-PL-12, anti-EJ, anti-OJ, anti-KS, anti-ZO, and anti-tyrosyl-tRNA synthetase antibodies. Patients usually do not have more than one of these anti-synthetase

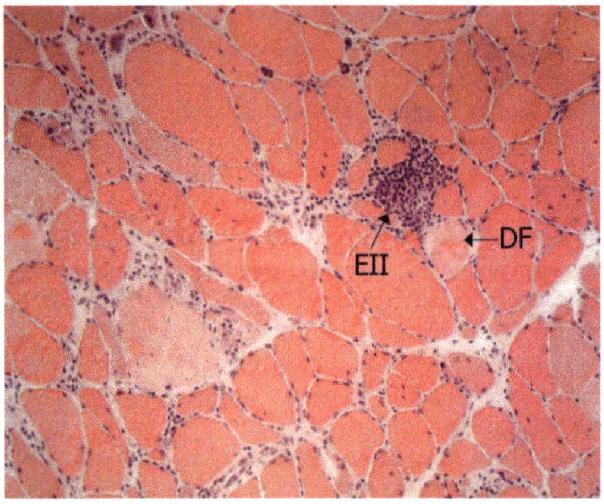

Fig. 26.10 Muscle biopsy of a patient with polymyositis. Note the variation in fiber size, degenerating muscle fibers (*DF*), and endomysial mononuclear inflammatory infiltrates (*EII*). (H&E)

antibodies. MSAs are present in around 40 % of PM patients. Anti Jo-1 is associated with the antisynthetase syndrome, a combination of interstitial lung disease, myositis, Raynaud phenomenon, and nonerosive arthritis. Patients with anti-SRP antibodies are clinically more diverse. They have a worse treatment effect and are associated with higher mortality. This antibody has lately become more frequently associated with necrotizing myopathy.

Polymyositis occurs as an isolated entity or in association with a connective tissue disease (CTD) or cancer. A retrospective study showed that fewer than 2 % of patients with an inflammatory myopathy had the histopathological features of definitive PM. Most patients have a histopathologically unspecified myositis, partly in conjunction with a CTD. PM is therefore considered an overdiagnosed entity. PM usually occurs sporadically, although familial clustering can occur, suggesting a genetic predisposition. PM is associated with the 8.1 HLA haplotype.

26.3.3 Histopathology

Polymyositis is histopathologically characterized by the presence of predominantly endomysial mononuclear infiltrates (Fig. 26.10) penetrating non-necrotic muscle fibers that express MHC-I molecules on the sarcolemma. These mononuclear infiltrates consist of mainly CD8-positive T cells, macrophages, and to a lesser degree B cells.

26.3.4 Clinical Presentation

Polymyositis presents with a subacute (weeks to months) onset of symmetrical weakness of proximal muscles, which can be accompanied by muscle pain, tenderness, fever, and nondestructive arthritis. It usually presents after the second decade of life. Onset before the age of 20 years should prompt a search for an alternative diagnosis, such as a muscular dystrophy with secondary inflammatory infiltrates (e.g., dysferlinopathy or facioscapulohumeral dystrophy). In about one-third of patients, PM is associated with a CTD according to the literature, but these groups most likely include patients with unspecified myositis. PM patients may have a higher chance of developing malignancy, but this is debatable. Accurate data are lacking because of the ill-defined entity of PM. If left untreated, the disease is progressive, leading to severe disability. Self-limiting disease has been reported in untreated patients. Often, however, it gives rise to severe chronic disability. MSA levels correlate with disease severity. Serum CK activity can be elevated to as high as 50 times the normal limit.

26.3.5 Imaging Findings

26.3.5.1 Magnetic Resonance Imaging

There are quite a few MRI studies on PM, especially those imaging the legs. However, a substantial number of these studies used the Bohan and Peter criteria and thus may have included IBM patients in their description of muscle involvement. Studies in which IBM patients are excluded show that inflammation and fatty infiltration are the most common findings in PM. Inflammation is far more common than fatty infiltration. Therefore, T2-weighted MRI with fat suppression provides the most useful sequences for detecting abnormalities in PM. As MRI findings in PM and dermatomyositis are similar, we refer the reader to the figures on dermatomyositis later in the Sect. 26.4.5.

Inflammation and fatty infiltration are both proximally and symmetrically located in the upper and lower extremities. Inflammation is frequently present in the vastus muscles, medial head of the gastrocnemius, and the tibialis anterior muscle. The gracilis muscles, extensor digitorum, tibial posterior muscle, flexor digitorum, flexor hallucis longus, and peroneal muscles are least affected. In contrast to IBM, there can be isolated inflammation in the absence of fatty infiltration, suggesting that inflammation seems to precede fatty infiltration.

The degree of fatty infiltration in the anterior part of the lower extremity is comparable to that in the posterior part. Preferentially, fatty infiltration can be observed in the vastus muscles, hamstrings, and gastrocnemius muscles. Relatively spared from fatty infiltration are the gracilis, rectus femoris, posterior tibial, and soleus muscles. These descriptions of fatty infiltration, however, should be interpreted cautiously, as wrongly included IBM cases may have corrupted these data.

Inflammatory changes have been reported to normalize after treatment, without a clinical correlation. However, this subject has not been investigated in large series.

For a final diagnosis, muscle biopsy is still the gold standard. However, it is not uncommon that a first muscle biopsy shows nonspecific changes, without the required inflammatory changes. Pathological sarcolemmal expression of MHC-I molecules may facilitate the diagnosis of PM. Weakness—in contrast to fatty infiltration—does not correlate with inflammatory changes on MRI. Sampling error may occur even in weak muscles because of the patchy distribution of the inflammation. Some authors advise muscle MRI scanning prior to biopsy to identify muscles that show inflammation and thus increase the yield of the muscle biopsy.

26.3.5.2 Ultrasonography

Although MRI is probably more sensitive for detecting inflammation than ultrasonography (US) because more muscles are investigated at once, and MRI imaging can better visualize the global pattern of muscle involvement, US can also be used to detect inflammation in muscles (see Chap. 2). Features in PM include increased muscle echo intensity and altered architecture of the fasciae/septa. Contrast-enhanced US is a way to measure blood flow in tissues. One study showed significantly higher blood flow velocity and blood volume in patients with PM and DM than in patients with comparable clinical characteristics who had a different myopathy or motor neuron disease.

26.3.6 Therapy

The initial goal of treatment is to improve muscle strength. Based on empirical data, high-dose prednisone for 6–8 weeks and then in tapering doses for approximately 1 year is the first-line treatment strategy. Alternatively, cycles of high-dose pulsed dexamethasone for 6 months can be given. Only 10 % of PM patients have an immediate remission after treatment with prednisone. In case of treatment failure, relapse, or unacceptable side effects, other immunosuppressive agents (e.g., azathioprine, methotrexate, cyclosporin A, cyclophosphamide) can be added. Treatment failure may be explained by a wrong diagnosis (see Differential Diagnosis, below), possibly due to a concurrent neoplasm or inadequate immunosuppressive treatment.

26.3.7 Differential Diagnosis

The differential diagnosis of PM includes DM and IBM. Chronic or treatment-resistant PM may have a clinical resemblance to sporadic IBM, apart from the histopathological overlap. It remains questionable whether these patients should be regarded as having sporadic IBM. DM is clinically similar but is distinguished by its cutaneous manifestations and different histopathology (discussed later in the chapter). Based on histopathology, muscular dystrophies such as the limb-girdle muscular dystrophies (see Chap. 19), facioscapulohumeral dystrophy (see Chap. 23), and dysferlinopathy (see Sect. 19.3)—which may show inflammatory changes suggestive of PM at first sight in the muscle biopsy—should be considered in the differential diagnosis. Pathological sarcolemmal MHC-I expression in the muscle biopsy may be helpful for discriminating between inflammatory myopathies and dystrophies. Endocrine, toxic, and infectious myopathies should also be considered in the differential diagnosis as they may have a clinical resemblance with subacute onset. Hypothyroid myopathy, for example, can resemble PM clinically. Infectious mimicking myopathies include human immunodeficiency virus (HIV)-related myopathy. Myopathies caused by toxins include corticosteroids, statins, antimalarials, and antipsychotics among others. Statins can cause rhabdomyolysis and nowadays are often linked to necrotizing myopathy (see Chap. 27). Autoimmune necrotizing myopathy is increasingly recognized as a separate disorder, different from PM.

Diseases of the neuromuscular junction, especially Lambert–Eaton myasthenic syndrome, can present with subacute proximal leg muscle weakness. Electrophysiological examination and the presence of antibodies against P/Q calcium channels lead to the correct diagnosis.

Inflammatory Myopathies: Polymyositis

Key Points

- Histopathologically definitive polymyositis is a rare disorder.
- MRI and ultrasound are of value in confirming the presence of inflammation.
- Abnormalities are proximal and symmetrical, with no preference for the anterior or posterior part of the upper leg.
- Inflammation seen on MRI scans can resolve with immunosuppressive treatment.

Suggestions for Further Reading

Bronner IM, van der Meulen MF, de VM, et al. Long-term outcome in polymyositis and dermatomyositis. Ann Rheum Dis. 2006;65:1456–61.

Dalakas MC. Inflammatory muscle diseases: a critical review on pathogenesis and therapies. Curr Opin Pharmacol. 2010;10:346–52.

Dion E, Cherin P, Payan C, et al. Magnetic resonance imaging criteria for distinguishing between inclusion body myositis and polymyositis. J Rheumatol. 2002;29:1897–1906.

Garcia J. MRI in inflammatory myopathies. Skeletal Radiol. 2000;29:425–38.

van der Meulen MF, Bronner IM, Hoogendijk JE, et al. Polymyositis: an overdiagnosed entity. Neurology. 2003;61:316–21.

van der Pas J, Hengstman GJ, ter Laak, HJ, et al. Diagnostic value of MHC class I staining in idiopathic inflammatory myopathies. J Neurol Neurosurg Psychiatry. 2004;75:136–9.

26.4 Dermatomyositis

26.4.1 Synonyms, Abbreviations

DM

26.4.2 Genetics and Pathophysiology

The pathogenetic molecular mechanisms leading to the initiation of autoimmunity in dermatomyositis (DM) remain unclear. DM is thought to be a complement-mediated microangiopathy. There is an association with cancer and with MSAs. Regenerating muscle fibers express high levels of MSAs, in contrast to normal muscle cells. MSAs are expressed in cancerous tissue as well. Possibly, an anticancer response not only targeting cancer cells but regenerating myofibers as well leads to an autoimmune attack against muscle tissue. The most common MSAs are anti-Mi-2 autoantibodies and anti-Jo-1 (associated with the antisynthetase syndrome), which are found in 25–30 % of DM patients. A more recently discovered autoantibody, anti-155/140, present in 13–21 % of DM patients, is associated with a markedly

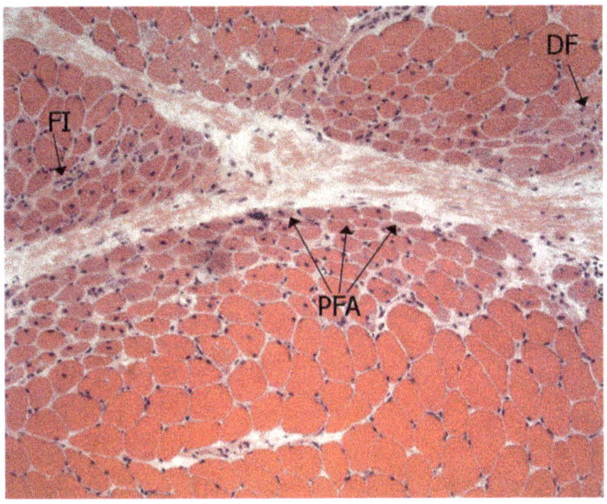

Fig. 26.11 Muscle biopsy of a patient with dermatomyositis. This biopsy shows perifascicular atrophy (*PFA*) with degenerating myofibers (*DF*) and scarce focal inflammation (*FI*). (H&E)

high risk of developing a malignancy. Melanoma differentiation-associated gene 5 is another MSA in DM patients, associated with only mild inflammation in the biopsy. DM is also associated with the 8.1 ancestral HLA haplotype.

26.4.3 Histopathology

Muscle biopsy may show a perifascicular distribution of atrophic, degenerating, and regenerating myofibers, especially in late stages of the disease (Fig. 26.11). The perifascicular location is probably due to destruction of capillaries in this region caused by a pathological deposition of immune complexes, such as membrane attack complex (MAC) of complement C5b-9. B cells are the predominant inflammatory cells found, together with plasmacytoid dendritic cells. They are part of the innate immune system, which plays an important role in antiviral and antitumor immune response. Skin biopsies reveal a cell-poor vacuolar interface dermatitis, where the inflammatory cells are located at the dermoepidermal junction as well as along vessel walls of the dermis. Because the immune response seen in muscle and skin biopsy specimens seems to be concentrated on the microvasculature, it is thought that capillaries are the primary target of the immune reaction in DM.

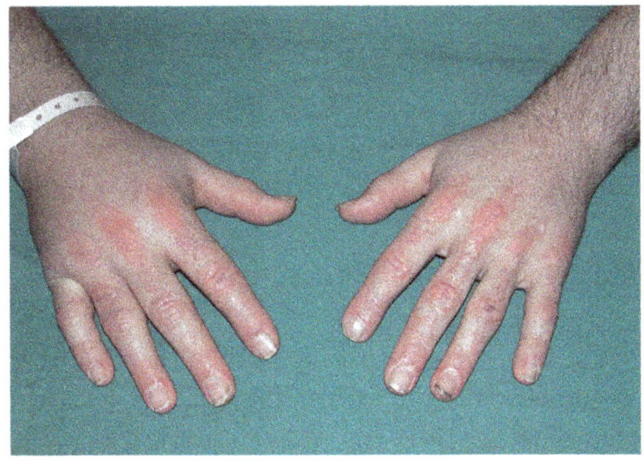

Fig. 26.12 Gottron's sign and papules in a patient with dermatomyositis

26.4.4 Clinical Presentation

The classic clinical presentation of DM is a subacute onset (weeks to months) of proximal and symmetrical muscle weakness. The first clinical manifestation can occur at any age, but peak incidence lies between 30 and 50 years of age. Women are affected twice as much as men. Muscle pain, especially exercise-induced pain, may be present. Characteristic for DM are the heliotrope rash: purplish discoloration around the eyes, sometimes with periorbital edema. Also characteristic is Gottron's sign, an erythematous or violet-colored symmetrical rash over the extensor surfaces of the metacarpophalangeal and interphalangeal joints, elbows, knees, and medial maleoli. This rash can evolve into a scaly eruption, called Gottron's papules (Fig. 26.12). Other characteristic skin abnormalities are a symmetrical rash in the neck area (the "shawl sign"); a rash on the cheeks, shoulders, back, or dorsal part of the extremities that is often aggravated by exposure to ultraviolet light; and poikiloderma atrophicans vasculare. Compatible other features are periungual erythema, skin ulcerations, lipodystrophy, alopecia, acanthosis nigrans, mechanics' hands, and livedo reticularis. The skin abnormalities may precede, occur in combination with, or appear after muscle involvement.

Dermatomyositis sine myositis, or amyopathic dermatomyositis, refers to a condition that shows the typical cutaneous manifestations of DM but no evidence of muscle weakness. However, when these patients are followed for up to 5 years, about 20 % of them are found to have developed muscle weakness. Patients who have muscle involvement based on evaluation of a muscle biopsy, electromyography, or MRI, but who have no apparent muscle weakness, are usually diagnosed as having hypomyopathic dermatomyositis.

Patients with DM have a higher risk of developing cancer compared to the general population, especially adenocarcinoma of the lung, colon, or rectum as well as ovarian and breast cancer. The overall risk of developing an associated cancer is highest during the first 3 years after the diagnosis, with a trend toward a decreased risk over time. Cancer can precede, occur simultaneously with, or appear after the diagnosis of DM. It is recommended that DM patients be screened for cancer at diagnosis and yearly thereafter for at least 3 years. Interstitial lung fibrosis and in rare cases cardiomyositis are also associated with DM.

In adults, the serum CK is slightly to moderately elevated (<10 times the upper limit of normal in 20–90 % of patients).

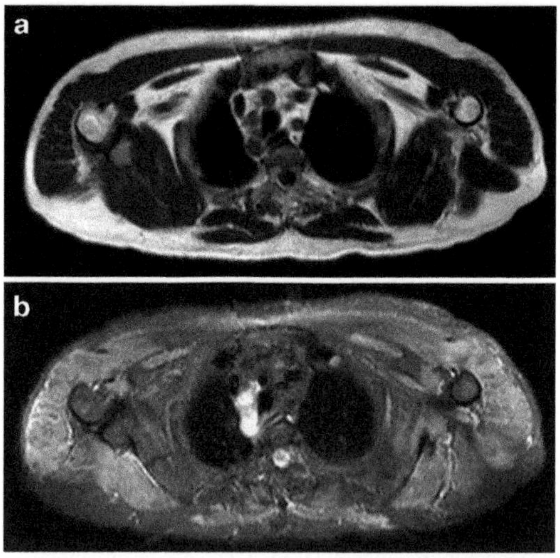

Fig. 26.13 Patient with dermatomyositis who complained of malaise, pain, and weakness lasting 7 weeks. (**a**) Axial T1-weighted MRI scans of the shoulder girdle show no signs of fatty infiltration. (**b**) Fat-suppressed T2-weighted images of the shoulder girdle show diffuse, symmetrical edematous abnormalities of all skeletal muscle groups including the pectoral muscles

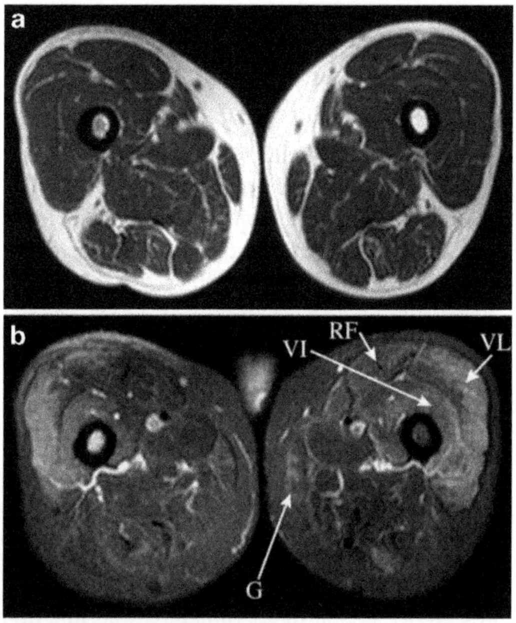

Fig. 26.14 Same patient as in Fig 26.13 with dermatomyositis. (**a**) Axial T1-weighted MRI scans of the upper leg show no signs of fatty infiltration. (**b**) Fat-suppressed T2-weighted images of the upper leg with more-or-less symmetrical edematous changes, compatible with inflammation, in the rectus femoris (*RF*), vastus intermedius (*VI*), vastus lateralis (*VL*), and gracilis (*G*) muscles

26.4.5 Imaging Findings

26.4.5.1 Magnetic Resonance Imaging

The published data on imaging findings in DM are limited. In general, MRI findings for DM are comparable to those found for PM. The most frequent abnormalities are areas with high signal intensities on fat-suppressed T2-weighted images, indicating edema suggestive of inflammation. These changes tend to be located proximally and are symmetrical (Figs. 26.13 and 26.14). Particularly, all four heads of the quadriceps femoris and the anterior part of the lower legs are involved. The thigh adductors, short head of the biceps femoris, pectineus, obturatorius, gracilis, soleus, and lateral head of the gastrocnemius are relatively spared. The inflammatory changes on MRI can be diffuse or focal. In the latter case, changes can be missed when only certain parts of the body are examined. Muscle calcification is rare in adults but more common after juvenile onset.

26.4.6 Therapy

Dermatomyositis can be treated with immunosuppressive agents such as corticosteroids. Immunosuppressive therapy should not always be the only therapeutic approach. As DM patients are at significant risk of having or developing a neoplasm, especially during the first 3 years after diagnosis, screening for cancer is mandatory. Such screening includes obtaining a thorough medical history, physical examination (including breast examination and rectal palpation), and laboratory testing. Age-appropriate cancer tests including CT of chest and abdomen, colonoscopy, and mammography are part of the screening. If DM is part of a paraneoplastic syndrome, surgical removal or pharmacological treatment of the primary neoplasm can result in disappearance of the clinical symptoms.

26.4.7 Differential Diagnosis

The differential diagnosis of DM includes PM (see Sect. 26.3) and IBM (see Sect. 26.2). The main clinical difference between PM/IBM and DM is the presence or absence of specific skin abnormalities. Also, the muscle biopsy shows discriminatory abnormalities, such as the mainly endomysial infiltrates in PM and IBM versus the mainly perimysial and perivascular infiltrates in DM. Systemic lupus erythematosus (SLE) may be difficult to discriminate on dermatological grounds. A skin biopsy can help differentiate between DM and SLE as the absence of immunoglobulin depositions at the dermoepidermal junctions makes SLE unlikely (although not impossible).

As for PM, other myopathies should also be considered, including muscular dystrophies and endocrine, toxic, and infectious myopathies.

Inflammatory Myopathies: Dermatomyositis

Key Points

- Dermatomyositis presents with proximal muscle weakness and characteristic cutaneous manifestations.
- Dermatomyositis is associated with malignancies, so screening for cancer is obligatory.
- Inflammation is the abnormality most commonly seen on MRI, possibly with a slight preference for the anterior thigh muscles in contrast to the posterior thigh muscles.

Suggestions for Further Reading

Dalakas MC. Review: an update on inflammatory and autoimmune myopathies. Neuropathol Appl Neurobiol. 2011;37:226–42.

Fujino H, Kobayashi T, Goto I, et al. Magnetic resonance imaging of the muscles in patients with polymyositis and dermatomyositis. Muscle Nerve. 1991; 14:716–20.

Mammen AL. Dermatomyositis and polymyositis: clinical presentation, autoantibodies, and pathogenesis. Ann N Y Acad Sci. 2010;1184:134–53.

Reimers CD, Schedel H, Fleckenstein JL et al. Magnetic resonance imaging of skeletal muscles in idiopathic inflammatory myopathies of adults. J Neurol. 1994;241:306–14.

Tomasová Studynková J, Charvát F, Jarosová K, et al. The role of MRI in the assessment of polymyositis and dermatomyositis. Rheumatology (Oxford). 2007;46: 1174–79.

Zampieri S, Valente M, Adami N et al. Polymyositis, dermatomyositis and malignancy: a further intriguing link. Autoimmun Rev. 2010;9:449–53.

Toxic and Drug-Induced Myopathies 27

Sören Peters and Rudolf Andre Kley

27.1 Introduction and Classification

Toxic and drug-induced myopathies as a group represent the most common form of myopathy with an estimated prevalence of more than 2,000 per 100,000 population in the Western Hemisphere. Patients with these myopathies often present to physicians who do not have the expertise of neuromuscular specialists. Failure to recognize the often iatrogenic nature of these disorders with ensuing continued exposure of the patient to the drug or toxin can unnecessarily prolong morbidity and lead to potentially fatal outcomes.

The clinical and morphological spectrum of toxic myopathies is almost as wide as the variety of drugs and toxins that can cause them. The clinical presentation may include weakness of varying intensity that is frequently proximally accentuated, mild-to-severe myalgias, exercise intolerance or cramps, elevated creatine kinase (CK) levels, and possible myoglobinuria. Symptoms occur mostly weeks to months after drug initiation or toxin exposure. In terms of clinical severity, the spectrum of possible clinical presentations ranges from asymptomatic hyperCKemia on one end of the scale to quadriplegic myopathy or acute rhabdomyolysis with concomitant myoglobinuria leading to renal failure and possible death from multiple organ failure on the other.

The myotoxic spectrum includes direct action on muscle cell organelles, induction of an inflammatory or autoimmune response, effects on neuromuscular transmission or peripheral nerve function, and systemic disturbances with secondary effects on muscle tissue or function (e.g., electrolyte imbalance, nutritional deficiencies) (see Table 27.1). Occupational and accidental exposure to industrial and environmental agents must also be taken into account. Also, additive myotoxic drug effects can occur in patients with preexisting muscle disease and have to be particularly considered in cases of otherwise inexplicable clinical deterioration.

In general, therapy of toxic myopathies is simple: discontinuation of drug exposure and/or removal of the toxin from the patients' environment (or the patient from the toxins' environment, whichever may be more feasible). If symptoms cease with time, a causative link to the offending drug or toxin is reasonable. Therapeutically, physical therapy can often be helpful, as physical inactivity has been postulated to increase susceptibility to toxic myopathy.

Magnetic resonance imaging (MRI) is an important paraclinical diagnostic tool, supplementing the information gained from the patient's

S. Peters (✉)
Berufsgenossenschaftliches Universitätsklinikum Bergmannsheil, Institut für Radiologische Diagnostik, Interventionelle Radiologie und Nuklearmedizin, Bürkle-de-la-Camp-Platz 1, Bochum 44789, Germany
e-mail: soeren.peters@rub.de

R.A. Kley
Department of Neurology, Neuromuscular Center Ruhrgebiet, University Hospital Bergmannsheil, Ruhr-University Bochum, Bochum, Germany
e-mail: rudolf.kley@rub.de

M.P. Wattjes and D. Fischer (eds.), *Neuromuscular Imaging*, DOI 10.1007/978-1-4614-6552-2_27,

Table 27.1 Spectrum of pathologies, clinical features, and respective agents causing drug-induced myopathy

Pathology	Histopathology	Typical clinical features	Main agents
Necrotizing myopathy	Scattered muscle fiber necrosis and degeneration, invasion by macrophages	Acute proximal weakness, myalgias, rhabdomyolysis, elevated CK	Alcohol, drugs, cyclosporine, ε-aminocaproic acid, fibrates, labetalol, propofol, statins, snake venoms
Inflammatory myopathy	Perimysial, endomysial or perivascular invasion by T-lymphocytes and macrophages, MHC-1-expression	Acute or gradual onset proximal and distal weakness, myalgias, dysphagia, elevated CK, myocarditis, conduction block	α-Interferon, cimetidine, D-penicillamine, hydroxyurea, imatinib, intramuscular gene therapy, L-dopa, L-tryptophan, lamotrigine, phenytoin, procainamide, statins, minocycline, toxic-oil-syndrome
Type II muscle fiber atrophy	Atrophy of type II fibers	Proximal weakness and atrophy, normal CK	Corticosteroids
Thick filament loss myopathy	Atrophy of muscle fibers, scattered necrotic fibers, focal or diffuse loss of thick filaments	Acute quadriplegic myopathy/critical illness myopathy, respiratory failure, normal or elevated CK	Corticosteroids, neuromuscular blocking agents (vecuronium, atracurium)
Mitochondrial myopathy	"ragged red"-, "ragged blue"-, COX-negative fibers, lipid accumulation, nemaline rods, cytoplasmic bodies, necrosis, fiber size variability, (inflammation)	Acute or gradual onset proximal and distal weakness, myalgias, painful sensorimotor neuropathy, rhabdomyolysis, normal or elevated CK	Fialuridine, germanium, zidovudine (AZT) and other nucleoside analogs, trichlorethylene (TCE)
Antimicrotubular myopathy	Lysosome accumulation, autophagic vacuoles/inclusions, MHC class I positive muscle fibers, myofibrillar disorganization	Acute or gradual onset proximal and distal weakness, myalgias, sensorimotor neuropathy, normal or elevated CK	Colchicine, vincristine
Ampiphilic drug myopathy	Myeloid storage in lysosomes, autophagic vacuoles, strong acid phosphatase staining	Acute or gradual onset proximal and distal weakness, myalgias, sensorimotor neuropathy, elevated CK	Amiodarone, chloroquine, emetine/ipecac, hydroxychloroquine, quinacrine, perhexiline, doxorubicin, chlorphenteramine, chlorcyclizine, triparanol, iprindol, local anesthetics
Emetine myopathy	Breakdown of myofilaments, accumulation of myofibrillar proteins, mitochondrial degeneration, muscle fiber necrosis and regeneration, motheaten muscle fibers	Acute or gradual onset proximal and distal weakness, myalgias, stiffness, elevated CK, rhabdomyolysis	Emetine/ipecac
Hyaline myopathy	Subsarcolemmal inclusions	Acute or gradual onset proximal and distal weakness, myalgias, elevated CK	Statins
Hypokalemic myopathy	Scattered necrotic fibers and vacuoles	Acute onset, proximal or generalized weakness, (myalgias), low potassium, elevated CK, myoglobinuria	Alcohol, amphotericin, corticosteroids, cottonseed oil, diuretics, laxatives, licorice, carbenoxolone, lithium, barium, methylxanthines (caffeine, theophylline), toluene
Fasciitis	Perimysial and perivascular inflammation (macrophages), thickening of fascia	Proximal weakness, myalgia, cramps, eosinophilia	L-tryptophan, toxic-oil-syndrome
Focal myopathy	Inflammation, fiber size variability, endomysial fibrosis	Indurated muscles, stiffness, mild muscle weakness	Injections of: heroin, penicillin, meperidine, pentazocine, diphenhydramine, piritramid, pethidine, triamcinolone

CK creatine kinase, *MHC-I* major histocompatibility complex type I and family history, laboratory and genetic work-up, and electrodiagnostic studies. For toxic myopathies, imaging the lower extremities in the transverse plane is sufficient, as this plane best lends itself to delineating muscle anatomy. T1-weighted sequences for anatomical imaging and detection of lipomatous muscle changes and fat-saturated T2 weighted sequences (e.g. short tau inversion recovery, or STIR) for depicting muscle edema are needed for examining cases of suspected toxic myopathy. Contrast medium is not mandatory except in cases where a neoplasm or infectious disease (e.g. abscess, fasciitis) is considered in the differential diagnosis.

MRI does not offer specific findings attributable to toxic myopathy per se, meaning that it does not facilitate identification of the responsible toxin or offending agent because there is no specific disease pattern in toxic myopathies. Muscle edema in proximal muscle groups is the MRI hallmark of acute toxic myopathy. It is especially pronounced in rhabdomyolysis. T1-weighted MRI often shows only subtle to moderate (if any) diffuse reticular lipomatous changes in muscle. Indeed, pronounced lipomatous muscle change is, as a rule, evidence against toxic myopathy. In cases of subsided rhabdomyolysis, however, lipomatous involution of necrotized tissue is a recognized effect. One must keep in mind also that in chronic cases of toxic myopathy, both T1- and fat saturated T2-weighted images can be completely unremarkable.

This chapter focuses on the drugs and toxins most commonly implicated in toxic myopathy: statins, steroids, and alcohol.

27.2 Statin-Induced Myopathy

27.2.1 Synonyms and Abbreviations

Statin myopathy

27.2.2 Introduction

Statins serve as competitive inhibitors of 3-hydroxy 3-methyl glutaryl coenzyme A (HMG-CoA) reductase, the rate-limiting enzyme in cholesterol synthesis, Their action ultimately leads to a decrease in serum cholesterol concentration. They are a mainstay of modern cardiovascular therapy, widely prescribed, and the most extensively examined causative agents of toxic myopathy. With statin monotherapy, a myopathy may manifest as muscle pain or soreness, weakness, and/or cramps with a >10-fold increase in the serum CK level, which is encountered at a prevalence of 0.1–0.5 %. The prevalence increases to 1–7 % in patients on polytherapy or with multiple risk factors.

As a group, lipophilic statins (atorvastatin, fluvastatin, lovastatin, simvastatin) have greater myotoxic potential than hydrophilic statins (pravastatin, rosuvastatin). Individually, simvastatin ranks as the most potentially myotoxic statin, followed by atorvastatin, lovastatin, pravastatin, and ending with fluvastatin.

27.2.3 Pathophysiology

As inhibitors of HMG-CoA reductase, statins restrict the production of mevalonate, an intermediary metabolite in cholesterol synthesis. Statins also restrict production of ubiquinone and coenzyme Q10 which are important intermediaries in the respiratory enzyme chain, needed for electron transport during oxidative phosphorylation. This latter effect is thought to constitute the underlying cause of statin-induced myopathy which manifests clinically as myalgia and exercise intolerance. Mitochondrial myopathy has been associated with statin use. In fact, it is statins' effect on the mitochondria and sarcoplasmic reticulum of type 2 muscle fibers that helps explain their myopathic potential: type 2 muscle fibers contain 30 % less fat than type 1 muscle fibers, rendering them more susceptible to a paucity of cholesterol for membrane synthesis.

As statins are metabolized by CYP3A4 to varying degrees (with the exception of pravastatin, which is cleared via the renal system), drugs that inhibit CYP3A4 can variably lead to elevated statin levels and exacerbate statin myotoxicity. These drugs include macrolide antibiotics (e.g., erythromycin), azole antifungals (e.g., ketoconazole), calcium channel blockers (e.g. verapamil), selective serotonin reuptake inhibitors (SSRIs), cyclosporin, and, do not forget, grapefruit juice, to name but a few. Of the 601 cases of rhabdomyolysis in patients taking simvastatin reported to the U.S. Food and Drug Administration from November 1997 to March 2000, 55 % were due to combination therapy. Furthermore, the elderly, diabetic patients, patients on a high-dose statin or combination statin-fibrate therapy, and patients with hypothyroidism, chronic renal failure, or hepatobiliary disease are particularly prone to statin-induced myopathy.

Genetics play a limited role in statin-induced myopathies, as elucidated in the SEARCH (Study of the Effectiveness of Additional Reductions in Cholesterol and Homocysteine) and STRENGTH (Statin Response Examined by Genetic Haplotype Markers) studies. Both studies demonstrated reduced-function single nucleotide polymorphisms of the *SLCO1B1* gene, which plays a role in the regulation of hepatic uptake of statins, in patients with atorvastatin-, pravastatin- and, especially, simvastatin-associated myopathies. Their findings stress the role of vulnerability to statin-induced myopathy as a drug-specific (rather than a drug-class effect) in genetically predisposed patients. These genetic insights have the potential to guide drug regimens according to genetic predisposition, i.e. individual risk profiles, for myopathic side-effects. Genetic polymorphisms in the CYP450 system are also thought to be at the root of some individual patients' susceptibility to statin-induced myopathy.

27.2.4 Histopathology

Histopathological findings in less severe cases of statin-induced myopathy include unspecific changes such as internal nuclei, fiber splitting, atrophic fibers, mild endomysial fibrosis, and a few necrotic fibers. Hyaline myopathy with subsarcolemmal inclusions has also been described. Neurogenic changes as fiber type grouping and small angular fibers may also occur indicating a supplementary statin-induced peripheral neuropathy. Uncommonly, statin-induced myopathy will present histologically as an immune-mediated inflammatory myopathy with autoinvasive T-cells and upregulation of MHC-1, akin to polymyositis. Rhabdomyolysis presents histologically as a necrotizing myopathy (Fig. 27.1).

27.2.5 Clinical Presentation

The most commonly reported finding is asymptomatic hyperCKemia, which is thought to occur in roughly 5 % of all patients taking statins. The most common clinical muscular side effect is myalgia, reported in 1.5–3 % of patients in randomized controlled trials and up to >10 % in day-to-day practice. In these cases, muscle strength is often normal and CK levels may be normal. More severe cases present with proximal muscle weakness and marked elevations of CK up to >10 times the upper limit of normal. Symptoms occur, as a rule, 1–3 months to 2 years after treatment initiation and abate days to weeks, rarely months, after drug cessation. As glutamic oxaloacetic transaminase, glutamate pyruvate transaminase and γ-glutamyl transferase are often elevated concurrently with CK, care must be taken not to confuse myopathy with liver toxicity, which is known to accompany statin treatment.

Rhabdomyolysis represents the most severe manifestation of statin-induced myopathy, and has been reported in 0.02–0.04 % of patients across all currently prescribed statins, with one fatal case per five million statin users. Concomitant medication may raise the prevalence of rhabdomyolysis to 0.22 %. Rhabdomyolysis manifests clinically as intense pain, muscle swelling with possible secondary compartment syndrome, and weakness developing within a period of up to 48 h. CK levels can reach 2000 times the upper limit of normal, and concurrent myoglobinuria can lead to oliguric renal failure.

27.2.6 Imaging Findings

Similar to toxic myopathy in general, statin-induced myopathy renders a non-specific pattern of myopathic changes without topical selectivity. In statin-induced myopathy, however, dorsal muscle groups of both thighs and legs tend to be more prone to pathological changes (Fig. 27.2g–i). STIR imaging will reveal edema in cases of acute

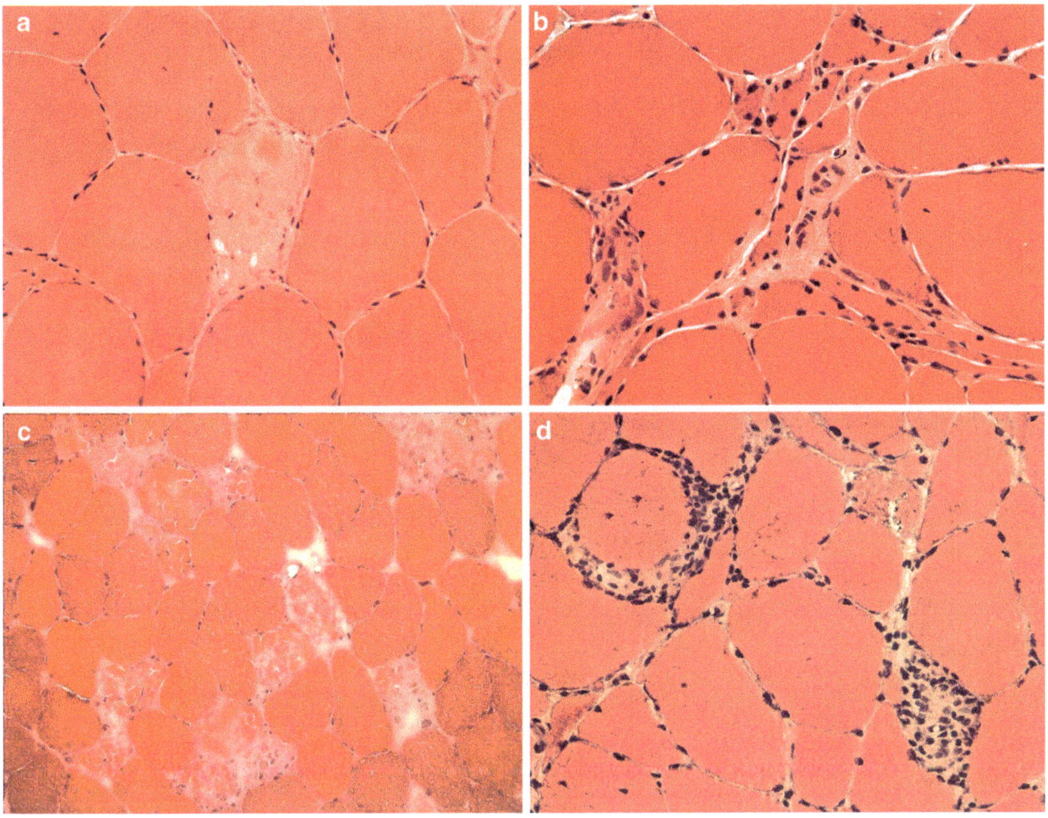

Fig. 27.1 Histological findings in statin-induced myopathy (H&E). (**a**) Necrotic fiber, atrophic fibers, and fiber splitting. (**b**) Fiber necrosis, degenerating and regenerating fibers, and endomysial fibrosis. (**c**) Rhabdomyolysis with scattered fiber necrosis. (**d**) Uncommon presentation with inflammatory cell infiltrates

toxic myopathy (Fig. 27.2a–c), especially rhabdomyolysis (Fig. 27.2d–f). If there is no edema on STIR imaging, there is no active myopathy.

Edema in rhabdomyolysis is often asymmetrical, patchy, and often centered on deep muscle groups, with relative sparing of superficial muscle groups, and associated with muscle swelling. Contrast enhancement of affected muscles is prominent in rhabdomyolysis in contrast to myositis. As a rule, MRI changes due to rhabdomyolysis regress 8–12 weeks after discontinuation of toxin exposure. Pathological imaging that persists more than 12 weeks after drug discontinuation should prompt a search for an alternative diagnosis.

T1-weighted MRI often shows only subtle to moderate, diffusely reticular lipomatous changes of muscle. Cases of subsided rhabdomyolysis demonstrate lipomatous involution of necrotized tissue.

27.2.7 Therapy

Drug discontinuation because of side effects must always be weighed against possible negative consequences to patients' health as patients with relevant cardiovascular or cerebrovascular risk factors undoubtedly benefit from statins. In patients with mild symptoms, a "wait-and-see" approach might be considered, as mild symptoms can disappear over the course of a few weeks. In some instances, switching to a less toxic member of the same class of drugs might be viable—i.e., switching from a lipophilic statin (e.g., simvastatin) to a hydrophilic statin (e.g., pravastatin). Alternate-day or once-a-week dosing can also help circumvent this problem, with studies demonstrating effective lowering of low-density lipoprotein cholesterol and triglyceride levels using alternative dosing schedules in patients with prior statin intolerance.

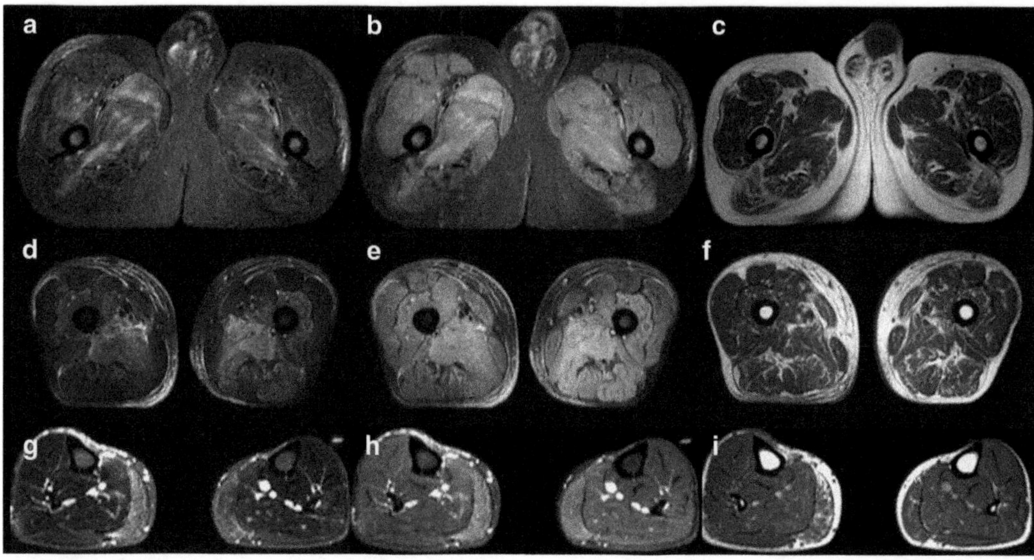

Fig. 27.2 Imaging spectrum of statin-induced myopathy. (**a–c**) A 56-year-old man with myalgia and moderately elevated creatine kinase (CK) after 12 months of simvastatin therapy. Short tau inversion recovery (STIR) MRI scans. (**a**) "Long" STIR. (**b**) "Short" STIR. Note the edema in the proximal adductors (m. adductor longus, m. adductor magnus)— more prominent on the right—and the right ventral thigh muscle group (m. vastus intermedius, m. vastus lateralis) with nonspecific subcutaneous edema of the ventrolateral thighs. (**c**) T1-weighted MRI reveals nonspecific, unrelated fatty changes of the dorsal thigh muscle groups but no corresponding lipomatous signal changes in edematous muscle. These findings are consistent with chronic inflammatory toxic myopathy. (**d–f**) A 67-year-old man with myalgia, muscle proximal weakness, myoglobinuria, and excessively elevated CK shortly after initiation of simvastatin therapy. STIR images (**d**, "long" STIR; **e**, "short" STIR) exhibit extensive edematous signal changes in the thigh musculature—more pronounced on the left (m. vastus intermedius, m. vastus lateralis, m. vastus medialis, m. adductor magnus, m. biceps femoris, m. semimembranosus)—with accompanying subcutaneous edema. (**f**) T1-weighted MRI shows unrelated extensive reticular lipomatous changes in all muscle groups, particularly the hamstrings. The imaging is compatible with the clinical presentation of rhabdomyolysis and a histological diagnosis of necrotizing myopathy. (**g–i**) A 62-year-old man after 24 months of ezetimibe and simvastatin therapy. He presented with myalgia, mildly elevated CK, and symptom duration of 20 months. STIR images (**g**, "long" STIR; **h**, "short" STIR) display edema in the dorsal leg muscle groups (m. soleus, m. gastrocnemius medialis)—more pronounced on the right. (**i**) T1-weighted MRI reveals circumscribed corresponding fatty changes, compatible with, but not prerequisite for, long-standing toxic myopathy. He had superficial varicoses and subcutaneous signal changes, particularly of the ventral right leg. The findings indicate a chronic, but active, inflammatory toxic myopathy. From Peters SA, et al (2010) MRI in lipid-lowering agent–associated myopathy: a retrospective review of 21 cases. AJR Am J Roentgenol. 194(4):W323–8. Reprinted with permission from American Roentgen Ray Society

If symptoms persist a few months after drug discontinuation, coenzyme Q10 supplementation can be considered. Trials using 100–200 mg of coenzyme Q10 daily showed varying positive effects or no benefit whatsoever, but this dosage may be too low. Based on empirical data, a daily dose up to 600–800 mg has been recommended. In cases of statin-induced inflammatory myopathy, steroids or intravenous immunoglobulin should be administered.

Rhabdomyolysis should entail immediate discontinuation of the offending agent and symptomatic and supportive therapy in an intermediate or intensive care unit, including nephrological support with close monitoring of renal function and electrolyte balance. Relevant muscle swelling and possible subsequent compartment syndrome should prompt intracompartment pressure monitoring and surgical intervention.

A diagnosis of hitherto unrecognized myopathy (e.g., inflammatory, mitochondrial) must be entertained and pursued if symptoms continue despite therapy. Muscle biopsy might be warranted to identify any underlying primary myopathy.

Key Points

- Statin-induced myopathy—defined by myalgia, weakness, and elevation in serum CK to more than 10 times the upper limit of normal—occurs in 0.1–0.5 % of patients on statin monotherapy. Rhabdomyolysis is the most severe manifestation of statin myotoxicity and constitutes a medical emergency.
- Simvastatin has the greatest myotoxic potential, followed by atorvastatin, lovastatin, pravastatin, and fluvastatin. Concomitant medication, use of high statin doses, old age, obesity, diabetes mellitus, hypothyroidism, renal failure, hepatobiliary disease, and genetic variation at the *SLCO1B1* gene locus can increase the risk of statin-induced myopathy
- Histological findings range from unspecific changes, hyaline myopathy or inflammatory myopathy to necrotizing myopathy.
- There are no disease-specific findings on MRI. MRI does demonstrate muscle edema on STIR images in the presence of acute statin myopathy, with a predilection for dorsal muscle groups of the legs and thighs. Edema is pronounced, patchy, and asymmetrical in rhabdomyolysis. T1-weighted images often show only subtle to moderate, diffusely reticular lipomatous changes in muscle.
- Therapy mainly consists of switching to another statin or an alternative lipid-lowering agent, alternate-day dosing, or drug discontinuation.

Suggestions for Further Reading

Bruckert E, Hayem G, Dejager S, et al. Mild to moderate muscular symptoms with high-dosage statin therapy in hyperlipidemic patients—the PRIMO study. Cardiovasc Drugs Ther. 2005;19(6):403–14.

Dalakas MC. Toxic and drug-induced myopathies. J Neurol Neurosurg Psychiatry. 2009;80:832–8.

El-Salem K, Ababneh B, Rudnicki S, et al. Prevalence and risk factors of muscle complications secondary to statins. Muscle Nerve. 2009;44(6):877–81.

Mastaglia FL. Drug induced myopathies. Pract Neurol. 2006;6:4–13.

Mor A, Mitnick HJ, Pillinger MH, et al. Drug-induced myopathies. Bull NYU Hosp Jt Dis. 2009;67(4):358–69.

Peters SA, Kley R, Tegenthoff M, et al. MRI in lipid-lowering agent-associated myopathy: a retrospective review of 21 cases. AJR Am J Roentgenol. 2010;194:W323–8.

Study of the Effectiveness of Additional Reductions in Cholesterol and Homocysteine (SEARCH) Collaborative Group; Armitage J, Bowman L, et al. (2010) Intensive lowering of LDL cholesterol with 80 mg versus 20 mg simvastatin daily in 12,064 survivors of myocardial infarction: a double-blind randomised trial. *Lancet* 2010;376(9753):1658–69.

SEARCH Collaborative Group; Link E, Parish S, et al. SLCO1B1 variants and statin-induced myopathy—a genome-wide study. N Engl J Med. 2008;359:789–99.

Valiyil R, Christopher-Stine L. Drug-related myopathies of which the clinician should be aware. Curr Rheumatol Rep. 2010;12:213–20.

Voora D, Shah SH, Spasiojevic I, et al. The SLCO1B1*5 genetic variant is associated with statin-induced side effects. J Am Coll Cardiol. 2009;54(17):1609–16.

27.3 Glucocorticoid-Induced Myopathy

27.3.1 Synonyms and Abbreviations

Steroid-induced myopathy, Steroid myopathy

27.3.2 Introduction

Given the fact that steroid treatment is used for a wide spectrum of diseases, glucocorticoid-induced myopathy is a particularly common myopathy. It was first recognized and described by Harvey Cushing in 1932. Whereas many of the other substances known to cause toxic myopathy do so in a limited number of patients, suggesting idiosyncratic vulnerability, glucocorticoids produce a dose-dependent myotoxic effect and induce myopathic symptoms in any individual patient treated with a sufficient cumulative dosage, akin to a stochastic effect. Myopathic side effects are particularly common with 9-α-fluorinated corticosteroids (dexamethasone, betamethasone, triamcinolone) compared to non-fluorinated corticosteroids (e.g. hydrocortisone, prednisone).

The incidence of myopathy during long-term therapy (ranging from weeks to years) has been reported to reach 60 %. Myopathy has clinically been observed during long-term treatment with doses of as little as 10 mg of prednisone or prednisone equivalents per day. More commonly, patients become symptomatic with a daily dose of 20–30 mg or more. Symptoms may present as soon as 1 month after treatment initiation. Cancer patients and the elderly are particularly at risk, and women are more susceptible than men (2:1).

27.3.3 Pathophysiology

Both chronic exogenous application and excess endogenous production of steroids, as in Cushing's disease, can induce myopathy. The underlying pathophysiological mechanism is thought to be reduced protein synthesis, enhanced catabolism and proteolysis, and induction of apoptosis. Glucocorticoids inhibit the stimulatory effects of insulin, insulin-like growth factor-I (IGF-I), and amino acids, especially leucine, on the protein synthesis machinery. They also impair myogenesis through downregulation of myogenin. Increased protein breakdown results from activation of the ubiquitin proteasome system (UPS), mediated through increased expression of UPS components and atrogenes such as atrogin-1 and MuRF-1, the lysosomal system, and calpains. The induction of transcription factor FOXO and increased expression of myostatin also play an important role in catabolism and downregulation of protein synthesis, leading to atrophy of muscle fibers. Apoptosis in glucocorticoid-induced myopathy seems to be triggered by Fas–Fas ligand signals and increased levels of pro-apoptotic proteins.

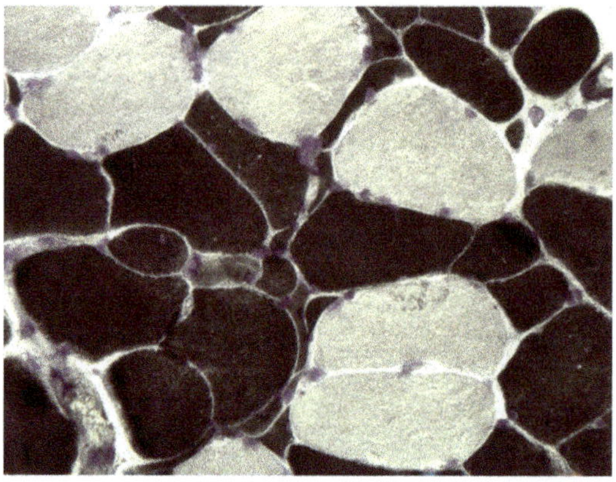

Fig. 27.3 Histological findings in glucocorticoid-induced myopathy (ATPase 9.4 stain). Selective atrophy of type 2 fibers (type 2 fibers are stained *dark* and type 1 fibers *light*)

27.3.4 Histopathology

The histological hallmark of glucocorticoid-induced myopathy is atrophy of type 2 fibers with little or no impact on type 1 fibers (Fig. 27.3). Additional findings may include vacuolization of muscle fibers and glycogen deposits, mitochondrial abnormalities, lipid bodies, and scattered necrotic fibers. In acute quadriplegic myopathy, electron microscopy may reveal a characteristic pattern of selective loss of myosin filaments in sarcomeres. Histological changes are nonspecific.

27.3.5 Clinical Presentation

The most common clinical presentation is chronic proximal muscle weakness and atrophy, particularly affecting the quadriceps muscles, with involvement of neck flexor muscles. Depending on the route of administration (oral, inhaled or parenteral), symptoms can focus on those organs most directly in contact with the applied corticosteroid, leading to dysphonia in laryngeal myopathy with use of inhaled steroids, for instance, and diaphragmatic myopathy especially in asthmatics. Pain is not a common clinical feature. Serum CK is usually normal. In cases of elevated CK, an alternative underlying cause of myopathy should be considered.

A particular problem in steroid-induced myopathy is exacerbation of a primary myopathy for which corticosteroids were initially prescribed. In inflammatory myopathies, a secondary steroid-induced myopathy can coexist, potentially worsening the clinical presentation. Rising CK levels and a florid myopathic pattern on electromyography favor a primary inflammatory disease as the main culprit, entailing an augmentation of the corticosteroid therapy. In unequivocal cases, muscle biopsy is often required to distinguish between the two entities. Clinically, a cushingoid habitus or other steroid-induced side effects may point to steroid-induced myopathy, as can the emergence of symptoms on chronic high steroid doses, rather than when the dose is being tapered, which in turn suggests exacerbation of a primary myopathy. Discontinuation of steroids should lead to symptom amelioration after 3–4 weeks for steroid-induced myopathy, but exacerbation of inflammatory myopathy.

A further serious variant of steroid-induced myopathy is acute quadriplegic myopathy, historically known as acute illness myopathy, acute steroid-induced myopathy, or critical care myopathy. Transplant recipients and severely affected asthmatics receiving high doses of intravenous glucocorticoids are particularly prone, as are patients under non-depolarizing neuromuscular blockade. Clinically, In addition to profound muscle weakness, which develops over a matter of days, depressed tendon reflexes, hypotonia and respiratory muscle weakness are clinical features. The latter can give rise to difficulty weaning the patient from assisted ventilation. CK levels are mildly elevated in around 50 % of patients. They are rarely excessively elevated. Mortality rates can reach 30 %. Death is due to sepsis and multiple organ failure.

27.3.6 Imaging Findings

The involvement pattern of steroid-induced myopathy on MRI is non-specific and comparable to those seen in other toxic myopathies. Fat-suppressed T2-weighted (e.g., STIR) MRI shows pathology in acute quadriplegic myopathy akin to that seen with rhabdomyolysis: edema that is often asymmetrical, patchy, and often centered on deep muscle groups with relative sparing of superficial muscle groups (Fig. 27.4c–e). Chronic cases may exibit diffuse, often reticular lipomatous alterations of muscle and generalized muscle atrophy (Fig. 27.4f–h).

Simultaneous presentation of steroid-induced myopathy and immune-mediated myopathy for which steroids may have been prescribed in the first place remains a diagnostic challenge (Fig. 27.4a, b). In this scenario, MRI can help detect any active myopathy, such as in exacerbated inflammatory myopathy. In most cases of toxic myopathy, symptoms abate after drug discontinuation, mirrored by improvement or resolution of MRI images within 1–6 months. If symptoms persist, an alternative diagnosis must be entertained.

27.3.7 Therapy

Drug discontinuation or dose reduction below a threshold level is the mainstay of treatment of steroid-induced myopathy. Drug discontinuation must always be weighed against possible negative consequences to the patient's health, as discontinuing corticosteroids in patients needing immunosuppression can lead to dramatic relapses. Alternate-day dosing can be considered. Amelioration of symptoms should become evident after 3–4 weeks. Fluorinated steroids (e.g., dexamethasone) should be

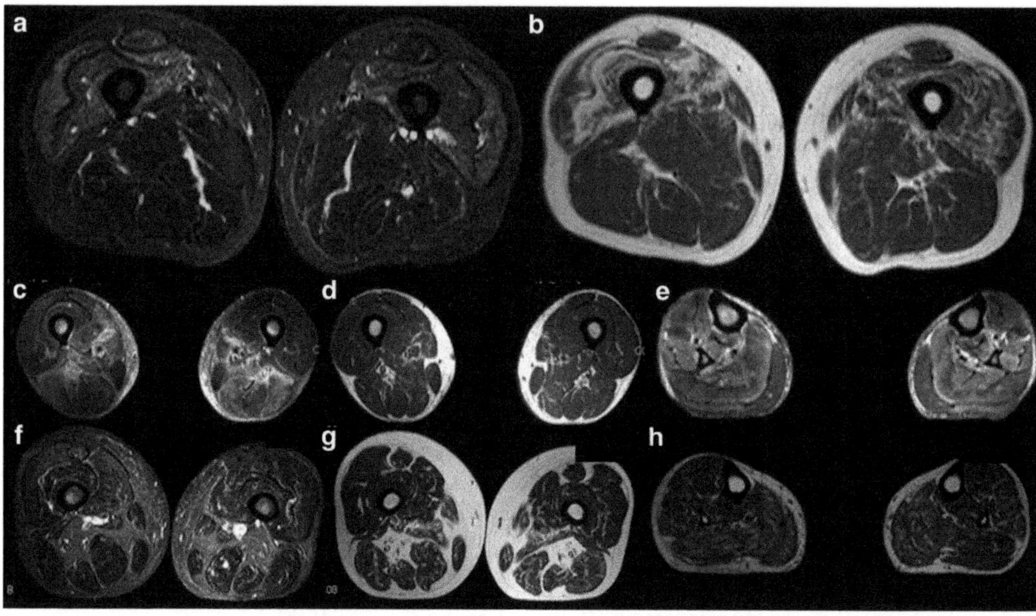

Fig. 27.4 Steroid-induced myopathy. Only "long" STIR images are presented. (**a, b**) A 66-year-old man undergoing corticosteroid-based treatment for inclusion body myositis presenting with proximal weakness, wasting of the ventral thighs, and unremarkable CK level. (**a**) STIR image discloses edema and atrophy of the ventral muscle groups of the thighs, particularly on the right, with sparing of other muscle groups. (**b**) T1-weighted image exhibits corresponding advanced lipomatous degenerative changes of the ventral muscle groups, most likely a result of long-standing disease than a toxic effect of medication. These images would, however, also fit the picture of type II muscle fiber atrophy resulting from chronic steroid medication. The fact that other muscle groups are inconspicuous on T1-weighted MRI does not eliminate a diagnosis of chronic toxic myopathy. The case serves to illustrate the difficulty occasionally encountered in differentiating a new toxic myopathy from exacerbation of an underlying inflammatory myopathy. (**c–e**) A 54-year-old man with recent induction of steroid therapy for chronic inflammatory demyelinating polyneuropathy (CIDP) presented with exacerbation of generalized weakness, newly arisen myalgia, and a markedly elevated CK level. STIR images of the thighs and legs (**c, e**) reveal extensive edematous changes of both muscles (**c**: m. vastus medialis, m. adductor longus et magnus, and m. sartorius especially on the right; m. biceps femoris and semimembranosus particularly on the left; **e**: general involvement with relative sparing of the gastrocnemius and tibialis anterior muscles) and subcutaneous fat tissue (**c**: medial thighs; **e**: medial and lateral legs). (**d**) T1-weighted MRI (legs not shown) discloses basically unremarkable findings. Although overlap with the underlying disease merits consideration, the imaging findings are compatible with an early case of acute quadriplegic myopathy. (**f–h**) A 50-year-old man with a long-standing history of steroid therapy for pulmonary disease presented with a normal CK level and persistent subjective leg weakness. (**f**) STIR MRI (legs not shown) does not reveal any hint of edema. (**g, h**) T1-weighted MRI reveals diffuse, reticular fatty changes, accentuated dorsally, particularly in the legs. These findings are consistent with chronic toxic myopathy

replaced with nonfluorinated steroids (e.g., prednisone). Aerobic and resistance exercises in a program of physical therapy have been shown to attenuate muscle atrophy in steroid-induced myopathy. Experimental approaches include application of IGF-1, branched-chain amino acids, creatine, androgens (DHEA, testosterone, nandrolone), and glutamine. In acute quadriplegic myopathy, avoidance of triggers, particularly nondepolarizing neuromuscular blockade, and optimal supportive care are the only available therapeutic options.

Key Points

- Given the fact that steroid treatment is used for a wide spectrum of diseases, steroid-induced myopathy is very common.
- Myopathic side effects are particularly common with 9-α-fluorinated corticosteroids (dexamethasone, betamethasone, and triamcinolone) compared to non-fluorinated corticosteroids (e.g. hydrocortisone, prednisone).
- Both chronic exogenous application and excess endogenous production of steroids, as in Cushing's disease, can induce myopathy. The most common clinical presentation is chronic proximal muscle weakness and atrophy, particularly affecting the quadriceps muscles, with involvement of neck flexor muscles.
- A serious variant of steroid-induced myopathy is acute quadriplegic myopathy. Transplant recipients and severely affected asthmatics receiving high doses of intravenous glucocorticoids are particularly prone, as are patients under non-depolarizing neuromuscular blockade.
- The pattern of disease on MRI is nonspecific. Acute quadriplegic myopathy displays pathology on fat-suppressed T2-weighted MRI (e.g., STIR) akin to that of rhabdomyolysis.
- Drug discontinuation or dose reduction below a threshold level is the mainstay for treating steroid-induced myopathy. Alternate-day dosing can be considered.

Suggestions for Further Reading

Dalakas MC. Toxic and drug-induced myopathies. J Neurol Neurosurg Psychiatry. 2009;80:832–8.

Decramer M, de Bock V, Dom R. Functional and histologic picture of steroid-induced myopathy in chronic obstructive pulmonary disease. Am J Respir Crit Care Med. 1996;153:1958–64.

Dirks-Naylor AJ, Griffiths CL. Glucocorticoid-induced apoptosis and cellular mechanisms of myopathy. J Steroid Biochem Mol Biol. 2009;117(1–3):1–7.

Mastaglia FL. Drug induced myopathies. Pract Neurol. 2006;6:4–13.

Mor A, Mitnick HJ, Pillinger MH, et al. Drug-induced myopathies. Bull NYU Hosp Jt Dis. 2009;67(4): 358–69

Pereira RMR, de Carvalho JF. Glucocorticoid-induced myopathy. Joint Bone Spine. 2011;78:41–44.

Schakman O, Gilson H, Thissen JP. Mechanisms of glucocorticoid-induced myopathy. J Endocrinol. 2008; 197(1):1–10.

Valiyil R, Christopher-Stine L. Drug-related myopathies of which the clinician should be aware. Curr Rheumatol Rep. 2010;12:213–20.

27.4 Alcohol-Induced Myopathy

27.4.1 Synonyms and Abbreviations

Alcoholic myopathy

27.4.2 Introduction

With alcohol being a socially more-or-less sanctioned drug, the prevalence of alcohol-induced complications are bound to be prominent. In industrialized countries, chronic alcohol-induced myopathy is one of the most prevalent muscle disorders, with about 2,000 cases per 100,000 individuals. It affects 40–60 % of alcoholics, making it more common than cirrhosis, neuropathy, intestinal disease, and cardiomyopathy.

27.4.3 Pathophysiology

Alcohol-induced myopathy is dose-dependent and related to lifetime alcohol consumption. It mainly affects fast-twitch muscle fibers (type 2). Ethanol consumption decreases protein synthesis and seems to accelerate specific protein degradation via the UPS. It also induces oxidative stress and cellular damage by reactive oxygen species. Direct toxic effects on ion channels, reduced expression of molecular chaperones, activation of apoptosis through various mechanisms, and impaired glycolysis and glycogenolysis may also play a role in the pathogenesis.

27.4.4 Histopathology

There is no unique or specific histological pattern of alcohol-induced myopathy. Nonspecific histological findings may include fiber-size variability with type 2 fiber atrophy, oxidative disturbances and non-inflammatory myocytolysis.

The histological picture for acute alcoholic myopathy is typically that of rhabdomyolysis, with extensive muscle fiber necrosis and intracellular edema followed by fiber degeneration, phagocytosis, and regeneration. Affected muscle fibers are typically depleted of glycogen and show oxidative disturbances. Acute hypokalemic myopathy shows vacuoles on biopsy, as with other hypokalemic conditions.

Chronic alcohol-induced myopathy typically leads to selective fiber type 2B atrophy. Infrequent findings include type 1 fiber predominance, internal nuclei, interstitial fibrosis, cytoplasmic or interstitial lipid deposition, and cytoplasmic tubular aggregates.

27.4.5 Clinical Presentation

Apart from asymptomatic hyperCKemia, the clinical spectrum of alcohol-induced myopathy includes acute necrotizing myopathy, acute hypokalemic myopathy and chronic alcoholic myopathy. About 50 % of patients with alcohol-induced myopathy complain of weakness and about 25 % describe muscle cramps. The severity of alcohol-induced myopathy is related to total lifetime consumption of alcohol. It is at least partially reversible with abstinence.

Binge drinking typically triggers acute necrotizing myopathy. Clinically, patients present with acute muscle pain, cramping, and swelling. The CK level is markedly elevated, and rhabdomyolysis and myoglobinuria can give rise to renal failure. Muscle cramps may resolve over a few days, but it can take weeks before the clinical picture improves.

Patients with acute hypokalemic myopathy develop painless but generalized weakness, even presenting with flaccid paralysis. Symptoms appear at potassium levels <2.5 mEq/L, although potassium levels may first decrease to as low as 2.0 mEq/L. CK can be markedly elevated. Weakness evolves over 1–2 days but may resolve quickly with judicious potassium substitution.

Finally, chronic alcohol-induced myopathy is characterized by general weakness, with predilection for the proximal lower limbs, and insidious muscle wasting. CK may be mildly elevated. Nutritional deficiency, sedentary lifestyle and concomitant neuropathic disease contribute to the clinical picture.

27.4.6 Imaging Findings

Alcohol-induced myopathy also renders a nonspecific pattern of myopathic changes without a specific distribution pattern. Pathological changes tend to be proximally accentuated. However, alcohol-induced myopathy is sometimes accompanied by more-distal changes in patient with concomitant neuropathy (Fig. 27.5a–d)

The findings of chronic alcohol-induced myopathy often comprise subtle to moderate diffuse reticular lipomatous changes on T1-weighted MRI without predilection for specific muscle groups. Generalized muscle atrophy is common.

Acute necrotizing myopathy shows the hallmarks of rhabdomyolysis: pronounced edema of the thighs and legs on fat-suppressed T2-weighted MRI that is often asymmetrical, patchy, and centered on deep muscle groups, with relative sparing of superficial muscle groups (Fig. 27.5e–h).

The MRI scans of acute hypokalemic myopathy are often unremarkable, although they may display discrete patchy and diffuse edema.

27.4.7 Therapy

Abstinence in combination with nutritional and physical therapy support is paramount to improving the clinical manifestations of alcohol-induced myopathy.

Acute alcoholic myopathy usually reverses within days or weeks of alcohol abstinence. Adequate correction of vitamin deficiencies, electrolyte disturbances and malnutritation promotes a

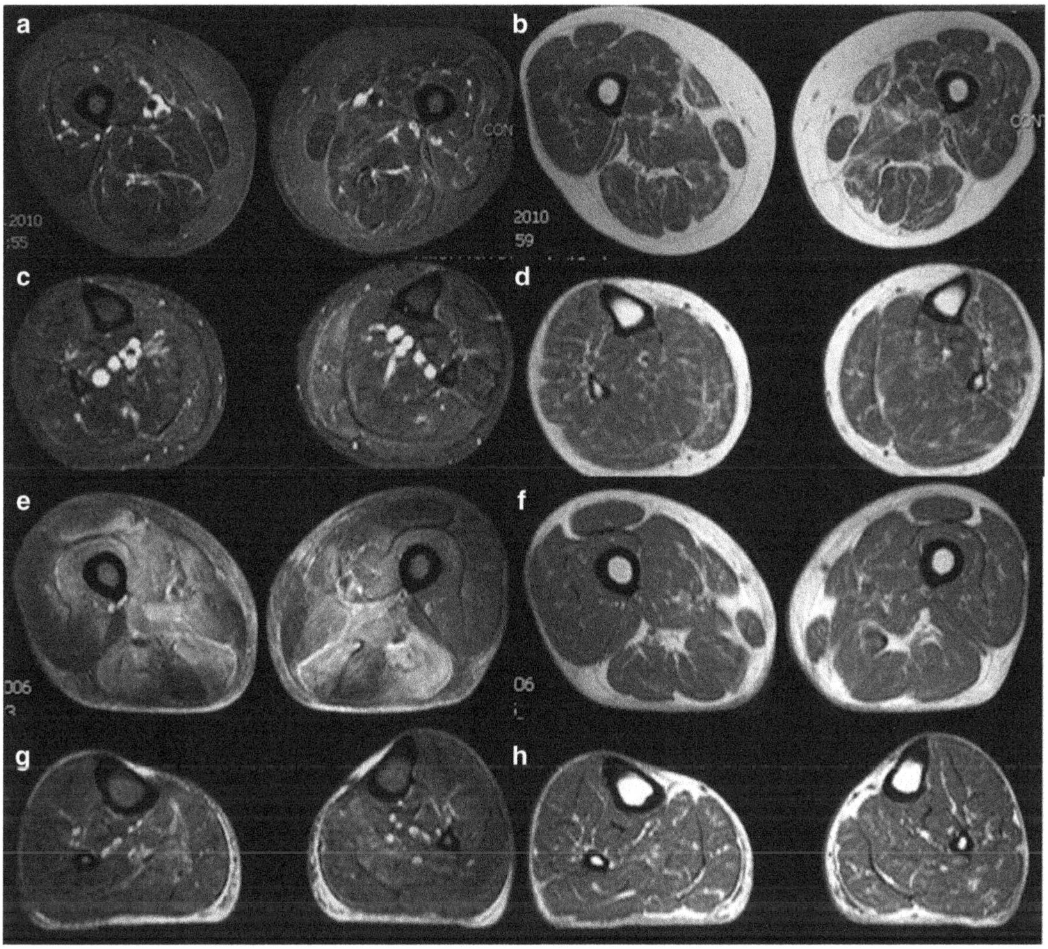

Fig. 27.5 Alcohol-induced myopathy. Only "long" STIR images are presented. (**a–d**) A 59-year-old man, a chronic alcoholic, displays the nonspecific changes of alcohol-induced myopathy. (**a**, **c**) STIR MRI identifies edema in the left vastus lateralis muscle, left m. adductor magnus, and the dorsal muscle groups of the legs, especially on the left, as a correlate of ongoing disease activity. (**b**, **d**) T1-weighted MRI show generalized reticular fatty changes in both thighs and legs as a consequence of long-standing disease. The effects of alcohol-induced neuropathy must also be taken into account, especially regarding changes in distal muscle groups. (**e–h**) A 41-year-old man after a bout of binge drinking presented with myalgia, proximally accentuated weakness, and a markedly elevated CK level. (**e**, **g**) STIR MRI shows extensive edema of the thighs involving the dorsal muscle groups (with relative sparing of the semitendinosus muscles), large adductors, and vastus medialis, vastus intermedius, and rectus femoris muscles, with a trace of edema in the soleus muscles. (**f**, **h**) T1-weighted MRI scans are essentially normal. The clinical and imaging findings are compatible with rhabdomyolysis secondary to necrotizing myopathy

prompt recovery. Acute hypokalemic myopathy requires prudent potassium substitution and supportive care.

Rhabdomyolysis calls for immediate abstinence, and symptomatic and supportive therapy in an intermediate or intensive care unit. Nephrological support include parenteral fluid supplementation and monitoring renal function and the electrolyte balance. In case of acute renal failure, renal function should be supported by temporary hemodialysis. Surgery is needed in cases of compartment syndrome.

Chronic alcoholic myopathy normally reverses within 2–12 months of alcohol abstinence.

Key Points

- Alcohol-induced myopathy is perhaps the most common form of myopathy, and the most prevalent complication of chronic alcohol consumption.
- Binge drinking typically triggers acute necrotizing myopathy. Rhabdomyolysis and myoglobinuria can give rise to renal failure.
- Acute hypokalemic myopathy arises at potassium levels <2.5 mEq/L.
- Nutritional deficiency, sedentary lifestyle and concomitant neuropathic disease can all contribute to the clinical picture of chronic alcohol-induced myopathy.
- Although alcohol-induced myopathy also renders a non-specific pattern of myopathic changes without a specific distribution pattern, pathological changes tend to be accentuated proximally. Alcohol-induced myopathy is sometimes accompanied by more distal changes in patients with concomitant neuropathy.

Suggestions for Further Reading

Dalakas MC. Toxic and drug-induced myopathies. J Neurol Neurosurg Psychiatry. 2009;80:832–8.

Fernandez-Solà J, Preedy VR, Lang CH, et al. Molecular and cellular events in alcohol-induced muscle disease. Alcohol Clin Exp Res. 2007;31(12):1953–62.

Mor A, Mitnick HJ, Pillinger MH, et al. Drug-induced myopathies. Bull NYU Hosp Jt Dis. 2009;67(4): 358–69.

Preedy VR, Ohlendieck K, Adachi J, et al. The importance of alcohol-induced muscle disease. J Muscle Res Cell Motil. 2003;14:55–63.

Urbano-Márquez A, Fernández-Solà J. Effects of alcohol on skeletal and cardiac muscle. Muscle Nerve. 2004;30(6):689–707.

Winkler G, Beese M. Toxische Myopathien. In: Beese M, Winkler G,editors. MRT der Muskulatur. New York: Thieme; 1997. p. 225–9.

27.5 Differential Diagnosis

As the clinical and imaging presentation of toxic myopathy are non-specific, the spectrum of differential diagnoses can be quite daunting, spanning the whole spectrum of muscle diseases.

Nutritional deficiencies, electrolyte imbalances, and concomitant neuropathy particularly must be considered in alcohol-induced myopathy. Inflammatory diseases, especially exacerbation of preexisting disease, need to kept in mind in regard to steroid- and statin-induced myopathies. The differential diagnosis for rhabdomyolysis (e.g., dyskinesias, seizures, neuroleptic malignant syndrome, muscle trauma with significant muscle injury, thermal or electrical injury, prolonged immobility with muscle compression) merits consideration especially in alcohol- and statin-induced myopathies.

A critical distinction must also be made between critical illness neuropathy and critical illness myopathy (acute quadriplegic myopathy), as the former carries a worse prognosis.

28 Muscle Neoplasms

Michèle Kind and Jean-Michel Coindre

28.1 Introduction and Classification

Soft tissue tumors are mesenchymal tumors for which the classification was established by the World Health Organization (WHO) in 2002. The classification is based on identifying the diseased tissue or on the line of differentiation of the tumor cells.

Muscle tumors are deep soft tissue tumors located beyond the superficial muscle fascia with a topography that is initially intermuscular or intramuscular. This group generally includes lesions such as myositis ossificans, a disorder of unknown etiopathogenesis and a pseudo-tumoral presentation.

Muscle tumors comprise a heterogeneous group of disease entities based on their clinical presentation and prognosis. They include approximately 150 histological types and subtypes, about 50 of which are sarcomas.

Muscle tumors are grouped into nine main classes according to the tissue differentiation expressed. Each class is subdivided into benign, intermediate malignancy (locally aggressive or with low metastatic potential), and malignancy categories (Table 28.1).

28.2 Etiology

In general, the etiology of muscle tumors is unknown. Certain predisposition factors have been identified that significantly increase the risk of developing a sarcoma, including exposure to ionizing radiation, chronic lymphedema, and certain genetic alterations (e.g., mutation of the *NF1* gene in neurofibromatosis, the *RB* gene in retinoblastoma, or the *P53* gene in Li Fraumeni syndrome).

28.3 Epidemiology

Benign tumors are 100 times more frequent than their malignant counterparts or soft tissue sarcomas (STSs). For tumors >5 cm diameter, the ratio becomes 7:1 (benign versus sarcoma). Sarcomas are rare, accounting for approximately 1 % of cancers in adults and 10–15 % in infants. Their exact incidence has probably been underestimated. If we refer to current publications by specialist oncology networks, the standardized incidence in relation to the European population is 5.6/100,000 population per year for both soft tissue and visceral sarcomas. The rate for STSs alone is 3.58/100,000 in males and 2.55/100,000 in females. Poorly differentiated sarcomas, liposarcomas, leiomyosarcomas, and desmoid tumors

M. Kind
Radiology Department, Institut Bergonie, Bordeaux Cedex, France
e-mail: kind@bergonie.org

J.-M. Coindre (✉)
Department of Pathology, Institut Bergonie, 229 cours de l'Argonne, 33076 Bordeaux Cedex, France
e-mail: coindre@bergonie.org

M.P. Wattjes and D. Fischer (eds.), *Neuromuscular Imaging*, DOI 10.1007/978-1-4614-6552-2_28,

Table 28.1 Soft tissue tumor classification (WHO 2002)

Tumors	Benign	Intermediate	Malignant
Adipocytic	Lipoma Lipomatosis Lipomatosis of nerve Lipoblastoma/lipoblastomatosis Angiolipoma Myolipoma of soft tissue Chondroid lipoma Spindle cell lipoma/pleomorphic lipoma Hibernoma	Atypical lipomatous tumor/well differentiated liposarcoma	Dedifferentiated liposarcoma Myxoid liposarcoma Pleomorphic liposarcoma Mixed-type liposarcoma
Fibroblastic Myofibroblastic	Nodular fasciitis Proliferative fasciitis and proliferative mysositis Myositis ossificans Elastofibroma Myofibroma/myofibromatosis Fibromatosis colli Fibroma of tendon sheath Desmoplastic fibroblastoma Calcifying fibrous tumor Angiofibroma Angiomyofibroblastoma Gardner fibroma Giant cell angiofibroma	*Intermediate (locally aggressive)* Superficial fibromatosis (plantar/palmar) Desmoid-type fibromatosis Lipofibromatosis *Intermediate (rarely metastasizing)* Solitary fibrous tumor hemangiopericytoma Myofibroblastic inflammatory T Myofibroblastic sarcoma	Adult fibrosarcoma Myxofibrosarcoma Low-grade fibromyxoid sarcoma
So-called fibrohistiocytic	Giant cell tumour of tendon sheath PVNS Benign fibrous histiocytoma	Plexiform fibrohistiocytic tumor Giant cell tumor of soft tissue	Pleomorphic malignant fibrous histiocytoma Giant cell malignant fibrous histiocytoma Inflammatory malignant fibrous histiocytoma
Smooth muscle	Angioleiomyoma Leiomyoma of deep soft tissue		Leiomyosarcoma
Pericytic (perivascular)	Glomus tumors (and variants)		Malignant glomus tumor
Skeletal muscle	Rhabdomyoma		Rhabdomyosarcoma Embryonal, alveolar Pleomorphic
Vascular	Hemangiomas Epithelioid hemangioma Angiomatosis Lymphangioma	Papillary intralymphatic angioendothelioma Hemangioendothelioma Kaposi sarcoma	Epithelioid hemangioendothelioma Angiosarcoma
Chondro-osseous	Soft-tissue chondroma		Mesenchymal chondrosarcoma Extraskeletal osteosarcoma
Uncertain differentiation	Intramuscular—juxta-articular myxoma Angiomyxoma	Angiomatoid fibrous histiocytoma Ossifying fibromyxoid tumor Mixed tumor/myoepithelioma/parachordoma	Synovial sarcoma Epithelioid sarcoma Alveolar soft part sarcoma Clear cell sarcoma of soft tissue Extraskeletal myxoid chondrosarcoma Malignant mesenchymoma Desmoplastic small round cell tumor PNET Ewing's sarcoma of soft tissue PEComa

PNET peripheral primitive neuroectodermal tumor, *PEComa* neoplasms with perivascular epithelioid cell differentiation
Classification according to: J C.Vilanova et al. (2007) Soft-tissue tumors update: MR imaging features according to the WHO classification. Eur Radiol. 17:125–138 and Fletcher CDM, Unni KK, Mertens F (2002) Pathology and genetics of tumours of soft tissue and bone. In: World Health Organization Classification of Tumours, IARC Press, Lyon

are the most frequent malignant or locally aggressive tumors of the limbs.

Benign tumors can occur at all ages and are ubiquitous: 60 % of all mesenchymal tumors are found in the limbs and trunk wall. Certain histological types have a slightly more specific distribution according to age or topography. For instance, alveolar rhabdomyosarcomas principally affect young children, epithelioid sarcoma develop more often in young adults (with 80 % in the wrist or hand), and synovial sarcomas, although ubiquitous, are generally found in the vicinity of the knee joint in adults <50 years of age.

28.4 Clinical Presentation and Diagnosis

The clinical presentations of benign and malignant tumors are similar. The patient spontaneously discovers a mass, which may be painful (or not), and the patient often relates it to a trauma. The painful nature is not a negative sign and can be found in inflammatory or similar conditions such as myositis ossificans or as part of an infectious process. A slowly progressive nature, unlike other situations, is not an argument for benignity. Certain low-grade sarcomas (e.g., liposarcoma) or even more aggressive tumors (e.g., synovial sarcoma) can develop over a number of years. The lesion size is not a good criterion for discriminating benign and malignant tumors.

For the diagnostic workup, ultrasonography (US) should be performed first. US can reveal certain tissue characteristics (e.g., the tissular or cystic nature of the lesion) and can help differentiate a tumor from a hematoma, which is important because trauma is almost always reported by the patient. Magnetic resonance imaging (MRI) is the modality of choice for analyzing musculoskeletal tissue. It should always be performed systematically—it must be standardized and the results reproducible—before, during, and after treatment of any muscular tumor. Orthogonal plane imaging is necessary with axial and longitudinal sequences for adequate coverage of the entire involved muscular compartment. Both T1- and T2-weighted sequences must be performed: the T1-weighted sequences for fat and/or hemorrhage characterization and the T2-weighted sequences for sensitive detection of lesions in the muscle. The administration of gadolinium-based contrast may be essential in distinguishing a cyst versus a myxoid or necrotic tumor. The routine use of fluorodeoxyglucose (FDG) positron emission tomography (^{18}F-FDG-PET) is currently unjustified. In particular cases, computed tomography (CT) could help assess the presence of calcifications in a mass of unclear origin or a zonal architecture of some lesion such as myositis ossificans.

Although imaging can narrow the differential diagnosis, the histopathological diagnosis after biopsy is still the gold standard and should be considered mandatory. It is currently well accepted that microbiopsies, image guided or not, can be performed routinely. However, this practice can pose problems with regard to tumor tissue sampling, diagnosis, grading because of the small quantity of material that is available in comparison with an open (surgical) biopsy. The low morbidity and reduced time before treatment can be started are, however, distinctly in favor of the microbiopsy—with the surgical biopsy being performed after failure of the microbiopsy. The French Federation of Cancer Centers Sarcoma Group and the Italian National Research Council reached a consensus on their clinical practice guidelines through the European Connective Tissue Cancer Network (CONTICANET). These guidelines recommend performing a biopsy routinely before any treatment of a deep tumor or a tumor >5 cm in diameter. The biopsy technique and procedure has to meet strict rules: (1) imaging (preferably MRI) is performed prior to the biopsy procedure; (2) the biopsy route is as direct as possible, perpendicular to the muscle fibers to avoid dissemination along the fascias or aponeurosis; (3) the biopsy route is chosen so that any possible tumor dissemination can be removed during surgery.

28.5 Histopathology

28.5.1 Principle

The final diagnosis of an intramuscular tumor is based on the histopathology, generally aided by immunohistochemical and molecular analysis, to provide a detailed classification of the tumor (e.g., sarcoma). Immunohistochemistry is used almost routinely except when a lipoma is evident. This technique is particularly valuable for identifying benign peripheral nerve sheath tumors (schwannoma, neurofibroma), a solitary fibrous tumor, and for classifying certain sarcomas (e.g., rhabdomyosarcoma, angiosarcoma, low-grade fibromyxoid sarcoma, clear-cell sarcoma, epithelioid sarcoma, soft part alveolar sarcoma).

28.5.2 Molecular Classification

Approximately 30–40 % of all sarcomas of the limbs are carriers of a molecular anomaly leading to a specific diagnosis. Specific translocations are present in several types of sarcomas including synovial sarcoma, mysoid liposarcoma, Ewing's sarcoma, alveolar rhabdomyosarcoma, low-grade fibromyxoid sarcoma, and clear-cell sarcoma. Amplification of the *MDM2* and *CDK4* genes are characteristic for atypical adipocytic tumors or well-differentiated and dedifferentiated liposarcomas. Therefore, the diagnosis of an atypical adipocytic tumor or a well-differentiated liposarcoma (WDLS) should be assigned only after demonstrating this amplification by fluorescence in situ hybridization (FISH) analysis.

28.5.3 Histological Grading and Prognostic Factors

The main prognostic factor for STSs is the histological grade of the tumor. The French sarcoma group grading system is a three-grade system (low, intermediate, and high risk groups) that uses the combination of three criteria: degree of differentiation, mitotic index, amount of tumor necrosis. The value of the histological grade diminishes because of the difficulty of assessing the mitotic index in material obtained by microbiopsy. This mitotic index can be replaced by the proliferation index (more easily obtained by immunohistochemistry) and the extent of tumor necrosis, which can also be evaluated by imaging. More recently a two-point molecular grading system ("poor" and "good" prognostic groups) has been reported based on a gene expression signature. The value of this molecular grade is superior to that of the histological grade. These grading systems enable prediction of the metastatic potential of a sarcoma. This prediction is aided by the size of the tumor, with a cutoff of 10 cm. On the other hand, prediction of local recurrence is based principally on the quality of the excision margins.

28.5.4 Difficulties and Rate of Discordance

The diagnosis of sarcomas is difficult, with rates of discrepancy among pathologists ranging from 8 % to 25 % depending on whether there is systematic reviewing or a second opinion is given. The lower rate is obtained when there is systematic reviewing of all cases. This rate rises to 25 % when the initial pathologist asks for a second opinion when the diagnosis is uncertain.

This interrater variability is further increased by the more systematic use of microbiopsy material as a first diagnostic approach, which increases the number of differential diagnoses to be envisaged.

28.6 Treatment Principles

The treatment strategy for each patient should always be discussed in a multidisciplinary setting. Surgery is the standard treatment for muscle tumors. In the case of soft tissue sarcoma, oncological surgery is recommended with healthy resection margins and wide resection into healthy tissue if possible. The definition of what is considered wide resection margins (1–5 cm) is still subject to discussion. It is accepted that fascia, an aponeurosis, or the periosteum constitutes a solid natural barrier and therefore permits more restricted margins. When surgery is ideally carried out in a specialized clinical setting, the local 5-year recurrence rate is about 10–15 % compared with 50 % in the case of inadequate surgery. Additional treatment by radiotherapy is always programmed after removal of an intermediate or high-grade sarcoma, thus improving local control. When there has no biopsy before surgery or an inadequate initial surgery, the feasibility of repeat surgery to obtain wide excision margins should be considered. It is well known that the quality of surgical removal is, along with the histological grade, one of the important prognostic factors. Surgical removal influences the local recurrence rate but does not affect overall survival of patients. In the case of an inoperable tumor or one with initial metastasis, neoadjuvant systemic treatment may be envisaged.

The overall 2-year survival rate is about 75 % for all types of sarcoma. The metastatic risk, based on the grading and the histological type, is about 50 %.

28.7 Differential Diagnosis

The first differential diagnosis to be excluded is a hematoma because it is a frequent occurrence, particularly when trauma has been reported. In the case of uncertainty, or with an atypical aspect on US (hematoma disproportionate to the reported trauma, without further regression, or vascularized on a Doppler image), MRI with and without fat signal suppression sequences can lead to the definitive diagnosis.

More rarely, a metastasis reveals a nonsarcomatous malignant tumor, principally a bronchogenic, mammalian, or renal carcinoma. Alternatively, it may indicate an unknown primary tumor, a melanoma, or a lymphoma.

28.8 Main Tumor Types

Data from imaging (US, radiography, CT, MRI) does not always enable a clear, definitive diagnosis, particularly in terms of differentiating between a benign or malignant nature of the tumor. A diagnosis based on imaging findings is correct in approximately 50 % of cases. However, there are certain imaging signs, principally on MRI, that suggest a specific tissue composition that is typical of certain histological tumor types or associated with malignancy (Fig. 28.1). Knowledge about these findings is therefore crucial for diagnosing sarcomas based on the hypothesis of a differential diagnosis and relevant therapeutic approach according to clinical practice guidelines.

This chapter gives an overview of the various types of muscular tumors according to established classification schemes based on MRI findings (Fig. 28.1).

28.8.1 Tumors with a Hyperintense Signal on T1-Weighted MRI

28.8.1.1 Adipocytic Tumors

Adipocytic tumors are grouped in the first category of the World Health Organization (WHO) classification and are broadly the most frequent muscle tumors because of the high incidence of lipomas and liposarcomas. Liposarcomas account for 24 % of all sarcomas and have an estimated prevalence of 2.5 cases per million in the Swedish population. Soft tissue WDLSs represent 13 % of sarcomas. Well-differentiated atypical adipocytic tumors and WDLSs are now grouped under a single entity called "atypical lipomatous tumors," which never lead to metastasis. Because of the high sensitivity of T1-weighted MRI for demonstrating fatty tissue, it is easy to diagnose adipocytic tumors.

Intramuscular Lipoma

Intramuscular lipoma represents a heterotopic variant of the subcutaneous lipoma. It is a well-encapsulated intramuscular tumor, containing only fat tissue, with no other visible tissue component. A virtually certain diagnosis can be made if the tumor is infiltrating, has poorly defined contours dissociating the muscle fibers, and consists exclusively of adipose tissue on MRI with no septa or tissue nodule (Fig. 28.2). Recently, however, it has been demonstrated that the presence of muscle fibers in an adipocytic tumor is not in itself a formal argument in favor of a diagnosis of lipoma.

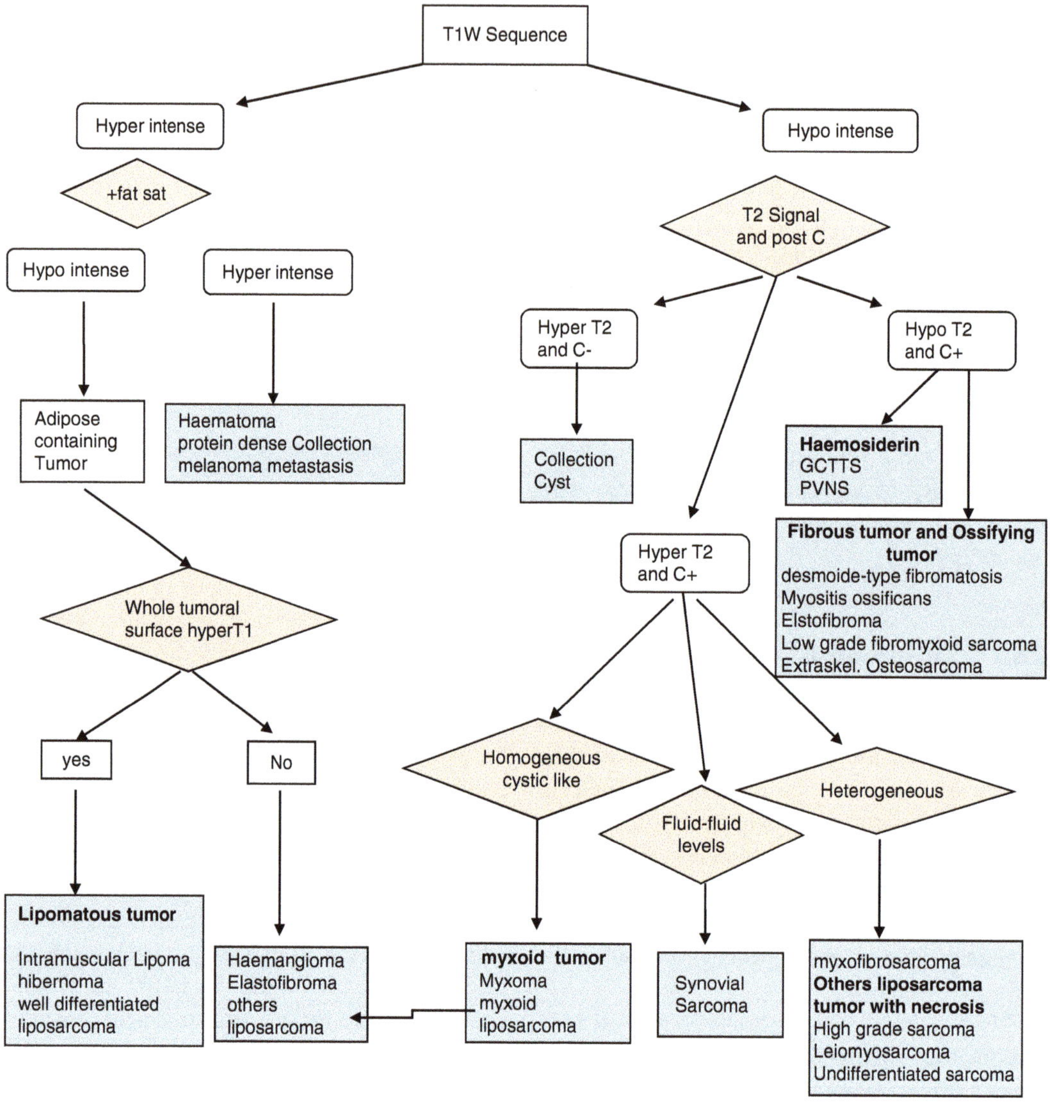

Fig. 28.1 Flow chart presenting a diagnostic approach according to MRI signal analysis

Histopathologically, the residual striated muscle retains its fasciculated architecture. Mature adipocytes can be seen between the striated muscle fibers. They are of regular size and shape, with no atypical nuclei.

In 30 % of cases, there are modifications of the imaging findings, including the presence of not strictly adipose signal zones inside the tumor. These zones are attributed to necrosis, inflammation, or the presence of heterologous tissue (chondroid, angiomatous, osseous) and intratumoral septa. These heterogeneous aspects of pathology underscore that a specific diagnosis relying solely on MRI is no longer possible. The lipoma variants are now, according to the WHO classification, within the group of atypical adipocytic tumors.

Hibernoma

The hibernoma is a relatively rare, benign, adipocytic tumor of brown fat. On MRI, the tumor is well delimited, with less T1 signal intensity than that of subcutaneous fat (Fig. 28.3) The tumor can be discretely heterogeneous with numerous vascular structures but no identifiable tissue component.

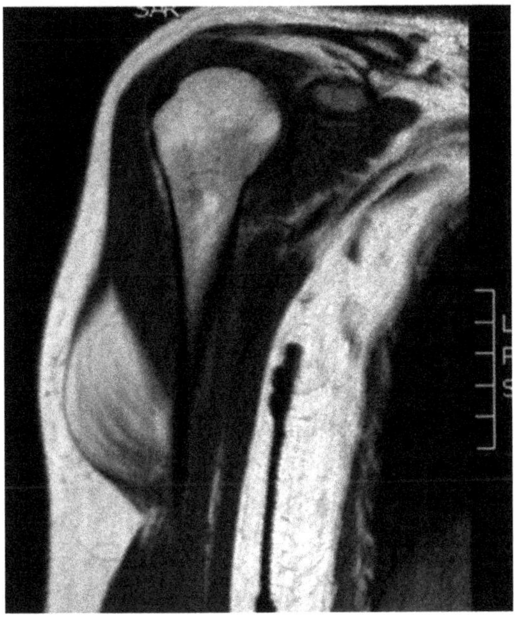

Fig. 28.2 Intramuscular lipoma in the right shoulder of a 50-year-old woman. The mass had been apparent for 6 months. Coronal turbo spin echo (TSE) T1-weighted MRI shows a uniformly hyperintense lesion infiltrating deltoid muscle fibers

Well-Differentiated Liposarcoma

The WDLS represents the most common liposarcoma, accounting for 40 % of all liposarcomas. It is the second most frequent tumor after the undifferentiated sarcomas and is found in adults most frequently during their sixth or seventh decade. Overall, 65–75 % of these liposarcomas develop in the extremities and 50 % in the thigh. The lesions are located both intra- and intermuscularly. They show local aggressiveness, with a high rate of recurrence in the case of incomplete removal. They do not metastasize. After multiple local relapses, a dedifferentiation occurs in 6–13 % of cases.

The tumor is histologically characterized by the presence of mature adipocytes, irregular in size, and partitioned by thick fibromyxoid septa containing characteristic cells. These cells have atypical nuclei, are hyperchromatic, and exhibit hyperexpression of *MDM2* and *CDK4* genes.

MRI shows on T1- and T2-weighted sequences a hyperintense deep mass containing more than 75 % adipose tissue with septa relatively thicker (>2 mm) than those observed in lipomas. There may also be nodules or small tissue areas (<1 cm) that enhance after intravenous contrast medium administration (Fig. 28.4). The main differential diagnoses are lipoma variants with secondary changes. These show on MRI either thin, regular (<2 mm thick) septa inside an adipocytic tumor, nonfatty signal zones corresponding to necrosis or inflammation, or heterologous tissue formations. Based on imaging, there are no formal criteria for distinguishing these lipoma variants from WDLS. Neither the evolution nor the size is a good criterion for distinguishing atypical lipoma from WDLS. Image-guided biopsies of the nonadipose areas are essential for diagnosis. Only a FISH analysis enables formal distinction of an atypical adipocytic tumor or WDLS from an atypical lipoma.

Dedifferentiated Liposarcoma

The dedifferentiated liposarcoma (DDLS) is a particular subtype of biphasic liposarcoma comprising two components, one being a WDLS and the other a high-grade or dedifferentiated sarcoma of nonadipose tissue. The incidence of DDLSs has been underestimated for a long time. In fact, they represent almost 40 % of all liposarcomas. The dedifferentiation arises de novo in 90 % of cases. In only 10 % of cases it occurs in a preexisting WDLS. The risk of dedifferentiation depends on location. It occurs preferentially in the retroperitoneal area and, more rarely, in the extremities. When the liposarcoma is localized in the retroperitoneum, the period of tumor development before diagnosis is much longer—hence, the greater chance of dedifferentiation.

Histopathologically, the tumor is characterized by the presence of two components: a WDLS-type and an undifferentiated sarcoma-type with spindle and/or pleomorphic cells without an identifiable line of differentiation or, more rarely, a rhabdomyosarcoma-, leiomyosarcoma-, osteosarcoma-, or chondrosarcoma-type component. The cells also show hyperexpression and amplification of the *MDM2* and *CDK4* genes.

On MRI, these lesions are easily recognizable by the presence of a well-differentiated hyperintense

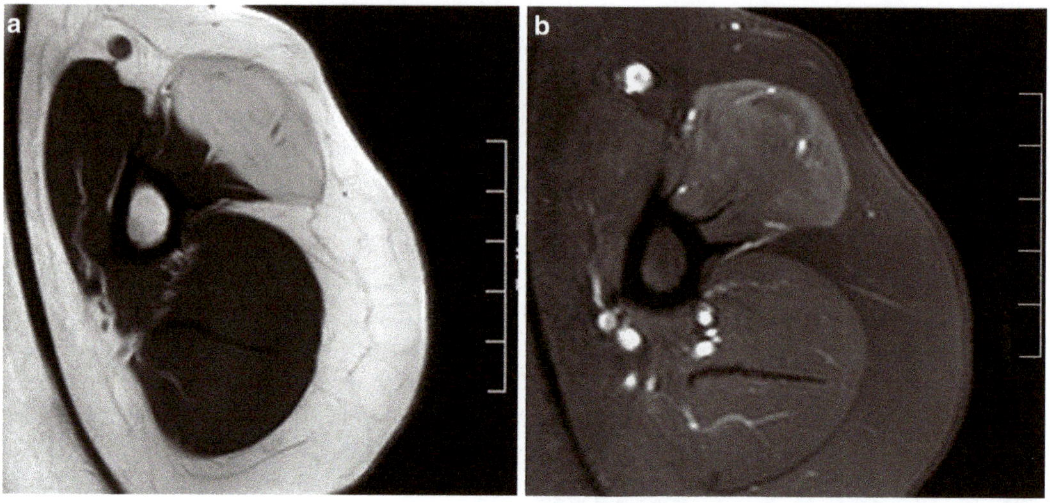

Fig. 28.3 Hibernoma of the left shoulder in a 66-year-old woman with a lesion of 3 years duration. (**a**) Axial T1-weighted MRI shows an adipose-like lesion with a homogeneous hyperintense signal that was not identical to the signal for fat. (**b**) Corresponding axial T1-weighted fat-suppressed contrast-enhanced MRI demonstrates numerous vascular structures within the mass

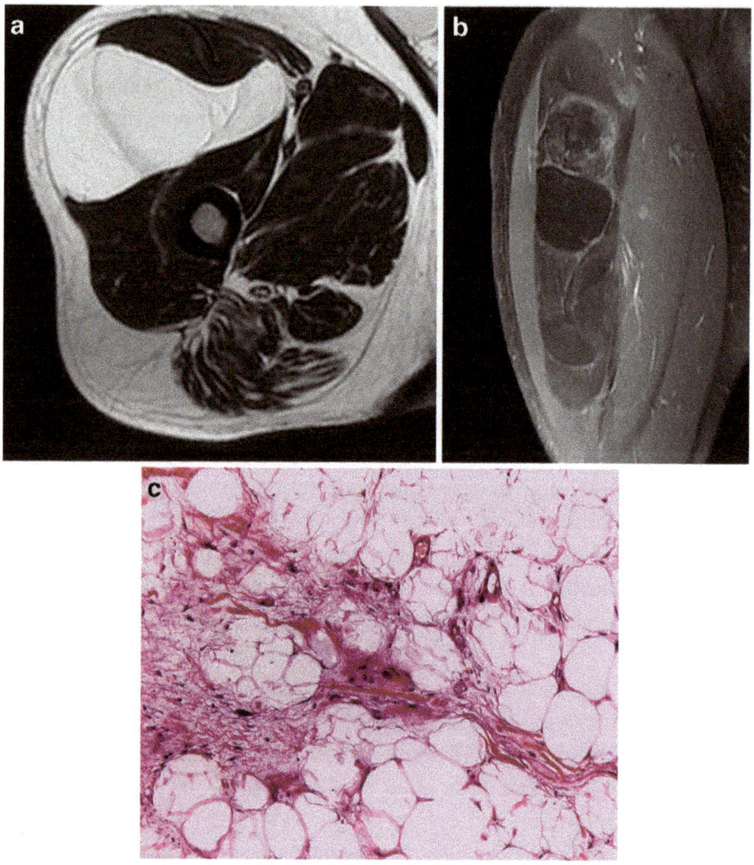

Fig. 28.4 Well differentiated liposarcoma (WDLS) of the right thigh in a 48-year-old man. (**a**) Axial TSE T2-weighted sequence shows a homogeneous hyperintense intermuscular lipoma-like lesion. (**b**) Postcontrast coronal TSE T1-weighted sequence with fat saturation shows signal saturation of lipomatous counterparts with enhancement of thin septa and tissue nodules, which is quite specific for liposarcoma. (**c**) Histology of the tumor shows mature adipocytes with fibromyxoid septa and cells with atypical nuclei

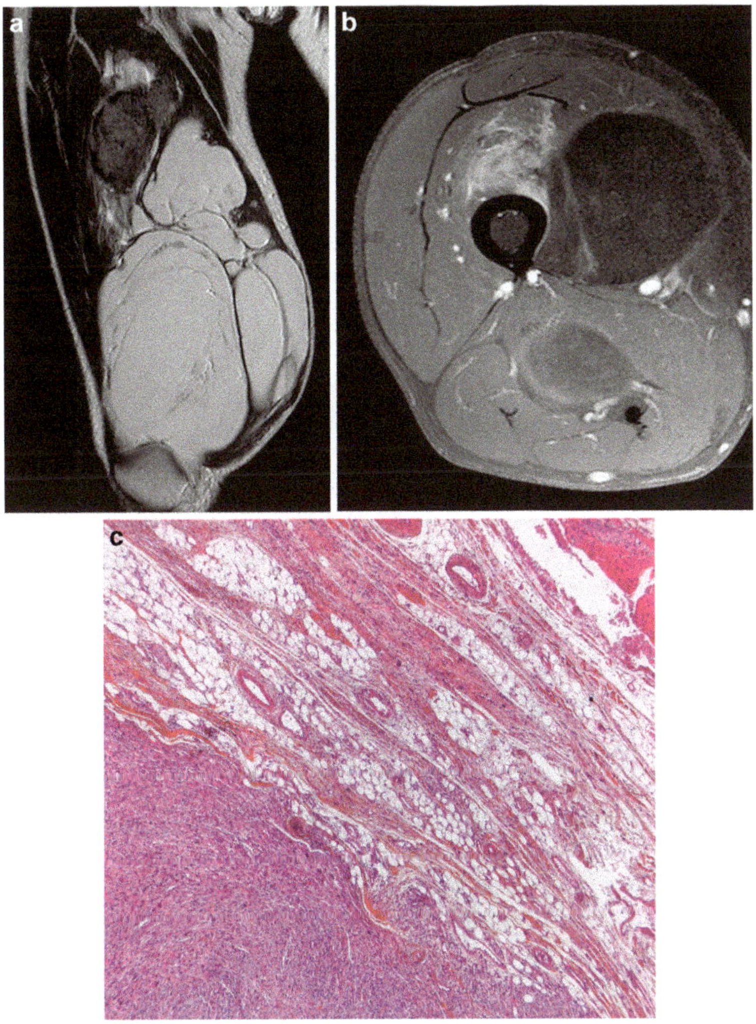

Fig. 28.3 Dedifferentiated liposarcoma (DDLS) of the right thigh in a 74-year-old man. His history showed resection of a lipoma 7 years previously and a recently growing painful mass. (**a**) Coronal T2-weighted TSE image shows a two-compartment tumor: one hyperintense with thick septa and one with nonspecific tissue signal. (**b**) Axial postcontrast T1-weighted with fat suppression showing enhancement only of the tissue component. (**c**) Tumor with two components: a well differentiated liposarcoma aspect and an undifferentiated fusiform cell sarcoma with no differentiation line

liposarcoma on T1-weighted sequences and a nonspecific tissue component signal that is >1 cm in diameter (Fig. 28.5). It is this tissular component that is important to biopsy with an image-guided technique because of the prognostic and therapeutic impact. This subtype of liposarcoma presents with metastases (lung, bone) in 15–20 % of cases. Surgery should always be performed in association with radiotherapy.

Pleomorphic Liposarcoma

Pleomorphic liposarcoma is the less common subtype of liposarcoma, representing approximately 5 % of all liposarcomas. The majority of the patients are older than 50 years of age, with men and women equally affected. The lower extremity is the most common site affected (60 %). In general, it is an aggressive sarcoma with an overall 5-year survival of about 50 %.

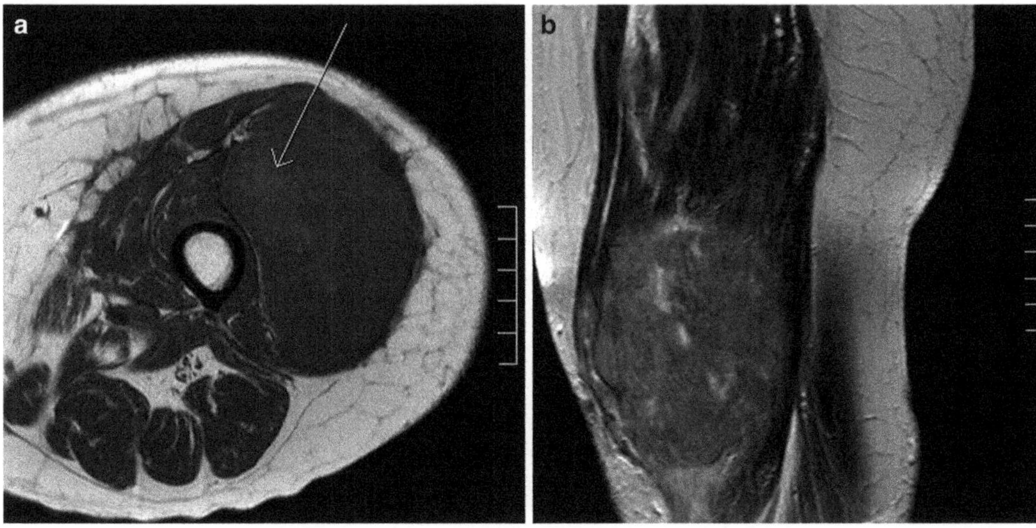

Fig. 28.6 Pleomorphic liposarcoma in a 73-year-old woman with a rapidly evolving painless mass in the left thigh. (**a**) Axial T1-weighted MRI shows a large anterior compartment intramuscular mass with a small focus of high signal similar to that of fat (*arrow*). (**b**) Sagittal T2-weighted MRI demonstrates a nonspecific intermediate intensity tissue signal

The most frequent histopathological picture is that of a fibrous histiocytoma-like spindle cell tumor with abnormal lipoblasts. Less than 5 % of the volume of the tumor contains adipose tissue.

On MRI, it appears as a nonspecific soft tissue mass. As the adipose component is the only one recognizable by MRI, the diagnosis is challenging. T1-weighted sequences in particular show rare hyperintense foci of fat that can be distinguished from hemorrhage on fat-saturation T1-weighted sequences (Fig. 28.6).

Adipocytic Tumors: Hyperintense on T1 and T2-Weighted Sequences

Key Points

- Lipoma
  - Intramuscular tumor
  - Normal muscular fibers visible inside the lesion
  - No septa
  - No tissular nodules
- Hibernoma
  - Intermuscular tumor
  - Less hyperintense on T1-weighted sequence than subcutaneous fat
  - No tissular nodules
- WDLS
  - Occurs during the sixth and seventh decades of life
  - Occurs frequently in the lower extremity
  - More than 75 % of the tumor is hyperintense on T1-weighted sequences
  - Thick septa (>2 mm) and tissular nodules
- DDLS
  - Dedifferentiation occurs more frequently de novo
  - Accounts for 40 % of liposarcomas
  - Tumor with two components: WDLS and nonspecific sarcoma
- Pleomorphic liposarcoma
  - Fewer than 5 % of the tumors present a high signal on T1-weighted sequence

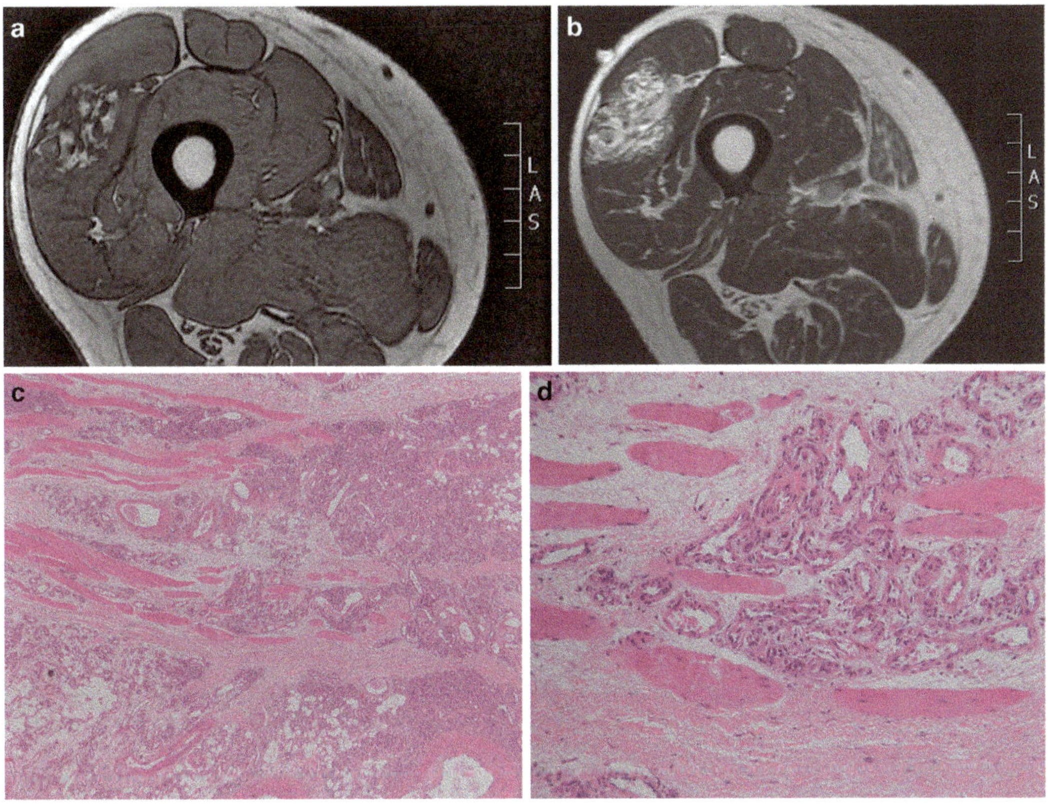

Fig. 28.7 Hemangioma of the right thigh in a 64-year-old man with significant sudden pain that had been present for 2 months. (**a**) Axial gradient echo T1-weighted MRI shows an intramuscular heterogeneous mass in the vastus lateralis muscle with a focal area of hyperintensity. (**b**) Axial TSE T2-weighted MRI demonstrates some signal-void vessels and the lobulated architecture described as a "bunch made up of clusters of grapes." (**c, d**) Histology shows proliferation made up of clusters of small capillaries infiltrating the muscular fibers

28.8.1.2 Nonadipocytic Tumors

Hemangioma

Along with lipomas, hemangiomas are the most frequent muscular tumors. They account for approximately 7 % of soft tissue tumors. Benign vascular tumors are classified according to the type of vessels: capillary, venous, arteriolar. They can be found at all ages but appear more frequently in children and young adults. Clinically, there may be changes in skin coloration, pain, and sometimes fluctuation in the size of the lesion over time. It is this variation that causes the patient concern and motivates the consultation. Hemangioma is the most frequent vascular tumor in the limbs, particularly in the lower limbs.

The histopathology consists of a persistence of striated muscle fibers between vessels of variable size, capillaries, or cavernous vessels, or mixed vascular tissue. It is also often associated with adjacent adipose tissue.

An MRI diagnosis is easier for its cavernous form than its capillary form. The signal intensity of the tumor on MRI is heterogeneous and difficult to interpret. The MRI features include a hypointense T1 signal from its serpiginous vascular structures and dissociating fibroadipocytic tissue. The existence of phlebolites or of intratumoral deposits of hemosiderin cause a drop in the MRI signal through perturbation of the magnetic field, which translates into intratumoral foci with signal loss. In addition, there are areas of T1 hyperintense signal corresponding to areas of adipose tissue. In general, the hemangioma is poorly circumscribed and spindle-shaped, with a more-or-less lobulated architecture in the shape of a bunch of grapes on T2-weighted images. There are also structures with no signal (Fig. 28.7).

As is often the case with slow-growing benign tumors, there is a peritumoral zone of T1 hyperintense signal that represents muscular atrophy or increased production of adipose tissue—the "fat split sign." Changes in neighboring bone structures, such as hypertrophia or periosteal reactions, are observed infrequently.

Non Adipocytic Tumors with Hyperintense Signal on T1-Weighted Sequence: Hemangioma

Key Points

- Hemangioma preferentially occurs during childhood and young adulthood.
- It is an ill-defined lesion.
- MRI features include the following: (1) coexisting adipose areas, signal void vessels, and tissue components; (2) heterogeneous T1 and T2 signal intensity; (3) lobulated architecture with a bunch of grapes appearance on T2-weighted imaging; (4) peripheral hyperintense signal rim separating the tumor from adjacent muscle-the "fat split sign."

28.8.2 Tumors with a Strong Hyperintense Signal on T2-Weighted MRI

Tumors with a strong hyperintense signal on T2-weighted MRI are characterized histopathologically by poor cellularity and a matrix that generally consists of hyaluronic acid or, more rarely, mucus, and a chondroid substance.

Deep myxoid tumors pose the problems of determining whether they are benign or malignant and of identifying the line of differentiation. The most common deep myxoid tumors are myxoid liposarcoma, myxofibrosarcoma, and intramuscular or juxta-articular myxoma. Other exceptionally rare tumors may also be observed, including extraskeletal myxoid chondrosarcoma and low-grade fibromyxoid sarcoma.

Myxoid tissue is recognizable on MRI based on its signal, which is identical to that of fluid on T1- and T2-weighted sequences. Intravenous injection of gadolinium-based contrast medium leads to enhancement of the tumor tissue and the tumor matrix, which is always vascularized—in contrast to cystic lesions.

28.8.2.1 Myxoma

Intramuscular myxoma is a benign mesenchymal tumor that mostly occurs in adults (median age 50 years). Myxomas generally affect women more frequently than men, with a ratio of 1.4:1.0. In 50 % of cases, myxomas are located in the thigh. The circumstances in which myxomas are discovered vary. They may be discovered incidentally as a slowly growing, nonpainful mass. Rarely, they are rapidly growing, painful lesions and become evident because of the symptoms they produce.

Bone involvement such as polyostotic fibrous dysplasia can be observed. In this case, it is part of Mazabraud's syndrome, suggesting a basic error in connective tissue metabolism.

Histolopathological analysis shows a relatively regular myxoid tissue that is finely fibrillated and with few vascular structures. There is also a scarce cell component consisting of elements with small nuclei and an absence of atypia.

The imaging features seen with US and particularly MRI are well described in the literature and in general enable a straightforward diagnosis. The myxoma is a tumor with sharp contours and has a cystic appearance on T1- and T2-weighted MRI sequences. A complete or partial capsule is identified with MRI in 55 % of the cases. The lesion may be lobulated, with thin internal septa. It characteristically presents a thin, bordered hyperintense T1 signal in the periphery corresponding to muscular atrophy. Its very intense signal on T2-weighted sequences is related to the rich content of mucopolysaccharides. There is an almost constant T2 hyperintense signal in adjacent muscles suggesting edema. Three enhancement pattern have been described after injection of contrast: peripheral; peripheral and in the septa; or peripheral and central with a punctuated contrast uptake in the central zone (Fig. 28.8).

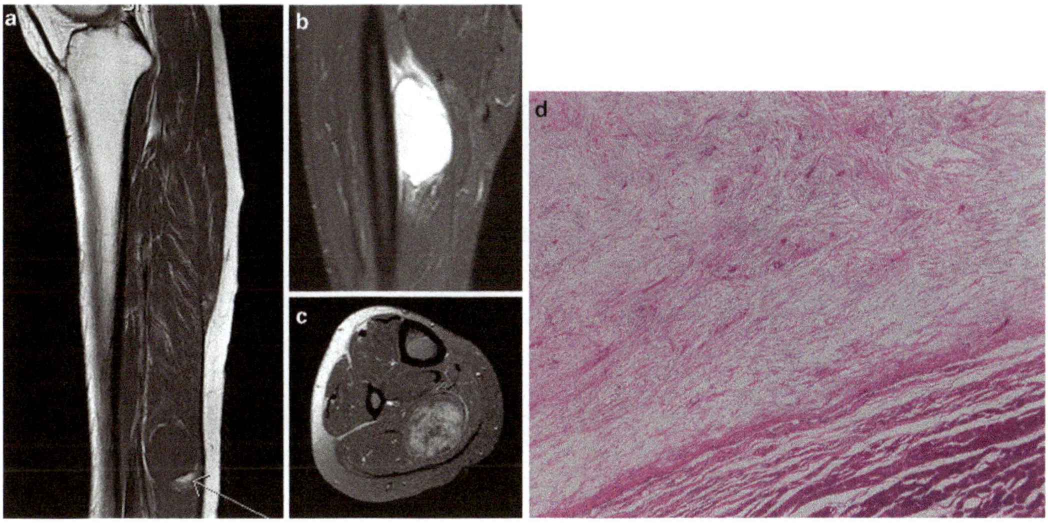

Fig. 28.8 Myxoma of the right leg of a 51-year-old woman. She had had the painful lesion for 2 years, but it was initially diagnosed as a hematoma. (**a**) Sagittal TSE T1-weighted MRI shows an intramuscular homogeneous isointense tumor with a peripheral hyperintense fat ring (*arrow*), described as the "split fat sign." (**b**) Sagittal TSE T2-weighted sequence with fat saturation MRI demonstrates a lesion with very high fluid-like signal intensity. There is also an ill-defined peripheral hyperintense signal in adjacent muscles. (**c**) Axial postcontrast TSE T1-weighted MRI shows internal and peripheral type III enhancement of the lesion. (**d**) Histological analysis shows a homogeneous fibrillated myxoid matrix with few vascular structures. There are small nuclei cells without atypia

The principal differential diagnoses include other tumors with a myxoid component. Intramuscular nerve sheath tumors are recognizable by their spindle shape with a parent nerve entering and exiting. This fairly specific target pattern on T2-weighted sequences is not found in myxomas. Other myxoid tumors, such as myxoid liposarcoma or myxofibrosarcoma, tend to have a more intermuscular topography. They are not associated with peritumoral edema or a peripheral fatty border. They present with a more heterogeneous matrix on T2-weighted images and more intense contrast enhancement.

28.8.2.2 Myxoid Liposarcoma

Myxoid liposarcoma and round cell liposarcoma are two variants of the same tumor (MRCLS). They represent about 10–20 % of all liposarcomas. Compared to the DDLSs, these tumors occur more frequently in the young adult population. In 80 % of the cases, they develop in deep soft tissue areas in the lower limbs, particularly in the thigh or the popliteal fossa.

The prognosis is also less favorable in terms of local recurrence but particularly in terms of metastatic dissemination. MRCLS differs from most sarcomas in its metastatic spread to extrapulmonary sites with frequent bone involvement. The poor prognosis is directly related to the percentage of round cells in the tumor. The 5 % cutoff value has been accepted as the most valuable. The Canadian multidisciplinary sarcoma team showed in a recent retrospective study of 418 patients that the 5-year metastasis-free survival drops from 84 % for myxoid liposarcomas to 69 % for round cell liposarcomas.

Histopathologically, this tumor consists of a regular myxoid matrix with rich vascularization consisting of thin-walled capillaries, often anastomosed, and the presence of small cells with round, regular nuclei predominantly around the capillaries. It is important to obtain a good sample of the tumor to identify any eventual round cell component, which would worsen the prognosis.

An MRI evaluation is fairly efficient because of the high sensitivity of the T1 sequences for detecting

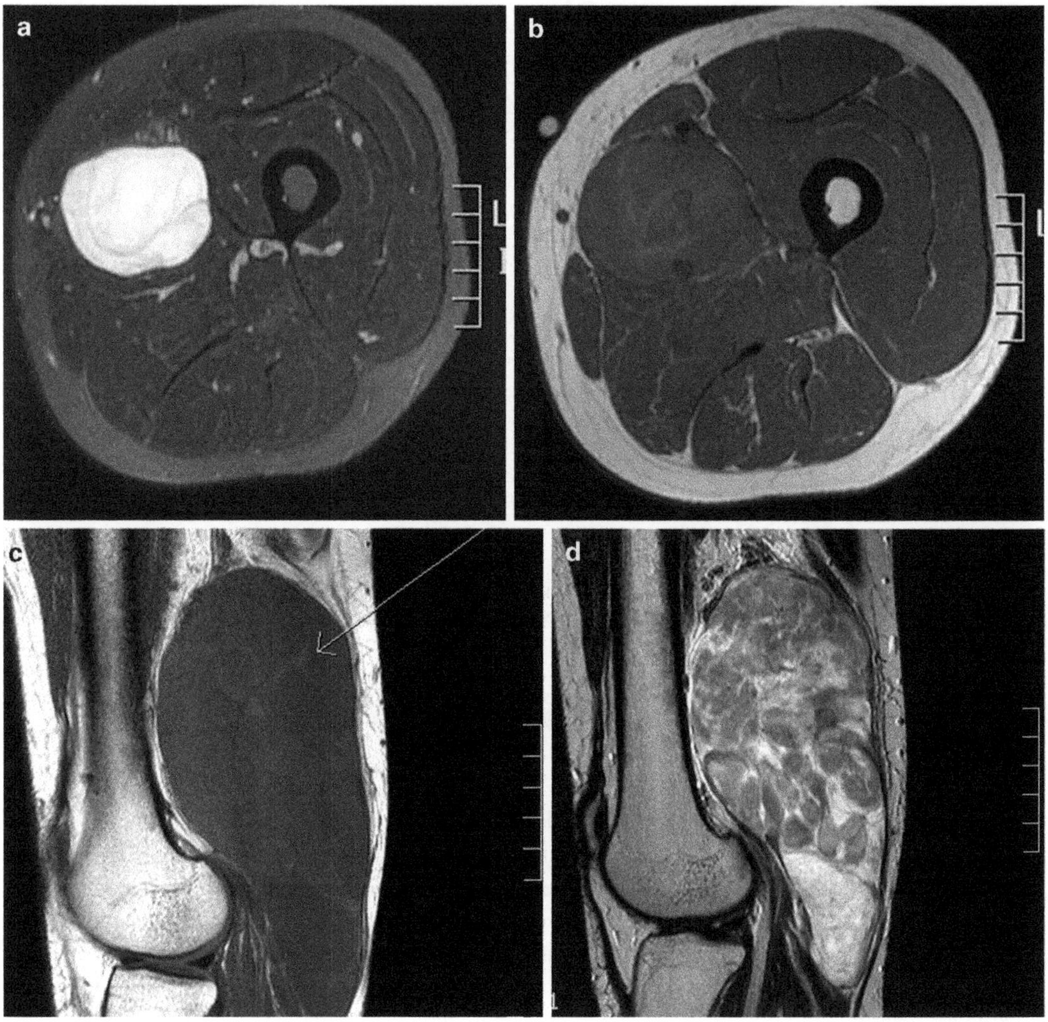

Fig. 28.9 Myxoid and round cell liposarcomas. (**a**, **b**) Myxoid liposarcoma in a 54-year-old man with a painless mass of the posterior right thigh and an initial diagnosis of hematoma. (**a**) Axial TSE T2-weighted MRI shows a well-defined tumor with a fluid-like signal. (**b**) Axial TSE T1-weighted MRI shows an isointense tumor but with fine hyperintense strands corresponding to adipose tissue, indicating a myxoid liposarcoma. (**c**, **d**) Myxoid liposarcoma with a prominent round cell component in a 41-year-old woman who had had an enlarging mass of the left popliteal fossa for 4 years. Sagittal T1-weighted (**c**) and corresponding sagittal T2-weighted (**d**) MRI demonstrate a 15-cm posterior mass with fine hyperintense areas on the T1-weighted image (adipose tissue) and nonspecific tissue signal on the T2-weighted image. The signal intensity is not as high as that for myxoid matrix on T2-weighted MRI

fatty tissue even in small amounts (generally <10 % of tumoral volume) and demonstrating the liquid-type signal of mxyoid tissue on T2-weighted sequences. Adipose tissue can be identified in the form of fine, hyperintense linear structures in T1-weighted images. These lesions are large, well delimited, and multi-lobulated, and they have an intermuscular topography. The tumors show heterogeneous enhancement after injection of contrast (Fig. 28.9). With this classic presentation, the differential diagnosis is limited and straightforward. However, there is a histological variant of this tumor that is the round cell liposarcoma with small, round tumor cells and no fatty tissue. In this particular subtype, because of the absence of a fatty component (and therefore a specific MRI cri-

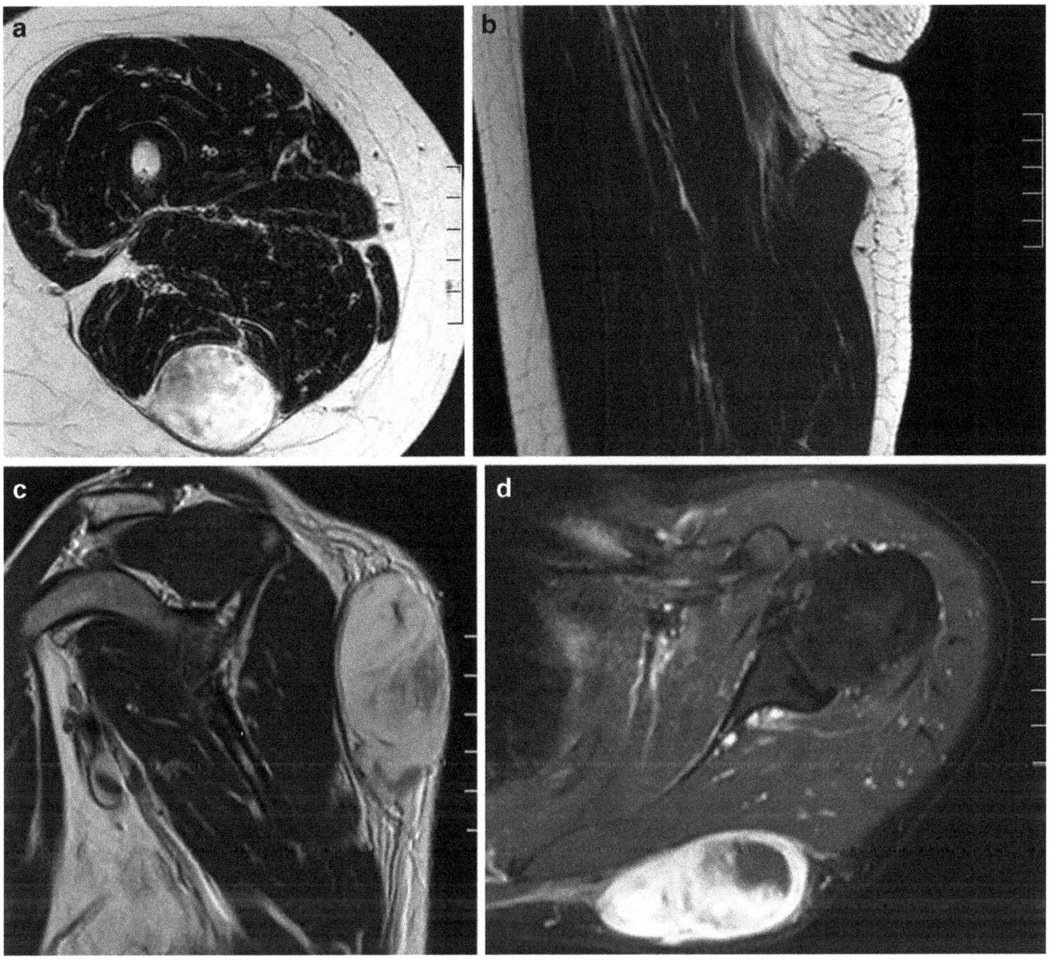

Fig. 28.10 Myxofibrosarcomas. (**a**, **b**) Myxofibrosarcoma of the left thigh. Axial T2-weighted MRI (**a**) demonstrates a high signal due to myxoid matrix, but there is no hyperintense area on the T1-weighted sequence because there is no fat in the lesion. This is the criterion used to differentiate myxofibrosarcoma from myxoid liposarcoma. (**c**, **d**) Myxofibrosarcoma of the left shoulder in a 53-year-old woman. (**c**) Sagittal T2-weighted MRI shows a relatively well-circumscribed hyperintense but heterogeneous mass. (**d**) Axial postcontrast T1-weighted MRI with fat saturation shows that the tumor spread along the fascial plane, which is relatively frequent for this soft-tissue tumor subtype

terion), imaging cannot contribute substantially to the correct diagnosis.

28.8.2.3 Myxofibrosarcoma

Myxofibromas are malignant tumors that mainly affect the elderly. They have a heterogeneous composition and present with a composite T2-weighted signal on MRI. The tumor is found most often in the thigh, progressing and infiltrating the surrounding soft tissue. The tumor is not well delimited, sometimes showing a multifocal presentation disseminating along the fascias. After injection of intravenous contrast material, the highly heterogeneous enhancement suggests a malignant tumor. Myxoid tissue can be identified on T2-weighted images, but unlike the myxoid liposarcoma adipose tissue is not found on T1-weighted images (Fig. 28.10) Metastasis is observed in 35 % of cases and therefore is less frequent compared to other pleomorphic sarcomas, formerly known as malignant fibrous histocytomas (MFHs).

> **Tumors with a Strong Hyperintense Signal on T2-Weighted MRI**
>
> **Key Points**
> - Myxoma
>   - It is a well-delimitated intramuscular lesion, lobulated with septa.
>   - It has a cystic-like appearance on T2-weighted MRI.
>   - The fat slit sign is apparent on T1-weighted imaging.
>   - Postcontrast image shows three types of enhancement: peripheral; peripheral and septa; punctuated internal matrix tumor enhancement.
> - Myxoid liposarcoma and round cell liposarcoma
>   - They occur in young adults.
>   - They are well-defined, multilobulated tumors.
>   - They contain a small amount of adipose tissue (<10 % of the tumor).
>   - There are fine hyperintense linear structures on T1-weighted images.
>   - These tumors have a cystic-like appearance on T2-weighted MRI.
>   - Postcontrast images show heterogeneous enhancement.
> - Myxofibrosarcoma
>   - It occur in elderly patients.
>   - It is ill-defined and often multifocal.
>   - It has a heterogeneous appearance on T1- and T2-weigjhted images
>   - Strongly hyperintense zones on T2-weighted MRI correspond to myxoid tissue.

28.8.3 Tumors with Hypointense Signal on T2-Weighted MRI

28.8.3.1 Tumor with T2 Hypointense Signal Corresponding to Fibrous Tissue

Elastofibroma

Elastofibromas are benign tumors that have distinctive imaging features on both CT and MRI based on the lesion's appearance and topography. These tumors are found in adults, usually women (female/male ratio 4:1). The lesion is infiltrating and not well delineated.

Histopathologically, elastofibromas contain fibrous tissue, including bundles of adipose tissue and particularly numerous elastic fibers, which constitutes the most characteristic element for diagnosis.

On MRI, elastofibromas are associated with a hypointense signal on T2-weighted images of striated adipose tissue. In 90 % of cases, the lesion is localized in the wall of the thorax, lying under the serratus anterior muscle or in the subscapular area. In many patients, the tumor appears bilaterally (Fig. 28.11).

> **Tumor with T2 Hypointense Signal Corresponding to Fibrous Tissue: Elastofibroma**
>
> **Key Points**
> - Elastofibromas preferentially occur in woman and are often bilateral.
> - They are located in the subscapular space at the scapula tip.
> - On imaging (CT or MRI), linear adipose strands are seen interspersed within tissue components, producing a striated appearance.

Myositis Ossificans

Myositis ossificans is an intramuscular tumor occurring in young adults. It is of unknown etiology, occurring occasionally after trauma. It can present clinically with pain during the initial phase. The histopathological diagnosis can be difficult, therefore imaging plays an essential role in diagnosis and in treatment decisions. The lesion evolves over time into a mass that calcifies after a number of weeks in centripetal fashion starting in the periphery. Initially flocculent, the calcifications become increasingly dense over time.

Histopathologically, myositis ossificans is easily diagnosed by demonstrating a zoning phenomenon characterized by relatively mature peripheral ossification and a lesion center

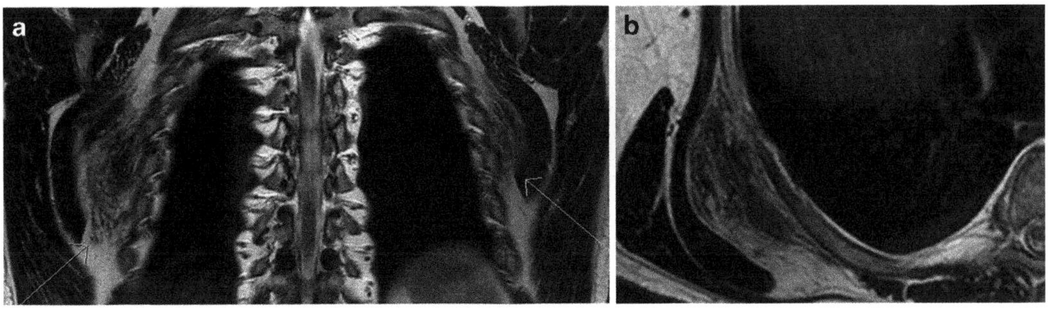

Fig. 28.11 Elastofibroma. Coronal (**a**) and axial (**b**) T2-weighted MRI show ill-defined bilateral lesions with linear interspersed adipose tissue. The location deep in relation to the scapular tip is almost specific for this tumor

comprising immature ossification and zones of myofibroblasts. At this stage, interpreting material from a microbiopsy specimen obtained from the center of the lesion without considering the radiological aspects of the lesion may lead to a wrong diagnosis. Immature ossification comprising numerous cells, often in mitosis, may be noted, which may suggest an erroneous diagnosis of osteosarcoma.

On MRI, the appearance may be heterogeneous and confusing during the early stage. It shows a poorly defined, heterogeneous lesion with non specific T2 hyperintensity. The diagnosis should be based on various aspects, including the clinical presentation and the presence of a perilesional hyperintense signal on T2-weighted images suggesting muscle and neighboring cancellous bone edema. It should be noted that there is never contiguous bone destruction and that a border of separation is always present between the mass and the underlying bone. At this stage, if a diagnosis of myositis ossificans is suggested, a CT scan, which is more sensitive for detecting calcifications, may assist in confirming the diagnosis by showing the zonal architecture of the tumor (Fig. 28.12). The differential diagnosis includes extraskeletal osteosarcoma, which generally presents with ossification of the central matrix of the tumor and tumor tissue proliferation on the periphery—an architecture that is different from that of myositis ossificans.

Tumor with T2 Hypointense Signal Corresponding to Fibrous Tissue: Myositis ossificans

Key Points

- Myositis ossificans occurs in young adults.
- It is a poorly defined and heterogeneous lesion.
- There may be neighboring bone and/or muscle edema.
- It is always separated from underlying bone.
- It is an evolving mass with zonal architecture marked by a calcified rim at the periphery, seen on CT.

Desmoid-Like Fibromatosis

Desmoid-like fibromatosis is a benign tumor that can be locally aggressive. It frequently occurs during the second to fourth decade of life and is seen more often in women (67 %). Its clinical presentation can be inconclusive and depends on the localization of the tumor. Although it appears in the abdominal wall in women, in 70 % of cases it is extra-abdominal. In more than one-third of cases it is located in upper or lower limbs and more frequently in the shoulder girdle. When the lesion is located deep in the abdomen, it can be associated with a mutation of the *APC* gene (adenomatous polyposis coli) in Gardner's syndrome. Surgical resection remains the gold standard. However, with these voluminous benign tumors, it can lead to complications and functional impairment. The time point at which surgery should be carried out is difficult to define. Surgery should be reserved for progressing tumors as some lesions can stabilize or even regress spontane-

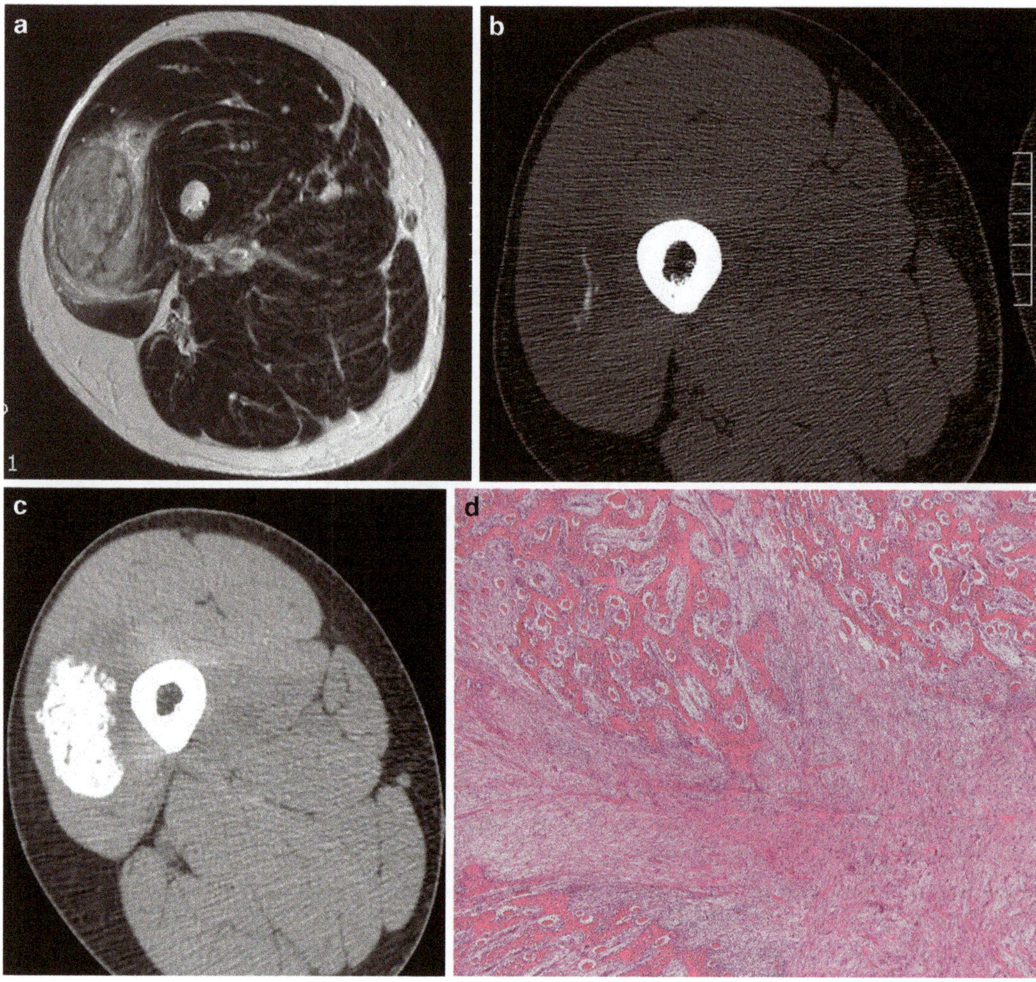

Fig. 28.12 Myositis ossificans in a 32-year-old man with a painful mass in the thigh. (**a**) Axial TSE T2-weighted MRI demonstrates a heterogeneous tumor in the vastus lateralis muscle associated with a hyperintense signal of the adjacent tissue that is edema-like. (**b**) Noncontrast computed tomography (CT) shows central calcifications in the lesion. (**c**) Noncontrast CT 5 months later shows that the entire lesion is calcified. (**d**) Histologically, the lesion has zonal architecture with newly formed trabecular bone that has a reactional aspect and a central zone with cells and myxoid matrix

ously after an initial phase of progression. The rate of local relapse is high (44 %) in those who undergo complete surgical tumor removal, compared with 66 % in cases of incomplete removal.

Histopathologically, the tumor consists of a low-density proliferation of cytologically benign myofibroblasts arranged in bundles within a collagen-rich matrix. A characteristic feature is the infiltration mode of the peripheral striated muscles. There is no necrosis. The histopathological diagnosis can be confirmed if necessary by demonstrating a mutation in the β-catenin gene, which is found in 85 % of extra-abdominal desmoid tumors.

On MRI (Fig. 28.13), the appearance is fairly characteristic on T1- and T2-weighted images. The tumor is either well delineated (>50 % of cases) or infiltrating (34 % of patients) along the fascias ("fascial tail sign") and demonstrates bundles with a marked hyposignal regardless of the sequence. These features are correlated with the presence of collagen, alternating with more vascularized tissue zones. This appearance is found in approximately 85 % of cases. The lesion develops on the surface of the muscle structures in the fascia or aponeurosis and can invade the underlying muscle over several anatomical compartments. This appearance is quite unusual in

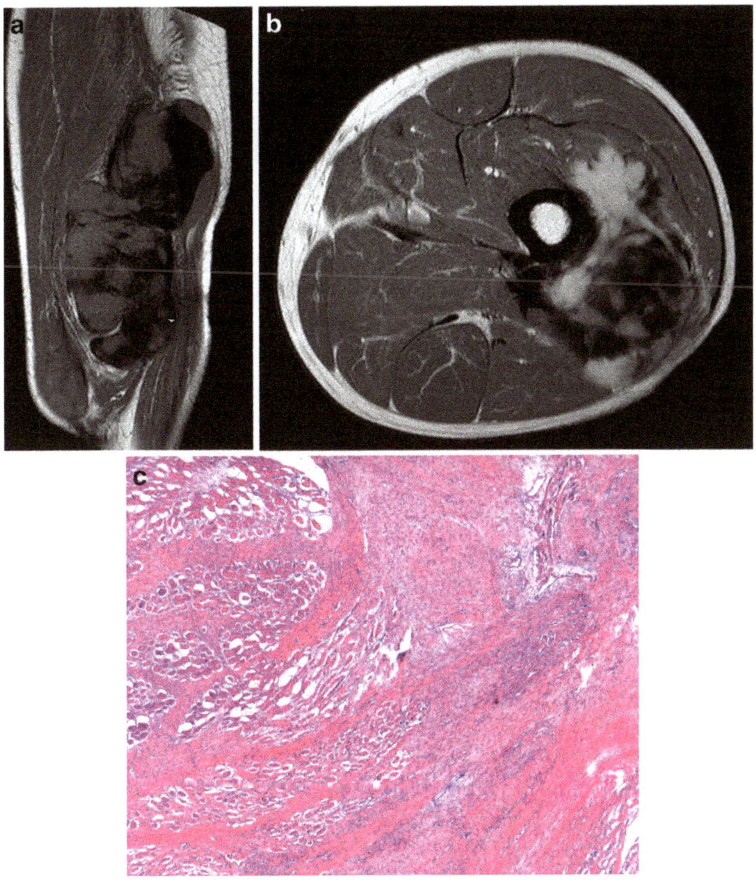

Fig. 28.13 Desmoid-like fibromatosis. (**a**) Sagittal TSE T1-weighted MRI shows a heterogeneous tumor with hypointense and isointense areas. (**b**) Postcontrast axial TSE T1-weighted MRI with fat saturation shows a deeply infiltrating tumor crossing over several compartments of the left thigh with strongly hypointense zones within the global tumor enhancement. (**c**) Histologically, the tumor contains fusiform cells with a fibrous matrix. It has infiltrated striated muscles that are partially destroyed

the case of a sarcomatous tumor. It may also show spicules with retraction of the skin.

Low-Grade Fibromyxoid Sarcoma

Low-grade fibromyxoid sarcoma is a rare tumor that occurs mainly in adults (during the fourth decade). The tumor is predominantly localized in the lower extremity and trunk wall. Clinically, it is a deep, slow-growing, painless tumor that produces metastases in the lungs and bone.

The histopathological diagnosis is often difficult, particularly when the material is obtained by microbiopsy. The tumor presents as a fibromyxoid matrix with a cell component of varying density. These cells tend to be arranged in short

Tumor with T2 Hypointense Signal Corresponding to Fibrous Tissue: Desmoid-like fibromatosis

Key Points

- Desmoid-like fibromatosis occurs during the second to fourth decade of life; 67 % of cases occur in women.
- It is an ill-defined benign tumor that develops at the muscle surface.
- The shoulder and neck are the most frequent locations.
- On MRI, there is a specific band-like

morphology of some areas and hypointensity on T1- and T2-weighted images.
- It exhibits linear extension along fascial planes (i.e., "fascial tail sign").
- There are subcutaneous spicules with cutaneous retraction.
- With fibrous dysplasia it constitutes Mazabraud's syndrome.
- It may be associated with *APC* gene mutation in Gardner's syndrome.

revolving bundles but exhibit little atypia. The diagnosis is now assisted by the recent discovery of an immunohistochemical marker, MUC4, which is highly sensitive and specific. In addition, the tumor has a specific genetic translocation t(7;16) with a chimeric gene *FUS-CREB3L2*.

The MRI evaluation reveals a well-delimited tumor with fairly intense areas on T2-weighted images alternating with areas showing a strong T2 hypointense signal intensity corresponding to myxoid and fibrous tissue, respectively. It contains neither necrosis nor hemorrhagic surfaces (Fig. 28.14). The differential diagnosis includes tumors containing myxoid tissue, in particular liposarcoma. However, liposarcoma is characterized by its fatty component, which is hyperintense on T1-weighted images. The main differential diagnosis is desmoid-like fibromatosis.

Tumor with T2 Hypointense Signal Corresponding to Fibrous Tissue: Low-grade fibromyxoid sarcoma

Key Points

- Low-grade fibromyxoid sarcoma preferentially occurs in young adults in their fourth decade of life.
- It is predominantly located in the lower extremity.
- On T2-weighted MRI, the lesion shows hyperintense areas alternating with large hypointense zones.

28.8.3.2 Tumors with T2 Hypointense Signal Corresponding to Hemosiderin or Ossification Matrix

Giant Cell Tumors of the Tendon Sheath and Pigmented Villonodular Synovitis

Pigmented villonodular synovitis (PVNS) is benign proliferation of the synovial membrane, that simulates tumoral proliferation. Giant cell tumor of the tendon sheath (GCTTS), is the tumoral counterpart of the same disorder.

Histopathologically, this tumor is generally well delimited, except in its diffuse forms. It consists of histiocytic cell types with mononucleic cells, giant multinucleic cells, macrophages, and siderophages. Immunohistochemical analysis with anti-CD163 highlights the histiocyic nature of visible cells. The stroma may be fibrous or hyalinized with an osteoid-like appearance. This histopathological appearance may be misleading and might suggest round-cell sarcoma or osteosarcoma.

On MRI, the appearances of the two pathologies are similar. Both show a hypointense signal on T1- and T2-weighted images, reflecting hemosiderin deposits. They can be observed more sensitively on T2-weighted gradient-echo sequences. The differential diagnosis is based on the lesion's location: intra-articularly (PVNS) or near a joint along a tendon (GCTTS) (Fig. 28.15). For the latter, the principal differential diagnosis includes malignant fibrous tumors or tumors with an osteogenic matrix, such as low-grade fibromyxoid sarcoma or the exceptionally rare extraskeletal osteosarcoma.

Tumor with T2 Hypointense Signal Corresponding to Hemosiderin or Ossification-Matrix

Key Points

- These two entities are predominantly located in the lower extremity: intra-articularly in the knee joint (PVNS) or along the tendons (GCTTS)
- On T2-weighted MRI, the lesions show hypointense lesions corresponding to hemosiderin deposits.

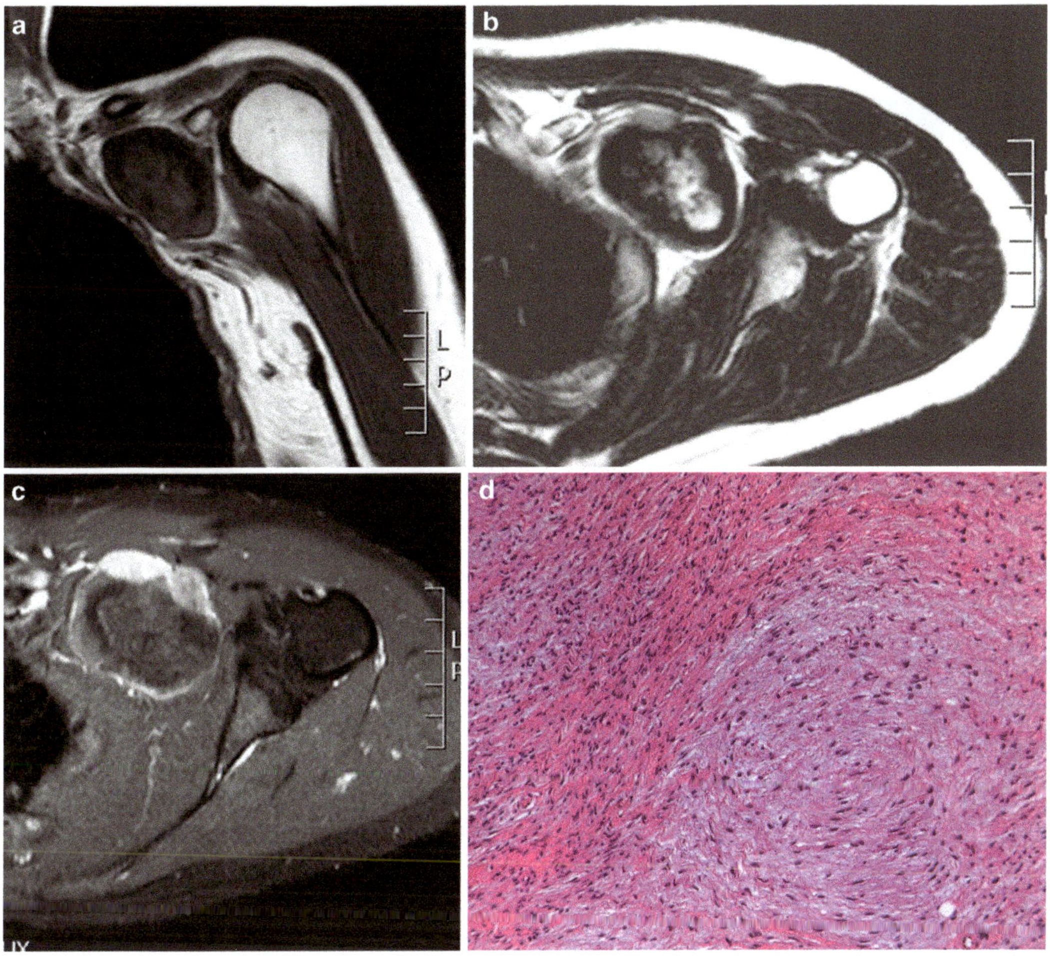

Fig. 28.14 Low-grade fibromyxoid sarcoma in a 35-year-old woman with an enlarging painful mass of the left shoulder girdle of 1-year duration. (**a**) Coronal TSE T1-weighted MRI shows a hypointense mass in the area of the left upper axilla. (**b**) Axial T2-weighted MRI demonstrates areas of low intensity. The main differential diagnosis is desmoid-like fibromatosis. However, the latter usually spreads along the fascia or aponeurosis and can affect several muscular groups. (**c**) Postcontrast axial TSE T1-weighted MRI with fat saturation shows poor heterogeneous, nonspecific enhancement with nonenhancing areas. (**d**) Histologically, it is a tumor with a fibromyxoid matrix. Fusiform cells tend to be arranged in short revolving bundles and exhibit atypia

Extraskeletal Osteosarcoma

Extraskeletal osteosarcoma is a rare tumor. On histopathology, the appearance is similar to that of conventional osteosarcomas with predominant ossification in the center, which is different from myositis ossificans.

The diagnosis is mainly based on the MRI evaluation, which shows a tumor with an osteogenic matrix and central calcifications and tumor tissue on the periphery. It presents as a heterogeneous lesion on T2-weighted images without the zonal architecture seen in myositis ossificans.

28.8.4 Tumors of Uncertain Differentiation with Specific MRI Features

28.8.4.1 Synovial Sarcoma

The synovial sarcoma is a malignant tumor found mainly in relatively young adults (<50 years). In almost 85 % of cases the tumor is located in the extremities, generally in the vicinity of the knee joint, although it is a ubiquitous tumor. The prognosis is poor as it is considered a high-grade sarcoma. It has a 5-year disease-free survival of about 60 %.

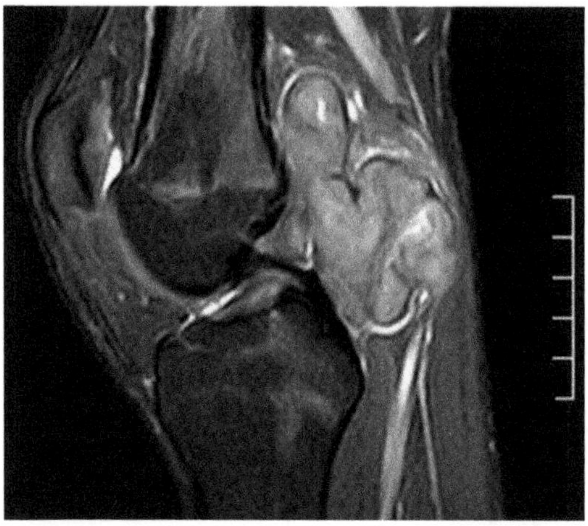

Fig. 28.15 Pigmented villonodular synovitis (PVNS) of the knee in a young boy. Sagittal T2-weighted MRI demonstrates a tumor-like lesion with an intra-articular origin. This pattern is quite unusual for a sarcoma, and PVNS should be suggested first

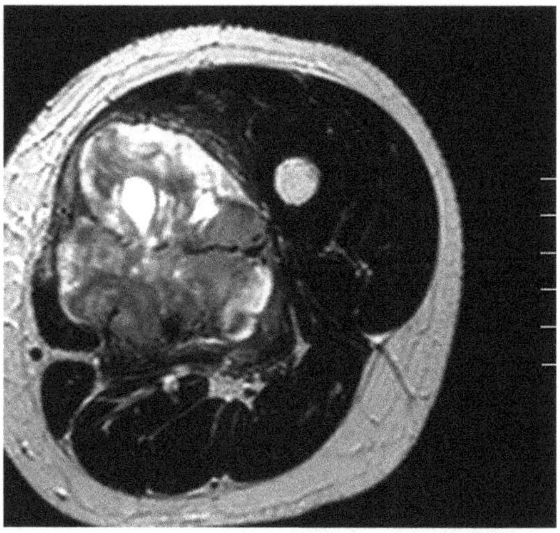

Fig. 28.16 Synovial sarcoma in a 56-year-old woman with a history of a rapidly enlarging mass in the left thigh. Axial T2-weighted MRI shows a lesion infiltrating the anterior compartment of the left thigh. It has a composite signal with low-, intermediate-, and high-intensity signal areas—the "triple sign"

Synovial sarcoma represents a densely cellular tumor consisting of small spindle cells associated with an epithelial-type component which may include calcifications, ossification, and zones of tumoral necrosis. Immunohistochemical analysis shows partially an epithelial phenotype, while molecular analysis shows a specific translocation t(X;18).

On MRI, the appearance may be deceptive, seemingly representative of a benign tumor. The tumor is sometimes slow-growing, well defined with a pseudo-capsule, and a pseudo-cystic appearance on T2-weighted images. Generally, it is a multiloculated tumor containing septa, with a heterogeneous appearance on T1- and T2-weighted images due to the presence of intratumoral hemorrhagic zones. Calcifications are present in one-third of cases. The heterogeneous appearance is rather unusual for a benign tumor, however. On T2-weighted images, the lesion presents with a heterogeneous aspect including areas with hypo-, iso-, and hyperintensity—generally described as "the triple sign." Fluid-fluid levels relating to intratumoral hemorrhage can also be observed (Fig. 28.16). The underlying bone is invaded through contiguity in approximately 20 % of cases.

Tumors of Uncertain Differentiation with Specific MR Imaging Features: Synovial sarcoma

Key Points

- The synovial sarcoma occurs preferentially in young adults <50 years of age.
- In all, 85 % of all tumors are located in the lower extremity near the knee joint.
- On MRI, the tumor has a well-defined and pseudo-cystic benign appearance.
- Heterogeneous signals on T1- and T2-weighted images provide the "triple sign."
- Fluid-fluid levels are present and are related to intratumoral hemorrhage.

28.9 Summary

Muscle tumors comprise a heterogeneous group of mesenchymal lesions for which the diagnosis and management can be complex. The treatment is radically different according to whether it is a benign lesion that can be removed simply, or it is a sarcoma requiring initial surgery in a specialized environment. Better knowledge of the molecular biology of these tumors and the improved imaging techniques enable a reduction in diagnostic hypotheses and provide optimum initial treatment for the patient.

Suggestions for Further Reading

Chibon F, Lagarde P, Salas S, et al. Validated prediction of clinical outcome in sarcomas and multiple types of cancer on the basis of a gene expression signature related to genome complexity. Nat Med. 2010;16:781–7.

Coindre JM. Molecular biology of soft-tissue sarcomas. Bull Cancer. 2010;97:1337–45.

Coindre JM, Pédeutour F, Aurias A. Well-differentiated and dedifferentiated liposarcomas. Virchows Arch. 2010;456:167–79.

Fletcher CDM. The evolving classification of soft tissue tumors: an update based on the new WHO classification. Histopathology. 2006;48:3–12.

Griffin N, Khan N, Thomas JM, et al. The radiological manifestations of intramuscular haemangiomas in adults: magnetic resonance imaging, computed tomography and ultrasound appearances. Skeletal Radiol. 2007;36:1051–9.

Kind M, Stock N, Coindre JM. Histology and imaging of soft tissue sarcomas. Eur J Radiol. 2009;72:6–15.

Luna A, Martinez S, Bossen E. Magnetic resonance imaging of intramuscular myxoma with histological comparison and a review of the literature. Skeletal Radiol. 2005;34:19–28.

Murphey MD. World Health Organization classification of bone and soft tissue tumors: modifications and implications for radiologists. Semin Musculoskelet Radiol. 2007;11:201–14.

Murphey MD, Arcara LK, Fanburg-Smith J. From the archives of the AFIP: imaging of musculoskeletal liposarcoma with radiologic-pathologic correlation. Radiographics. 2005;25:1371–95.

Murphey MD, Ruble CM, Tyszko SM, et al. From the archives of the AFIP: musculoskeletal fibromatoses: radiologic-pathologic correlation. Radiographics. 2009;29:2143–73.

O'Sullivan PJ, Harris AC, Munk PL. Radiological features of synovial cell sarcoma. Br J Radiol. 2008;81: 346–56.

Robinson E, Bleakney RR, Ferguson PC, et al. Oncodiagnosis panel: 2007: multidisciplinary management of soft-tissue sarcoma. Radiographics. 2008;28: 2069–86.

Stoeckle E, Coindre JM, Kind M, et al. Evaluating surgery quality in soft tissue sarcoma. Recent Results Cancer Res. 2009;179:229–42.

Toro JR, Travis LB, Wu HJ, et al. Incidence patterns of soft tissue sarcomas, regardless of primary site, in the surveillance, epidemiology and end results program, 1978–2001: an analysis of 26,758 cases. Int J Cancer. 2006;119:2922–30.

Van Vliet M, Kliffen M, Krestin GP, et al. Soft tissue sarcomas at a glance: clinical, histological, and MR imaging features of malignant extremity soft tissue tumors. Eur Radiol. 2009;19:1499–511.

Vilanova JC, Woertler K, Narváez JA, et al. Soft-tissue tumors update: MR imaging features according to the WHO classification. Eur Radiol. 2007;17:125–38.

Walker EA, Song AJ, Murphey MD. Magnetic resonance imaging of soft-tissue masses. Semin Roentgenol. 2010;45: 277–97.

Wu JS, Hochman MG. Soft-tissue tumors and tumor like lesions: a systematic imaging approach. Radiology. 2009;253:297 316.

Part V

Clinical Applications in Motor Neuron Disorders and Peripheral Nerve Imaging

Motor Neuron Diseases

29

Susana Quijano-Roy, Daniela Avila-Smirnow, Robert-Yves Carlier, Mike P. Wattjes, and Dirk Fischer

29.1 Introduction

Motor neuron diseases (MNDs) represent a group of neurological diseases characterized by progressive deterioration of the motor neurons in the brain, brain stem, and spinal cord, leading to muscle weakness and wasting. Genetic MND may be caused by mutations in genes that are widely expressed. Although our understanding of the pathophysiology has increased substantially over the years, the selective vulnerability of motor neurons in this context remains unexplained. In addition to genetic MND, sporadic amyotrophic lateral sclerosis is the most common and devastating motor neuron disorder in adults, with rapid progression leading to a severely impaired life and early death.

S. Quijano-Roy (✉)
Garches Neuromuscular Center (GNMH),
Pediatric Division, Raymond Poincare Hospital,
Paris Ile-de-France Ouest University Hospitals (APHP),
Versailles Saint-Quentin-en-Yvelines University
(UVSQ), 104 boulevard R. Poincare,
92380 Garches, France
e-mail: susana.quijano-roy@rpc.aphp.fr

D. Avila-Smirnow
Servicio de Pediatría, Unidad de Neurología, Complejo Asistencial Dr. Sótero del Río, Red de Salud UC,
Santiago, Chile
e-mail: avidaniela@gmail.com

R.-Y. Carlier
Pole Neuro-Locomoteur, Service d'imagerie Medicale,
Hopital Raymond Poincare, Garches, France
e-mail: robert.carlier@rpc.aphp.fr

M.P. Wattjes
Department of Radiology, Nuclear Medicine & PET
Research, VU University Medical Center,
De Boelelaan 1117, 1081 HV Amsterdam,
The Netherlands
e-mail: m.wattjes@vumc.nl

D. Fischer
Division of Neuropaediatrics, University Childrens
Hospital Basel, 4056 Basel, Switzerland

Department of Neurology, University Hospital Basel,
4031 Basel, Switzerland
e-mail: Dirk.fischer@ukbb.ch

29.2 Spinal Muscular Atrophy

Susana Quijano-Roy, Daniela Avila-Smirnow, and Robert-Yves Carlier

29.2.1 Synonyms and Abbreviations

Hereditary motor neuron disease; Spinal muscular atrophy (SMA); Survival motor neuron (SMN) gene; Werdnig–Hoffmann disease; Kugelberg–Welander disease

29.2.2 Introduction

Spinal muscular atrophy (SMA) is the most common degenerative disease of the nervous system in children. It is the second most common disease inherited in an autosomal recessive pattern (after cystic fibrosis) that affects children and it the

M.P. Wattjes and D. Fischer (eds.), *Neuromuscular Imaging*, DOI 10.1007/978-1-4614-6552-2_29,

most common cause of death during infancy. SMA is caused by deficient survival of motor neuron (SMN) protein, which leads to progressive degeneration of anterior horn cells in the lower brain stem and spinal cord. It produces flaccid weakness in the bulbar, respiratory, trunk, and limb musculature. There is a continuum of phenotypes in terms of clinical severity, ranging from a rapidly lethal course presenting at birth or during the first months of life to adult onset of proximal progressive weakness. Patients usually present during infancy or early childhood with progressive proximal muscular atrophy and weakness. The proximal muscles are more severely affected than the distal and facial muscles. Cognitive function is not impaired. In addition to motor dysfunction, the most severe complications are progressive respiratory insufficiency and spinal deformity due to weakness of the intercostal and paravertebral muscles. The younger the patient at onset, the worse the prognosis and bulbar and cranial nerve involvement is observed. Death may occur as a consequence of respiratory compromise.

Based on historical clinical reports, patients are usually classified into three subtypes. In type I SMA (Werdnig–Hoffmann disease, OMIM#253300), symptoms are present at birth or occur during the first months of life. Patients never sit or walk independently and usually die owing to respiratory failure before the age of 2 years. Patients with type II SMA (OMIM#253550) present after 6 months of age but never walk unaided. In type III (Kugelberg–Welander disease, OMIM#253400), symptoms appear after 2 years of age, sometimes even during late adulthood. In addition to these three groups, a type 0 (neonatal form) and a type IV (adult form) are described. These classifications are based on the age of onset and the maximum function achieved. It is important to observe the clinical course before classifying a patient definitively as an atypical static course lacking the usual rapid initial deterioration may be seen. In most populations, SMA occurs at an incidence of 1/10,000 births and a carrier rate of approximately 2 %. Prevalence is 1.5/10,000.

29.2.3 Genetics and Pathophysiology

The genetics of SMA is complex and not yet completely understood. Independent of the clinical severity, most patients with SMA have a homozygous deletion of the telomeric *SMN1* (survival motor neuron 1) gene found on chromosome 5q13. Small-scale genetic mutations (point mutations, insertions, deletions, small frameshift mutations) in this gene are found in the remaining 5 % of patients. The *SMN1* gene encodes for most of the mRNA for the SMN protein, and SMA patients show a decrease in full-length SMN protein. *SMN2* is an almost identical centromeric homologue of *SMN1* that is located in the same region and, because of alternative splicing, expresses predominantly truncated SMN protein. In fact, *SMN1* and *SMN2* differ in their coding sequences only by a synonymous point mutation in exon 7. The single nucleotide difference does not affect the protein sequence but reduces the splicing efficiency of exon 7. Most SMN2 transcripts are inactive, lacking exon 7; but a small fraction is normal. Patients with homozygous deletion of *SMN1* but high *SMN2* copy number have a milder clinical phenotype than expected, presumably because of this fraction of normal transcripts. Phase 1 trials using compounds expected to optimize SMN2 transcripts or increase production of SMN protein are ongoing.

The SMN protein allows normal apoptosis in the developing fetus, and when the fetus matures it becomes active in stabilizing the neuronal population. In the absence of SMN, programmed cell death seems to persist. SMN is part of a multiprotein complex required for the biogenesis of small nuclear ribonucleoproteins (snRNPs). It is expressed in all mammalian tissues. Presumably, altered snRNPs result in the missplicing of transcripts that are important for motor neuron survival but less crucial for other cells. In addition, recent data support the conclusion that changes in SMN-deficient muscle do not result solely from motor neuron degeneration. SMN is transported along the cytoskeleton in neurons, suggesting a function for SMN in the axon distinct from its role in snRNP biogenesis. Cytoskeletal dynamics and cellular trafficking are critical in muscle and motor neurons, which may explain why both could be involved in the pathology. The fact that muscle weakness and degeneration occur before motor neuron loss and the increased serum creatine kinase (CK) levels (which are higher than normally observed in other diseases causing denervation) supports also the hypothesis that defects intrinsic to the muscle and neuromuscular junction (NMJ) may contribute to disease manifestations. There is evidence that impaired transmission hinders maturation of the NMJ and contributes to the SMA phenotype. Also, data from human tissue and model organisms indicate that SMN deficiency causes intrinsic muscle defects and that muscle tissue may modulate the SMA phenotype through indirect effects on motor neurons.

29.2.4 Histopathology

The disease shows abnormalities mostly confined to motor neurons in the lower brain stem and the anterior horn cells of the spinal cord, as revealed by postmortem examination. With the advent of molecular diagnosis, muscle biopsy is less frequently used for the diagnosis of SMA. SMA I and II in the affected muscles exhibit round, atrophic type I and II fibers. The entire fascicles or groups of fascicles are atrophied. Other fascicles are composed of markedly hypertrophied fibers. The majority of the hypertrophic fibers are type I, and individual hypertrophic type I fibers may be scattered among the atrophic fibers. Fiber-type grouping, when present, is not often marked in SMA type I, particularly if the biopsy is done at a very early stage of the disease. In type III SMA, large- and small-group atrophy of both fiber types can be present. Atrophic fibers may be more angular than the infantile and intermediate forms. Fiber-type grouping is also a more prominent feature in this form of SMA. Occasionally in advanced stages of type III SMA, secondary "myopathic"-appearing changes—fiber size variability, fiber splitting, fibrosis, internal nuclei—may be observed on muscle biopsy.

29.2.5 Clinical Presentation

Clinical findings in SMA types I–III are illustrated in Fig. 29.1. In SMA type I, most mothers report abnormal inactivity of the fetus during the later stages of pregnancy. The newborn or infants with type I SMA are floppy and inactive, and they usually have a weak cry. Facial muscles are only mildly affected, giving these children an alert and interactive expression. Extraocular eye movements are always normal. However, bulbar musculature weakness makes feeding laborious. Aspiration pneumonia is a potentially life-threatening complication. The hips are flexed, abducted, and externally rotated in a "frog-like" position at rest. The knees are flexed. The arms assume a similar posture, with abduction and external rotation of the shoulders and flexion of the elbows. Because the distal musculature is relatively spared, the fingers and toes can be moved. Infants cannot control or lift the head. Areflexia is universal. These children are unable to roll over or sit. The clinical course is progressive deterioration. Death usually results from respiratory failure before the age of 2 years. A subgroup of patients who gain the ability to hold the head up and have partial trunk control may develop a less severe course with preserved cranial nerve function at the end of the first year (no major swallowing disorder and relatively preserved facial expression). At this point, multidisciplinary proactive therapy as that used for SMA type II (positive-pressure or mechanical ventilation, trunk orthosis with braces not harming pulmonary function, oral or enteral nutrition via gastrostomy) may significantly improve.

Patients with SMA type II show normal development during the first 4–6 months of life. They are able to sit independently, but they are never able to walk independently. Muscular weakness is more severe in the lower than the upper extremities. The patellar reflex is absent, while biceps and triceps tendon reflexes may be preserved. Tongue fasciculations are present as well as upper extremity tremors. Scoliosis is a constant finding, and most patients develop hip dislocation, either unilateral or bilateral, before the age of 10 years. All patients require a wheelchair for locomotion.

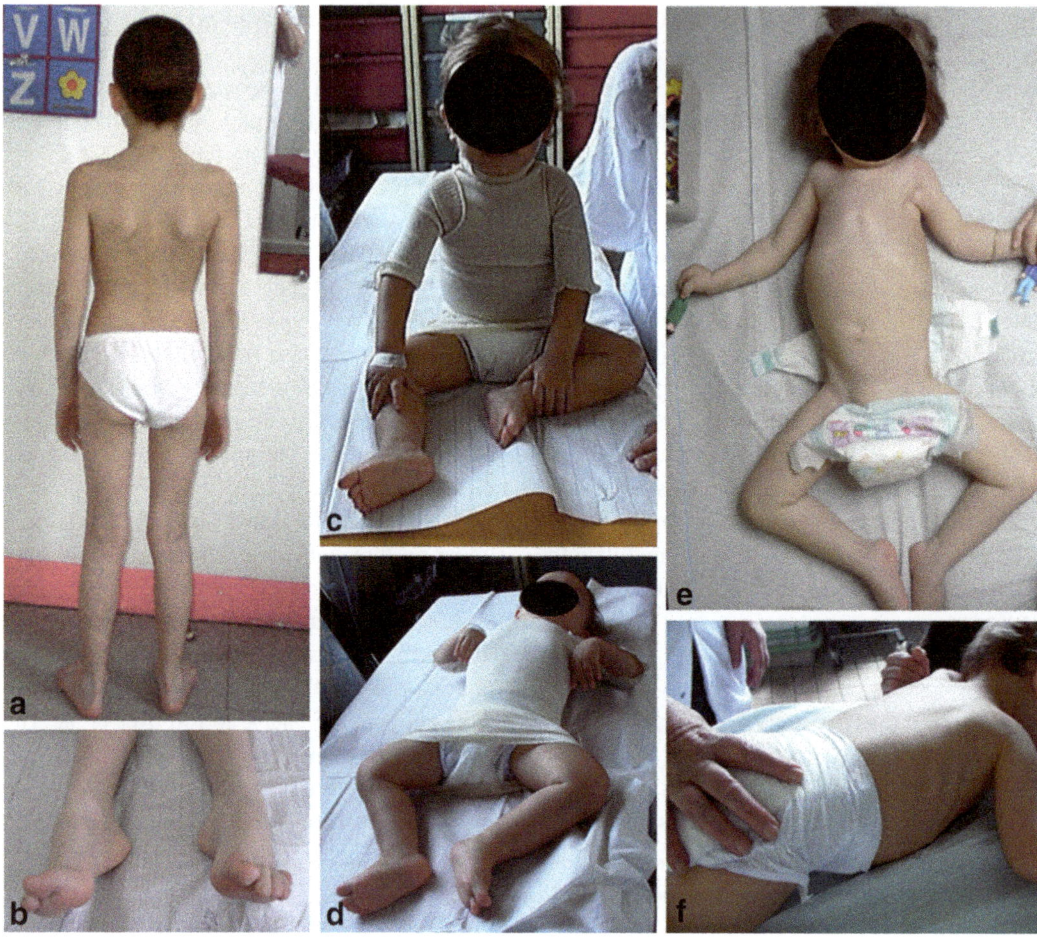

Fig. 29.1 Clinical features of spinal muscular atrophy (SMA) type III (**a**, **b**), type II (**c**, **d**, **f**), and type I (**e**). (**a**, **b**) Type III SMA. There is mild diffuse amyotrophy predominantly in the thighs and mild scapula alata (**a**), and pes cavus (**b**). (**c**, **d**, **f**) Type II SMA. Note the sitting position with axial hypotonia (**c**), diffuse hypotonia in the lying position with hip abduction and flat feet (**d**), intercostal depression on inspiration in a child in ventral decubitus and signs of intercostal muscles weakness (**f**). Type I SMA: typical findings in a child with a Werdnig–Hoffman disease. Note the generalized hypotonia with "frog-like" positions of the lower limbs, absent antigravitatory movements, and the thoracic deformity (bell-shaped) due to paralysis of intercostal muscles, while diaphragmatic function is preserved (**e**)

Patients with SMA type III walk early in life and maintain their ambulatory capacity into adolescence. Their leading clinical presentation includes difficulty climbing stairs or getting up from the floor (because of hip extensor weakness). Weakness may cause foot drop, and patients have limited endurance. One-third of the patients becomes wheelchair-bound as adults (mean age 40 years). Lifespan is almost normal.

Electrophysiological studies are supportive, but genetic studies are needed to confirm the diagnosis of SMA. Sensory nerve conduction studies are uniformly normal. Compound motor action potentials may have reduced amplitude, reflecting motor fiber depletion. Motor nerve conduction velocities are generally normal, and needle electrode examination demonstrates abnormal spontaneous activity, including fibrillation potentials, positive sharp waves, and rarely fasciculations. Even with maximal effort, motor unit potentials are poorly recruited and units fire rapidly.

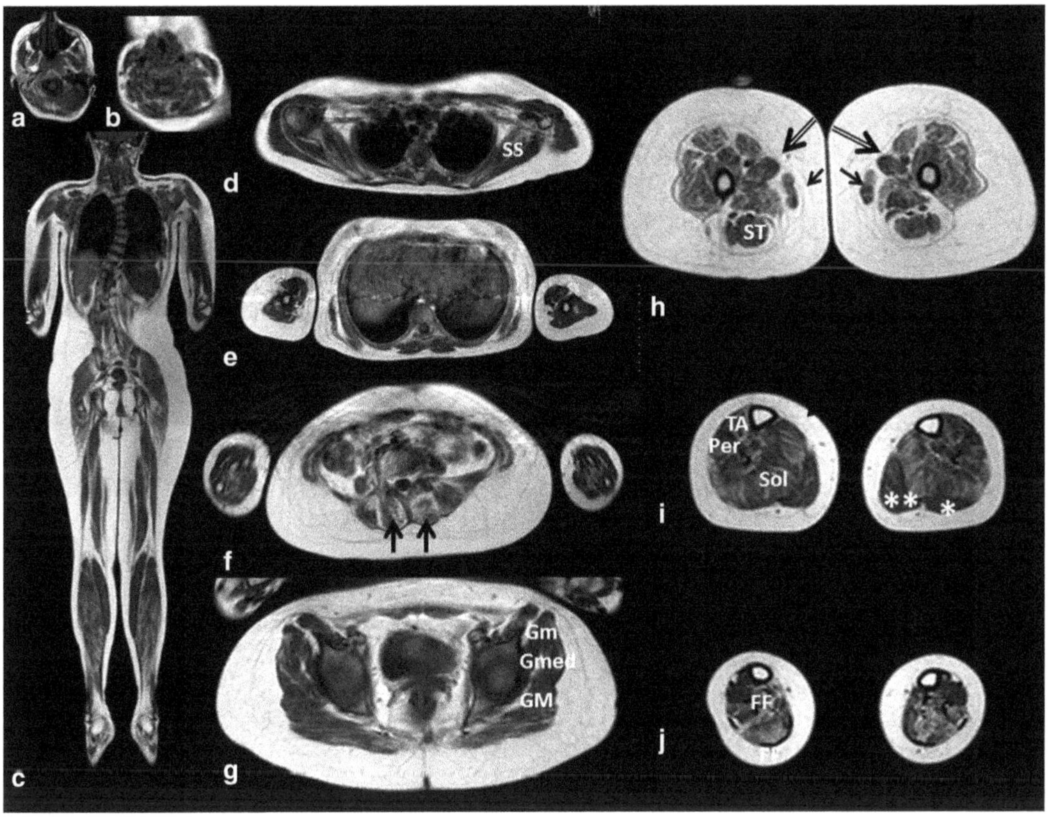

Fig. 29.2 Magnetic resonance imaging (MRI) findings in SMA type III (**a**–**j**). (**a, b**) Spared facial, head and neck muscles. (**b**) Mild involvement of neck extensors. (**c**) Frontal view shows scoliosis, thigh atrophy, and involvement of the distal lower limbs. (**d**) Mild involvement of subscapular (*SS*) muscles. (**e**) Normal findings in arms and dorsal upper trunk region. (**f**) Moderate to severe infitration of lumbar paravertebral muscles (*black vertical arrows*). (**g**) Mild involvement of the gluteal muscles (*GM* gluteus maximus, *Gme* medius, *Gm* minimus). (**h**) Thighs show diffuse moderate to severe involvement. Muscle signal shows fine striations. There is relative preservation of the gracilis (*small black arrows*), hypertrophic adductor longus (*large black arrows*), and semitendinous (ST) muscles. (**i**) In the lower legs there is moderate involvement of the soleus (Sol) and peroneus (Per) muscles with relatively preserved tibialis anterior (TA) and gastrocnemii (*white stars*) muscles. (**j**) Distal leg and fingers show involvement of the flexor (FF) and extensor digitorum muscles

29.2.6 Muscle Imaging

Muscle MRI findings of patients with SMA are shown in Fig. 29.2. The few reports describing muscle MRI features in SMA patients have focused mainly on children with type II disease. Whole-body magnetic resonance imaging (MRI) results have been reported for only two patients, both of whom had SMA type III. They were initially suspected to have a myopathy because of proximal weakness and "myopathic" or "nonspecific" changes in the muscle biopsy. Muscle imaging showed, in both patients, mild to moderate abnormalities in various muscles of the body, sparing the head and upper limbs. Interestingly, compared to the myopathies, the MRI signal contained fine hyperintense striations, giving a heterogeneous aspect to the abnormal muscle. The most affected muscles were the paravertebral (lumbar more than dorsal), psoas, and abdominal muscles. The gluteal region was mildly to moderately affected, with the gluteus medius and minimus muscles being more involved than the gluteus maximus muscle. The lower limbs were also predominantly involved, and findings were in accordance with previous reports of SMA type II patients using sequential muscle MRI, with slight differences. The thigh showed selective abnormalities in the adductor magnus and quadriceps muscles, sparing the gracilis, semitendinosus, and adductor longus muscles, the latter being strikingly enlarged. In the lower leg, the most severe changes were observed in the soleus, peroneus, and the flexor and extensor digitorum muscles, with relative preservation of gastrocnemii and tibialis anterior muscles. The mildest abnormalities were observed in the neck and periscapular muscles, with mild involvement of the longus colli, neck extensors, and the subscapular, suprascapular, and serratus anterior muscles. Sequential studies of lower limbs in children affected with SMA II have shown a similar pattern, with the difference being that the sartorius muscle was relatively spared. Also, the hamstrings, including the semitendinosus muscles, were severely affected.

29.2.7 Differential Diagnosis

Diagnosing SMA types I and II is usually straightforward because SMA is more common than other neuromuscular disorders, which are much rarer at young age, and because of their characteristic clinical presentation with rapidly regression of motor skills in an alert, cognitively unimpaired infant. The differential diagnosis of SMA type I includes disorders of the cerebrum, spinal cord, motor neurons and peripheral nerves, NMJ, and muscle. In particular, congenital muscular dystrophies and myopathies may show overlapping features, especially when serum CK levels are slightly elevated. Central nervous system (CNS) dysfunction and seizures are uncommon in SMA and point toward hypotonia due to central nervous system disease. Macroglossia, relatively organomegaly, and cardiac enlargement are typical of Pompe's disease (see Sect. 14.2.1). Mitochondrial diseases (see Sect. 14.3), such as synthesis-of-cytochrome oxidase 2 (*SCO2*) gene mutations, can present as atypical SMA type I, although lactic acidosis and cardiomyopathy are often associated. A mitochondrial DNA depletion syndrome associated with thymidine kinase 2 (*TK2*) can manifest with an SMA phenotype. In the milder SMA II and III, the differential diagnosis includes other disorders of motor neurons, myasthenia gravis, muscular dystrophies (see Chaps. 16, 17, 19), inflammatory myopathies (see Chap. 26), and a variety of congenital (see Chap. 15), metabolic (see Chap. 14), and endocrine myopathies. These disorders are usually easily distinguished by their clinical, laboratory, and muscle biopsy features.

29.2.8 Therapy

Symptomatic, respiratory, orthopaedic and nutritional treatments are indicated to treat respiratory insufficiency and scoliosis in children with type 2 SMA and in some cases with intermediate 1-2 subtype without an early severe progressive course. In the absence of a curative treatment, there is not consensual indication for invassive supportive treatment in the most severe type. Promissing therapies directed to enhance SMN2 transcripts are currently under development and a number of other molecules have been or are currently included in therapeutic trials.

Motor Neuron Diseases: SMA

Key Points

- SMA is a neurodegenerative disorder that affects lower motor neurons.
- There is a continuum of severity in the phenotypes of SMA: type I, patients cannot sit; type II, patients are unable to walk; type III, patients acquire walking ability.
- Most affected patients have a homozygous deletion of exon 7 in the *SMN1* gene. Differences of severity are thought to be due to modifying genes, such as *SMN2*.
- Distinct muscle MRI features observed are as follows.
  - Type III: there is often diffuse fine striation of the muscle signal. *In the*

thigh, there is diffuse involvement, sparing the gracilis, semitendinosus, and adductor longus muscles (the adductor longus often shows striking hypertrophy). *In the leg*, soleus and flexor and extensor digitorum muscles are selectively affected. Other severely involved muscles are the paravertebral, gluteal, psoas, and abdominal muscles. The head and upper limbs seem to be preserved.
– Type II: The thigh has findings similar to those of SMA type III, although the hamstrings are more affected.

Suggestions for Further Reading

Bürglen L, Lefebvre S, Clermont O, et al. Structure and organization of the human survival motor neurone (SMN) gene. Genomics 1996;32:479–82.

Ioos C, Leclair-richard D, Mrad S, et al. Respiratory capacity course in patients with infantile spinal muscular atrophy. Chest 2004;126:831–7.

Lewelt A, Newcomb TM, Swoboda KJ. New therapeutic approaches to spinal muscular atrophy. Curr Neurol Neurosci Rep. 2012;12:42–53.

Liu GC, Jong YJ, Chiang CH, et al. Spinal muscular atrophy: MR evaluation. Pediatr Radiol. 1992;22:584–6.

Quijano-Roy S, Avila-Smirnow D, Carlier. Whole body muscle MRI protocol: pattern recognition in early-onset neuromuscular disorders. Neuromuscul Disord. 2012;22 Suppl 2:S68–84.

Ueno T, Yoshioka H, Iwasaki N, et al. MR findings of spinal muscular atrophy type II: sibling cases. Magn Reson Med Sci. 2003;31:195–8.

Vitte J, Attali R, Warwar N, et al. Spinal muscular atrophy. Adv Exp Med Biol. 2009;652:237–46.

29.3 Amyotrophic Lateral Sclerosis

Mike P. Wattjes, and Dirk Fischer

29.3.1 Synonyms and Abbreviations

Amyotrophic lateral sclerosis (ALS); motor neuron disease (MND); motoneuron disease; Lou Gehrig's disease

29.3.2 Introduction and Classification

Amyotrophic lateral sclerosis (ALS) is a neurodegenerative disorder that belongs to the group of MNDs. Jean-Martin Charcot first described the disease in 1869. In its classic form, ALS is characterized by degeneration of the first and second motor neurons, leading to sclerosis of the ventral and mediolateral horn. This, in combination with the atrophic aspect of the striated muscles, led to the term "amyotrophic lateral sclerosis."

The incidence in Europe is about 2–3/100,000 persons per year. In the vast majority of patients (90–95 %), ALS occurs sporadically. In about 5–10 %, it is familial, exhibiting Mendelian inheritance associated with certain target genes.

29.3.3 Genetics and Pathophysiology

The disease ALS is defined by degeneration of the upper and lower motor neurons located in the brain, brain stem, and spinal cord. The cause of the isolated involvement and degeneration of motor neurons remains unsolved. However, before cell death occurs, intraneuronal protein inclusions containing ubiquitin, superoxide dismutase (SOD1), and TAR DNA-binding protein (*TARDBP*) have been observed. Also, the genetic background and pathophysiology are complex and still not fully understood. Several risk factors have been described, including smoking, physical exertion, chronic traumatic encephalopathy, and neurotoxins. The most important risk factor is age. A well-established model to explain the pathogenesis is the concept of glutamate-induced excitoxicity leading to neurodegeneration. Several pathways have been postulated, including activation of calcium-dependent enzymes and generation of free radicals. In addition, abnormalities of cell organelles and ion pumps may play a role in the pathophysiological process. Based on these pathophysiological concepts, it has been shown that certain genetic defects are associated with ALS. Mutations of the *SOD1* gene (21q22.1), encoding for an enzyme acting as an antioxidant, are present in 20 % of familial and 5 % of sporadic ALS patients. Other target genes that show alterations associated with ALS are *TARDBP* (1p36.2), *FUS* (16p11.2), and *ANG* (14q11.2).

29.3.4 Histopathology

Muscle biopsy is rarely performed in patients with ALS as it is usually not needed to confirm the diagnosis. Pathological findings include those of neurogenic denervation changes, such as atrophy of both main muscle fiber types. Also, atrophic muscle fibers are often small and angulated and might be clustered in small groups (Figs. 29.3 and 29.4).

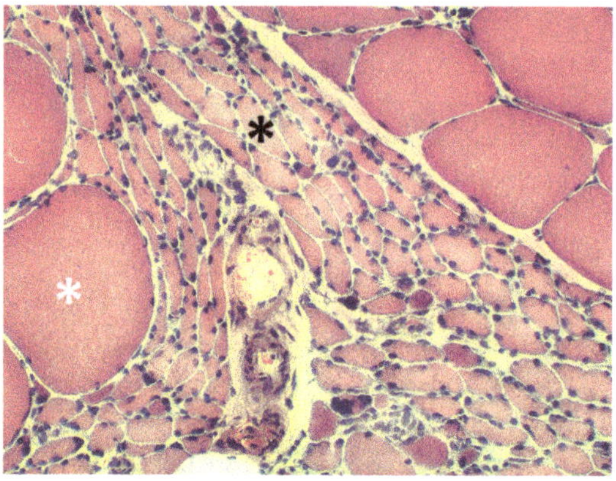

Fig. 29.3 Muscle biopsy findings in amyotrophic lateral sclerosis. Neurogenic changes show "large group atrophy" with a large number of grouped atrophic fibers (*black stars*) surrounded by a few normal muscle fibers (*white stars*)

29.3.5 Clinical Presentation

Although age has been discussed as the most important risk factor for ALS, the disease may start at any age. ALS is characterized by the occurrence of slowly progressive painless motor symptoms that may begin in any region of the body, starting in the legs, arms, or bulbar muscles depending on the motor neurons most severely affected (Fig. 29.5). Sensory symptoms are usually absent or unrelated. Positive motor symptoms include fasciculations, cramps, stiffness,

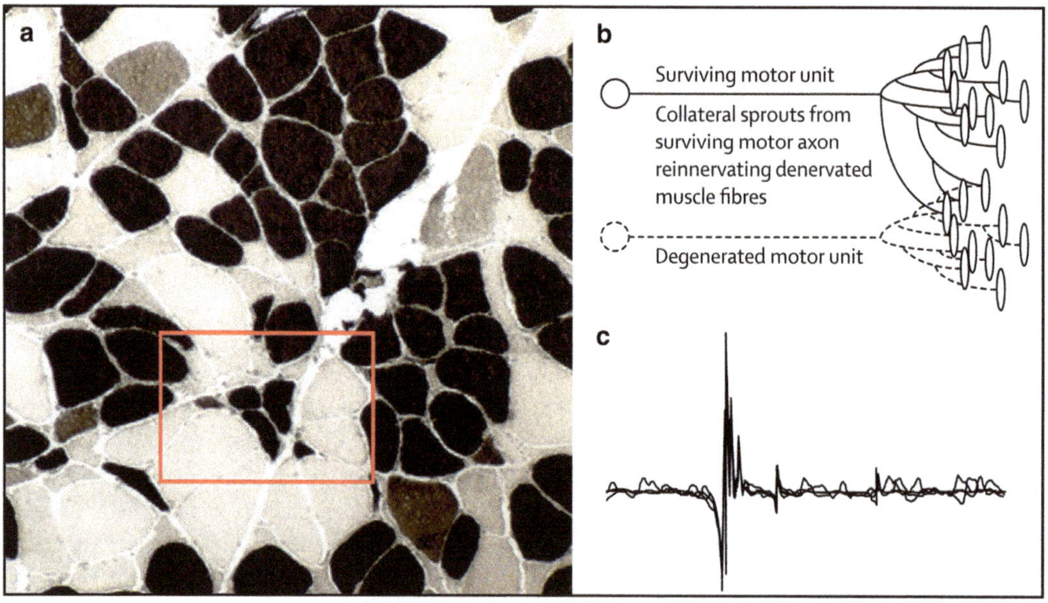

Fig. 29.4 (**a**) Muscle biopsy material obtained from the left vastus lateralis muscle from a patient with ALS. The tissue shows the grouped atrophic fibers with type I and type II fibers (*red box*) (ATPase ph 9.4 stain). (**b**) Pathophysiology of motor unit degeneration and reinnervation showing superimposition (**c**) of ten traces. Note the typically large, polyphasic, unstable (complex) motor units observed in ALS with late components, suggestive of reinnervation. From Kiernan MC, et al (2011) Lancet 377:942–55. Reprinted with permission from Elsevier

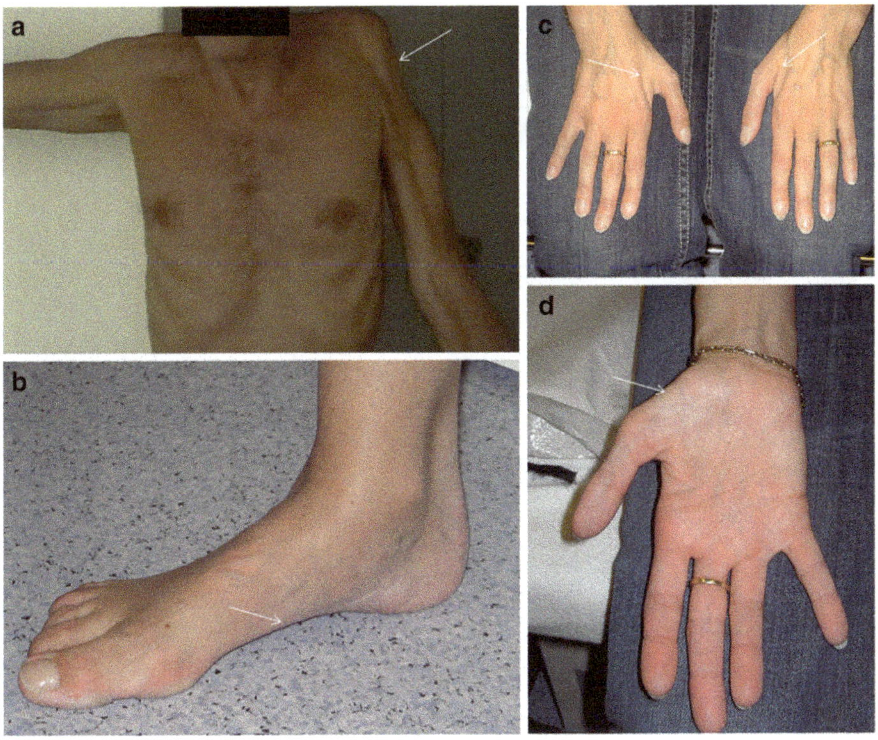

Fig. 29.5 Clinical features of ALS in two patients. Often there is marked asymmetry of involvement as demonstrated in a male patient with severe proximal atrophy and weakness of the shoulder and upper arm muscles on the left. The photograph was obtained when the patient was trying to abduct both arms (**a**, *arrow*). Female patient with motor neuron disease presenting with atrophy of the distal small foot muscles on the right (**b**, *arrow*), the first interosseal spatium on both hands (**c**, *arrows*), and the thenar muscles on the right (**d**, *arrow*).

and/or spasticity. Negative symptoms include muscle weakness and atrophy. Onset is often asymmetrical. In about 75 % of patients the disease starts in one limb. In about 25 % of patients it begins in the bulbar region, resulting in dysphagia or dysarthria. During its relentless course other regions usually become affected, finally resulting in a mixture of generalized muscular atrophy (second motor neurons) and spasticity (first motor neurons). Often, patients are ultimately unable to use their hands, walk, wash themselves, or talk. Disease progression can vary, but death usually occurs after 2–3 years, resulting from respiratory muscle weakness or aspiration pneumonia.

In addition to the classic type (affecting both motor neurons), there is a subtype that predominantly affects the upper motor neuron. It is called primary lateral sclerosis. The progressive muscular atrophy variant predominantly affects the lower motor neurons. ALS can be associated with other neurodegenerative diseases, such as frontotemporal dementia (FTD). In fact, a familial clustering has been observed that shows a common gene locus on chromosome 9.

29.3.6 Imaging Findings

29.3.6.1 Muscle Imaging

Ultrasonography (US) has a diagnostic value for ALS. Particularly, it can help to differentiate ALS from some mimics with relatively high sensitivity and specificity (see Chap. 2). US is not valuable for monitoring muscle changes in ALS (muscle thickness, echo intensity, fasciculations) because the involvement pattern is highly variable and does not correlate with any functional

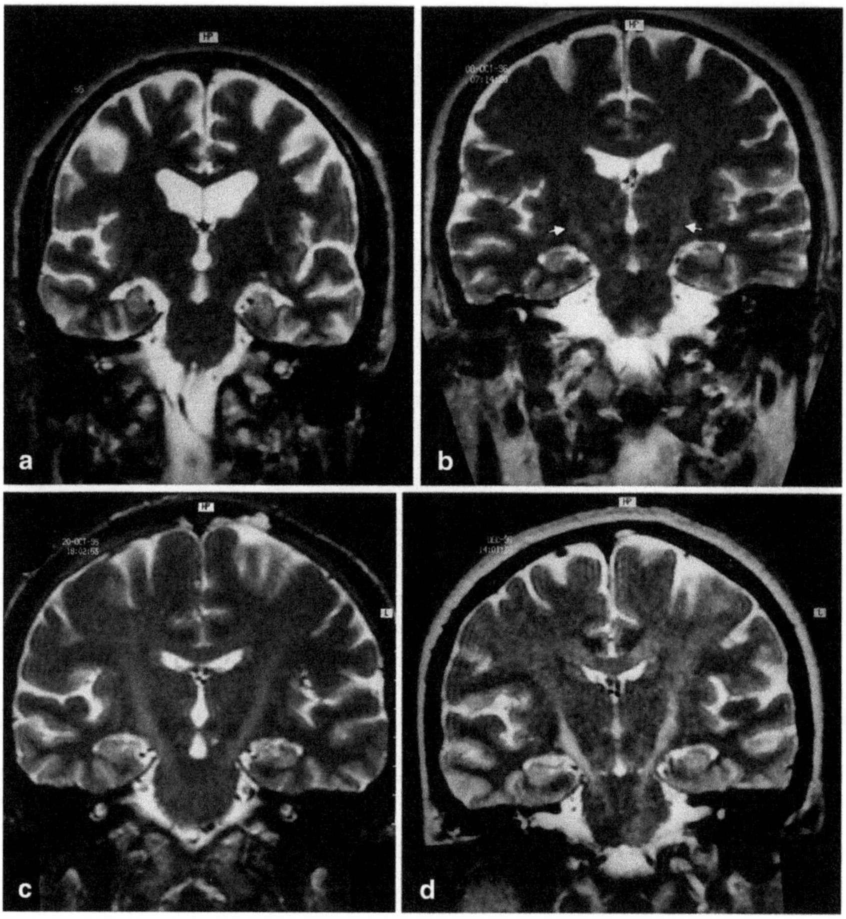

Fig. 29.6 Coronal T2-weighted turbo (fast) spin echo MRI demonstrates varying degrees of high signal hyperintensity in the corticospinal tracts in ALS patients. Grade 0 (**a**) shows no abnormalities; grade 1 (**b**) shows mild changes (*white arrows*); grade 2 (**c**) demonstrates moderate changes involving the corona radiata and the pons; grade 3 (**d**) shows severe high signal changes from the corona radiata to the pons. From Peretti-Viton P, et al (1999) Neuroradiology 41:744–9. Reprinted with permission from Springer Verlag

measures, such as muscle strength or scores based on the ALS functional rating scale (ALSFRS). However, muscle US baseline measures can have predictive value for patient survival.

In contrast to brain MRI, data and experience in muscle MRI in ALS patients is rather limited. Changes due to chronic denervation can be detected particularly in later disease stages, including atrophy and fatty replacement of muscle tissue. These findings can also be detected on MRI, showing muscle edema in acute stages of denervation and fatty replacement and atrophy in chronic stages.

29.3.6.2 Structural Brain and Spinal Cord Imaging

Brain and spinal cord imaging, preferably using MRI, is routinely performed in patients with clinical findings suggestive of ALS to rule out possibly treatable diseases in the differential diagnosis. Structural brain MRI can show hyperintense signal abnormalities on T2-weighted and fluid-attenuated inversion recovery (FLAIR) sequences in the corticospinal tract of ALS patients (Fig. 29.6). These abnormalities are more frequently found in young ALS patients with greater disability. Corticospinal tract changes can also be

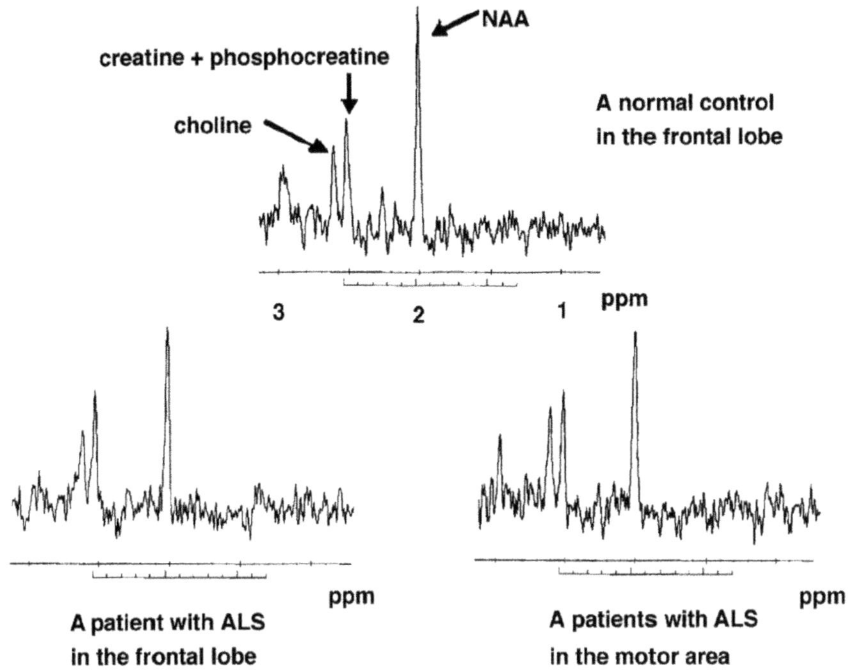

Fig. 29.7 ^{1}H-MRS spectra obtained from a control subject and an ALS patient. Please note the decreased *N*-acetylaspartate (NAA) levels, particularly in the motor area of the ALS patient. From Abe K, et al (2001) Neuroradiology 43: 537–41. Reprinted with permission from Springer Verlag

observed in healthy controls and in patients who underwent hepatic transplantation. These changes are therefore not specific for ALS (specificity is < 70 %) but can be observed in some ALS patients. In other words, the absence of these findings does not rule out ALS. A T2 hypointense rim can be observed ("ribbon-like hypointensity") in the precentral cortex.

In the spinal cord, T1 hyperintensities in the anterior and mediolateral column of the cervical spinal cord and decreased T2 hyperintensities over time have been observed. However, because spinal cord MRI is more challenging than brain MRI, these changes should not be considered as key imaging findings in ALS.

29.3.6.3 ^{1}H-MRS Proton Magnetic Resonance Spectroscopy

N-Acetylaspartate (NAA) and *N*-acetylaspartylglutamate (NAAG) are markers of neuronal function and integrity in many inflammatory and neurodegenerative CNS diseases. In ALS, it has been conclusively shown that neuronal damage in terms of decreased NAA and NAAG concentrations can be observed in the motor cortex, along the corticospinal tracts in the supratentorial brain, and the brain stem (Fig. 29.7). Regarding the primary motor cortex, the assessment of decreased NAA levels can be useful for distinguishing between typical ALS patients and progressive muscular atrophy. The degree of neuronal damage is associated with the severity of the clinical presentation in ALS patients (particularly in the brain stem of patients with bulbar symptoms) and with clinical progression during follow-up. Lower NAA/creatinine (Cr) ratios have been observed in the premotor area, primary sensory cortex, and nonmotor cortices. Concentrations of myoinositol (Ins), a marker of glial cell activity, are increased in areas of the motor cortex that show an abnormal signal on T2-weighted images.

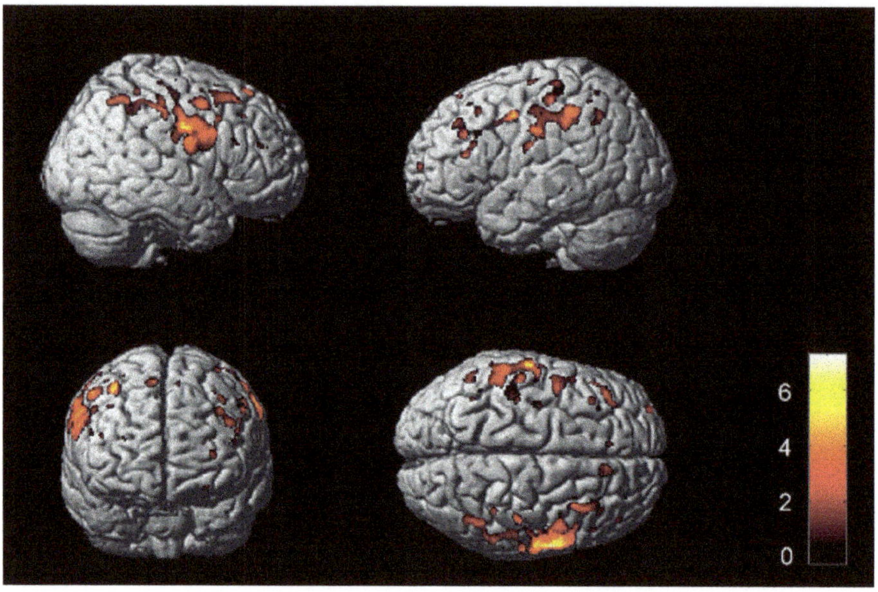

Fig. 29.8 Voxel-based morphometry was used to compare 17 ALS patients and 17 healthy controls. It demonstrates regional gray matter loss in the precentral and postcentral gyrus of both hemispheres in the ALS patients. The changes extended from the bilateral primary motor cortex to the premotor, parietal, and frontal regions. The *color bar* represents the *T*-score. From Grosskreutz J, et al (2006) BMC Neurol.6:17. Reprinted with permission from BioMedCentral

29.3.6.4 Diffusion Tensor Imaging

Based on the anisotropic tissue organization in white matter, diffusion tensor imaging (DTI) is able to measure the direction of water molecules in the brain. Reduced anisotropy is expressed by reduced fractional anisotropy (FA) and/or increased mean diffusivity (MD) values. Decreased FA values along the corticospinal tracts are observed in ALS patients and seem to be related to clinical and electrophysiological manifestations. MD values have been linked to disease duration. Applying voxel-based analysis, it has been shown that the FA decrease is not limited to the corticospinal tract, but has also been observed in the corpus callosum, in premotor area white matter, and temporal white matter. Longitudinal DTI studies have not been able to monitor disease progression conclusively.

Recent advances in DTI methods allow evaluation of the cervical spinal cord. ALS patients show substantially lower FA but normal MD values in the spinal cord compared to healthy controls. These values are associated with disease severity. During follow-up, the FA values further decrease and MD values increase significantly.

29.3.6.5 Atrophy Measurements

Data on measurements of gray and white matter volumes in patients with ALS are inconclusive. White matter changes were observed in ALS patients with cognitive decline—both frontal and temporal. Using voxel-based morphometric analysis, extended gray matter atrophy in precentral and postcentral gyrus could be found involving also other parts of the frontal and parietal lobes (Fig. 29.8). Prominent changes were visible in the frontal lobes of patients presenting with ALS and with ALS/FTD overlap.

29.3.7 Differential Diagnosis

The differential diagnosis of ALS is important because it is crucial to exclude all possible

Table 29.1 Differential diagnosis of ALS

Differential diagnosis of ALS
Motor neuron disorders
Spinal muscular atrophy
Kennedy's disease
Poliomyelitis, postpoliomyelitis syndrome
Distal motor nerve disorders
Neuropathies
Multifocal motor neuropathy
Chronic inflammatory demyelinating neuropathy
Hereditary motor neuron myopathy
Cramp–fasciculation syndrome
Plexus pathology: tumors, traumatic changes, inflammation
Intoxication: heavy metal, organic solvents
Diseases of the neuromuscular junction
Myasthenia gravis
Lambert–Eaton syndrome
Muscle diseases
Myositis
Channelopathies
Myopathies
CNS pathologies
Inflammatory diseases (e.g., multiple sclerosis, Lyme disease)
Infectious diseases (e.g., tabes dorsalis)
Syringomyelia, syringobulbia
Neoplastic (e.g., lymphoma, glioma)
Systemic diseases
Endocrine disorders (e.g., thyroid, parathyroid)
Metabolic (e.g., vitamin deficiencies)
Inflammatory bowel disease

differential diagnoses before ALS is finally diagnosed. The process must exclude a complex whole battery of diseases including other motor neuron disorders; diseases of the peripheral nerves, the NMJ, the muscle itself; and systemic diseases. Table 29.1 gives on overview of the differential diagnosis that should be considered in patients with suspected ALS.

There is no definitive test for diagnosing ALS. The presence of lower (fasciculations, atrophy) and upper (pathological brisk reflexes, Babinski sign) motor signs in various limbs and regions of the body is, however, highly suggestive of ALS. Additional nerve conduction tests and electromyography studies are usually performed to exclude other treatable conditions such as multifocal motor neuropathy and to support the diagnosis of ALS by searching for lower motor neuron involvement in clinically unaffected limbs or regions.

29.3.8 Therapy

Currently, there is no curative treatment for ALS. Symptomatic treatment to improve quality of life and limit morbidity is the mainstay of management. So far, riluzole is the only available treatment that has been demonstrated to slow the disease progression slightly and to improve survival by a few months. Supportive care may include medical treatment for cramps, stiffness, spasticity; physical, occupational, and speech therapy; and ventilatory assistance for patients with nocturnal hypoventilation.

Motor Neuron Diseases: ALS

Key Points

- ALS is a rapidly progressing neurodegenerative motor neuron disease affecting the upper motor neurons (located in the brain and brain stem) and lower motor neurons (in the spinal cord), often causing death within 3 years after onset.
- ALS presents with negative (weakness, atrophy) and positive (fasciculations, cramps, stiffness, spasticity) motor symptoms.
- Onset can be at any age, and symptoms may start in any limb or (bulbar) region.
- There is no definitive diagnostic test. Structural imaging of the brain and spinal cord and electrophysiological examinations are usually undertaken to exclude other (possibly treatable) conditions and to support the diagnosis.
- Muscle US can detect fasciculations and high echo intensities in affected muscles and has predictive value in terms of survival.
- Advanced MRI techniques are still mainly experimental.
- There is no cure available. Riluzole slows the disease progression slightly and improves survival by a few months. Symptomatic treatment that improves quality of life is most important.

Suggestions for Further Reading

Arts IM, Overeem, Pillen S, et al. Muscle ultrasonography to predict survival in amyotrophic lateral sclerosis. J Neurol Neurosurg Psychiatry. 2011a;82:552–4.

Arts IM, Overeem, Pillen S, et al. Muscle changes in amyotrophic lateral sclerosis: a longitudinal ultrasonography study. Clin Neurophysiol. 2011b;122:623–8.

Arts IM, Overeem, Pillen S, et al. Muscle ultrasonography: a diagnostic tool for amyotrophic lateral sclerosis. Clin Neurophysiol. 2012;123:1662–7.

Filippi M, Agosta F, Abrahams S, et al. EFNS guidelines on the use of neuroimaging in the management of motor neuron diseases. Eur J Neurol. 2010;17: 526–33.

Kiernan MC, Vucic S, Cheah BC, et al. Amyotrophic lateral sclerosis. Lancet 2011;377:942–55.

Turner MR, Modo M. Advances in the application of MRI to amyotrophic lateral sclerosis. Expert Opin Med Diagn. 2010;4:483–96.

Turner MR, Kiernan MC, Leigh PN, et al. Biomarkers in amyotrophic lateral sclerosis. Lancet Neurol. 2009;8: 94–109.

Imaging of the Peripheral Nerves: Clinical Applications and Diagnostic Relevance

30

Arnold Kang and Michel Kliot

30.1 Introduction

The diagnosis of peripheral nerve problems has traditionally been based on "three pillars": clinical history, physical examination, and corroborative electrodiagnostic test findings.

The clinical history should elicit patient age, pertinent symptoms, known genetic disorders (e.g. neurofibromatosis 1 or 2), and any previous malignancy or radiation therapy. The physical examination should detect relevant skin abnormalities (e.g., café au lait spots), palpable mass lesions (e.g., neurofibromas) and any alteration of sensory, motor or autonomic neural function. Electrodiagnostic tests may include: (1) electromyography (EMG), to detect fibrillations and positive short waves; (2) nerve conduction studies, to detect motor and sensory latencies; and (3) intraoperative electrophysiological monitoring to grade nerve injury (neurapraxia vs. axonotmesis vs. neurotmesis) and differentiate functioning nerve from non-functioning tissue such as tumor.

A. Kang
Division of Neuroradiology, Department of Radiology, University of Washington, 1959 NE Pacific St, Seattle, WA 98195-7115, USA
e-mail: akang79@uw.edu

M. Kliot (✉)
Department of Neurological Surgery, University of California San Francisco, 500 Parnassus Avenue, M780, San Francisco, CA 94143-0112, USA
e-mail: kliotm@neurosurg.ucsf.edu

30.2 Diagnostic Applications of Peripheral Nerve Imaging

Although the well-accepted "three pillar" workup algorithm remains the gold standard of peripheral nerve assessment, the supplementary role of imaging as a tentative "fourth pillar" has recently started to expand beyond that of tumor evaluation alone. Technological improvements in the visualization of small peripheral nerves now mean that imaging can assist in the diagnosis of peripheral nerve entrapments (particularly when clinical suspicion is high but electrodiagnostic tests are either negative or equivocal), peripheral nerve injuries (e.g., contusion or compression versus laceration) and post-surgical problems (e.g., failed carpal or cubital tunnel release).

Magnetic resonance imaging (MRI) and high-resolution ultrasonography (US) have been used to assist in the diagnosis of peripheral nerve conditions that can be broadly categorized as (1) traumatic injuries, (2) tumor and tumor-like conditions, and (3) entrapment syndromes. The use of MRI neurography for hereditary myopathies will is also discussed albeit briefly.

30.2.1 Traumatic Injury

Mechanisms of nerve injury include compression, traction, ischemia, and laceration. Contusion secondary to blunt closed trauma is the most common, and nerves that have a superficial course

M.P. Wattjes and D. Fischer (eds.), *Neuromuscular Imaging*, DOI 10.1007/978-1-4614-6552-2_30,

over bone are most vulnerable (e.g., peroneal nerve adjacent to a fibular head). Stretch or traction injuries may result from manipulation, abnormal limb positioning, dislocations/fractures, and surgical interventions. Impaired intraneural microvascular flow resulting in local ischemia may then produce segmental demyelinization, axonal degeneration, and loss of nerve function. Penetrating injuries may directly lacerate or transect a nerve.

Peripheral nerve injuries are graded as neurapraxic, axonotmetic or neurotmetic:

1. *Neurapraxia*: Injury to the *myelin sheath* with axonal sparing; nerve conduction studies show conduction block or delay; no EMG abnormality or MRI evidence of muscle denervation; loss of nerve function is temporary, management usually conservative.
2. *Axonotmesis: Axonal injury* with distal Wallerian degeneration but preserved myelin sheath; causes acute muscle denervation appreciated on MRI as increased signal as early as 4 days after injury and on EMG as fibrillation potentials some 2–3 weeks later (usually reversible); generally managed conservatively, but may require surgical exploration and intraoperative electophysiological evaluation.
3. *Neurotmesis*: Disruption of *both the myelin sheath and axonal components* of the nerve with physical discontinuity that is either partial or complete; associated muscle denervation and subsequent fibrosis; recovery cannot occur spontaneously and surgery is required to remove scar tissue and re-establish axonal continuity (either *with or without* an interposed nerve graft); improved outcomes possible with early surgical intervention.

30.2.1.1 Imaging of Nerve Injuries

Early imaging can be used to confirm the exact location and, in some cases, the degree of nerve injury. This may be important as the window of time available for conservative management shortens with a more proximal level of nerve injury. The main issue with serial MRI and US is that it is difficult to distinguish regenerating nerve from chronically degenerating nerve secondary to the inflammatory products of Wallerian degeneration. Surgical exploration with intraoperative electrophysiological monitoring therefore remains the gold standard of management for peripheral nerve lesions that are failing to recover.

Injured nerve segments in both neurapraxia and axonotmesis demonstrate intraneural edema and consequently appear swollen and hyperintense on MRI [using short tau inversion recovery (STIR), fat-suppressed T2-weighted or fat-suppressed proton-density (PD) weighted images] or swollen and hypoechoic on US (Figs. 30.1, 30.2, and 30.3). On MRI, it is important to distinguish intraneural hyperintensity created by a "magic angle" artifact from that reflecting true pathology. In the case of axonotmesis, the nerve may also show loss of the normal "fascicular" appearance, and muscles supplied by the nerve distal to the site of injury may show features of denervation.

On MRI, an extended field of view is often needed to detect relevant muscle denervation changes. Normal muscle demonstrates intermediate signal intensity on T1-weighted imaging and low signal intensity on T2-weighted imaging. In contrast to EMG studies which take 10–14 days to demonstrate denervation changes, MR can demonstrate increased signal intensity on STIR or fat-suppressed T2/PD-weighted images in muscle 3–4 days after axonotmetic or neurotmetic injury. This is due to fluid shift into the extracellular compartment and increased blood volume secondary to an enlarged capillary bed. These changes persist into the subacute stage (days to weeks). During the chronic stage (usually many months), there is muscle atrophy with high signal on T1-weighted images, indicating fatty infiltration/replacement and resolution of the earlier hyperintense signal on fat-suppressed T2 or STIR imaging.

With complete nerve transection injuries, terminal neuromas may develop as small or large masses in continuity with the proximal stump of the severed nerve (Figs. 30.4 and 30.5). They appear hyperintense on fluid-sensitive MRI sequences and markedly hypoechoic on US. Both MRI and US can measure the gap between nerve ends and the cross-sectional diameter of the nerve at the injury site. However, neither MRI nor US

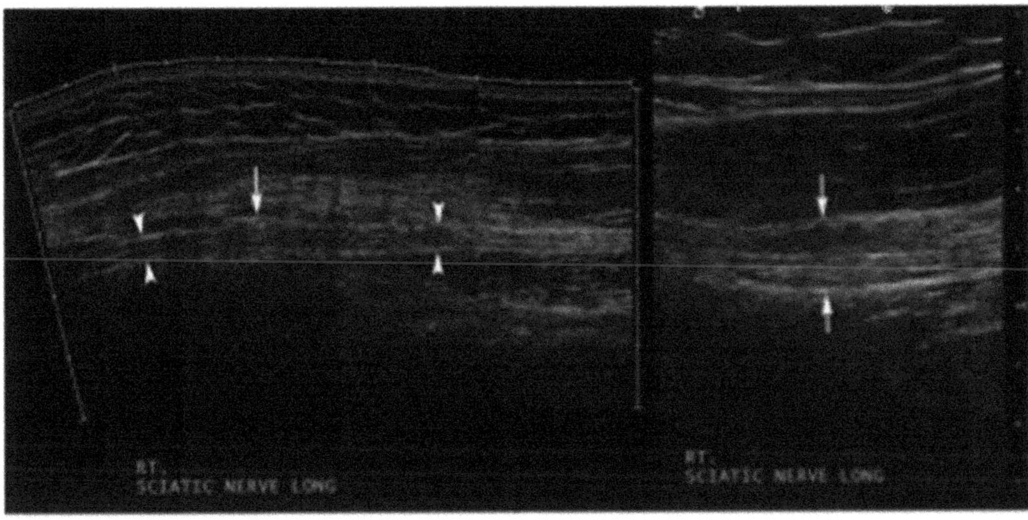

Fig. 30.1 Longitudinal US image of the sciatic nerve in the upper thigh. *Left image*: Panoramic overview of sciatic nerve in the upper thigh level; right image: detail view of abnormal sciatic nerve segment; *arrowheads*: normal sciatic nerve above and below abnormal segment; *arrows*: focal fusiform hypoechoic swelling of nerve at site of contusional injury (courtesy Dr John W Read, Castlereagh Imaging, Sydney)

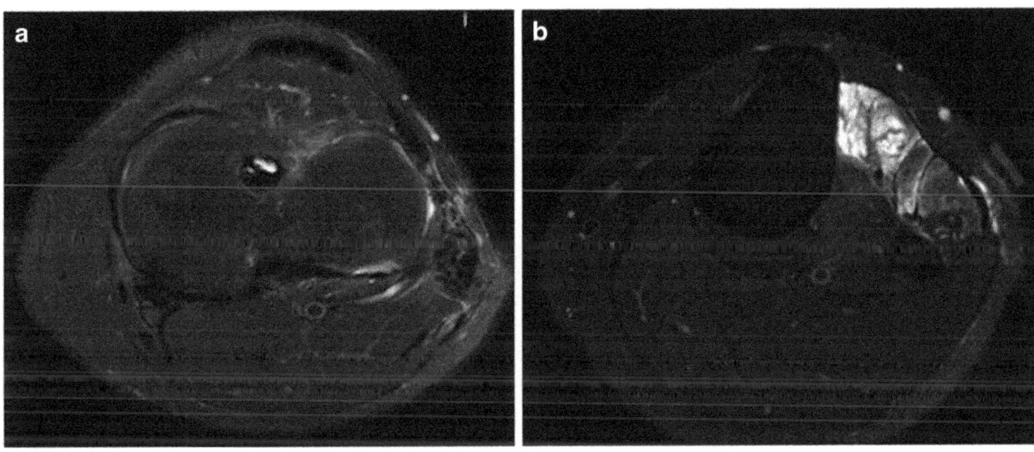

Fig. 30.2 (**a**, **b**) MR neurogram of the knee region in a 27-year-old male status post left knee injury with common peroneal nerve palsy approximately 1 year prior. *Top image*: axial T2 with fat saturation demonstrates increased T2 signal intensity and thickening of the common peroneal nerve superior to the region where it crosses over the medial aspect of the fibula. *Bottom image*: axial T2 with fat saturation demonstrates high signal intensity in the anterolateral muscular compartment consistent with denervation injury (*source*: University of Washington PACS)

can be relied on to predict the functional outcome and time to recovery.

30.2.1.2 Muscle Denervation Changes

Given that this section of the chapter deals with traumatic nerve injury, it is appropriate that denervation changes also be discussed. An extended field of view is often needed to detect muscle changes because of the muscle supply being distal to the actual site of nerve pathology. Normal muscle demonstrates intermediate signal intensity on T1-weighted imaging and low signal intensity on T2-weighted imaging (Fig. 30.2b). In contrast to EMG studies, which take 10–14 days to demonstrate denervation changes, MRI can demonstrate increased signal intensity on

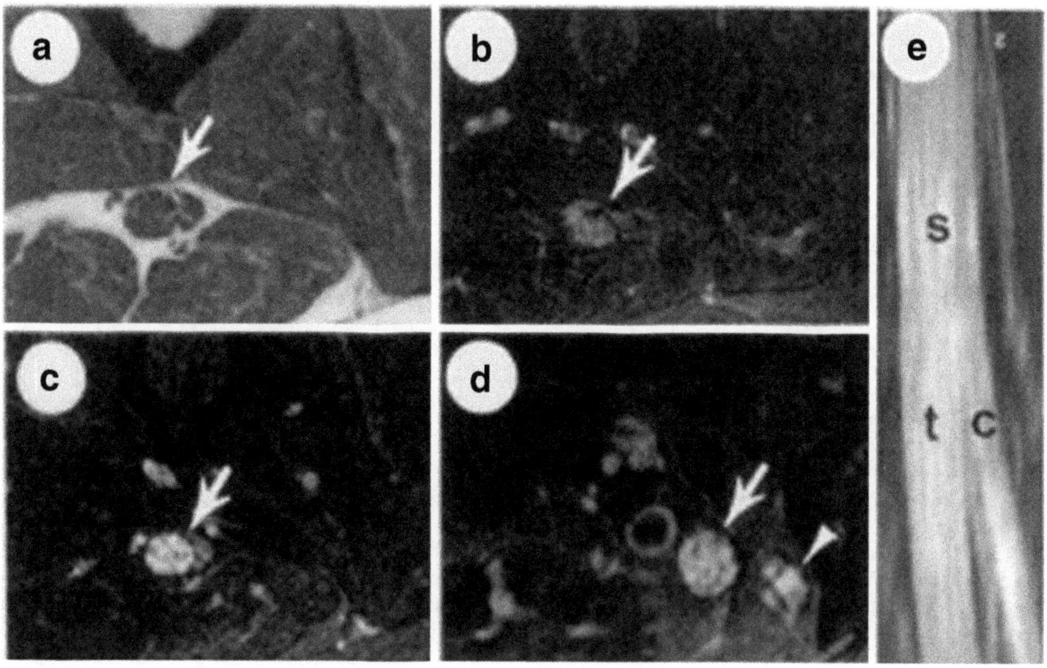

Fig. 30.3 MR images of the distal left thigh. MRN images of a 36-year-old female patient with a compression neuropathy involving the distal left sciatic nerve. (**a**) Axial T1 SE image showing the normal fascicular structure of the sciatic nerve (*arrow*) in the proximal thigh. (**b**) Axial T2 FSE image showing the normal signal intensity of fascicles within the sciatic nerve (*arrow*) in the proximal thigh. (**c**) Axial T2 FSE image showing increased signal and size of fascicles within the sciatic nerve (*arrow*) in the distal thigh. (**d**) Axial T2 FSE image showing increased signal and size of fascicles within the more distal tibial (*arrow*) and common peroneal (*arrowhead*) nerve branches. (**e**) Coronal T2 FSE maximum intensity projection showing the distal sciatic (s) nerve splitting into tibial (t) and common (c) peroneal nerve branches

T2-weighted or STIR images in muscle 3–4 days after nerve injury involving disruption of axons (an axonotmetic or neurotmetic grade of injury). This is due to fluid shift into the extracellular compartment and increased blood volume secondary to an enlarged capillary bed. These changes persist into the subacute stage (days to weeks). During the chronic stage (usually many months), there is muscular atrophy, high signal on T1-weighted images consistent with fatty infiltration/replacement and normalization of the hyperintense signal on T2-weighted and STIR imaging.

30.2.2 Tumor-Like Conditions

30.2.2.1 Peripheral Nerve Sheath Tumors

MRI and US are useful modalities for assessing peripheral nerve tumors and cysts (e.g., intraneural gangliomas). The two main peripheral nerve tumors are the schwannoma and neurofibroma. The schwannoma arises from Schwann cells of the nerve sheath, develops eccentrically, and is covered by perineurium, making it well encapsulated. It accounts for approximately 5 % of soft tissue neoplasms. Schwannomas commonly occur in the 20- to 50-year age group. They are usually benign, asymptomatic, and an isolated finding without association with neurofibromatosis. They often grow to a certain size and then become stable over a long period of time. Neurofibromas are usually not as well encapsulated as schwannomas and are often seen in patients with neurofibromatosis type 1. They are often asymptomatic and exhibit slow or no growth. A small subset of these tumors may become malignant.

Schwannomas and the more localized type of neurofibromas are difficult to differentiate on MRI and US as they have similar imaging appearances. Ultimately, the diagnosis is obtained by

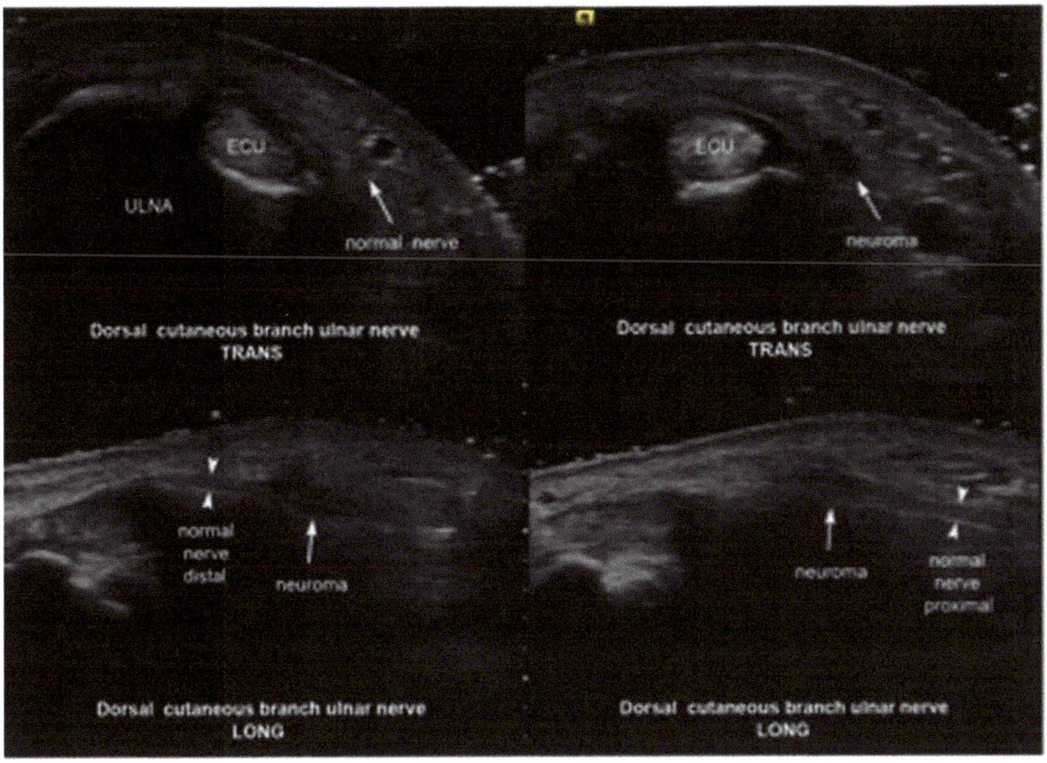

Fig. 30.4 US cross-sectional image of post-traumatic neuroma involving the dorsal cutaneous branch of the ulnar nerve at the wrist. A 50-year-old male with pain and paraesthesia radiating along dorsoulnar aspect of hand persisting many months after a direct blow to the ulnar border of wrist. The trigger point to palpation was over the medial aspect of ulnar styloid. *Upper left*: demonstrates transverse image of the normal appearing dorsal cutaneous branch of the ulnar nerve at the wrist (*arrow*). Upper right: transverse image of the neuroma of the dorsal cutaneous branch of the ulnar nerve (*arrow*). *Lower left*: longitudinal image demonstrates the normal nerve distally and fusiform hypoechoic dilatation (*arrow*) consistent with a neuroma. *Lower right*: longitudinal image demonstrates the normal nerve proximally and fusiform hypoechoic swelling (*arrow*) consistent with a neuroma (courtesy Dr John W Read, Castlereagh Imaging, Sydney)

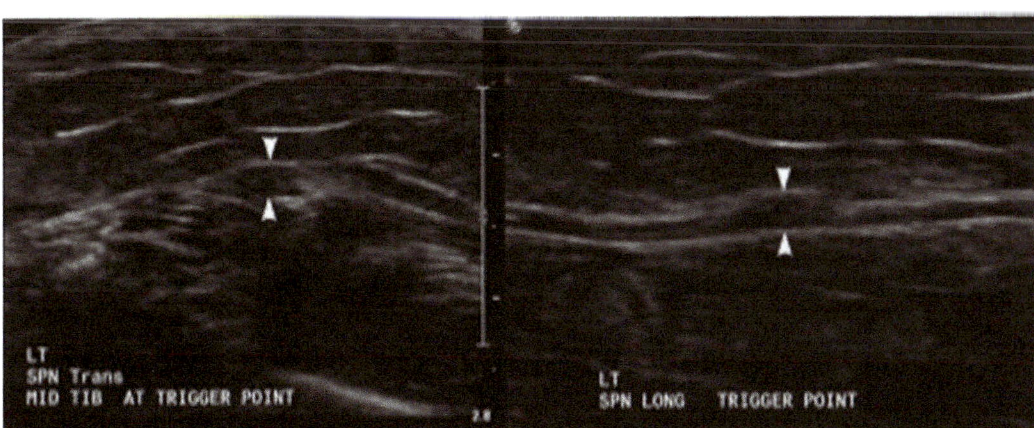

Fig. 30.5 US longitudinal image through the upper portion of the lower leg US obtained years after a penetrating knife injury to the superficial peroneal nerve at the mid to distal tibial shaft level demonstrate a focal tender swelling of neuroma (between arrowheads: left image is a transverse view and right image is a longitudinal view) (courtesy Dr John W Read, Castlereagh Imaging, Sydney)

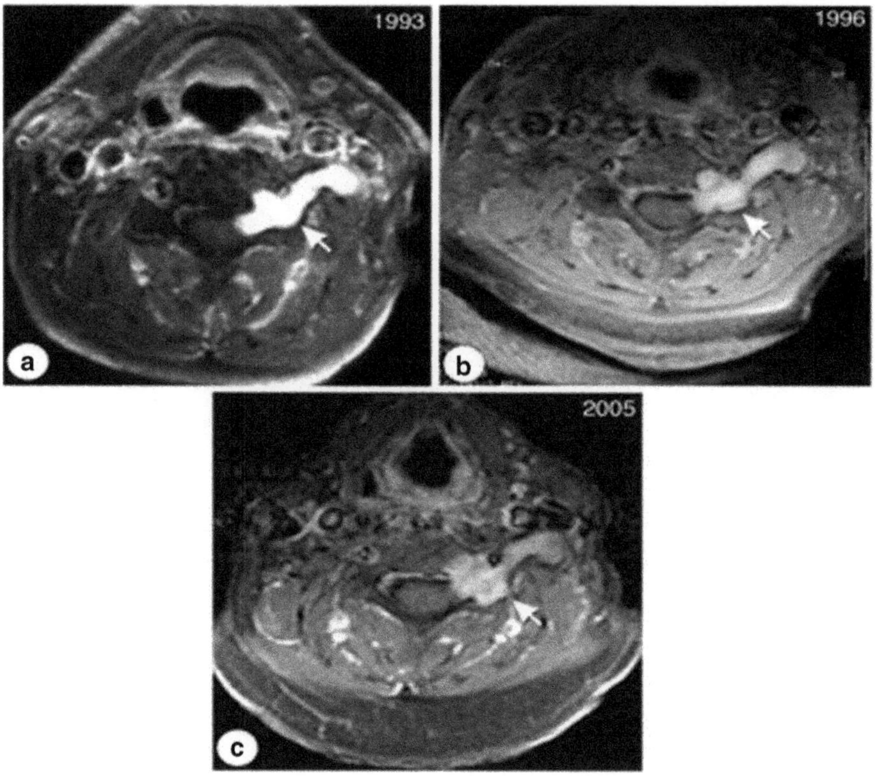

Fig. 30.6 a, b and c are axial T1 fat saturated with contrast MR images of the cervical spine in a patient imaged from 1993 to 2005. The arrows demonstrate a left C6 nerve schwannoma with a typical dumb bell shaped appearance. Note that the tumor has not significantly changed in size over a period of 12 years. This demonstrates the natural history of schwannomas (*source*: University of Washington, PACS)

biopsy or resection. They appear as fusiform masses that are usually <5 cm in diameter. They are isointense or slightly hyperintense on T1-weighted imaging and hyperintense to muscle and fat on T2-weighted imaging. Two specific signs have been well described regarding these tumors. The "split fat sign" appears when an intermuscularly located tumor is surrounded by a rim of fat. The "target sign" appears as T2 hyperintensity in the periphery of the tumor with low to intermediate signal intensity centrally. In both cases, the tumors demonstrate enhancement following the gadolinium administration (Figs. 30.6, 30.7, 30.8, and 30.9). Small tumors are sometimes difficult to distinguish from a hyperplastic lymph node.

In fewer than 10 % of cases, these tumors become malignant. It may occur de novo or reflect malignant transformation, with the former being more likely. Although ultimately a pathological diagnosis is required, imaging features that suggest malignancy include >5 cm in size, rapid documented growth, metastases, and increased metabolic activity on positron emission tomography. A prior history of malignant peripheral nerve tumor is also helpful.

A subtype of neurofibroma that requires brief mention is the plexiform neurofibroma. It is pathognomonic of neurofibromatosis 1 (NF1) and is included in the clinical diagnostic criteria for NF1. It has an up to 10 % risk of malignant transformation. It usually expands and distorts a large segment of nerve and insinuates itself into adjacent structures, including soft tissue, muscles, and other nerves and vessels. It is commonly seen in the head and neck region.

The fundamental purpose of peripheral nerve tumor imaging is to provide a roadmap for the

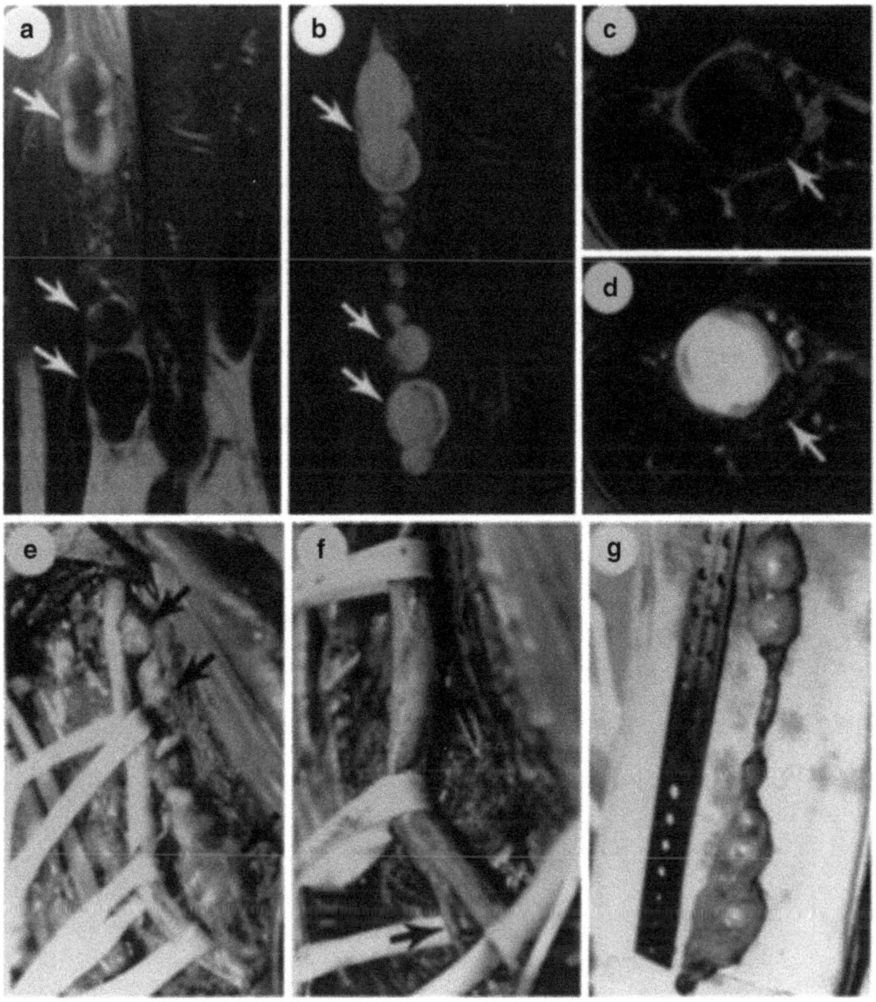

Fig. 30.7 MR images in correlation with intraoperative findings demonstrating a surgically cooperative neurofibroma (easily separable from the adjacent sciatic nerve). MR images of a 69-year-old female patient with a right sciatic neurofibroma in the lower thigh. (**a**) Coronal fat-suppressed T1 image after administration of gadolinium showing heterogeneous enhancement of a multilobulated and cystic mass lesion (*white arrows*) in the posterior thigh. (**b**) Coronal STIR image showing high signal within the multilobulated lesion (*white arrows*). (**c**) Axial T1 MR image after administration of gadolinium. (**d**) Axial T2 MR image showing discrete demarcation of the fascicular structure of the sciatic nerve (*white arrow*) along the posteromedial circumference of the tumor. (**e**) Intraoperative photograph showing Penrose loops elevating the sciatic from the multilobulated neurofibroma (*black arrows*). (**f**) Intraoperative photograph after removal of the neurofibroma. Note the splitting of the distal sciatic nerve into common peroneal and tibial (*black arrow*) nerve branches. (**g**) Photograph of the resected neurofibroma oriented as shown in (**a**) and (**b**)

neurosurgeon. Peripheral nerve masses need to be imaged in two orthogonal planes—longitudinal and cross sectional. The important information to describe based on MRI or US findings comprise the site, size, and shape of the lesion; its relations to the fascicles (often functional) from the nerve from which it arises and other important adjacent structures; evidence of invasion into adjacent structures; and its rate of growth (by comparison to previous images).

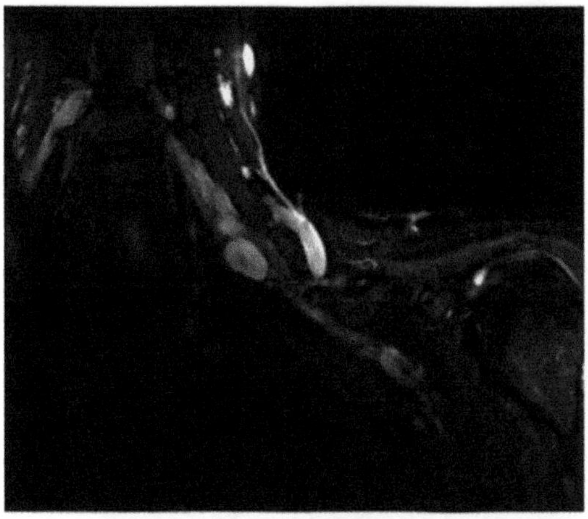

Fig. 30.8 Coronal STIR image demonstrates a plexiform neurofibroma involving the roots, trunks, divisions and cords of the left brachial plexus. Note the diffuse hyperintensity, enlarged and lobulated appearance of the neurofibroma. The patient had known neurofibromatosis 1. This tumor due to its diffuse and complex configuration is less likely to be cooperative in terms of its surgically resectability (*source*: University of Washington, PACS)

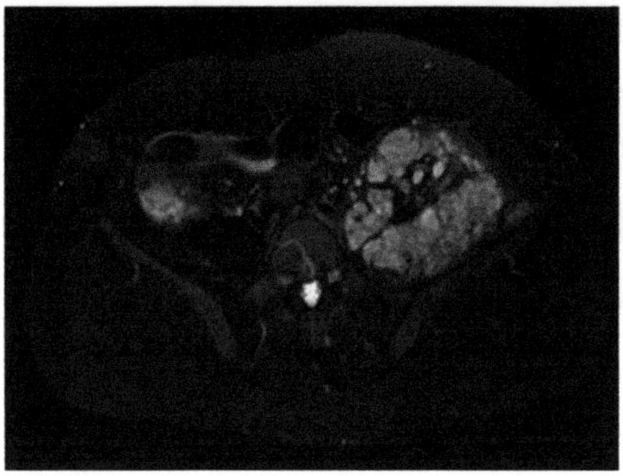

Fig. 30.9 Axial STIR image of the lumbosacral plexus demonstrates a plexiform neurofibroma. The plexiform neurofibroma involves the left lumbosacral plexus and iliopsoas muscle. Note the diffuse hyperintensity, enlargement and lobulated appearance. This patient also had a known history of neurofibromatosis 1 (*source*: University of Washington, PACS)

30.2.2.2 Radiation-Induced Plexopathy vs. Recurrent Tumor

Recurrent tumor is usually the first diagnosis to exclude in a patient who has undergone tumor treatment. Tumors, especially if they are invasive or malignant, are usually >5 cm, have central necrosis (nonenhancing central component), and demonstrate invasion of adjacent structures. Radiation plexopathy is especially common in the brachial plexus in the setting of breast carcinoma. It can present weeks to years after radiation therapy with symptoms that are usually sensory in nature. The severity is dose-dependent and often seen if doses are >60 Gy. MRI is the modality of choice as it can demonstrate the lack of the characteristic features of a tumor mass. Instead, the involved plexus is usually hyperintense on T2-weighted or STIR imaging and demonstrates minimal linear and usually sharply demarcated enlargement corresponding to the radiation field (Fig. 30.10).

30.2.2.3 Intraneural Perineurinoma (Localized Hypertrophic Neuropathy)

Intraneural perineurinomas are considered a type of benign neurogenic tumor. They are usually seen in children and young adults. The lesion commonly involves a single nerve—sciatic nerve, part of the brachial plexus, ulnar and radial nerves—with fusiform localized enlargement over 2–3 cm. It is thought not to have malignant potential, and its size is stable over many years. MRI demonstrates a thickened nerve with preserved fascicles and nonspecific low T1 and high T2 signal intensity. There may be secondary signs on MRI, including denervation edema in the acute to subacute stages or muscle atrophy and fatty degeneration in the chronic stage (Fig. 30.11).

Other tumor-like conditions include neurolymphomatosis or lymphomatous invasion of nerves in a patient with known non-Hodgkin's lymphoma. This causes enlargement of the involved nerve, alteration of its course, and T2 hyperintensity and heterogeneous enhancement.

Fibrolipomatous hamartoma commonly involves the median nerve, causing it to become thick and tortuous. There is no evidence of enhancement. Amyloidosis is a systemic condition that can cause mixed neuropathy and autonomic dysfunction. It causes nerve enlargement with course alteration and focal masses.

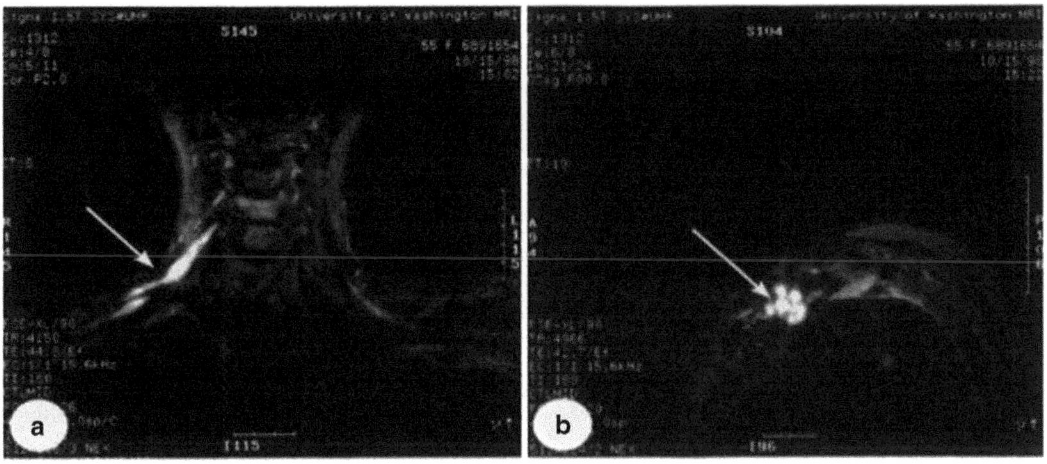

Fig. 30.10 Coronal (**a**) and sagittal (**b**) MRI STIR sequence images through the brachial plexus in a patient with a radiation induced right brachial plexopathy for treatment of breast cancer. Abnormal signal involves the spinal nerves and trunks [*white arrow* in (**a**)] as well as the divisions and cords more distally [*white arrow* in (**b**)]. No evidence of tumor recurrence was found (*source*: University of Washington, PACS)

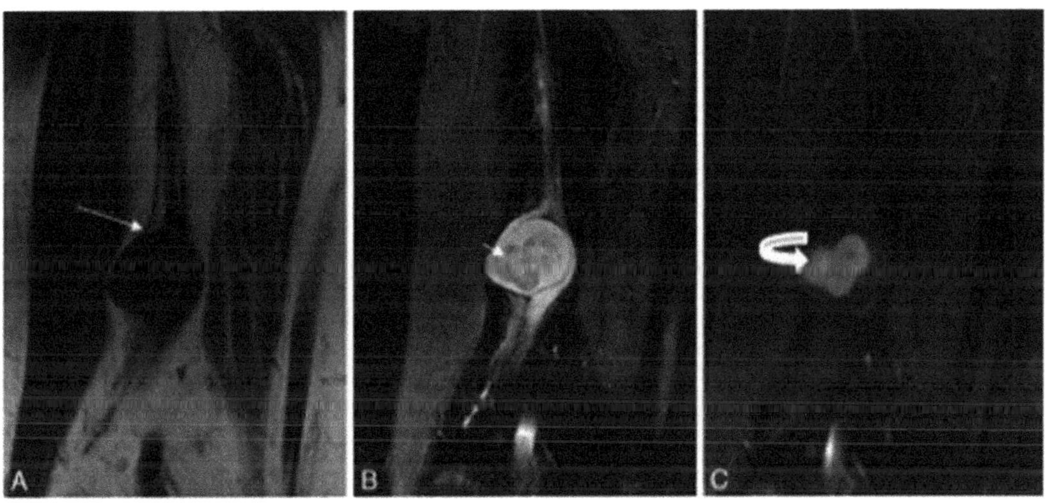

Fig. 30.11 Benign peripheral nerve sheath tumor of the sciatic nerve shows: (**a**) the typical split fat sign (*arrow*) on coronal T1, (**b**) target sign (*short arrow*) on coronal STIR nodular enhancement (**c**) (*curved arrow*) on a post-contrast coronal T1 fat-saturated image

30.2.3 Ganglion Cysts

Extraneural ganglions cysts are quite common (e.g., Bible cyst of the wrist). Intraneural ganglion cysts are less common and most commonly involve the common peroneal nerve and its branches near the fibular head, although other nerves can be involved. Until recently, the pathophysiology of these cysts and how they become intraneural was unknown. Recently, however, Spinner and colleagues showed quite convincingly how these cysts arise from an adjacent joint space by means of an articular twig that transmits the gelatinous material of the joint space intraneurally. In addition to providing an explanation about how they become intraneural, it provided a way to prevent recurrence of these intraneural cysts once they are surgically drained

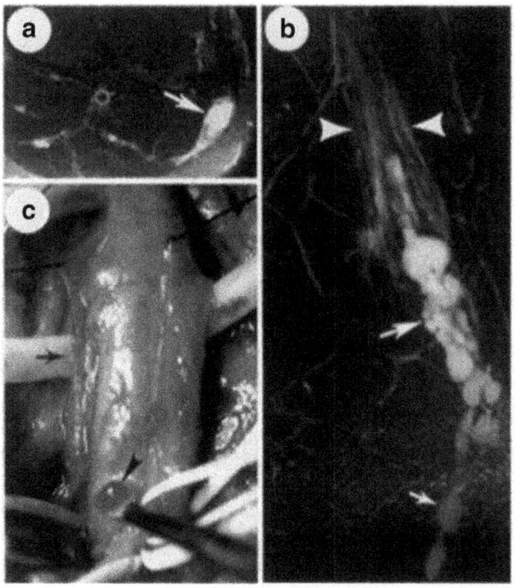

Fig. 30.12 MRN images of a 40-year-old male patient with multiple intraneural cysts involving the left common peroneal nerve and its deep peroneal nerve branch. (**a**) Axial T2 FSE image showing high signal cystic lesions (*white arrow*) within the common peroneal nerve. (**b**) Coronal T2 FSE multiplanar reconstruction showing multiple high signal intraneural cysts within the distal common peroneal nerve (*large white arrow*) that extend into the deep peroneal nerve branch (*small white arrow*). Note the abnormally bright nerve fascicles (between *white arrowheads*) splayed apart by the cysts. (**c**) Intraoperative photograph demonstrating abnormal enlargement of the common peroneal nerve (*black arrow*). Note the extrusion of gelatinous material from a surgically ruptured cyst (*black arrowhead*)

by identifying and then cutting the articular twig that transmits the joint space material retrogradely into the nerve (Figs. 30.12, 30.13, and 30.14).

30.2.4 Entrapment Neuropathies

Nerve entrapment syndromes, which involve various fibro-osseous "tunnels," are the most common form of chronic nerve injury. Less commonly, entrapment may be due to mass lesions that compress or infiltrate a nerve. Systemic diseases that contribute to soft tissue swelling can also contribute to nerve entrapment (e.g., renal failure, hypothyroidism, diabetes mellitus, gout, amyloidosis). Symptoms include paraesthesia, pain, and partial or complete loss of motor or sensory function. Nerves most vulnerable to entrapment often have anatomical features conducive to that problem, such as a superficial location, constrained position, or exposed path (e.g., crossing a joint). There are numerous entrapment or "tunnel" syndromes, the most common of which are discussed here.

30.2.4.1 Carpal Tunnel Syndrome

Physical examination and electrodiagnostic tests are the mainstays for diagnosing carpal tunnel syndrome (CTS), but it is not uncommon for nerve conduction studies to be falsely negative. The problem with imaging is that abnormal findings are common and do not alone predict a symptomatic disorder. In CTS, the median nerve on both MRI and US appears compressed and flattened at the point of entrapment (most often at the mid-to-distal carpal tunnel level) and swollen proximal (sometimes also distal) to the point of entrapment (Figs. 30.15, 30.16, 30.17, and 30.18). The transverse cross-sectional area of the nerve at the proximal carpal tunnel level is usually >10 mm^2. On MRI, the nerve within the carpal tunnel shows increased signal intensity, best appreciated on fat-suppressed T2-weighted images. The transverse carpal ligament may be seen to bulge volarly (>4 mm from a line drawn between the tip of the hook of hamate and the tubercle of the trapezium). Imaging can also be used to exclude a space-occupying lesion and to detect alignment abnormalities, but it cannot grade the severity of CTS—and electrodiagnostic studies can. US can be used to guide injection of corticosteroids into the flexor tendon sheath in the carpal tunnel.

30.2.4.2 Neurogenic Thoracic Outlet Syndrome

Neurogenic thoracic outlet syndrome (TOS) involves entrapment of the brachial plexus at any of three defined spaces in the thoracic outlet: the interscalene, costoclavicular, and retropectoralis minor spaces. Entrapment is usually exacerbated with arm abduction and external rotation. The causes are multiple and include muscle hypertrophy in athletes, cervical ribs, fibrous bands, accessory muscles, post-traumatic fibrosis, and clavicular fractures. Clinically, the patient may present with hand weakness or arm paraesthesia. If there is associated compression of the subclavian

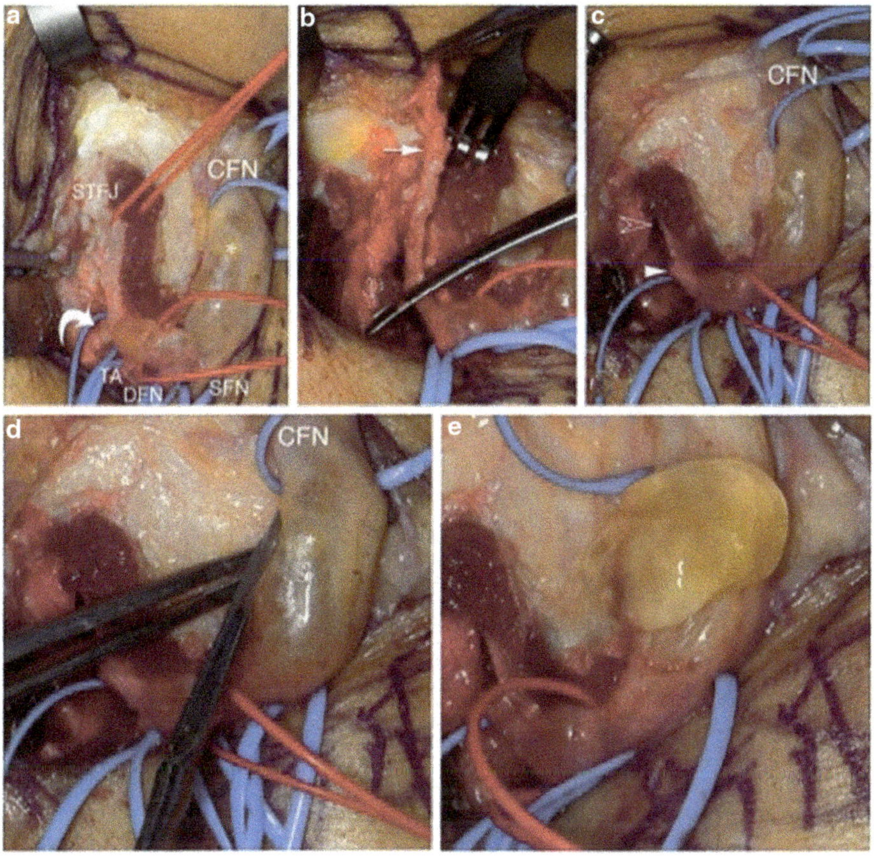

Fig. 30.13 Operative appearance. (**a**) The fibular intraneural cyst (*asterisk*) is seen extending from the superior tibiofibular joint (STFJ) along the U-shaped articular branch to the common fibular nerve (CFN). The take-off of the enlarged terminal branch to the patellar ligament (*curved arrow*) is seen as is the tibialis anterior (TA) proximal motor branch, deep fibular nerve (DFN), and the superficial fibular nerve (SFN). (**b**) The articular branch to the superior tibiofibular joint (*arrow*) was resected just above the terminal branch to the patellar ligament. (**c**) The superior tibiofibular joint was resected (*open arrowhead*). The stump of the articular branch after its resection (*arrowhead*) is seen. (**d**) A small slit is made in the cystic expansion of the common fibular nerve (CFN) away from its fascicles. The intraneural ganglion cyst is decompressed but not resected. (**e**) Gelatinous material is drained, decompressing the common fibular nerve

artery (vascular TOS), pallor may also be evident. EMG studies are often nondiagnostic.

In some cases MRI may be helpful. US cannot provide an accurate assessment for TOS because of the surface contour, presence of bone (i.e., the clavicle), and air in the lung apices. Chest radiography may be helpful in identifying cervical ribs as a potential cause.

Sagittal T1-weighted imaging is usually the procedure of choice, with narrowing of the costoclavicular space most commonly demonstrated. Coronal T1- and T2-weighted images may also show abnormal deviation of brachial plexus nerve elements by connective tissue bands, an enlarged transverse process, or a cervical rib. On T2-weighted imaging, one may see abnormally increased signal of the brachial plexus (Fig. 30.19), which can be accentuated by dynamic maneuvers. MRI demonstrates effacement of the fat planes around the brachial plexus and secondary features such as muscle atrophy and fatty infiltration.

30.2.4.3 Botulinum Toxin and Entrapment Neuropathies

Botox is a commercial product prepared from a toxin made by the bacterium *Clostridium botulinum*. Its mechanism of action is to produce muscle

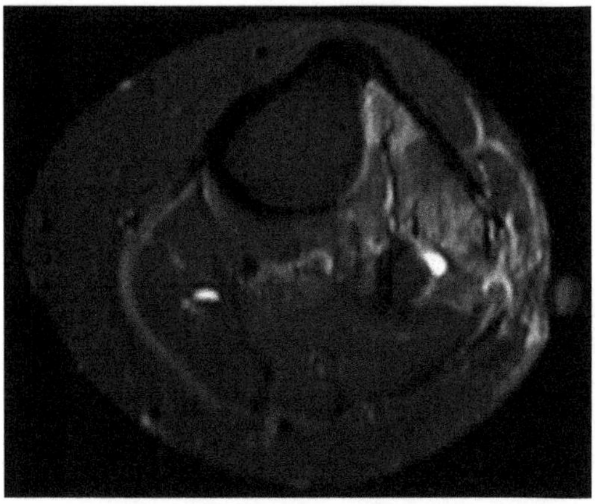

Fig. 30.14 Axial STIR image demonstrates the presence of a very high signal intensity lesion near the neck of the fibula consistent with an intraneural cyst. The patient had previous surgery but suboptimal recovery due to the residual/recurrent intraneural cyst. Overlying skin marker is present

paralysis via blocking release of acetylcholine by synaptic nerve terminals, thereby creating chemical denervation of muscle that lasts for several months. This potentially toxic effect is being used clinically for cosmetic purposes and to address a variety of medical problems such as hard-to-control muscle spasticity. A recent clinical application has been to help diagnose, and even treat if only for several months, peripheral nerve disorders thought to be due, at least in part, to compression of nerves by adjacent muscles that may have abnormally increased activity. Two such clinical applications are thoracic outlet and piriformis syndromes. In the former, the scalene muscles are injected with Botox under imaging guidance to relieve pressure on the brachial plexus. In the latter case, the piriformis muscle is

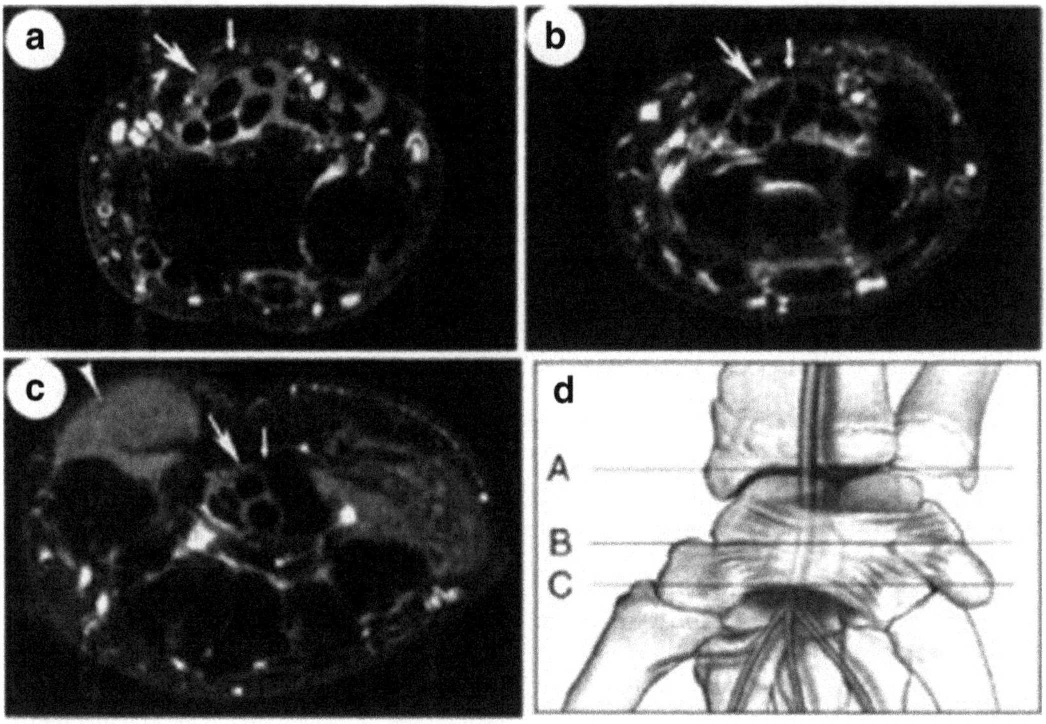

Fig. 30.15 MR images of the wrist, carpal tunnel, and thenar muscles, using a STIR sequence, demonstrating configurational changes in the median nerve (*large white arrows*) as it traverses the carpal tunnel, flexor retinaculum (*small white arrows*), and thenar muscles (*arrowhead*) and a schematic representation of the median nerve traversing the carpal tunnel. (**a**) MR image of the wrist at the level of the distal radius, showing an oval, enlarged median nerve. (**b**) MR image of the carpal tunnel at the level of the pisiform bone, showing mildly increased signal in a flattened median nerve. (**c**) MR image of the carpal tunnel at the level of the hook of the hamate, showing a flattened and smaller median nerve, with normal signal of the thenar muscles. (**d**) schematic representation of the median nerve traversing the wrist and carpal tunnel at the level of the distal radius (**a**), pisiform bone (**b**), and hook of the hamate (**c**)

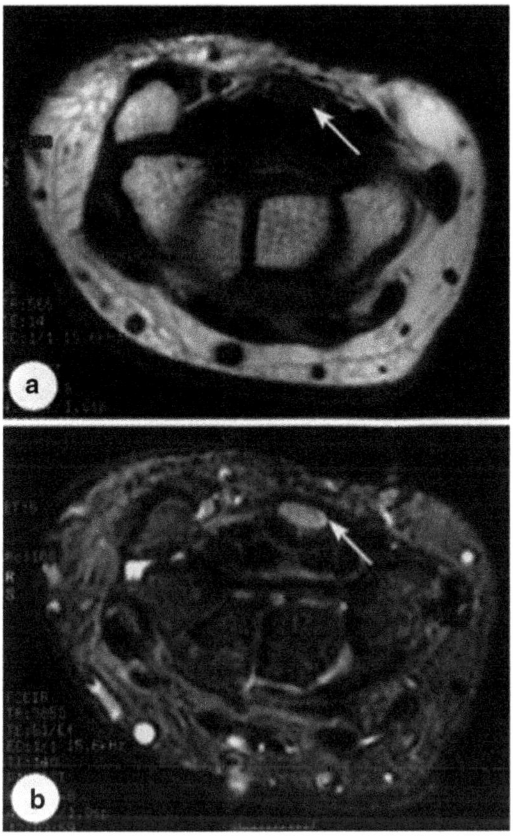

Fig. 30.16 Axial MR images through the palm of a patient with CTS at the level of the pisiform bone using T1-weighted (**a**) and STIR (**b**) pulse sequences. The median nerve (*white arrow*) has abnormally increased STIR signal (**b**) in comparison to the median nerve of an asymptomatic person (see Fig. 1**b**). Note the prominent fascicular structure of the nerve seen best in (**b**)

injected with Botox to relieve pressure on the sciatic nerve. Symptom relief may indicate that these muscles are contributing to the patient's symptoms by compressing adjacent peripheral nerves. Treatment may consist of repeated Botox injections at several-month intervals combined with physical therapy to help stretch the denervated muscles. Alternatively, if Botox reduces symptoms, a more definitive surgical approach may be taken in which the muscles thought to be compressing symptomatic nerves are cut to relieve pressure on the nerves. Some studies are using MRI to visualize muscles injected with Botox, as it can demonstrate denervation changes several weeks after the injections.

30.2.4.4 Brachial Neuritis or Parsonage Turner Syndrome

Brachial neuritis affects the brachial plexus at the thoracic outlet. It is an idiopathic condition that results in shoulder pain and marked muscle weakness that can last for years but usually recovers. There may be a history of antecedent viral illness but no trauma. The differential diagnosis includes rotator cuff, labral tears, trauma, and myositis. EMG findings are often nonspecific. On MRI, there is usually diffuse high signal intensity in the suprascapular, axillary, long thoracic, and subscapular nerves. However, on T2/STIR MRI scans, marked hyperintensity of the supraspinatus, infraspinatus, deltoid, and teres minor muscles, which becomes evident within 2–4 days, is much more common (Fig. 30.20). MRI allows localization of the involved nerve directly or indirectly by the muscle pattern involved. It also allows assessment of the rotator cuff tendons and labrum, especially for paralabral cysts, which may cause similar denervation changes.

30.2.4.5 Ulnar Nerve Entrapment at the Elbow

Ulnar nerve entrapment at the elbow is the second most common upper limb neuropathy. It is caused by compression of the ulnar nerve in the cubital tunnel in turn causing blunt trauma, accessory muscle (anconeus epitrochlearis), bony osteophytes, laxity of the ulnar collateral ligament and synovitis. Both MRI and US can over estimate entrapment and be "false positive" because of the high frequency of asymptomatic nerve changes in the general population. However, in the appropriate clinical context, findings of nerve swelling with hyperintensity and fascicular distortion on fluid sensitive MRI sequences become significant. Less commonly, there may be distal denervation changes. US usually shows a swollen, hypoechoic nerve proximal to the site of compression (Figs. 30.21, 30.22, and 30.23). Dynamic assessment during full elbow flexion may demonstrate marked indentation of the nerve by an overlying thickened cubital tunnel retinaculum or subluxation of the nerve around the medial humeral epicondyle (*with or without* an accompanying snapping sensation).

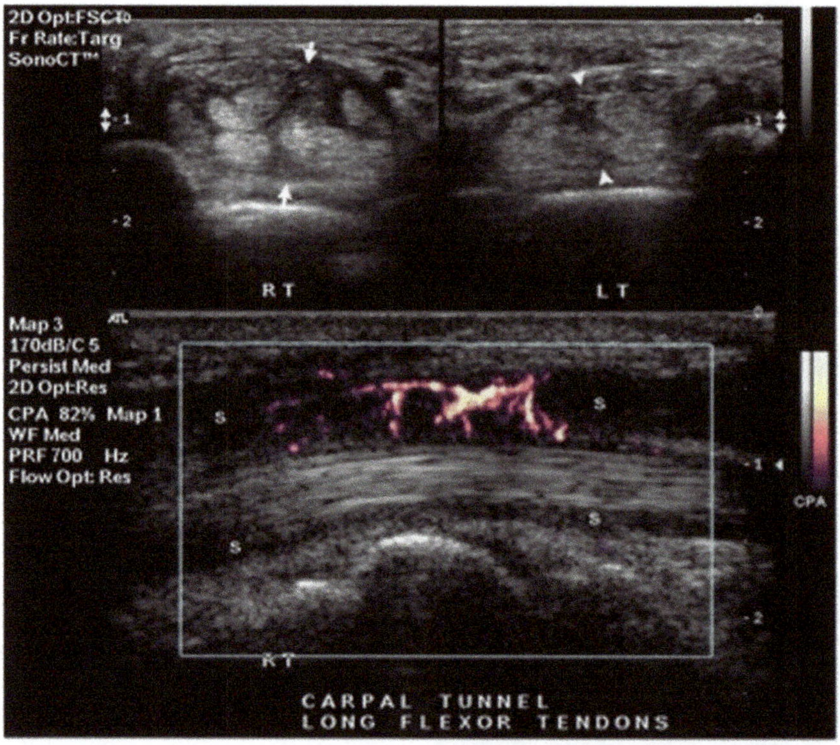

Fig. 30.17 US demonstrates carpal tunnel syndrome secondary to flexor tenosynovitis. *Upper left image*: *arrows* indicate increased AP diameter of carpal tunnel on the right. *Upper right image*: *arrowheads* indicate normal AP diameter of carpal tunnel on the left. *Bottom image*: hypoechoic synovial thickening(s) within the common flexor tendon sheath of carpal tunnel shows associated hyperemia on Power Doppler imaging

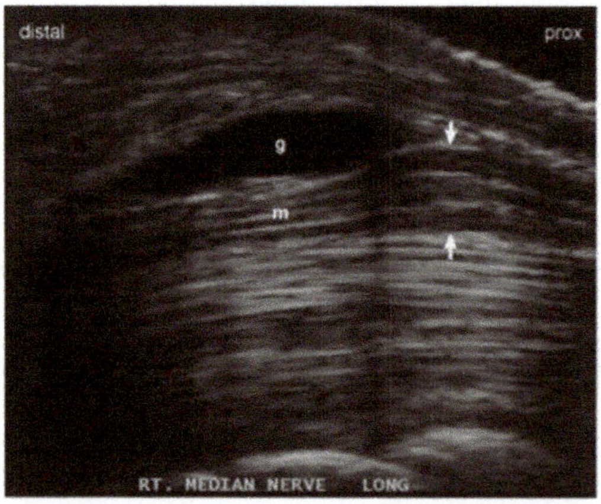

Fig. 30.18 US demonstrates CTS secondary to a ganglion (g) cyst. MRI more convincingly showed this to arise from the STT joint. The arrows demonstrate swelling of the median nerve immediately proximal to the ganglion. Note fascicular appearance of median (m) nerve (courtesy Dr John W Read, Castlereagh Imaging, Sydney)

30.2.4.6 Distal Ulnar Tunnel Entrapment

The ulnar nerve can be entrapped at the level of the in Guyon's canal where is passes through a confined space and is susceptible to external compression (most commonly by a ganglion arising from the pisotriquetral joint). MRI can demonstrate ganglia as a cause for entrapment. If the ulnar nerve is entrapped in Guyon's canal, it becomes swollen (>3 mm) and demonstrates hyperintensity on fluid-sensitive MRI sequences (Fig. 30.24).

30.2.4.7 Posterior Interosseous Syndrome

The radial nerve at the level of the elbow joint divides into superficial sensory and deep motor branches, with the deep branch being the posterior interosseous nerve (PIN), which courses between the superior and deep heads of the supinator muscle. Entrapment at this level is described as

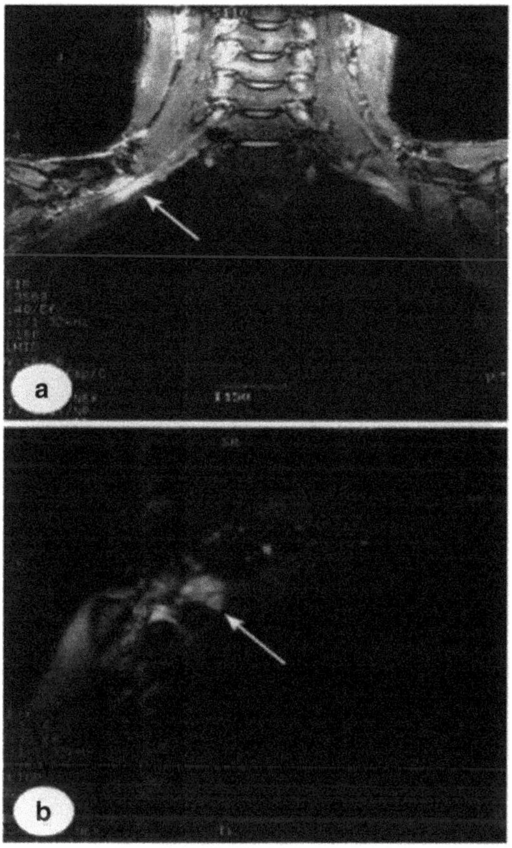

Fig. 30.19 Coronal (**a**) and sagittal (**b**) STIR MR images through the brachial plexus. The patient had clinical and electrodiagnostic evidence of thoracic outlet syndrome. Increased signal is visualized in peripheral nerve elements of the brachial plexus in both planes that is maximal in the lower trunk (*white arrows*)

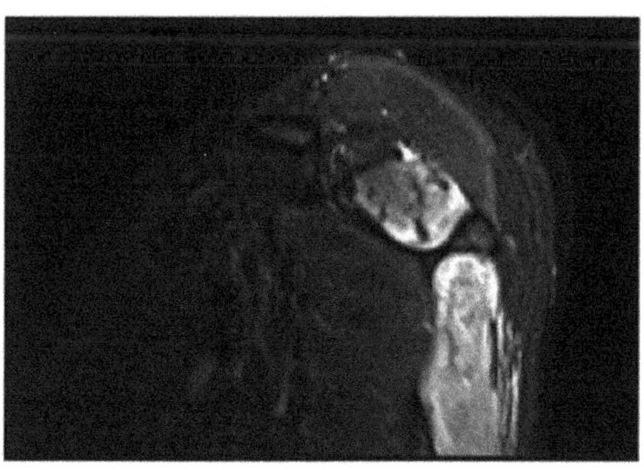

Fig. 30.20 Sagittal MR T2-weighted image with fat saturation of the rotator cuff muscles. This demonstrates T2 hyperintensity in the supraspinatus and infraspinatus muscles. No mass or cyst was identified in the suprascapular notch. The final diagnosis was brachial neuritis (*source*: University of Washington, PACS)

supinator syndrome or PIN entrapment. It causes lateral elbow/forearm pain and weakness of the finger and thumb extensors. Causes of PIN entrapment include trauma, space-occupying lesions, fibrous bands (up to 50 %), and a thickened arcade of Frohse. MRI can exclude a mass lesion, such as a ganglion cyst or intramuscular lipoma compressing the PIN. Denervation hyperintensity involving the supinator or extensor muscles of the forearm may be seen on fluid-sensitive sequences. US may demonstrate hypoechoic swelling of the PIN at the proximal (occasionally also the distal) end of the supinator tunnel (Fig. 30.25).

30.2.4.8 Meralgia Paresthetica

Meralgia paresthetica is entrapment of the lateral femoral cutaneous nerve at the level of the inguinal ligament. The small size of the nerve makes visualization of any abnormal signal difficult on MRI. Careful assessment with US, however, can show hypoechoic fusiform nerve swelling (Fig. 30.26).

30.2.4.9 Tarsal Tunnel Syndrome

Posterior tibial nerve compression can occur in the tarsal tunnel due to trauma, masses including ganglia, foot deformities e.g. pes planus and tarsal coalition and systemic disease such as diabetes mellitus. However, 40 % do not have an identifiable cause. The nerve is swollen, hyperintense on fluid sensitive MRI sequences, and hypoechoic on US.

30.2.4.10 Common Peroneal Nerve Compression

Peroneal nerve compression is the most common mononeuropathy in the lower extremity. The common peroneal nerve is fixed and superficial as it winds around the neck of the fibula to enter the peroneal tunnel. This is the location where it is vulnerable to compression, although it can also be compressed as it travels under the origin of the peroneus longus muscle. Causes of compression include direct trauma, short leg cast, prolonged immobilization, extended lithotomy position, or a mass such as a ganglion. Indirect signs of compression on MRI include increased signal intensity on T1- and T2-weighted imaging in the anterior and lateral compartments of the leg (Fig. 30.27). US may demonstrate swelling, decreased echogenicity, and tenderness over the nerve (Fig. 30.28).

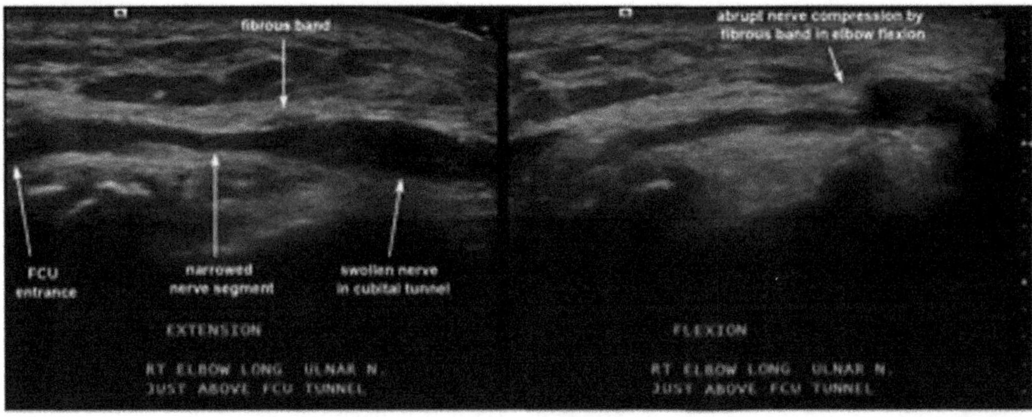

Fig. 30.21 US of the ulnar nerve at cubital tunnel level. *Left image*: longitudinal image demonstrates fusiform swelling of the ulnar nerve in the cubital tunnel. *Right image*: longitudinal image in flexion demonstrates abrupt angular indentation of the swollen ulnar nerve segment by the overlying fibrous band of thickened cubital tunnel retinaculum. The dynamic capabilities of US also allow the assessment of ulnar nerve and medial head triceps tendon stability (courtesy Dr John W Read, Castlereagh Imaging, Sydney)

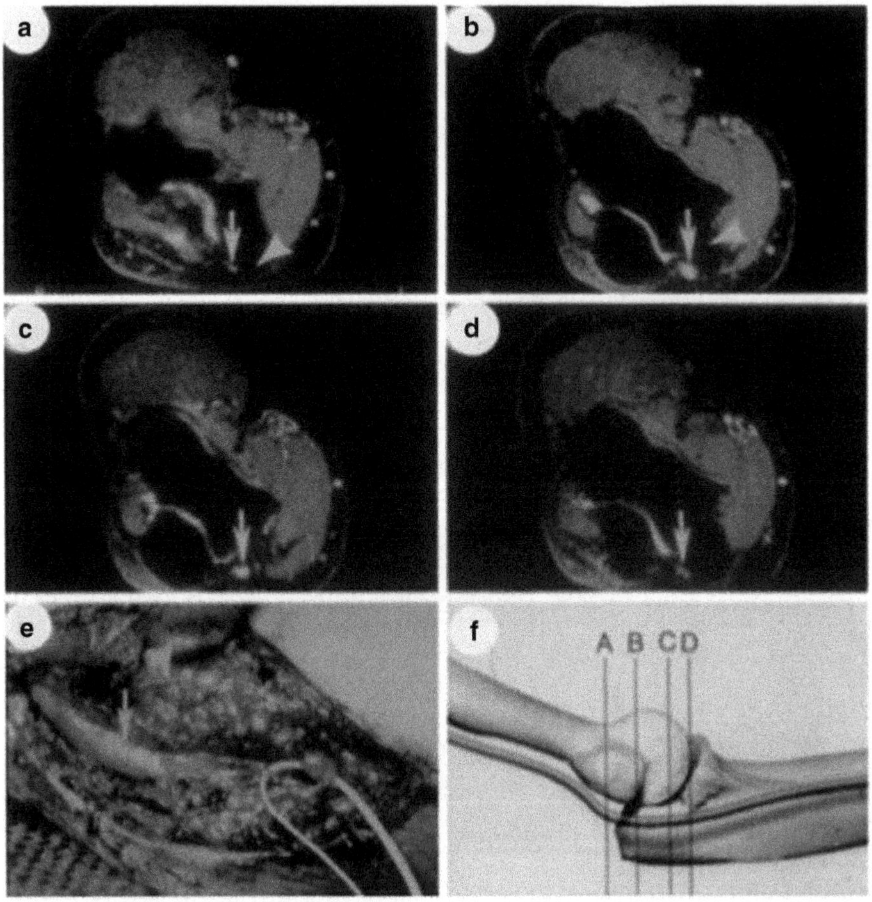

Fig. 30.22 (**a**–**d**) MRI axial sections using a STIR pulse sequence across the elbow at levels demonstrated schematically in figure **f** a patient with left cubital tunnel syndrome. The ulnar nerve (*white arrows*) is posterior to the medial epicondyle (*white arrowheads*). Note the increase in signal and size of the ulnar nerve across the cubital tunnel (**b**, **c**) and then a decrease in signal and size both proximally (**a**) and distally (**d**). (**e**) An intraoperative photograph showing exposure of the enlarged segment of the left ulnar nerve (*white arrow*) posterior to the medial epicondyle (*white arrowhead*)

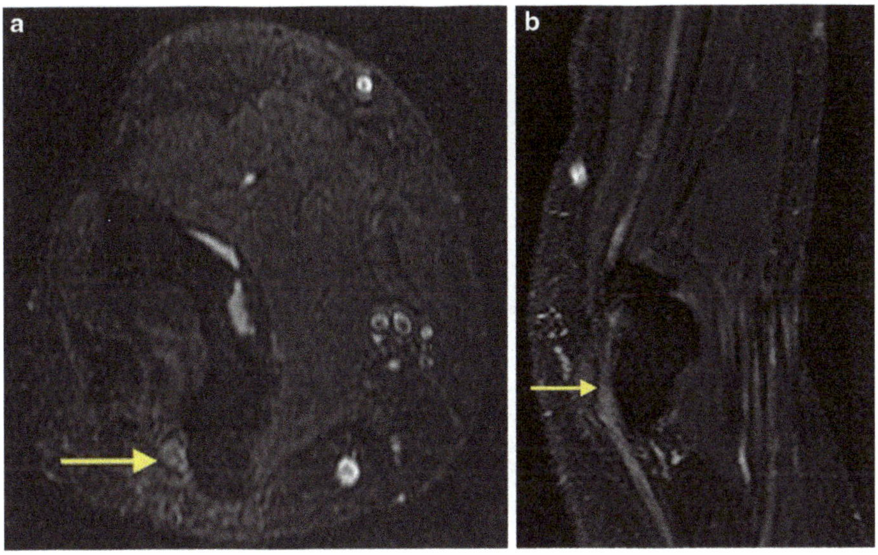

Fig. 30.23 (**a**) Axial STIR image demonstrates high signal intensity of the ulnar nerve within the cubital tunnel consistent with ulnar nerve neuropathy (UNN). (**b**) Sagittal STIR image confirms high signal intensity within the course of the ulnar nerve, again consistent with UNN

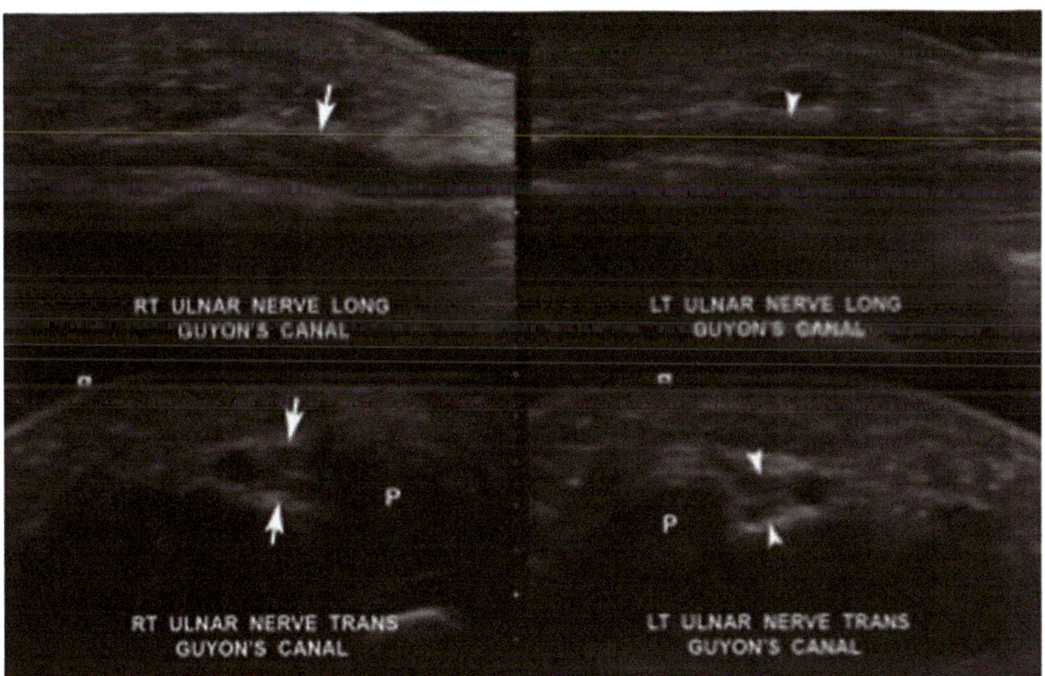

Fig. 30.24 US images of the right and left ulnar nerves in Guyon's canal in a 5-year-old girl with ulnar neurapraxia following blunt trauma to wrist. *Top left image*: longitudinal image of the right ulnar nerve in Guyon's canal demonstrate focal fusiform swelling (*arrow*). *Top right image*: *arrowhead* demonstrates a normal left ulnar nerve. Bottom left image: transverse image of the right ulnar nerve in Guyon's canal demonstrate focal fusiform swelling (*arrows*). *Bottom right image*: *arrowheads* demonstrate a normal left ulnar nerve. *P* unossified pisiform (courtesy Dr John W Read, Castlereagh Imaging, Sydney)

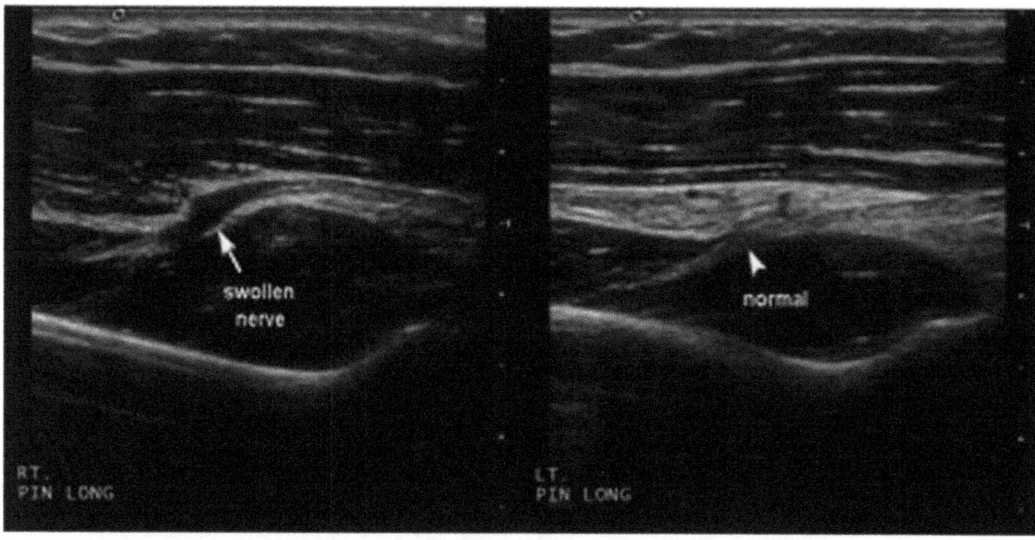

Fig. 30.25 US images of right posterior interosseous nerve entrapment. *Left image*: longitudinal image shows a hypoechoic swollen posterior interosseous nerve (*arrow*) at the level of entrance to supinator tunnel. This was present in both supination and pronation. *Right image*: comparison longitudinal image demonstrates the normal contralateral side (courtesy Dr John W Read, Castlereagh Imaging, Sydney)

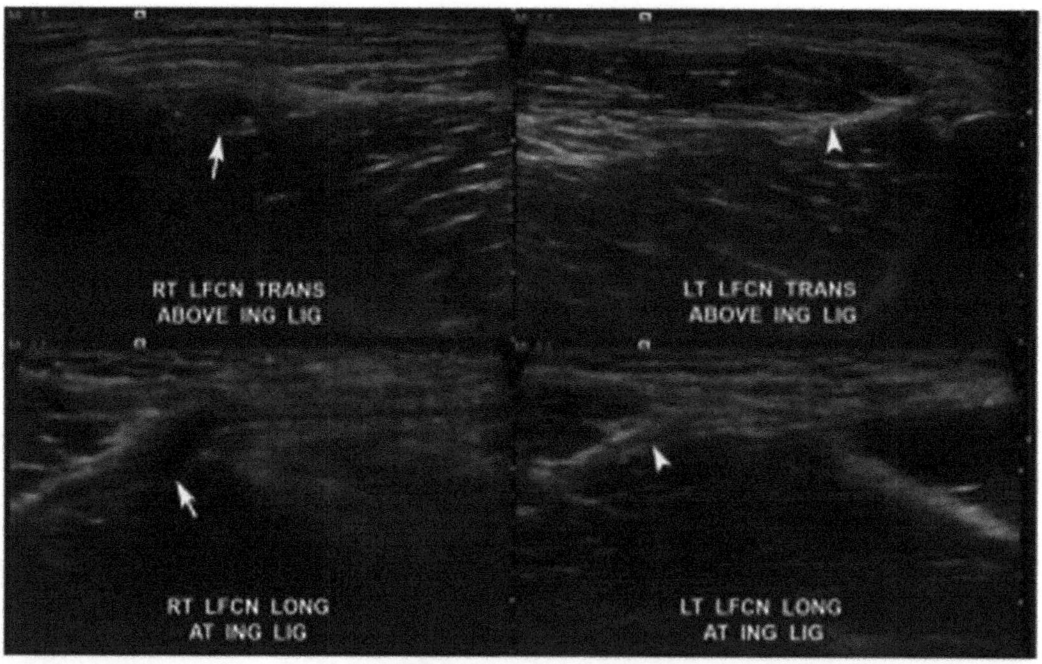

Fig. 30.26 US of meralgia paresthetica. *Top left*: transverse US image demonstrates a swollen right lateral femoral cutaneous nerve (LFCN) above the inguinal ligament (*arrow*). *Top right*: transverse US image demonstrates a normal left lateral femoral cutaneous nerve (LFCN) above the inguinal ligament (*arrowhead*). *Bottom left*: longitudinal US image demonstrates a swollen right lateral femoral cutaneous nerve (LFCN) at the inguinal ligament (*arrow*). *Bottom right*: longitudinal US image demonstrates a normal left lateral femoral cutaneous nerve (LFCN) at the inguinal ligament (*arrowhead*) (courtesy Dr John W Read, Castlereagh Imaging, Sydney)

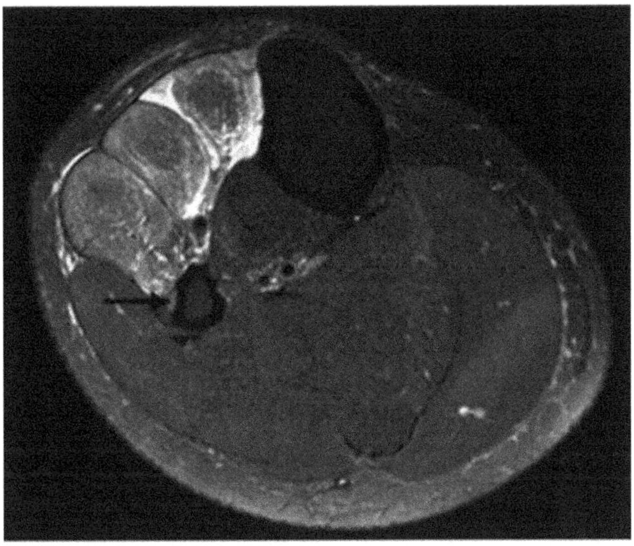

Fig. 30.27 Axial T2-weighted image with fat saturation MR at the level of the upper right leg. The MR demonstrates hyperintensity in the anterolateral muscles or peroneal compartment consistent with acute denervation changes. (*source*: University of Washington, PACS)

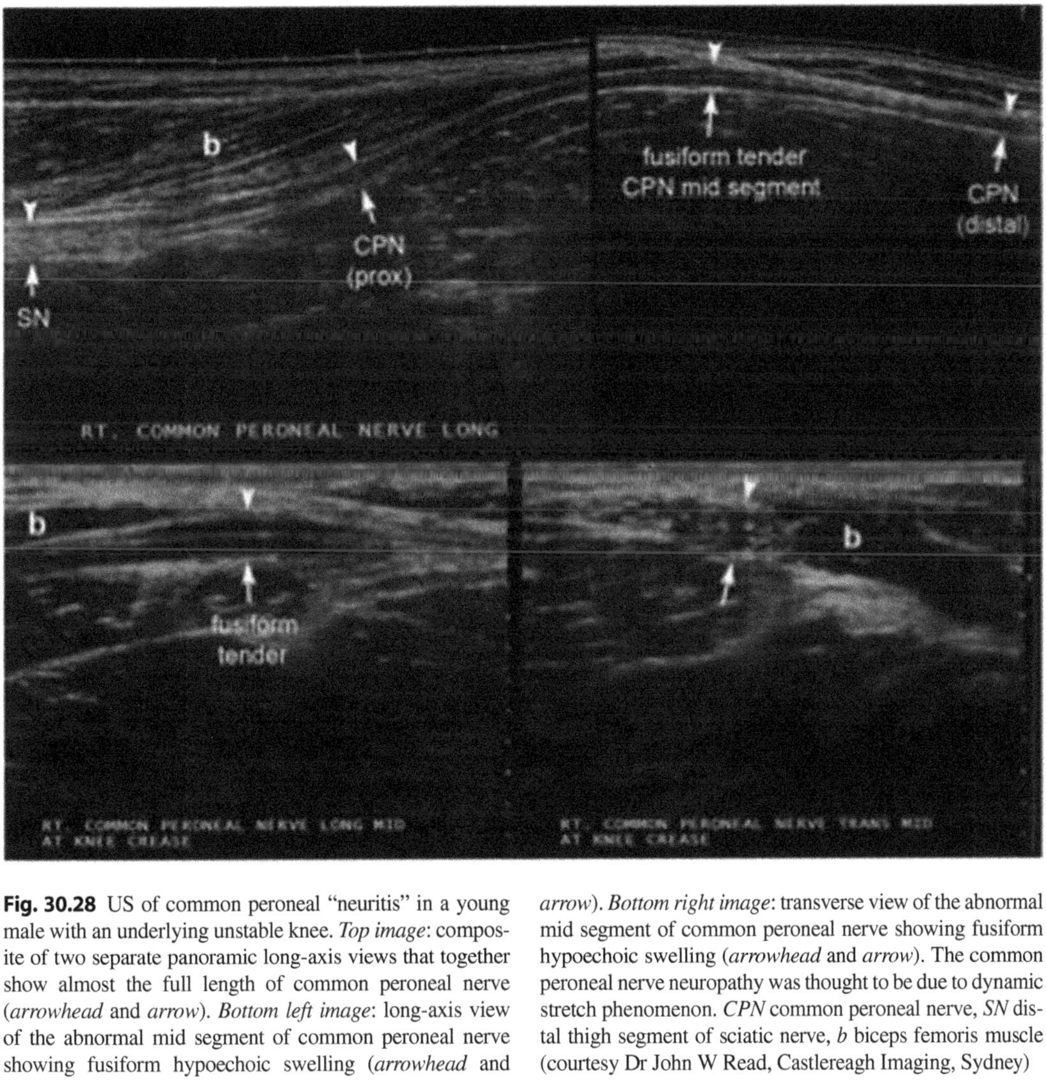

Fig. 30.28 US of common peroneal "neuritis" in a young male with an underlying unstable knee. *Top image*: composite of two separate panoramic long-axis views that together show almost the full length of common peroneal nerve (*arrowhead* and *arrow*). *Bottom left image*: long-axis view of the abnormal mid segment of common peroneal nerve showing fusiform hypoechoic swelling (*arrowhead* and *arrow*). *Bottom right image*: transverse view of the abnormal mid segment of common peroneal nerve showing fusiform hypoechoic swelling (*arrowhead* and *arrow*). The common peroneal nerve neuropathy was thought to be due to dynamic stretch phenomenon. *CPN* common peroneal nerve, *SN* distal thigh segment of sciatic nerve, *b* biceps femoris muscle (courtesy Dr John W Read, Castlereagh Imaging, Sydney)

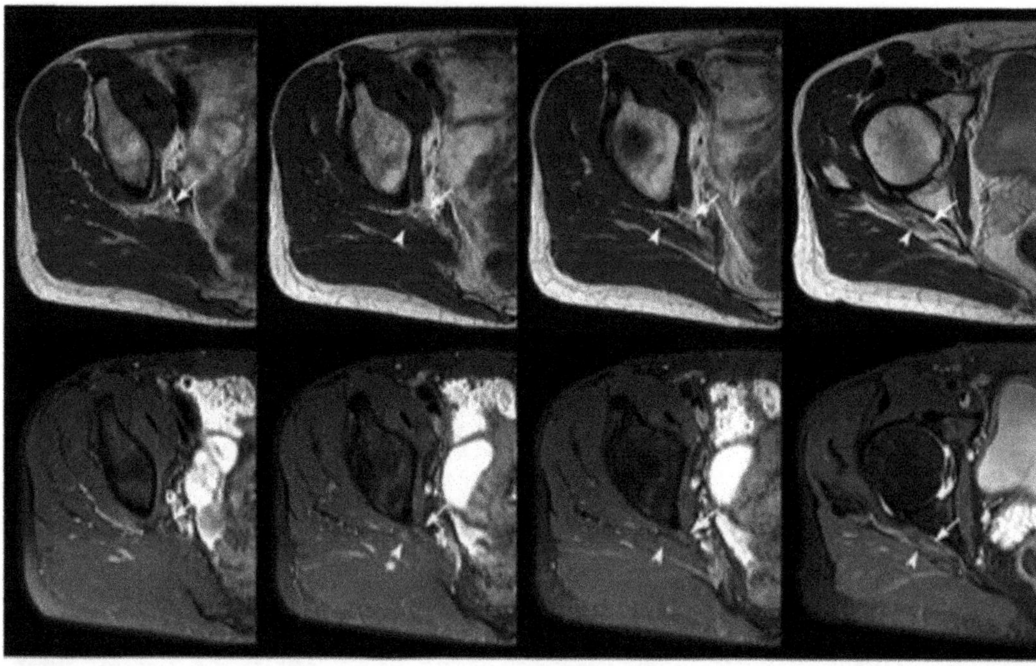

Fig. 30.29 *Top row*: axial T1-weighted MR of the right piriformis muscle demonstrates atrophy and fatty infiltration of the right piriformis muscle (*arrowhead*). The sciatic nerve is seen (*arrow*). *Bottom row*: axial T2-weighted image with fat saturation at the same level demonstrates hyperintensity within the right piriformis muscle consistent with subacute denervation change. Muscle bulk is again reduced (*arrowhead*). The sciatic nerve is mildly hyperintense likely reflecting neuropathy (*arrow*)

30.2.4.11 Piriformis Muscle Syndrome

Piriformis muscle syndrome is difficult to diagnose because of the nonspecific symptoms and the deep-seated location of the nerve. MRI is the investigation of choice. This syndrome is usually initiated by trauma and is the endpoint where the piriformis muscle compresses the sciatic nerve due to a combination of hypertrophy, inflammation, and scarring. On MRI, the muscle occasionally exhibits either hypertrophy or atrophy (Fig. 30.29). Recent studies with injection of botulinum toxin into the piriformis muscle to both diagnose and treat this syndrome are under way.

30.2.5 Genetic Neuropathies

The technique of MRI neurography has been used to as an investigative tool for possible diagnosis and monitoring of disease progression in a series of patients with Charcot–Marie–Tooth (CMT) neuropathy (Fig. 30.30). Case series were described in which, for the first time, a peripheral nerve disorder had been genetically subtyped and correlated with findings of electrophysiological studies and a nerve imaging technique (MR neurography). The authors concluded that MR neurography was able to characterize phenotypic features and disease

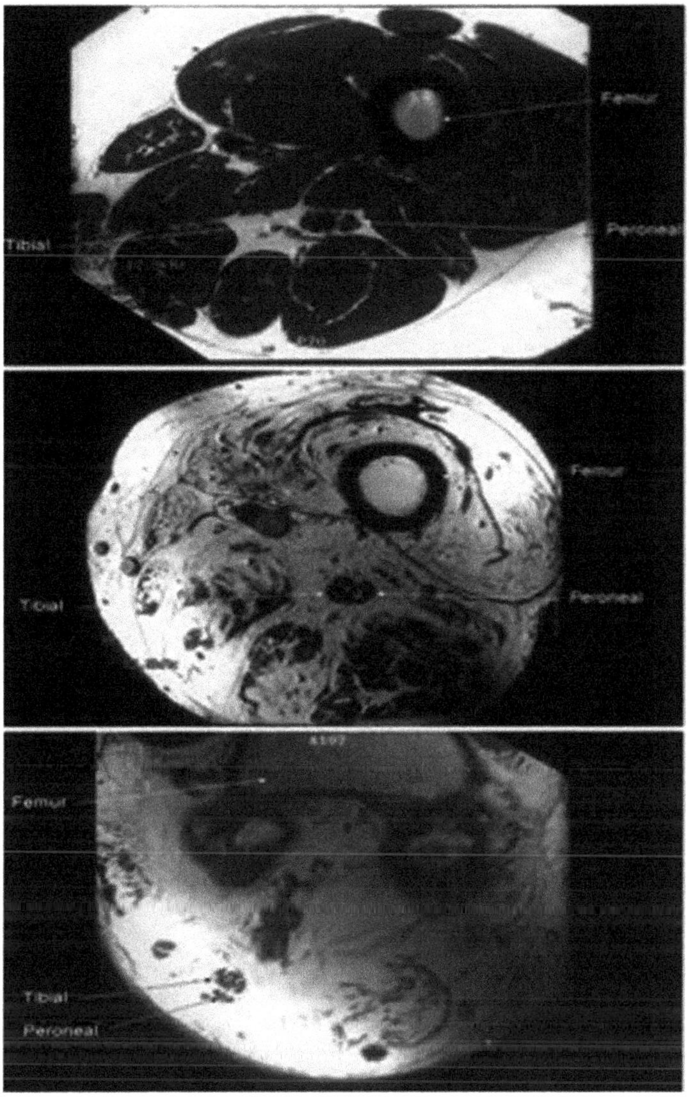

Fig. 30.30 Magnetic resonance T1-weighted neurograms obtained in a 34-year-old patient (*upper*), a 65-year-old patient (*center*), and an 84-year-old patient (*lower*) all of whom have CMT1A, revealing the progression of tissue changes (more fat infiltration of muscle) with the duration of the disease

progression noninvasively in patients with some subtypes of CMT disease. Therefore, in conjunction with nerve conduction velocity measurements, the imaging technique of MR neurography may be useful for diagnosing CMT neuropathy and monitoring disease progression.

Key Points

- Peripheral nerve sheath tumors exhibit variable patterns of growth. For some of these tumors the size remains stable over many years. In the setting of incidental asymptomatic peripheral nerve sheath tumors, one viable treatment option is to follow lesions with serial imaging examinations using MRI or US.
- In the near future, with continuing advancements in US and MRI technology, imaging may be able to prognosticate nerve injuries. In the meantime, rapid imaging is imperative to allow the neurosurgeon to evaluate the need for surgical repair.
- Each of the imaging techniques, US and MRI, has advantages and disadvantages. More often than not, the two techniques are complementary.
- Fundamental knowledge of anatomy and the appearance of "normal" peripheral nerves is the key to interpreting MR neurograms and peripheral nerve US scans.
- Imaging may be regarded as the fourth "pillar" in the diagnosis of peripheral nerve pathology.
- All imaging findings must be interpreted appropriately in the given clinical context.

Acknowledgements A special "thank you" to Dr. John Read for providing many of the US images and helping with editing the US sections. The authors also thank Aaron Filler and Cecil Hayes for their pioneering work in the development and refinement of MR neurography.

Suggestions for Further Reading

Aagaard BD, Maravilla KR, Kliot M. MR neurography. MR imaging of peripheral nerves. Magn Reson Imaging Clin N Am. 1998;6:179–94.

Aagaard BD, Maravilla KR, Kliot M. Magnetic resonance neurography: magnetic resonance imaging of peripheral nerves. Neuroimaging Clin N Am. 2001;11(1):viii, 131–46.

Anderson J, Read J. Atlas of Imaging in Sports Medicine. 2nd ed. McGraw Hill; 2008.

Britz GW, Haynor DR, Kuntz C, Goodkin R, Gitter A, Kliot M. Carpal tunnel syndrome: correlation of magnetic resonance imaging, clinical, electrodiagnostic, and intraoperative findings. Neurosurgery 1995;37(6): 1097–103.

Britz GW, Haynor DR, Kuntz C, et al. Ulnar nerve entrapment at the elbow: correlation of magnetic resonance imaging, clinical, electrodiagnostic, and intraoperative findings. Neurosurgery 1996;38:458–65; discussion 465.

Donovan A, Rosenberg ZS, Cavalcanti CF. MR imaging of entrapment neuropathies of the lower extremity. Part 2. The knee, leg, ankle, and foot. 2010;30(4): 1001–19.

Ellegala DB, Monteith SJ, Haynor D, Bird TD, Goodkin R, Kliot M. Characterization of genetically defined types of Charcot–Marie–Tooth neuropathies by using magnetic resonance neurography. J Neurosurg. 2005; 102(2):242–45.

Grant GA, Goodkin R, Kliot M. Evaluation and surgical management of peripheral nerve problems. Neurosurgery. 1999;44(4):825–39; discussion 839–40.

Grant GA, Britz GW, Goodkin R, Jarvik JG, Maravilla K, Kliot M. The utility of magnetic resonance imaging in evaluating peripheral nerve disorders. Muscle Nerve. 2002;25(3):314–31.

Grant GA, Goodkin R, Maravilla KR, Kliot M. MR neurography: diagnostic utility in the surgical treatment of peripheral nerve disorders. Neuroimaging Clin N Am. 2004;14(1):115–33.

Jacobson JA, Fessell DP, Lobo Lda G, Yang LJ. Entrapment neuropathies I: upper limb (carpal tunnel excluded). Semin Musculoskelet Radiol. 2010;14(5):473–86.

Kamath S, Venkatanarisimha N, Walsk MA, Hughes PM. MRI appearance of muscle denervation. Skeletal Radiol. 2008;37:397–404.

Kermarrec E, Demondion X, Khalil C, Le Thuc V, Boutry N, Cotten A. Ultrasound and magnetic resonance imaging of the peripheral nerves: current techniques, promising directions, and open issues. Semin Musculoskelet Radiol. 2010;14(5):463–72.

Klauser AS, Faschingbauer R, Bauer T, et al. Entrapment neuropathies II: carpal tunnel syndrome. Semin Musculoskelet Radiol. 2010;14(5):487–500.

Kuntz Ct, Blake L, Britz G, et al. Magnetic resonance neurography of peripheral nerve lesions in the lower extremity. Neurosurgery 1996;39(4):750–56; discussion 756–7.

Linda DD, Harish S, Stewart BG, Finlay K, Parasu N, Rebello RP. Multimodality imaging of peripheral neuropathies of the upper limb and brachial plexus. Radiographics. 2010;30(5):1373–400.

Petchprapa CN, Rosenberg ZS, Sconfienza LM, Cavalcanti CF, Vieira RL, Zember JS. MR imaging of entrapment neuropathies of the lower extremity. Part 1. The pelvis and hip. Radiographics 2010;30:983–1000.

Singh T, Kliot M. Imaging of peripheral nerve tumors. Neurosurg Focus. 2007;22:E6.

Spinner RJ, Puffer RC, Skinner JA, Amrami KK. The MRI appearance and importance of the "very" terminal branches of the recurrent articular branch in fibular intraneural ganglion cysts. Clin Anat. 2011;24(2): 268–72.

Thawait SK, Chaudhry V, Thawait GK, et al. High-resolution MR neurography of diffuse peripheral nerve lesions. AJNR Am J Neuroradiol. 2011;32(8):1365–72.

Woertler K. Tumors and tumor-like lesions of peripheral nerves. Semin Musculoskelet Radiol. 2010;14(5): 547–58.

Index

M.P. Wattjes and D. Fischer (eds.), *Neuromuscular Imaging*, DOI 10.1007/978-1-4614-6552-2,

GPSR Compliance
The European Union's (EU) General Product Safety Regulation (GPSR) is a set of rules that requires consumer products to be safe and our obligations to ensure this.

If you have any concerns about our products, you can contact us on

ProductSafety@springernature.com

In case Publisher is established outside the EU, the EU authorized representative is:

Springer Nature Customer Service Center GmbH
Europaplatz 3
69115 Heidelberg, Germany

www.ingramcontent.com/pod-product-compliance
Ingram Content Group UK Ltd.
Pitfield, Milton Keynes, MK11 3LW, UK
UKHW050227160926
475607UK00005B/113
* 9 7 8 1 4 6 1 4 6 5 5 1 5 *